# PHOSPHATE AND MINERALS IN HEALTH AND DISEASE

# ADVANCES IN EXPERIMENTAL MEDICINE AND BIOLOGY

### Recent Volumes in this Series

# PHOSPHATE AND MINERALS IN HEALTH AND DISEASE

Edited by

## Shaul G. Massry

University of Southern California
Los Angeles, California

## Eberhard Ritz

University of Heidelberg
Heidelberg, German Federal Republic

and

## Henri Jahn

Louis Pasteur University
Strasbourg, France

PLENUM PRESS • NEW YORK AND LONDON

Library of Congress Cataloging in Publication Data

International Workshop on Phosphate and Other Minerals, 4th, Strasbourg, 1979.
  Phosphate and minerals in health and disease.

  (Advances in experimental medicine and biology; 128)
  Includes bibliographical references and index.
  1. Phosphorus in the body — Congresses. 2. Phosphates — Metabolism — Con-
gresses. 3. Phosphorus metabolism disorders — Congresses. 4. Minerals in the
body — Congresses. I. Massry, Shaul G. II. Ritz, Eberhard. III. Jahn, Henri. IV. Ti-
tle. V. Series. [DNLM: 1. Minerals — Metabolism — Congresses. 2. Phosphates —
Metabolism — Congresses. W1 AD559 v. 128/QV285 I61 1979p]
QP535.P1I57  1979              612'.3924                    80-14464
  ISBN-13: 978-1-4615-9169-6      e-ISBN-13: 978-1-4615-9167-2
  DOI:  10.1007/978-1-4615-9167-2

Proceedings of the Fourth International Workshop on Phosphate and Other Minerals,
held in Strasbourg, France, June 22–24, 1979.


©1980 Plenum Press, New York
Softcover reprint of the hardcover 1st edition 1980
A Division of Plenum Publishing Corporation
227 West 17th Street, New York, N.Y. 10011

TO OUR WIVES

**MEIRA MASSRY**
**CHRISTINA RITZ**
**MARTINE JAHN**

PREFACE

We are pleased to present to our readers the Proceedings of the Fourth International Workshop on Phosphate and Other Minerals which was held in Strasbourg during June 22-24, 1979. It was hosted by Professor Henri Jahn, Professor of Medicine and Chief, Department of Nephrology at the University of Strasbourg.

These Workshops have become a tradition in the scientific scene of mineral metabolism. The meetings have been providing a unique framework for close interaction between scientists from various disciplines, such as nephrologists, endocrinologists, biochemists, nutritionists, and those dealing with bone metabolism. The Workshops also created a forum for the delivery of original information, as well as state-of-the-art presentations on exciting topics of current interest in this evergrowing field of phosphate and mineral homeostasis.

The Fourth International Workshop was attended by three-hundred scientists from 15 countries including Austria, Canada, Denmark, England, France, Germany, Holland, Israel, Italy, Japan, Sweden, Switzerland and the United States of America. The topics discussed included those dealing with the renal handling of phosphate, calcium and magnesium, intermediary phosphate metabolism and phosphate homeostasis in health and disease. Two symposia were also presented: one dealt with nephrolithiasis and its relation to phosphate and the other with bone metabolism. In addition to 22 presentations by invited speakers, the Workshop provided 46 oral and 93 poster presentations selected from over 250 abstracts submitted to the Organizing Committee.

The Fifth International Workshop on Phosphate and Other Minerals will be held during September 24-27, 1981 in New York City, U.S.A. It will be hosted by Dr. Joseph Letteri, Chief, Division of Nephrology, Nassau County Medical Center and Professor of Medicine at the State University of New York at Stoney Brook. The theme of this coming Workshop will continue to focus on the pathophysiology of phosphate homeostasis and the metabolism of other minerals.

      We would like to express our thanks and appreciation for all
those who have stimulated, encouraged and supported us to hold the
Fourth International Workshop in Strasbourg.  This endeavor could
not have been possible without the generous financial support of
the National Institute of Arthritis, Metabolism, and Digestive
Diseases of the National Institutes of Health (USA), University
Louis Pasteur (Strasbourg), Ciba Geigy (France), Eli Lilly (France),
Gambro (France), Groupe Parcor (France), Hellige (France), Hoechst
(France), Hoffmann La Roche (USA), Hospal (France), Kahi Vitrum
(France), Laboratoires Leo (France), Laboratoires Pech (France),
Laboratoires Roche (France), Marion Laboratories, Inc. (USA),
Merrell (France), Organon Teknika (France), Pharmindustrie (France),
Plenum Publishing Corporation (USA), Pegie Renault (France),
Roger Bellon (France), Servier (France), Proctor and Gamble Company
(USA), Upjohn Company (USA), Travenol (France) and Zyma S.A.
(Switzerland).

      A special tribute goes to Dr. Rene Schmitt for her tremendous
contribution to the local organization of the Workshop.  Her dedi-
cation, devotion and tireless efforts were essential for the success
of the Workshop.  We also are indebted to Ms. Gracy Fick and Ms.
Carla Schoenmakers for their invaluable assistance and help in the
organization of the Workshop.

                              Shaul G. Massry, M.D.
                              Eberhard Ritz, M.D.
                              Henri Jahn, M.D.

CONTENTS

III. PHOSPHATE DEPLETION

## IV. INTESTINAL ABSORPTION OF PHOSPHATE AND CALCIUM

## VII. TOPICS ON BONE AND VITAMIN D

# RENAL HANDLING OF PHOSPHATE,
# CALCIUM AND MAGNESIUM

# THE CONTROL OF PHOSPHATE UPTAKE BY THE ISOLATED RENAL TUBULE

Louis V. Avioli and Sook Won Lee

Department of Medicine and Division of Bone and
Mineral Metabolism, The Jewish Hospital of St. Louis
and Washington University School of Medicine, St.
Louis, Missouri

In studies detailing the effect of PTH on Pi accumulation
in vitro using kidney slices, Geary and Cousins (1) demonstrated
enhanced $^{32}PO_4$ uptake. However, in contrast to the results of
Egawa and Neuman (2) these investigators noted a significant delay
in the accumulation of $^{32}PO_4$ by the slice preparations. Since
convoluted renal tubular preparations devoid of stroma obtained by
preincubation of renal cortex with collagenase, appear to be
superior to renal slices as an experimental in vitro model (3), we
decided to evaluate factors which might condition or regulate
phosphate uptake by intact tubules isolated from rat renal cortex.
The accumulated data support the presence of an energy dependent
and ouabain-sensitive uptake mechanism which is stimulated by both
parathyroid hormone (PTH) and cyclic AMP (cAMP).

## Methods

Young male Holtzman rats weighing 60-70 grams were maintained
on a diet of Purina laboratory chow and fasted overnight prior to
use and renal tubule suspensions prepared according to a modification of the technique of Nagata and Rasmussen (4). 0.5 ml of the
suspension was added to 0.5 ml of KRB solution containing albumin,
penicillin, streptomycin, 2.0 mM glucose and 0.1 μCi/ml $^{32}PO_4$.
Incubations were performed at 37°C in the presence of 95% oxygen
and 5% carbon dioxide at pH 7.4. The incubation was terminated
by the addition of 4 ml iced KRB containing 3.0 mM phosphate and
then centrifuged at 50 x g at 4°C for one minute. The isolated
tubules were then resuspended and washed five times, and both
supernatant and washes pooled. Tubules were subjected to osmotic
shock by the addition of 2 ml distilled water. Aliquots of "shocked
tubules" were solubilized in a tissue solubilizer TS-1 and counted

3

in 10 ml of scintillating solution (2 mg of 2,5 diphenxyloxazole
and 0.1 gm B-Bis [2-(5-phenyloxazolyl] Benzene.  Aliquots of pooled
supernatant and washes were counted in 10 ml of Bray's solution.
Percent phosphate uptake was calculated by dividing the counts in
the tubules by the sum of the counts in the tubules, supernatant
and washes and multiplying by 100.  The amount of radioactivity
which accumulated in the tubules was converted to moles of Pi by
analysis of changes in specific activity.

     cAMP was determined by radioimmunoassay, by the method of
Steiner, Parker and Kipnis (5).  Tubules were incubated in the
presence of 10 mM theophylline.  The pH of the incubated media
prior to and following incubation ranged between 7.35 and 7.45.
Protein was determined by the method of Lowry (6) using BSA as
the standard.  Samples of the protein suspensions were solubilized
in 0.5% sodium lauryl sulfate prior to determination of protein
content.  Statistical analysis was by the paired "t" test (7).

## Results

     Metabolism of $^{14}$C-glucose by the tubule preparation  was
linear during a 20 min. incubation period and in ten separate
experiments, recovery of the $^{14}$C-inulin added to the samples prior
to incubation was 101% (range 98-103%).  The "inulin space" remained constant under the incubation conditions used in this study.
Studies designed to evaluate the dependency of Pi uptake on media
glucose, sodium, calcium and magnesium concentration revealed:
(i) no effect of altering glucose concentration from 0.5 - 2.5 mM
although in the absence of glucose, Pi uptake was decreased by
5.4 $\pm$ 1.2%; (ii) maximal Pi uptake with media calcium concentration
of 0.5 - 2.0 mM with a 14-20% decrease in uptake when the tubular
preparation was preincubated with 0.5 mM EGTA; (iii) no significant
effect of varying medium magnesium concentrations from 0.5 - 2.0 mM;
(iv) complete inhibition of Pi accumulation when lithium was sub-
stituted for sodium in the media, with uptake restored with sodium
concentrations greater than 50 mM.

     Table 1 summarizes the effects of 2,4 dinitrophenol (DNP) and
ouabain, at low (0.7 mM) and high (4.0 mM) Pi concentrations.
Significant inhibition occurred with both inhibitors at all Pi
concentrations studied.

     Studies of the effect of PTH, cAMP and theophylline were all
done in 0.7 mM Pi; the tubules were preincubated with the test
substance 10 minutes prior to labeling with $^{32}$PO$_4$.  As noted in
Table 2, cAMP either in the presence or absence of theophylline,
caused significant enhancement of Pi entry.  In the absence of
theophylline, enhancement occurred at concentrations of $10^{-3}$M and
$10^{-4}$M, while in the presence of theophylline significant enhancement occurred at $10^{-5}$M cAMP.

TABLE 1

EFFECTS OF DINITROPHENOL AND OUABAIN
ON PHOSPHATE ACCUMULATION BY ISOLATED RAT RENAL TUBULES

% INHIBITION OF CONTROL

| | Low phosphate concentration | | High phosphate concentration | |
|---|---|---|---|---|
| Dinitrophenol | | | | |
| 0.25 mM | $76.7 \pm 0.8$ | (6) | $55.8 \pm 2.4$ | (5) |
| 0.75 mM | $74.2 \pm 2.0$ | (7) | $67.6 \pm 7.3$ | (7) |
| | | | | |
| Ouabain | | | | |
| 1.0 mM | $35.1 \pm 4.7$ | (9) | $28.0 \pm 3.3$ | (9) |
| 2.0 mM | $35.5 \pm 6.5$ | (7) | $32.1 \pm 3.6$ | (7) |

Each value represents the mean $\pm$ S.E.. Values in parenthesis
denote number of individual experiments in each study. All
results were significantly different from controls with $p<0.001$
in each instance.

TABLE 2

EFFECT OF CYCLIC AMP ON PHOSPHATE ACCUMULATION
BY ISOLATED RAT RENAL TUBULES

| | | Percent Change from control | P |
|---|---|---|---|
| cAMP | | | |
| $1 \times 10^{-3}$M | (7) | $+ 15.4 \pm 2.4$ | $< 0.001$ |
| $1 \times 10^{-4}$M | (7) | $+ 12.9 \pm 4.1$ | $< 0.001$ |
| $1 \times 10^{-5}$M | (8) | $- 4.1 \pm 5.4$ | N.S. |
| | | | |
| Theophylline ($1 \times 10^{-3}$M) | | | |
| Plus | | | |
| cAMP | | | |
| $1 \times 10^{-3}$M | (17) | $+ 18.4 \pm 6.6$ | $< 0.001$ |
| $1 \times 10^{-5}$M | (12) | $+ 8.0 \pm 2.9$ | $< 0.001$ |

Values in parenthesis denote number of experiments in each
instance. Data recorded as mean $\pm$ S.E.

In order to assess the integrity of the renal tubular membrane receptors to PTH, PTH stimulation of cAMP formation by the tubular preparation was also quantitated. A progressive increment in cAMP was observed with PTH concentrations of $6.5 \times 10^{-9}$M, $6.5 \times 10^{-8}$M and $2.6 \times 10^{-7}$M (Table 3). Studies were performed in the presence of $10^{-2}$M theophylline with 15 minutes of pre-incubation with theophylline and 10 minutes of incubation with PTH. Stimulation of cAMP was observed at PTH concentrations of $6.5 \times 10^{-9}$M, the lowest concentration tested.

TABLE 3

EFFECT OF SYNTHETIC BOVINE (I-34) PTH ON cAMP CONTENT
OF ISOLATED RAT RENAL TUBULES

|  |  | cAMP (pmoles/mg protein) |
|---|---|---|
| Control | (9) | $21.9 \pm 3.2$ |
| PTH |  |  |
| $6.5 \times 10^{-9}$M | (5) | $34.9 \pm 4.2$** |
| $6.5 \times 10^{-8}$M | (6) | $53.7 \pm 4.8$** |
| $2.6 \pm 10^{-7}$M | (4) | $73.1 \pm 3.1$** |

** Significantly different from control with $p < 0.01$.
Values in parenthesis denote number of experiments in each instance.
Data recorded as means $\pm$ SE.

When a maximal-stimulating dose of PTH in the presence of $10^{-3}$M theophylline or cAMP alone was incubated with tubules in the presence of dinitrophenol or ouabian, both agents caused significant inhibition of Pi uptake. Whereas DNP abolished the effects of both PTH and cAMP, the stimulating effect of PTH and cAMP on Pi uptake were not totally suppressed by 1.0 mM ouabain. Thus it appears that both PTH and cAMP stimulate Pi uptake via energy-dependent mechanism(s) and that the PTH-cAMP stimulation of Pi uptake by the rat renal tubule is mediated in large part, by a ouabain-inhibitable mechanism.

Discussion

The renal handling of phosphate has been examined repeatedly in the past with emphasis on the hormonal control of phosphate reabsorption by kidney tubules (8,9) and the characteristics and site(s) of phosphate transport across luminal membranes (10,11). Recently the effect of PTH on cellular transport processes has been localized to an adenylate cyclase in the contra-luminal membrane of the tubular cell (12). There are in addition, reports defining peritubular uptake for biologically active PTH preparations (13), and a PTH-dependent peritubular phosphate system in the rat (14).

The oxygen-temperature-dependent nature of Pi entry into the renal tubule cell and the inhibition of Pi uptake observed in the dinitrophenol experiments constitute good evidence for the existance of a carrier-mediated ATP-dependent active Pi transport process which requires glycolytic and citric acid cycle activities for maximal efficiency. The uptake of Pi by the dispersed tubules was also $Na^+$-dependent and ouabain inhibitable, an observation consistent with active transport across an electrochemical gradient. Since renal cell phosphate concentration is high and the potential within the cell is negative (15), our observations are also consistent with a membrane transport system for Pi which is $Na^+$-dependent and actively transports phosphate into the renal tubular cell against an electrochemical gradient (10,15).

The observed effects of PTH, cAMP and theophylline confirm previous findings made by Biddulph and Wrenn (16) and Leland et al (17) in isolated renal cortical tubules, and Marcus and Aurbach in renal cortical tissue (18). While it is generally accepted that the physiological effects of PTH on phosphate transport by the renal tubule are mediated by cAMP (16-19), the cellular events which mediate this interaction are still virtually unknown.

Both ouabain and DNP inhibited the stimulating effect of PTH and cAMP on Pi uptake by the tubules. Whereas the effect of DNP in inhibiting PTH- or cAMP-induced increments in Pi accumulation was virtually complete, the ouabain inhibitory effect was blunted by PTH. These combined data suggest that: (i) oxidative phosphorylation is essential for the PTH effect; and (ii) PTH stimulates Pi transport in this in vitro preparation by at least two mechanisms, one of which is dependent on active sodium transport.

In summary, an in vitro isolated tubular model is presented which appears to have many characteristics of an active transport system in that Pi accumulation by the preparation is sodium- and temperature-dependent, stimulated by PTH and cAMP and is also conditioned by the metabolic integrity of the tissue. The relationship between the observations made in the dispersed convolutal tubule preparation in the present study and the mechanisms by which PTH affects phosphate transport in isolated perfused tubules and in vivo has not yet been ascertained.

References

1.    Geary, C.P. and Cousin, F.B., 1971, Effect of parathyroid extract and glycerol on $^{32}P$ uptake in rat renal tissue. Aust. J. Exp. Biol. Med. Sci. 49: 463.

2.    Egawa, J. and Neuman, W.F., 1964, Effects of parathyroid
      extract on the metabolism of radioactive phosphate in kidney.
      Endocrinology 74: 90.
3.    Burg, M.B. and Orloff, J., 1962, Oxygen consumption and active
      transport in separated renal tubules. Am. J. Physiol. 203: 327.
4.    Nagata, N. and Rasmussen, H., 1970, Renal glyconeogenesis:
      Effect of $Ca^{+2}$ and $H^+$. Biochem. Biophys. Acta 215: 1.
5.    Steiner, A.L., Parker, C.W. and Kipnis, D.M., 1972, Radio-
      immunoassay for cyclic nucleotides, J. Biol. Chem. 247: 1106.
6.    Lowry, O.H., Rosebrough, N.J., Fan, A.R. and Raudull, R.J.,
      1951, Protein measurement with the folin phenol reagment.
      J. Biol. Chem. 193: 265.
7.    Lewis, A.E., 1966, Biostatistics, Reinhold Publ. Corp., New
      York.
8.    Baumann, K., Chan, Y.L., Bode, F. and Papavassiliou, F., 1977,
      Effect of parathyroid hormone and cyclic adenosine 3'5'-
      monophosphate on isotonic fluid reabsorption: polarity of
      proximal tubular cells. Kid. Int'l. 11: 77.
9.    Lang, F., Greger, R., Marchand, G.R. and Knox, F.G., 1977,
      Stationary micro-perfusion study of phosphate reabsorption
      in proximal and distal nephron segments. Pflugers Arch.
      368: 45.
10.   Dennis, V.W. and Brazy, P.C., 1978, Sodium, phosphate, glucose,
      bicarbonate and alanine interactions in the isolated proximal
      convoluted tubule of the rabbit kidney. J. Clin. Invest. 62:
      387.
11.   Dennis, V.W., Bello-Reuss, E. and Robinson, R.R., 1977,
      Response of phosphate transport to parathyroid hormone in
      segments of rabbit nephron. Am. J. Physiol. 233: F29.
12.   Marx, S.J., Fedak, S.A., and Aurbach, G.D., 1972, Preparation
      and characterization of a hormone-respinsive renal plasma
      membrane fraction. J. Biol. Chem. 247: 6913.
13.   Martin, K.J., Hruska, K.A., Lewis, J., Anderson, C. and
      Slatopolsky, E., 1977, The renal handling of parathyroid
      hormone. Role of peritubular uptake and glomerular filtration.
      J. Clin. Invest.  60: 808.
14.   Weinman, E.J. and Suki, W.N., 1978, Evidence for phosphate
      secretion in the rat kidney. Min. Electro. Metab. 1: 92.
15.   Tanaka, Y. and DeLuca, H.F., 1973, The control of 25-hydroxy-
      vitamin D metabolism by inorganic phosphate. Arch. Biochem.
      Biophys. 154: 566.
16.   Biddulph, D.M. and Wrenn, R.W., 1977, Effects of parathyroid
      hormone on cyclic AMP, cyclic GMP, and efflux of calcium in
      isolated renal tubules. J. Cyclic Nucleo Res. 3: 129.
17.   Melson, G.L., Chase, L.R., and Aurbach, G.D., 1970, Parathy-
      roid hormone-sensitive adenyl cyclase in isolated renal
      tubules. Endocrinology 86: 511.
18.   Marcus, R. and Aurbach, G.D., 1969, Bioassay of parathyroid

hormone in vitro with a stable preparation of adenyl cyclase
from rat kidney. Endocrinology 85: 801.
19. Butlen, D. and Jard, S., 1972, Renal handling of 3'5' cyclic
AMP in the rat. Pflugers Arch.  331: 172.

# SODIUM-DEPENDENT TRANSPORT OF INORGANIC PHOSPHATE

# ACROSS THE RENAL BRUSH BORDER MEMBRANE

Heini Murer, Hardy Stern, Gerhard Burckhardt,
Carlo Storelli, and Rolf Kinne

Max-Planck-Institut für Biophysik
6000 Frankfurt (Main) 70
Germany

Studies using intact tissue preparations have documented that transepithelial transport of inorganic phosphate is dependent on the presence of sodium[1]. Physiological studies also revealed that the inorganic phosphate transport rate in the proximal tubule is subject to regulation by various factors such as parathyroid hormone, dietary intake, chronic administration of diphosphonates and chronic application of 1.25 $(OH)_2$ calciferol[2-5].

We present in this contribution a summary of experiments performed with brush border membrane vesicles with the aim to define the transport steps involved in transepithelial transport of inorganic phosphate. As specific aspects the sodium dependence, pH dependence, regulatory phenomena as well as the possible involvement of alkaline phosphatase will be discussed.

## BRUSH BORDER MEMBRANE ISOLATION

During the past several years various methods were developed for the isolation of brush border membranes which subsequently were used for the study of transmembrane movement of different solutes[6]. More recently brush border membrane vesicles were mainly isolated by the so-called $Ca^{2+}$ $(Mg^{2+})$ precipitation method[7]. Morphological as well as immunological studies have indicated that the brush border membrane vesicles are oriented right side out[8]. Transmembrane transport of different solutes is analyzed by incubating the membrane with different tracer substrates and separating the membranes from the incubation media by a rapid filtration technique[9].

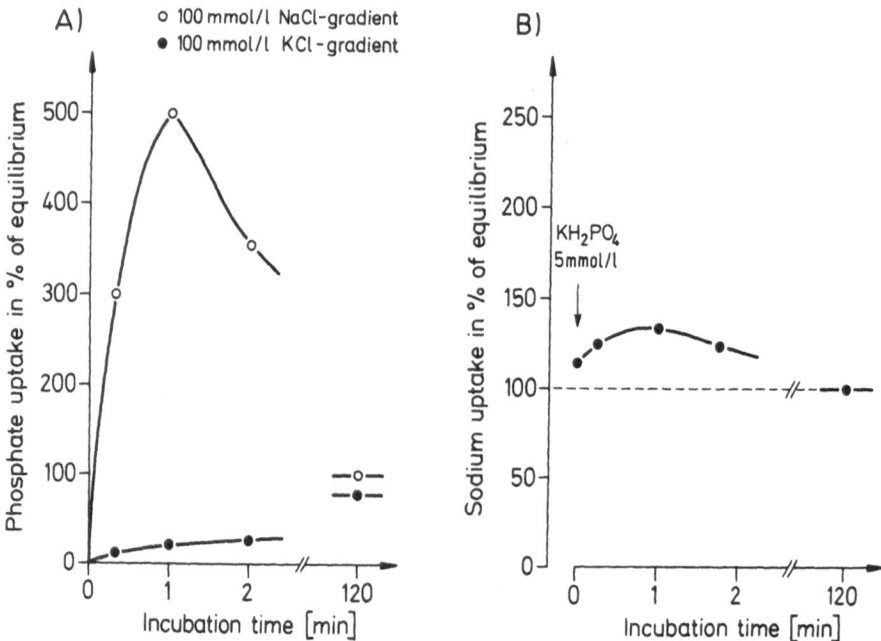

Fig. 1.   Effect of sodium gradient (A) on inorganic phosphate
transport and effect of phosphate gradient (B) on
sodium uptake by rat renal brush border vesicles.
Brush border membrane vesicles isolated by a $Ca^{2+}$ precipitation method[7] were suspended in 100 mmol/1 mannitol,
20 mmol/1 HEPES-Tris (pH 7.4). A) 20 µl of membrane suspension were incubated in 100 µl of a medium containing
in addition 100 mmol/1 NaCl (o) or 100 mmol/1 KCl (●)
and 0.1 mmol/1 $KH_2{}^{32}PO_4$. The results are expressed in percentage of the amount taken up by the vesicles in the
sodium containing medium after 120 min. Equilibrium uptake was 343 pmoles/mg protein. B) Membranes were preincubated for 1 h with 5 mmol/1 ${}^{22}NaSCN$ and 95 mmol/1 KSCN.
The experiment was started by adding 5 µl of an identical
solution containing in addition 100 mmol/1 $KH_2PO_4/K_2HPO_4$
(at pH 7.4) to 100 µl preequilibrated membrane suspension.
The results are expressed in % of the new equilibrium
value reached after 2 h. Equilibrium uptake was 13.2
nmoles/mg protein.

BASIC MECHANISM INVOLVED IN SODIUM-DEPENDENT TRANSPORT OF INORGANIC
PHOSPHATE ACROSS THE BRUSH BORDER MEMBRANE

A strong sodium dependence of transmembrane transport of inorganic phosphate was first described by Hoffmann et al. using
brush border membrane vesicles isolated by the free-flow electro-
phoretic method[10,11]. Similar characteristics of transmembrane
phosphate transport were obtained in studies with membrane vesicles isolated by the calcium precipitation method. In contrast to
any other monovalent cation gradient only a sodium gradient was
able to stimulate uptake of inorganic phosphate against its concentration gradient (Fig. 1A, overshoot). Furthermore, as expected
for a mechanism responsible for a cotransport or flux coupling, a
phosphate gradient was also able to stimulate sodium uptake (Fig.
1B). These stimulatory effects could also be observed under conditions of "short circuited" membrane potential conditions (potassium + valinomycin), i.e. the observed effects represent direct
coupling phenomena rather than indirect effects due to different
diffusion potentials exerted by the different salt gradients.

In contrast to sodium-dependent D-glucose transport sodium-
dependent phosphate transport is potential-insensitive at pH values
where predominantly secondary phosphate is present. As it is seen
from Table 1 potassium-valinomycin induced increased inside nega-
tivity of the transmembrane electrical potential difference stimulates sodium-dependent D-glucose transport but is without comparable effect on sodium-dependent transport of inorganic phos-

Table 1.  Effect of Potassium-Valinomycin Induced
          Diffusion Potentials on Sodium-Dependent
          Phosphate Uptake

|  | phosphate uptake<br>( pmoles / mg protein / 20 s ) | glucose uptake<br>( pmoles / mg protein / 20 s ) |
|---|---|---|
| without valinomycin | 1550 | 480 |
| plus valinomycin | 1750 | 1600 |

Membranes were prepared by the $Ca^{2+}$ precipitation method and
loaded with 100 mmol/1 mannitol, 50 mmol/1 KCl, 2 mmol HEPES-
Tris, pH 7.4, 20 µl membranes were added to 100 µl of an incubation medium containing 100 mmol/1 mannitol, 150 mmol/1
NaCl, 20 mmol HEPES-Tris, pH 7.4, 0.1 mmol/1 $K_2HPO_4$ and 0.1
mmol/1 $^3$H-D-glucose. Valinomycin concentration was approx.
10 µg/mg protein.

phate. This means that the negative charge(s) of the transported
phosphate ion is (are) compensated by the accompanying sodium
ion(s). Assuming that the phosphate transport system accepts either
ion species and at pH 7.4 predominantly secondary phosphate is
transported, one can conclude that stoichiometry is two sodium ions
per transported phosphate ion. This conclusion is in agreement with
the result obtained by Hoffmann et al. in studies on the sodium
concentration dependence of transmembrane phosphate flux using
brush border membranes isolated by free-flow electrophoresis[10].

Electrophysiological studies by Frömter (unpublished observations) have shown that addition of phosphate to the tubular lumen
at low pH values causes depolarization of the cell potential[28].
Assuming that also at low pH, stoichiometry is not altered - as it
is suggested by the experiments of Hoffmann et al.[10] - the electrophysiological data seem to indicate that also primary phosphate is

Table 2.   Effect of Medium pH on Kinetic Parameters
of Sodium-Dependent Phosphate Uptake

|  | $V_{max}$ (nmoles/10s/mg protein) | $K_{m(P_i)}$ (mmol/l) |
|---|---|---|
| medium pH 6.3 | $1.23 \pm 0.35$ | $0.66 \pm 0.02$ |
| medium pH 6.9 | $4.13 \pm 0.39$ | $1.47 \pm 0.04$ |
| medium pH 7.4 | $5.49 \pm 0.34$ | $1.44 \pm 0.08$ |

The $K_a$ ($H_2PO_4^- / HPO_4^{--}$) experimentally determined at the ionic
strength used was 6.86

Membranes were prepared by the $Ca^{2+}$ precipitation method in
100 mmol/l mannitol, 2 mmol/l HEPES-Tris, pH 7.4, and preincubated for 0.5 h with 20 mmol/l MES-Tris, pH 6.3, or 20
mmol/l HEPES-Tris, pH 6.9 and 7.4, respectively. Uptake was
started by adding 1 volume of 1 mol/l NaCl containing the
appropriate concentration of $KH_2^{32}PO_4$ to 9 volumes preequilibrated membrane suspension. Incubation time was 10 s.
The equilibrium space as calculated from the equilibrium
values (2 h) was identical for all the different experimental conditions. $V_{max}$ values and $K_m$ values were derived
from Eadie-Hofstee kinetic plots. 7 different phosphate concentrations in the range between 0.1 and 3.0 mmol/l phosphate
were used. In linear regression analysis correlation coefficient was always higher than 0.9.

transported. Depolarization would therefore be provoked by a cotransport of two sodium ions with primary phosphate. Evidence that
primary phosphate and secondary phosphate are accepted by the transport system is also obtained from experiments at different pH
values on the apparent kinetic parameters of the transport system
(Table 2). The apparent $V_{max}$ of the transport system is augmented
by a factor of 3.5 by increasing pH from 6.3 to 6.9 and by a factor of 4.5 by increasing pH from 6.3 to 7.4. There is also an increase in the apparent $K_m$, i.e. a decrease in the affinity of the
transport system for phosphate by a factor of about 2. If the
nature of the ionic species to be preferentially transported would
be the main determinant for the kinetic parameters, one would expect an alteration predominantly in the apparent $K_m$. Thus a decrease in the apparent $K_m$ values with increasing pH would be expected in a kinetic analysis based on total phosphate concentrations, if secondary phosphate would be the preferentially
accepted species. The observed increase in the apparent $K_m$ value,
however, does not support the view that secondary phosphate is the
preferentially accepted substrate. Stimulation of total phosphate
uptake by increasing pH – as observed also by Hoffmann et al.[10] –
seems to be caused predominantly by an alteration in the apparent
$V_{max}$. The alteration in the apparent $V_{max}$ of the system at a given
constant sodium concentration might reflect a pH-dependent alteration in the apparent affinity of the transport system for its
cosubstrate sodium. This for the following two reasons: 1) As
shown by Evers et al. sodium affects the $V_{max}$ of the phosphate
transport system[16]; 2) As shown by Hoffmann et al. the apparent
$K_m$ for sodium is strongly pH-dependent ranging from 129 mmol/l at
pH 6.0 to 60 mmol/l at pH 7.4[10]. Therefore the difference in the
apparent $V_{max}$ might just reflect a difference in the "saturation"
of the transport system with sodium. An alternate explanation
would be a pH sensitivity of the "carrier molecule" similar to
pH optima in enzyme systems. No attempt was thus far made to
distinguish between these two possibilities. The increase in the
apparent $K_m$ by increasing pH might also reflect different phenomena: 1) If the system would show a preference for primary phosphate an increase in the apparent $K_m$ should be observed if analyzed on the basis of total phosphate. However, the observed increase (factor 2) does not correlate with the decrease in primary
phosphate concentration (pH 6.3 to 7.4 about 10-fold). 2) Affinity
could be decreased due to protonation of cationic groups necessary
for binding of the substrate anion. Again no attempt was made to
distinguish among the two possibilities.

On the basis of the experiments summarized above it seems to
be quite certain that translocation of sodium across the brush
border membrane involves cotransport of two sodium ions with one
phosphate ion. Although it is not yet finally proven, it seems
that secondary as well as primary phosphate are transported according to their availability.

REGULATION OF SODIUM-DEPENDENT TRANSPORT OF INORGANIC PHOSPHATE
ACROSS THE BRUSH BORDER MEMBRANE

During the past two to three years extensive studies on the
regulation of the sodium-dependent transport system for inorganic
phosphate located in the brush border membrane were carried out.
Thereby it was observed that alterations in the handling of inorganic phosphate, as observed in the intact kidney *in situ*, are
expressed on the level of the brush border membrane.

As an example for these studies an experiment on the effect of
dietary phosphate on sodium-dependent transport of inorganic phosphate across the brush border membrane is given in Figure 2. As
compared to sodium-gradient dependent transport of inorganic phosphate by brush border membrane vesicles isolated from rats fed
for a period of 5 to 7 weeks on a standard diet (0.8g%), phosphate
uptake into brush border vesicles isolated from low phosphate diet

Table 3.    Kinetic Parameters of the Sodium-Dependent
            Phosphate Transport System and of Alkaline
            Phosphatase Activity

| | $P_i$ transport | | alkaline phosphatase | |
|---|---|---|---|---|
| | $V_{max}$ (nmoles / 10s / mg prot.) | $K_{m(P_i)}$ (mmol/l) | $V_{max}$ (mU / mg prot.) | $K_m$ (mmol/l) |
| low $P_i$ diet (0.15g %) | 5.46 ± 1.66 | 0.91 ± 0.10 | 19.61 ± 2.04 | 1.58 ± 0.18 |
| high $P_i$ diet (2.0g %) | 2.00 ± 1.48 | 0.92 ± 0.20 | 13.71 ± 2.06 | 1.46 ± 0.07 |

$V_{max}$ values and $K_m$ values were derived from Eadie-Hofstee
kinetic plots. 6 - 8 different substrate concentrations
were used in a range between 0.1 - 10 mmol/1 p-nitro-
phenylphosphate for the enzyme activity and in a range
between 0.1 and 1.5 mmol/1 $P_i$ for transport activity.
Incubation time for uptake measurements was 10 s. The values
represent means ± S.D. from 4 experiments involving 5 ani-
mals/preparation. The p-value for the differences in the
$V_{max}$ was < 0.01. In linear regression analysis correlation
coefficient was always higher than 0.9.

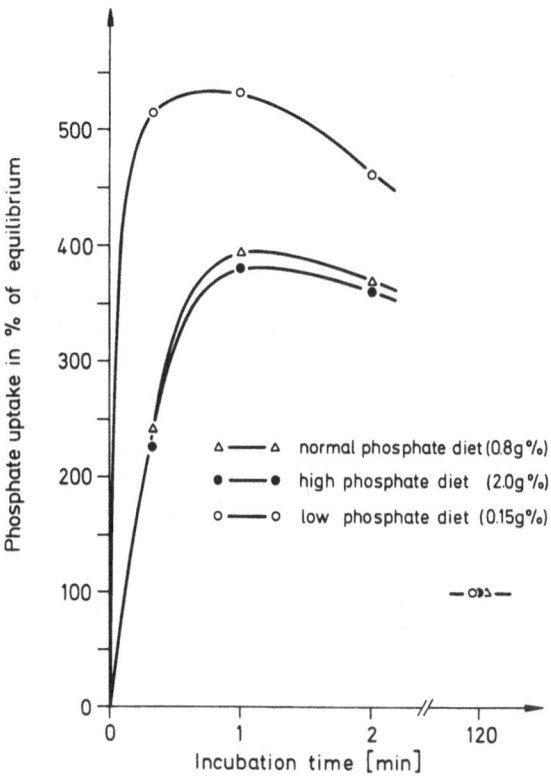

Fig. 2. Effect of dietary intake on sodium-dependent transport of phosphate by renal brush border membrane vesicles. Brush border membrane vesicles isolated by the $Ca^{2+}$ precipitation method were loaded with a buffer containing 100 mmol/l mannitol and 20 mmol/l Hepes-Tris (pH 7.4). 20 µl of membrane suspension were incubated in 100 µl of a medium containing 100 mmol/l NaCl, 100 mmol/l mannitol, 20 mmol/l Hepes-Tris and 0.1 mmol/l phosphate. Phosphate uptake is expressed in percentage of the amount taken up by the vesicles after 120 minutes of incubation. The equilibrium values (120 minutes) for the phosphate uptake by the brush border membrane vesicles amounted to 325 ±12 pmoles/mg protein (mean ± S.D. of the 3 different experimental conditions carried out as triplicate experiments).

animals (0.15g%) is drastically stimulated. Practically no difference, however, could be observed between the standard diet group
and high phosphate diet groups. No significant differences were
observed for the sodium-dependent D-glucose transport using the
same membrane preparations[13]. This suggested dietary induced specific alteration of the sodium-dependent transport of inorganic
phosphate. Similar experiments were also reported by Kempson and
Dousa and by Sacktor and Cheng[14,27]. Recently, we were able to
demonstrate that the increased transport rate in brush border
membrane vesicles isolated from low phosphate diet animals is due
to an increase in the apparent $V_{max}$ of the transport system, the
apparent $K_m$ remaining unaltered (Table 3)[15].

A summary of the studies performed thus far with isolated
brush border vesicles on the regulation of proximal tubular phosphate transport is presented in Table 4. Decrease in sodium-dependent transport of inorganic phosphate by brush border vesicles
is observed after acute administration of parathyroid hormone or
dibutyryl c-AMP, after chronic application of 1.25 $(OH)_2$ calciferol at physiological doses or chronic application of diphosphonates (the inhibitors of bone mineralization) as well as in brush
border membranes isolated from genetically defective hypophosphataemic male mices. Increase in sodium-dependent transport of inorganic phosphate is observed after chronic or acute parathyroidectomy as well as after adaptation to low phosphate diet. Also
resistance to parathyroid hormone in low phosphate diet animals,
which can be abolished by acute phosphate loading, could be demonstrated on the level of isolated brush border membranes. Similar to the effect of dietary adaptation, acute parathyroid hormone
provoked an alteration in the apparent $V_{max}$ of the transport system. It should be mentioned that in all these studies on regulatory phenomena with isolated vesicles the alterations had to be
introduced in the intact animal prior to sacrifice and membrane
isolation. These experiments seem to document that the final
event in the regulation of proximal tubular phosphate transport
occurs at the level of the sodium-dependent transport system for
inorganic phosphate. This could be nicely documented in the studies where phosphate reabsorption was measured by in vivo micropuncture or clearance studies and with vesicles isolated from
rats which have been prepared under identical physiological conditions[19,20]. In view of this parallelism between the handling
of phosphate in the intact proximal tubule and the transport in
isolated membrane vesicles, it is evident that studies with brush
border membrane vesicles might provide a most useful tool in defining biochemical processes involved in these regulatory phenomena.

Table 4. Studies with Isolated Brush Border Vesicles on the Regulation of Proximal Tubular Phosphate Transport

| Status of the animals | Handling of inorganic phosphate in the intact nephron | Observation with vesicles on sodium-dependent transport of inorganic phosphate | Alteration of kinetic parameters | Reference |
|---|---|---|---|---|
| acute parathyroid hormone administration | decreased reabsorption | decreased transport | decreased $V_{max}$ | 2, 16 |
| acute dibutyryl-c-AMP-infusion | decreased reabsorption | decreased transport | – | 16,17,18 |
| chronic administration of diphosphonates | decreased reabsorption | decreased transport | – | 4,19 |
| chronic administration of physiological dosis 1.25 $(OH)_2$ calciferol | decreased reabsorption | decreased transport | – | 5,20 |
| hypophosphataemic male mouse | decreased reabsorption | decreased transport | – | 21 |
| acute (thyro)para-thyroidectomy | increased reabsorption | increased transport | – | 13,18 |
| chronic (thyro)para-thyroidectomy | increased reabsorption | increased transport | – | 5,20 |
| low phosphate diet adaptation | increased reabsorption | increased transport | increased $V_{max}$ | 2,5,13,14, 15,19,20 |
| resistance to para-thyroid hormone | response after $PO_4^{2-}$ load | response after $PO_4^{2-}$ load | – | 13,22 |

POSSIBLE INVOLVEMENT OF ALKALINE PHOSPHATASE IN TRANSMEMBRANE
MOVEMENT OF INORGANIC PHOSPHATE

Several groups reported that the brush border membrane-bound
enzyme alkaline phosphatase is increased in low phosphate diet
animals as compared to high phosphate diet animals[23,24,25]. This
finding led to the speculation that alkaline phosphatase activity
might be associated with a mechanism responsible for phosphate
reabsorption. Recently Kempson and Dousa reported that alkaline
phosphatase activity and inorganic phosphate transport activity
correlates also at the level of the brush border membrane isolated
from rats adapted to different dietary inorganic phosphate contents[14]. However, in their experiments the initial rate of sodium-
dependent phosphate transport in brush border membrane vesicles
isolated from low phosphate diet rats (0.07g%) was about 4 times
higher than in membrane vesicles isolated from high phosphate diet
animals (1.3g%). Stimulation of alkaline phosphatase activity was

Table 5.   Effect of Zinc and EDTA on Alkaline Phos-
           phatase Activity and on Sodium-Dependent
           Transport of Inorganic Phosphate

|  | alkaline phosphatase ( mU/ml ) | phosphate transport ( pmoles/mg protein/20s ) |
|---|---|---|
| control | 483 | 340 |
| 0.2 mmol/l EDTA | 48 | not determined |
| 0.5 mmol/l EDTA | not measurable | 338 |
| control | 510 | 345 |
| 0.5 mmol/l zinc | 145 | 342 |

Membranes were prepared from normal diet animals in 100
mmol/l mannitol, 20 mmol/l Tris/HCl, pH 7.4. The incubation contained in addition 100 mmol/l NaCl and 0.083
mmol/l inorganic phosphate. In addition a final concentration of 0.5 mmol/l EDTA or $Zn^{2+}$ was present. The
values of one typical experiment (in triplicate)
are shown. Alkaline phosphatase activity was measured
in the same membrane preparation in the presence of the
inhibitors EDTA (0.2–0.5 mmol/l) or $Zn^{2+}$ (0.5 mmol/l).

only 1.5-fold, i.e. moderate compared to the stimulation observed in transport. In similar experiments Storelli and Murer[15] observed that alkaline phosphatase activity was not increased in the low phosphate diet group (0.15g%) as compared to the standard phosphate diet group (0.8g%). The group on high phosphate diet (2.0g%), however, showed a drastic decrease in activity if compared with the other two groups. Sodium-dependent transport of inorgnic phosphate was increased 2 to 3-fold in the low phosphate diet group as compared to the standard phosphate diet group, whereas transport activity was only unsignificantly decreased in the high phosphate diet group. By comparing the kinetic parameters of the transport system with that of the enzyme activity in the two extreme dietary groups, high vs low phosphate diet, reduced $V_{max}$ and practically unaltered $K_m$ were found. The difference in the $V_{max}$ of the transport system, however, was much larger than the difference of the $V_{max}$ of the enzyme activity (Table 3)[15].

Alkaline phosphatase activity and transport of phosphate in brush border membrane vesicles were also compared in the presence of EDTA or $Zn^{2+}$ at concentrations which inhibit alkaline phosphatase activity. Transport of inorganic phosphate was not affected by the inhibitors even when alkaline phosphatase was inhibited by more than 70% (0.5 mmol/l $Zn^{2+}$) or completely (0.5 mmol/l EDTA) (Table 5). Comparing kinetic parameters unaltered $K_m$ or $V_{max}$ for the enzyme activity was observed in the presence of EDTA or zinc[15]. Furthermore, the group of Sacktor was able to dissociate alkaline phosphatase activity from transport activity by proteolysis of brush border membrane vesicles isolated from rabbit kidney[26]. All these studies do not support the notion that alkaline phosphatase is involved in transport of inorganic phosphate across the brush border membrane.

## ACKNOWLEDGEMENTS

The authors are grateful to Professor K.J. Ullrich for his encouragement and critical reading of the manuscript.

## REFERENCES

1.  Baumann, K., de Rouffignac, C., Roinel, N., Rumrich, G., and Ullrich, K.J.: Renal phosphate transport: inhomogeneity of local transport rates and sodium dependence. Pflügers Arch. 356: 287 (1975).
2.  Ullrich, K.J., Rumrich, G., and Klöss, S.: Phosphate transport in the proximal convolution of the rat kidney. I. Tubular heterogeneity, effect of parathyroid hormone in acute and chronic parathyroidectomized animals and effect of phosphate diet. Pflügers Arch. 372: 269 (1977).
3.  Tröhler, U., Bonjour, J.P., and Fleisch, H.: Inorganic phosphate homeostasis. Renal adaption to the dietary intake in

intact and thyroparathyroidectomized rats. J. Clin. Invest.
57: 264 (1976).

4.  Bonjour, J.P., Tröhler, U., Preston, C., and Fleisch, H.:
    Parathyroid hormone and renal handling of $P_i$: effect of
    dietary $P_i$ and diphosphonates. Amer. J. Physiol. 234: F497
    (1978).

5.  Bonjour, J.P., Preston, C., and Fleisch, H.: Effect of 1.25
    dihydroxyvitamin $D_3$ on the renal handling of $P_i$ in thyropara-
    thyroidectomized rats. J. Clin. Invest. 60: 1419 (1977).

6.  Kinne, R., and Schwartz, I.L.: Isolated membrane vesicles in
    the evaluation of the nature, localization and regulation of
    renal transport processes. Kidney Int. 14: 547 (1978).

7.  Evers, C., Haase, W., Murer, H., and Kinne, R.: Properties
    of brush border membranes isolated from rat kidney cortex by
    calcium precipitation. J. Membrane Biochem. 1: 203 (1979).

8.  Haase, W., Schäfer, A., Murer, H., and Kinne, R.: Studies on
    the orientation of brush border membrane vesicles. Biochem. J.
    172: 57 (1978).

9.  Berner, W., Kinne, R., and Murer, H.: Phosphate transport in-
    to brush border membrane vesicles isolated from rat small in-
    testine. Biochem. J. 160: 467 (1976).

10. Hoffmann, N., Thees, M., and Kinne, R.: Phosphate transport
    by isolated renal brush border vesicles. Pflügers Arch. 362:
    147 (1976).

11. Kinne, R., Berner, W., Hoffmann, N., and Murer, H.: Phos-
    phate transport by isolated renal and intestinal plasma mem-
    branes. in: Phosphate Metabolism, S.G. Massry, E. Ritz, Eds.
    p. 265. Plenum Press, New York (1977).

12. Ullrich, K.J., Rumrich, G., and Klöss, S.: Phosphate trans-
    port in the proximal convolution of the rat kidney. III. Ef-
    fect of extracellular and intracellular pH. Pflügers Arch.
    377: 37 (1978).

13. Stoll, R., Kinne, R., and Murer, H.: Effect of dietary phos-
    phate intake on phosphate transport by isolated rat renal
    brush border vesicles. Biochem. J. 180, in press (1979).

14. Kempson, S.A., and Dousa, T.P.: Phosphate transport across
    renal cortical brush border membrane vesicles from rats
    stabilized on a normal, high or low phosphate diet. Life
    Sci. 24: 881 (1979).

15. Storelli, C., and Murer, H.: On the correlation between al-
    kaline phosphatase and phosphate reabsorption in proximal
    cortex tubule of rat kidney: studies with isolated brush
    border membrane vesicles. Pflügers Arch., submitted for
    publication.

16. Evers, C., Murer, H., and Kinne, R.: Effect of parathyroid
    hormone on the transport properties of isolated renal brush
    border vesicles. Biochem. J. 172: 49 (1978).

17. Rasmussen, H., Pechet, M., and Fast, D.: Effect of dibutyryl
    c-AMP, theophylline, and other nucleotides upon calcium and

phosphate metabolism. J. Clin. Invest. 47: 1843 (1968).

18.  Kuntziger, H., Amiel, C., Roinel, N., and Morel, F.: Effects of parathyroidectomy and cyclic AMP on renal transport of phosphate, calcium and magnesium. Amer. J. Physiol. 227: 905 (1974).

19.  Stoll, R., Murer, H., Fleisch, H., and Bonjour, J.P.: Effect of diphosphonate treatment on phosphate transport by renal brush border vesicles. Amer. J. Physiol., submitted for publication.

20.  Stoll, R., Kinne, R., and Murer, H.; Bonjour, J.P., and Fleisch, H.: Phosphate transport by rat renal brush border membrane vesicles: Influence of dietary phosphate, thyropara-thyroidectomy and 1.25-dihydroxyvitamin $D_3$. Pflügers Arch. 380: 47 (1979).

21.  Tenenhouse, H.S., Scriver, C.R., Mc Innes, R.R., and Glorieux F.H.: Renal handling of phosphate in vivo and in vitro by the X-linked hypophosphataemic male mouse: Evidence for a defect in the brush border membrane. Kidney Int. 14: 236 (1978).

22.  Sutton, R.A., Quamme, G., O'Callighan, T., Wong, N.L.M., and Dirks, J.H.: Renal tubular phosphate reabsorption in the phosphate depleted dog. in: Homeostasis of Phosphate and other Minerals, S.G. Massry, E. Ritz, A. Rapado, Eds. p. 405. Plenum Press, New York (1978).

23.  Kempson, S., Knox, F.G., and Dousa, T.: Enzyme changes in the renal cortex induced by low phosphate diet. Kidney Int. 12: 563 (1977).

24.  Melani, F., Ramponi, G., Farnararo, M., Cocucci, E., and Guerritore, A.: Regulation by phosphate of alkaline phos-phatase in rat kidney. Biochim. Biophys. Acta 138: 411 (1967).

25.  Plante, G.E., Erian, R., Nawar, T., and Peticlerc, C.: Renal transport of phosphate: role of alkaline phosphatase. in: Abstracts VIIth Int. Congress Nephrol., Montreal, E-13, June 1978.

26.  Noroaha-Blob, L.: Effects of papain on enzymic and transport functions of isolated rabbit renal brush border vesicles. Fed. Proc. 38: 838 (1979).

27.  Sacktor, B., and Cheng, L.: Phosphate transport in rabbit renal proximal tubule membrane vesicles, and its regulation. Fed. Proc. 38: S5, 110 (1979).

28.  Frömter, E., and Ullrich, K.J.: Effect of inhibitors and the mechanisms of anion transport in the proximal renal tubule of rats. Ann. New York Acad. Sci., submitted for publication.

# PHOSPHATE TRANSPORT IN ISOLATED AND PERFUSED RENAL TUBULES

Vincent W. Dennis, Peter C. Brazy and J. Wade McKeown

Division of Nephrology
Duke University Medical Center
Durham, North Carolina

## INTRODUCTION

The isolated perfused renal tubule technique has been adapted to study a number of questions regarding the renal handling of phosphate. The purpose of this review is to describe the observations made thus far relative to four areas of interest; segmental localization of phosphate reabsorption, structural-functional heterogeneity for phosphate transport, cellular mechanisms of phosphate reabosrption, and factors regulating epithelial phosphate reabsorption rates. Although our presentation will emphasize data obtained using the isolated perfused renal tubule technique, these observations need to be viewed, of course, in the context of the important information obtained using clearance, micropuncture and membrane vesicle techniques. This information has been reviewed previously.[1]

## METHODS

The basic methods used to study phosphate transport in isolated segments of the nephron have been described previously in detail.[2] Briefly, specific segments of the rabbit nephron are dissected and perfused in vitro with fluids of known but variable composition. In our laboratory, unidirectional fluxes of phosphate from lumen to bath and from bath to lumen are measured simultaneously by use of the two radioactive isotopes of phosphate, $^{32}P$ and $^{33}P$. Alternatively, others[3] measure net phosphate transport by electron probe microanalysis of the phosphate concentration in the perfusate and collected fluids.

LOCALIZATION OF PHOSPHATE REABSORPTION

Table 1 lists the values for phosphate reabsorption observed for various segments of the nephron. Only the rabbit nephron has been examined thus far and for this species every classical segment has been studied except the distal convoluted tubule. As noted in Table 1, and as demonstrated by micropuncture studies,[4] the highest rates of phosphate reabsorption occur in proximal convoluted tubules. Significant reabsorption of phosphate also occurs in the proximal straight tubule. Because phosphate reabsorption clearly occurs in the proximal straight tubule and because this segment lies beyond the point of late proximal micropuncture, there can be little doubt that the proximal straight tubule contributes, at least in part, to the so-called distal or loop component of phosphate reabsorption described by some micropuncture studies.[5,6,7] No phosphate reabsorption is detectable in the thin or thick limbs of Henle as examined in vitro.[8] It seems likely, therefore, that any reabsorption of phosphate that may occur between the points of late proximal-distal micropuncture occurs in the pars recta of the proximal tubule rather than specific portions of the loop of Henle.

On the other hand, as also noted in Table 1, there is clearly a distal component of phosphate reabsorption. Both Shareghi and Agus[9] and Peraino[10] have demonstrated small but measurable rates of phosphate reabsorption in cortical collecting tubules perfused under conditions that provide electrochemical gradients for phosphate from lumen to bath. We had demonstrated earlier that no measurable net transport of

Table 1.    Localization of Phosphate Absorption

| Segment | Rate<br>pmol/mm·min | Reference |
|---|---|---|
| Proximal convoluted | 6.60+1.41 | 2 |
| Proximal straight | 2.20+0.48 | 2 |
| Thin descending limb | undetectable | 8 |
| Thin ascending limb | undetectable | 8 |
| Thick ascending limb | undetectable | 8 |
| | undetectable | 9 |
| Cortical collecting tubule | undetectable | 11 |
| | 0.3 | 9 |
| | 0-1.2 | 10 |

phosphate occurred in this segment during perfusion with symmetric fluids.[11] The physiological impact of this small but significant component of phosphate reabsorption is uncertain. It appears to be independent of the direct effects of parathyroid hormone (PTH) in vitro and therefore differs perhaps from phosphate reabsorption that occurs in vivo in the distal convoluted tubule of the rat.[12] This component is inhibited by PTH.

HETEROGENEITY OF PROXIMAL REABSORPTION OF PHOSPHATE

It is clear from the data in Table 1 that the major portion of phosphate reabsorption occurs in the proximal convoluted and straight tubules. There is increasing recognition, however that subdivision of the proximal tubule on the basis of external configuration alone is an imperfect reflection of important ultrastructural and physiological differences that may exist along the length of externally similar segments. Thus, the proximal tubule of the rabbit may be subdivided on the basis of cell types into three sequential segments, $S_1$, $S_2$ and $S_3$. Woodhall et al[13] demonstrated that these three segments transport para-aminohippurate (PAH) at markedly different rates and we have used this observation to characterize proximal convoluted tubules as being early or late. That is, convoluted tubules that secrete PAH at relatively high rates may be expected to have originated from a later portion of the proximal convoluted tubule than convoluted segments that secrete PAH at lower rates. On the basis of our own observations,[14] we arbitrarily designate proximal convoluted tubules that secrete PAH at rates less than 300 fmol/mm·min as being early and those that secrete PAH at higher rates as being late. Using these criteria, we observed that twenty early proximal convoluted tubules reabsorbed phosphate at rates that averaged 11.05+1.15 pmol/mm·min and twenty late but convoluted segments averaged 3.82+0.48 pmol/mm·min (P < 0.001). All tubules were perfused with the same fluids and thus we conclude that phosphate reabsorptive rates in the early portions of the proximal convoluted tubule are 2-3 times the rates in later convolutions. Said in another way, there is heterogeneity for phosphate transport along the longitudinal axis of the proximal tubule (axial heterogeneity).

On the other hand, twenty proximal convoluted segments obtained from superficial nephrons reabsorbed phosphate at the same rate as twenty proximal convoluted tubules derived from juxtamedullary nephrons (7.19+1.34 versus 7.67+1.05 pmol/mm·min, respectively). Accordingly, there is no evidence from these data to support the presence of internephronal heterogeneity.

CELLULAR MECHANISMS

At this time, investigations of cellular mechanisms involved in transepithelial movement of phosphate have been

limited primarily to the proximal convoluted tubule. The
earliest studies[2] demonstrated that phosphate reabsorption by
the proximal convoluted tubule resulted primarily from the
unidirectional flux from lumen to bath and that little backflux
occurred.  The ratio of lumen-to-bath over bath-to-lumen fluxes
of phosphate exceeds 10:1 and thus the lumen-to-bath flux may
generally be regarded as absorption or net transport of phosphate.  Phosphate reabsorption in the isolated proximal tubule
is also saturated at the usual perfusion rates of 10-15 nl/min
and the usual phosphate concentrations of 1.5-1.8 mM in the
perfusate.

Two basic theories have been proposed to relate the reabsorption of phosphate to cellular metabolism.  The first
proposes that monovalent phosphate may be more permeant than
divalent phosphate and that phosphate is reabsorbed as a result
of acidification of the luminal fluid.[15]  Three lines of evidence
have been offered against this proposal.[11]  First, phosphate
reabsorption rates in vitro do not correlate with proximal
acidification rates as estimated by the increase in chloride
concentration in the collected fluids.  Second, phosphate reabsorption rates do not increase when bicarbonate is removed from
the perfusate even though intraluminal phosphate would then
represent the major intraluminal buffer for secreted hydrogen
ions.  Third, decreases in the pH of the ambient fluids by
changes in $PCO_2$ and bicarbonate concentration result in decreases in phosphate transport rather than increases as might be
expected if monovalent phosphate was more permeant. Thus, although
none of these arguments is conclusive, there is no support in
these observations for the theory that proximal phosphate reabsorption results from acidification of the luminal fluid.

The second major theory relates phosphate reabsorption to
metabolically-dependent sodium  transport.  Sodium transport by
the proximal convoluted tubule is a multifactorial process
involving cellular and paracellular pathways.  Figure 1 presents
schematically some of the components of sodium transport that
have been identified and that can be modified experimentally.
Sodium entry  at the luminal surface involves elements dependent
on the presence of glucose and of alanine. These sodium entry
steps contribute to the transepithelial electrical potential
difference[16] and thus may be designated as electrogenic (E).
Glucose entry is inhibited by phlorizin. Bicarbonate-dependent
sodium transport  in the rabbit is apparently electroneutral (N)
and may be inhibited by carbonic anhydrase inhibitors (CAI).  At
the basolateral surfaces, sodium extrusion is metabolically-
dependent and may be inhibited by ouabain and by removal of
potassium from the bath.

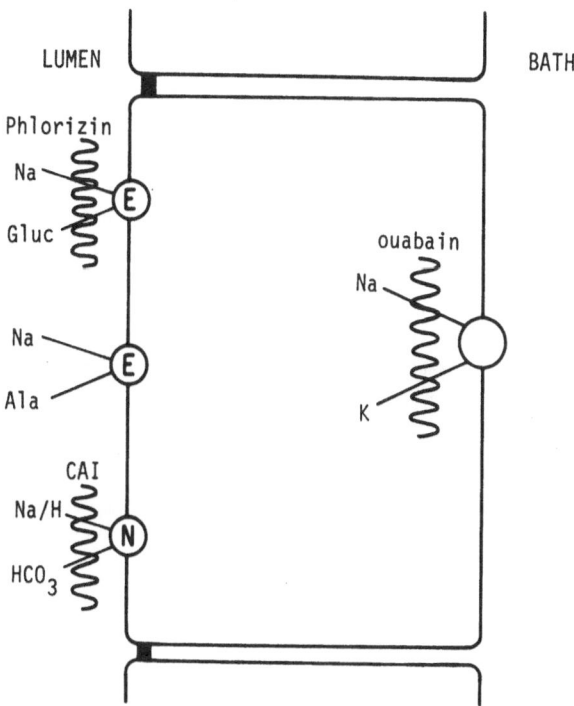

Figure 1.   Schematic representation of some sodium-related
transport processes proposed for the proximal renal tubule.


We performed studies to examine to what extent phosphate
transport may be related to each of these components of sodium
transport.[17]  First, the addition of $10^{-4}$ M ouabain to the bath
or the removal of potassium from the bath completely eliminated
the net transport of both sodium and phosphate.  Second, the
partial replacement of sodium chloride in the perfusate with
choline chloride resulted in proportional reductions in both
sodium and phosphate reabsorption.  These data indicate that
phosphate reabsorption by the proximal convoluted tubule is
related to some function of sodium transport.

Selective elimination of the glucose-, alanine-, or bicarbonate-dependent components of sodium transport had different
effects, however.  Removal of alanine from the perfusate, or
removal of glucose, or inhibition of glucose transport by
phlorizin each caused an increase in phosphate reabsorption of

about 60 percent although sodium uptake may  be expected to be
decreased by these maneuvers.  Inhibition of bicarbonate transport
by $2x10^{-4}$M acetazolamide in  the lumen and bath or by removing
bicarbonate from the perfusate had no effect on phosphate
reabsorption (Figure 2).  Phosphate reabsorption was inhibited
only if bicarbonate was removed from both the perfusate and the
bath, conditions that caused marked reductions in fluid  absorption
or net sodium transport.  Thus, at the luminal surface, phosphate
transport was inhibited by glucose and alanine transport but not
by bicarbonate transport.  This may  relate to the observation
that glucose and alanine transport result in changes in transmembrane
electrical potential differences whereas bicarbonate transport
may not.  That is, phosphate uptake appears to be sensitive to
changes in the transmembrane electrical potential difference

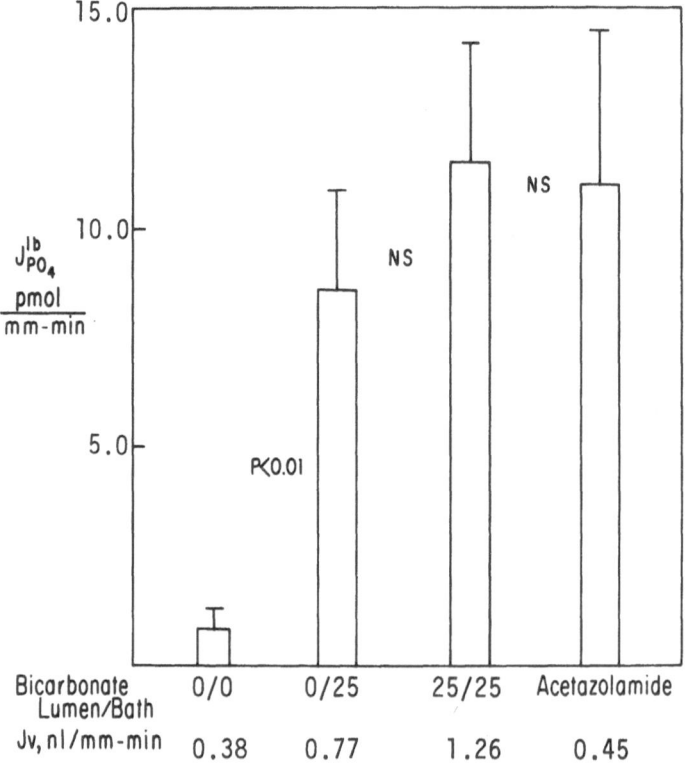

Figure 2.  Effects on phosphate and fluid absorption rates of
modifications in bicarbonate transport.  Bicarbonate when absnet
was replaced with chloride in artificial solutions that resemble
glomerular ultrafiltrate and rabbit serum.

that are presumed to result from the luminal uptake of glucose
and alanine.

These observations lead us to the working hypothesis
illustrated schematically in Figure 3.  Phosphate reabsorption
appears to result from the sodium-dependent uptake of phosphate
at the luminal surface (site 1).  This site is clearly different
from that involved in phlorizin-sensitive glucose uptake. Site 2
indicates the interaction beyond the brush border receptor sites
between phosphate transport and glucose or alanine transport.
The nature  of this interaction is unclear but may involve
indirect effects of transmembrane potentials or of changes in
cellular metabolism.  Ultimately, the net transport of phosphate,
glucose, alanine and bicarbonate depends on sodium extrusion at
the basolateral surface (site 3). In this schema, bicarbonate
transport at the luminal surface does not interact with phosphate
reabsorption, perhaps because it is electroneutral.[18]  Paracellular transport of phosphate has not been examined sufficiently at
this time.

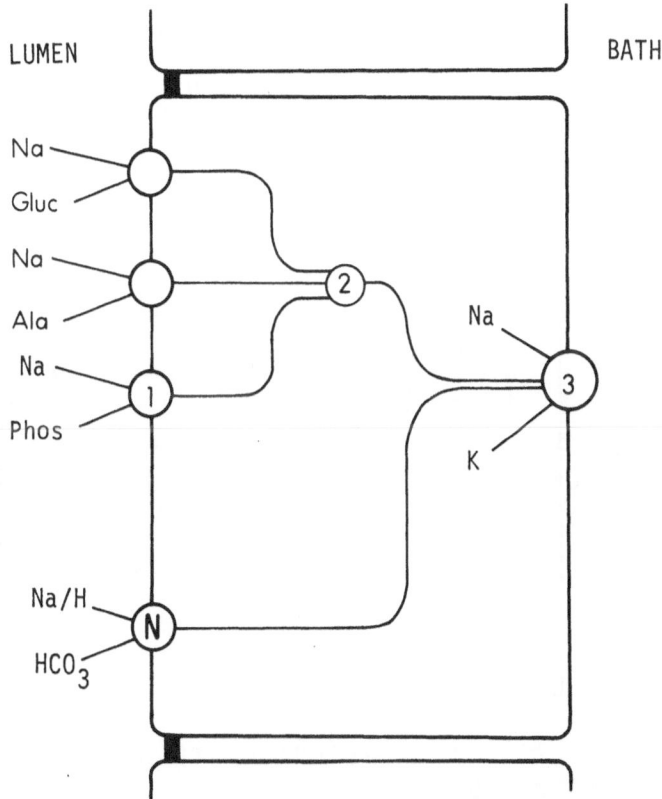

Figure 3.   Schematic representation of interactions among
phosphate transport and various components of sodium transport
in the proximal renal tubule.

FACTORS THAT REGULATE PHOSPHATE TRANSPORT

The two major factors that regulate phosphate excretion rates are PTH and the dietary uptake of phosphate. Figure 4 depicts the acute effects on fractional clearance of phosphate of bovine PTH, 1.0 unit/kg·min administered intravenously to anesthetized rabbits. The rabbits received mechanical respiratory ventilation to maintain $PCO_2$ constant and normal. As noted in Figure 4, the fractional clearance of phosphate increased significantly within 10 minutes after infusion of the PTH. Absolute rates of phosphate excretion increased from 0.128+0.020 to 0.152+0.018 mg/min, P < 0.01). Thus, PTH is clearly phosphaturic in these rabbits.

The effects of PTH on fluid and phosphte reabsorption by isolated proximal tubules have been described in detail.[19] Briefly, PTH at concentrations exceeding 0.01 units/ml bath inhibits bicarbonate-dependent sodium transport in proximal convoluted and straight tubules. On the other hand, phosphate reabsorption was inhibited by PTH only in the pars recta or late

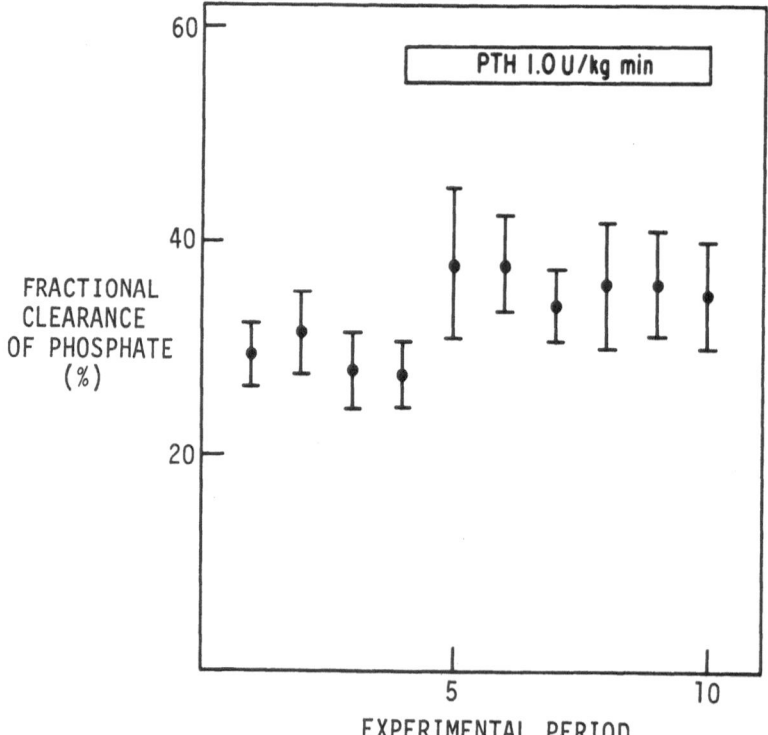

Figure 4. Effect of bovine PTH on fractional clearance of phosphate in anesthetized, ventilated rabbits. Each experimental period was about 10 minutes.

portion of the proximal tubule.  Thus, the inhibitory effects of PTH on bicarbonate transport appear to be distributed more generally along the length of the proximal tubule than are the inhibitory effects of PTH on phosphate reabsorption.  Also, the late proximal tubule appears to be the site of the effect of PTH on phosphate transport, at least in the rabbit.  Thus, important heterogeneity exists along the proximal tubule with regard to phosphate transport and its sensitivity to PTH.

The second major factor that affects the phosphate excretion rate is the dietary intake of phosphate.  The recommended minimum dietary content for phosphate for the rabbit is 0.22%.  Standard rabbit chow usually contains about 0.45%.  Preliminary data from our laboratory indicate that proximal convoluted tubules derived from rabbits maintained on a low phosphate diet (0.07%) reabsorb phosphate at rates that are significantly higher (11.07+1.30 pmol/mm·min) than rates observed for tubules from rabbits maintained on normal phosphate intake (7.23+1.02 pmol/mm·min; P < 0.02). These differences in phosphate transport rates occurred despite perfusion of all tubules with ultrafiltrate and serum obtained from normal rabbits. Thus, the changes in proximal tubule phosphate transport that occur  in response to differences in phosphate content of the diet persist in vitro and are largely independent of the composition of the ambient fluids. Further investigation of this adaptative phenomenon is clearly indicated.

SUMMARY

In summary, studies of phosphate transport by isolated renal tubules perfused in vitro confirm many of the data obtained by other techniques with regard to localization.  The major contributions of the technique revolve around studies of segments not accessible to micropuncture techniques and around studies of epithelial transport processes that are difficult to examine in vivo.

REFERENCES

1.  V.W. Dennis, W.W. Stead and J.L. Myers, Renal handling of phosphate and calcium, Ann. Rev. Physiol. 41:257 (1979).

2.  V.W. Dennis, P.B. Woodhall and R.R. Robinson,  Characteristics of phosphate transport in isolated proximal renal tubule. Am. J. Physiol. 231:979 (1976).

3.  G.R. Shareghi and Z.S. Agus, Magnesium transport in the rabbit cortical thick ascending limb.  Clin. Res. 27:430A (1979).

4.  J.C. Strickler, D.D. Thompson, R.M. Klose and G. Giebisch.
    Micropuncture study of inorganic phosphate excretion in the
    rat. J. Clin. Invest. 43:1596 (1964).

5.  C. Amiel, H. Kuntziger and G. Richet, Micropuncture study
    of handling of phosphate by proximal and distal nephron in
    normal and parathyroidectomized rat. Evidence for distal
    reabsorption. Pfluegers Arch. 317:93 (1970).

6.  H. Kuntziger, C. Amiel and C. Gaudebout, Phosphate handling
    by the rat nephron during saline diuresis. Kidney Internat.
    2:318 (1972).

7.  R.F. Greger, F. Lang, G. Marchand and F. G. Knox, Site of
    renal phosphate reabsorption-micropuncture and microinfusion
    study. Pfluegers Arch. 369:111 (1977).

8.  A.S. Rocha, J.B. Magaldi and J.P. Kokko, Calcium and
    phosphate transport in isolated segments of rabbit Henle's
    loop. J. Clin. Invest. 59:975 (1977).

9.  G.R. Shareghi and Z.S. Agus, Phosphate transport in the
    light segment of the rabbit cortical collecting tubule.
    Clin. Res. 27:430A (1979).

10. R.A. Peraino, Preliminary  study of phosphate transport by
    the cortical collecting tubule of the rabbit. Abstracts of
    the Eleventh Annual Meeting of the American Society of
    Nephrology 11:8A (1978).

11. V.W. Dennis, E. Bello-Reuss and R.R. Robinson, Response of
    phosphate transport to parathyroid hormone in segments of
    rabbit nephron. Am. J. Physiol. 233:F29 (1977).

12. E. Pastoriza-Munoz, R.E. Colindres, W.E. Lassiter and C.
    LeChene, Effect of PTH on phosphate transport in the  rat
    distal convolution. Am. J. Physiol. 235:F321 (1978).

13. P.B.  Woodhall, C.C.  Tisher, C.A. Simonton and R.R. Robinson,
    Relationship  between para-aminohippurate sectetion and
    cellular morphology in rabbit proximal tubules. J. Clin.
    Invest. 61:1320 (1978).

14. J.W. McKeown, P.C. Brazy and V.W. Dennis, Intrarenal hetero-
    geneity for fluid, phosphate and glucose absorption in the
    rabbit. Am. J. Physiol. (in press).

15.  N. Bank, H.S. Aynedjian and S.W. Weinstein, A microper-
     fusion study of phosphate reabsorption by the rat proximal
     renal tubule. J. Clin. Invest. 54:1040 (1974).

16.  J.P. Kokko, Proximal tubule potential difference:  dependence
     on glucose, $HCO_3$ and amino acids. J. Clin. Invest. 52:1362
     (1973).

17.  V.W. Dennis and P.C. Brazy, Sodium, phosphate, glucose,
     bicarbonate and alanine interactions in the isolated
     proximal convoluted tubule of the rabbit kidney. J. Clin.
     Invest. 62:387 (1978).

18.  M. Burg and N. Green, Bicarbonate transport by isolated
     perfused  rabbit proximal convoluted tubules. Am. J.
     Physiol. 233:F307 (1977).

19.  V.W.  Dennis, Influence of bicarbonate on parathyroid
     hormone-induced changes in fluid absorption by proximal
     tubule. Kidney Internat. 10:373 (1976).

# CALCIUM TRANSPORT IN THE PARS RECTA AND THE LOOP OF HENLE

Wadi N. Suki, M.D.

Renal Section, Department of Medicine
Baylor College of Medicine, & The Methodist Hospital
Houston, Texas   77030

In 1963 Lassiter et al[1] concluded from micropuncture studies that approximately 60% of the filtered calcium was reabsorbed in the proximal tubule and 35% was absorbed by more distal segments. Since only about 10% of the filtered calcium remains at the early distal convoluted tubule,[2] the loop of Henle must absorb about 30% of the filtered load.  Comparing the findings at the hairpin bend of the loop of Henle in the hamster to those in the distal tubule of the rat, Lassiter et al[1] concluded that the thick ascending limb (TAL) was the major site of calcium absorption.  Five different laboratories, including our own, have investigated calcium transport in this segment directly using the isolated rabbit renal tubule perfused in vitro by the method of Burg et al.[3]

The unidirectional fluxes of calcium from lumen-to-bath ($J_{lb}^{Ca}$) and from bath-to-lumen ($J_{bl}^{Ca}$) were measured in segments of TAL using $^{45}Ca$ in the perfusate and in the bath respectively.  Exhaustively dialyzed $^3H$-inulin was added to the perfusate as a volume marker.  The tubules were perfused with a bicarbonate-free solution, and bathed with an artificial ultrafiltrate of rabbit serum with 5% by volume calf serum added.

There are two methods to measure $J_{lb}^{Ca}$ with this technic:  one, by the difference between perfused and collected counts of $^{45}Ca$, and the other, by the counting of $^{45}Ca$ appearing in the bath.  In a series of tubules perfused with a bicarbonate free solution we found a very close correlation between these technics and, therefore, utilized the former technic in the studies to be presented.

Because of the known morphologic, enzymatic and functional heterogeneity of the TAL we studied calcium transport in both

medullary (mTAL) and cortical (cTAL) portions of this nephron segment.  In the mTAL furosemide in a concentration of $5 \times 10^{-5}$M
reversibly inhibited the transtubular potential difference (P.D.)
from 4mV to 1.5mV and back to 4mV.  Concomitantly $J_{1b}^{ca}$ fell from
12.8 to 5.5 and recovered to 11.8 peq·min$^{-1}$·cm$^{-1}$ when the diuretic
was removed.  These observations suggest a passive mechanism for
calcium efflux in this segment.  By contrast, in the cTAL furosemide
which also reversibly inhibits P.D. (3.3mV to 1.7mV and back to
2.7mV) was without effect on $J_{1b}^{ca}$ (9.7, 13.0 and 9.7 peq·min$^{-1}$·cm$^{-1}$).

    To study the differences between these two segments further,
we have measured $J_{1b}^{ca}$ & $J_{b1}^{ca}$ sequentially and randomly and calculated
the apparent permeabilities corrected for the P.D.  The ratio of
$P_{1b}/P_{b1}$ was calculated and compared to that predicted from the P.D.
for passive diffusion using the Ussing equation.  In the cTAL the
premeability ratio was more than twice that predicted, while in
the mTAL the ratio was not significantly different from that predicted from the P.D.  These results clearly demonstrate intrinsic
differences between mTAL and the cTAL but they do not in and of
themselves indicate active calcium transport in the cTAL.  Taken
together with the studies using fursemide,  however, our studies
lead  us to the conclusion that a component of active calcium
transport exists in the cortical thick ascending limb of Henle's
loop.

    Our studies are both in agreement and in conflict with those
of others, all of whom studied only the cTAL.  Both Rocha et al.[4]
and Imai[5] concluded that active calcium transport exists in this
segment.  Shareghi and Stoner[6] and Bourdeau and Burg[7], however,
concluded that calcium transport was purely passive, although
the latter authors[7] proposed an interaction between the ions as
they traverse the pores in opposing directions, the so-called single-
file diffusion.  The reasons for these differences are not clear
but methodological differences and the heterogeneity of the TAL
may well be responsible.  These differences not withstanding, there
is general agreement that the TAL contributes significantly to
calcium absorption in the loop of Henle.

    Earlier studies by Jamison et al[8] have suggested that a seg-
ment prior to the hairpin bend of the loop of Henle may also
contribute to calcium absorption in the loop.  They observed that
at the bend of the loop of Henle TF/UF ratio for calcium was lower
than the TF/P sodium, whereas these ratios were similar in the
superficial proximal tubule.  Also, the fractional delivery of
calcium to the bend of the loop was less than that of sodium,
suggesting absorption of calcium in excess of sodium in the descending limb of Henle.  Since the proximal straight tubule is known
to perform a variety of important transport functions, we investigated its possible role in calcium transport.

Utilizing the technics described earlier we studied unidirectional and net ($J^{Ca}_{net}$) calcium flux in superficial straight proximal
tubules. $J^{Ca}_{net}$ was measured by perfusing the tubule and bathing it
with ultrafiltrate and rabbit serum, respectively, of identical ul-
trafiltratable calcium concentration and $^{45}Ca$ specific activity.
The superficial origin of the tubules was ascertained by imposing a
50 mEq/l NaCl gradient (bath < lumen) and observing a positive P.D.
of at least 3mV. Because rabbit serum ultrafiltrate was used in
these experiments, the perfusate by necessity contained 25mM bicarbonate.

The results of these studies demonstrate a $J^{Ca}_{bl}$ of 8.0, and
$J^{Ca}_{lb}$ of 22 pEq min$^{-1}$ mm$^{-1}$. Calculated $J^{Ca}_{net}$ of 13 compared favorably
with the directly measured value of 11 pEq/min$^{-1}$ mm$^{-1}$. These values
of $J^{Ca}_{net}$ are three or four-fold net calcium absorption which can be
attributed to convectional forces. As expected, therefore, calcium
concentration in the effluent fluid was lowered by 18%. This out-
ward transport of calcium against a concentration and an electrical
(lumen-to-bath P.D.-1mV) gradient suggests an active mechanism for
calcium absorption in this segment. This transport process was not
saturated but appeared to increase with load; $J^{Ca}_{net}$ increased significantly at higher perfusion rates in a series of 20 tubules studied.

To further characterize this transport process, ouabain $10^{-5}M$
was added to the bath. While it caused a profound depression of
water absorption ($J_v$) and P.D., largely reversed by its removal
from the bath, ouabain did not significantly inhibit $J^{Ca}_{net}$. These
studies, however, do not completely exclude a relationship between
calcium and sodium transport in this segment. The tubules were
exposed to ouabain for a maximum period of 50 minutes, a period
conceivably insufficient for intracellular sodium to have risen.

Unlike ouabain, perfusion of the tubules at 25°C was associated
with insignificant calcium efflux. Warming the tubules to 37°C,
however, resulted in a steady rise of $J^{Ca}_{net}$ over a period of two
hours to values approximately half those observed in tubules that
were heated promptly after dissection. These studies suggest that
calcium transport in the superficial proximal straight tubule is
dependent upon an energy-producing metabolic process.

To validate further the above findings six thin descending
limb segments were studied in a manner identical to that used for
studying the superficial proximal straight tubule. Unlike the
latter segment, Jv, $J^{Ca}_{lb}$ and $J^{Ca}_{net}$ did not differ signficantly from
zero. The permeability, $P_{lb}$, was 0.64 x $10^{-5}$cm sec$^{-1}$, a value
comparable to that reported by Rocha et al[4], and twenty times
smaller than that of the superficial pars recta (12-14 x $10^{-5}$cm
sec$^{-1}$). These data clearly indicate that the thin descending limb
of Henle's loop is incapable of calcium absorption. Further, they

lend support and verification to the findings observed with
identical techniques in the superficial pars recta. The preliminary
report of data very similar to ours by Almeida, Kudo and Rocha[9]
lends further support to our observations.

In summary, studies in isolated rabbit renal tubular segments
perfused in vitro point to an important role for the proximal
straight tubule and the thick ascending limb, but not the thin
descending limb, in calcium transport.

## Acknowledgment

The author is deeply indebted to the diligent work of Ms. Diane
Rouse and Dr. Roland C. K. Ng. Work supported by research grant
# AM-21394 from the National Institute of Arthritis, Metabolism
and Digestive Diseases, National Institute of Health.

## REFERENCES

1.  W. E. Lassiter, C. W. Gottschalk, and M. Mylle, Micropuncture
    study of renal tubular reabsorption of calcium in normal rodents,
    Am. J. Physiol. 204:771 (1963).
2.  L. S. Costanzo, and E. E. Windhager, Calcium and sodium trans-
    port by the distal convoluted tubule of the rat, Am. J. Physiol.
    235:F492 (1978).
3.  M. B. Burg, J. Grantham, M. Ahramow, and J. Orloff, Preparation
    and study of fragments of single rabbit nephrons, Am. J. Physiol.
    210:1293 (1966).
4.  A. S. Rocha, J. B. Magaldi, and J. P. Kokko, Calcium and phos-
    phate transport in isolated segments of rabbit Henle's loop,
    J. Clin. Invest. 39:975 (1977).
5.  M. Imai, Calcium transport across the rabbit thick ascending
    limb of Henle's loop perfused in vitro, Pflugers Arch. 374:255
    (1978).
6.  G. R. Shareghi, and L. C. Stoner, Calcium transport across
    segments of the rabbit distal nephron in vitro. Am. J. Physiol.
    235:F367 (1978).
7.  J. E. Bourdeau, and M. B. Burg, Voltage dependence of calcium
    transport in the thick ascending limb of Henle's loop. Am. J.
    Physiol.  236:F357 (1979).
8.  R. L. Jamison, N. R. Frey, and F. B. Lacy, Calcium reabsorption
    in the thin loop of Henle, Am. J. Physiol. 227:745 (1974).
9.  A. L. J. Almeida, L. H. Kudo, and A. S. Rocha, Calcium transport
    in isolated perfused pars recta of proximal tubule.  Abstracts
    VIIth Int. Congress Nephrol. E-16 (1978).

RENAL MAGNESIUM TRANSPORT AND THE EFFECTS OF HYPERMAGNESEMIA,

HYPERCALCEMIA, BODY MAGNESIUM STORES AND PARATHYROID HORMONE

J. H. Dirks and G. A. Quamme

Department of Medicine and
G. F. Strong Laboratory for Medical Research
University of British Columbia
Vancouver, Canada

Handling of magnesium by the mammalian kidney is normally characterized by a filteration-reabsorptive system with little evidence for secretion (1). Despite considerable recent interest in the mechanism of renal magnesium reabsorption it has been difficult to characterize the system fully because of the very different processes occurring along the various nephron segments. Thus the sole use of urinary excretion rates may lead to mistaken interpretations as to cellular mechanisms.

Micropuncture investigations in all species studied to date (2-6) have indicated similar patterns of magnesium handling along the nephron. Direct micropuncture of surface glomeruli of the Munich-Wistar rat (7,8) indicate some 70-80% of the plasma magnesium is filtered at the glomerular membrane. Free flow micropuncture studies in rodents (2-5) and dogs (6) have demonstrated the tubular fluid to ultrafilterable (TF/UF) ratio for magnesium increases along the proximal tubule. This is in contrast to the concentration ratios of other major cations which remain close to unity as water is abstracted. This results in tubular fluid entering the loop with a magnesium concentration greater than glomerular filtrate. Tubular fluid obtained from the early distal tubule contains significantly less magnesium than does the glomerular filtrate, indicating that the loop of Henle is the major nephron segment reclaiming a significant portion of the filtered load. Comparison of samples taken from the bend of the loop with the early distal tubule (4,5) implicate the important role of the thick ascending limb in magnesium handling. The terminal segments of the nephron, i.e. distal convoluted tubule and beyond, demonstrate very little additional

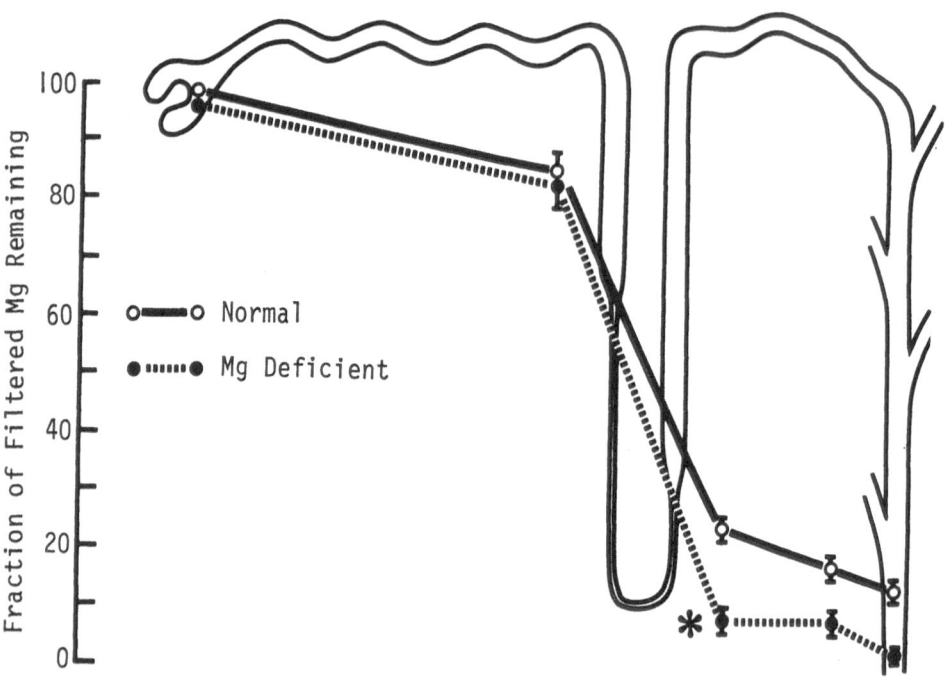

Fig. 1.   The fraction of ultrafilterable magnesium remaining
          along the superficial nephron and final urine in normal
          thyroparathyroidectomized rats and in rats pair-fed with
          a magnesium deficient diet (see text for details).


magnesium reabsorption (9-6), although this may be important in
some states (3,7,8).  Figure 1 summarizes the handling of
magnesium along the rat nephron.

     A large number of factors have been shown to affect urinary
magnesium excretion.  These have been summarized in Fig. 2 with
an indication of the nephron site affected.  Proximal magnesium
reabsorption, albeit relatively less than sodium and calcium,
amounts to about 20-30% of the filtered load.  Moreover, proximal
reabsorption is dependent on sodium reabsorption (9,10), thus
inhibition of sodium transport by extracellular volume expansion
or conversely an increase in sodium reabsorption by volume
contraction is accompanied by parallel changes in magnesium
reabsorption.  These changes result in alteration in distal
magnesium delivery with concomitant changes in the final urine.
Mannitol, on the other hand, results in inhibition of sodium
chloride and water reabsorption with litle or no change in

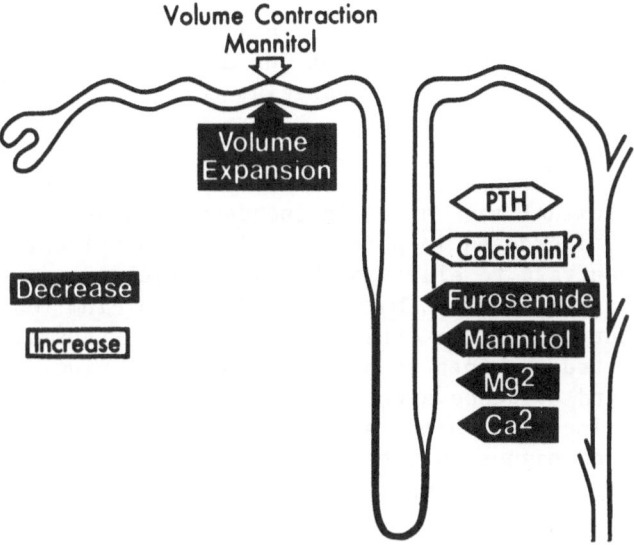

Fig. 2.   Factors affecting magnesium reabsorption along the
nephron.

proximal magnesium handling (11).  This presumably reflects the
lack of bidirectional flux of magnesium in contrast to sodium
(12).  Thus osmotic diuretics such as mannitol inhibit net
proximal sodium reabsorption by increasing the backflux of sodium
into the lumen.  As there is little or no magnesium backflux, net
magnesium reabsorption is not changed.  The coupling of proximal
net magnesium reabsorption with sodium transport requires further
investigation.

Diuretics including the organic mercurials, furosemide and
ethacrynic acid (13), osmotic diuretics such as mannitol (11) and
urea (14), and calcium and magnesium ions (3,15,16) result in
marked increases in urinary magnesium excretion.  These factors
all inhibit magnesium reabsorption within the loop of Henle.  The
mechanisms, however, are not quantitatively similar.  Loop
diuretics (mercurials, furosemide, ethacrynic acid) inhibit

active chloride transport within the thick ascending limb of
Henle which is the major site of magnesium reabsorption.
Inhibition may result from either a decrease of the
transepithelial potential difference which could provide the
driving force for magnesium reabsorption or alternatively a
direct effect may be postulated such as an inhibition of active
magnesium transport or a change in the cellular permeability.
The osmotic diuretics, mannitol (11) and urea (14), decrease the
contact time-concentration gradient for magnesium within the loop
of Henle, thus presenting more magnesium to the distal tubule
which appears in the final urine. Hypermagnesemia markedly
inhibits loop magnesium reabsorption. The major effect appears
to be on the contraluminal site of the epithelial membrane as
elevation of luminal magnesium, independent of plasma
concentration, increases loop reabsorption proportional to
delivery in contrast to elevation of extracellular magnesium
(12). Hypermagnesemia also markedly reduces calcium reabsorption
in the loop but has little effect on sodium. Furthermore,
hypercalcemia reduces both loop calcium and magnesium
reabsorption and evidence suggests this also occurs at a
contraluminal location in the ascending limb of the loop (17).
Thus calcium and magnesium interact at this site, perhaps at a
specific membrane carrier which modulates overall kidney
reabsorption.

    Parathyroid hormone (18,19) and calcitonin (20,21) have been
reported to affect urinary magnesium excretion. Acute
administration of parathyroid hormone to thyroparathyroidectomized dogs (18) and rats (22,23) has little effect on magnesium
transport but significantly increases reabsorption in
hypermagnesemic animals (18,23). In addition, parathyroid
hormone significantly increases magnesium reabsorption in
thyroparathyroidectomized hamsters (19). These effects appear to
be located in segments beyond the proximal tubule.
Calcitonin-responsive adenylate cyclase activity has been
demonstrated (24) in rabbit tubular fragments obtained from the
medullary portion of the thick ascending limb of Henle. Although
there appear to be species differences (25), the presence of
receptors for calcitonin in these nephron segments may suggest a
functional role for this hormone. The roles that parathyroid
hormone and calcitonin normally play in magnesium homeostasis
remain to be determined. Various other factors such as acid-base
disturbances, readily metabolizable substances such as
carbohydrates and alcohol, vitamin D, growth hormone and
mineralocorticoid steroids influence magnesium excretion, however
the mechanisms of action are imprecisely known at this time.

    High dietary magnesium augments renal magnesium excretion in
association with very little change in intracellular magnesium
concentration (26). Dietary magnesium deprivation, on the other

hand, results in a fall in urinary excretion which asymptotes towards immeasurable levels with a fall in filtered load or plasma concentration. The mechanism for this regulation is unknown. We have investigated renal handling of magnesium at the tubular level in magnesium deficient rats (7). Dietary restriction in rats resulted in a significant fall in fractional urinary excretion (15% to 3%) as plasma magnesium fell from 1.4 to 0.7 meq/l, respectively. The micropuncture results are summarized in Fig. 1. This data demonstrated the importance of the loop of Henle in renal magnesium homeostasis in deficient states. The transport capacity for magnesium, however, was less in deficient rats than control pair-fed animals. Further studies were done to test the transport capacities of the nephron by means of modest magnesium chloride infusions. Absolute magnesium reabsorption increased with acute infusions but was always less in magnesium deficient rats than control rats for any given filtered load, suggesting a dependence on filtered load rather than on adaptive change in a carrier system as observed for other electrolytes including sodium, potassium, calcium and phosphate.

Further speculation on cellular aspects of magnesium reabsorption: Although magnesium transport has not received the same intensive study as has calcium transport, magnesium constitutes a significant fraction of the total ion transport across the renal tubular cell and there are significant parallels between calcium and magnesium movements. As with calcium, transcellular flux may comprise a) influx across the luminal membrane, b) binding by intracellular organic ligands (eg. ATP, aspartate, citrate, etc.), c) uptake and release from mitochondria and d) efflux across the basal membrane (Fig. 3). Although very little is known about these various steps in renal cells, a number of possibilities are suggested by studies of other cells. As the thick ascending limb of the loop of Henle is the important reabsorptive site of magnesium we shall consider this segment. Magnesium may cross the luminal membrane down an electrical potential gradient but against a rather steep concentration gradient. Intraluminal magnesium concentration is 0.1 to 0.3 mM at this site. Intracellular concentrations are not known for the renal epithelial cell, but range from 5-20 mM for many other cells (1,27,28). No data exist as to the form in which magnesium crosses the cell membrane but it may be in association with an anion as either a monovalent or neutral species similar to that proposed for calcium. In addition, it is necessary to know the form in which magnesium exists in the cytosol to attempt to characterize the entry of magnesium into the cell. The true fraction of magnesium which is bound to various intracellular constituents is far from settled (1); however, it may be presumed that variations in intracellular-free magnesium concentration exert an immportant control on the transepithelial transport and that factors which alter this would

change the transport kinetics.  Mitochondria have been shown to
contain approximately three times as much magnesium as calcium (29).
The role of the mitochondria in magnesium transport is not known
but they could act as a large intracellular pool from which magnesium may be made available for transport.

Active extrusion of magnesium ions from the basolateral
membrane has not been demonstrated, although the basal,
pericapillary membrane has been shown to possess magnesium
activated ATPase activity (30).  The role of this enzyme system
in transepithelial flux of magnesium remains to be elucidated.
Alternatively, magnesium may be exchanged for sodium at the
contraluminal membrane as has been postulated for calcium
extrusion.  The influx of sodium down an electrochemical gradient
into the cell would provide the driving force for magnesium
extrusion as postulated in Fig. 3.  There is also a superficial
resemblance between calcium transport and magnesium transport and
the possibility exists that both calcium and magnesium may be
extruded by the same transport system (28).

Active chloride transport has been demonstrated in the thick
ascending limb of the loop.  Whether the avid reabsorption of
magnesium in this segment is independent or coupled to that of
chloride remains to be determined.  Fig. 3 summarizes some of the
factors which affect magnesium transport across the renal cell of
the loop of Henle.

In summary, magnesium reabsorption occurs throughout the
proximal, loop and distal segments of the nephron.  The proximal
tubule is less permeable to magnesium than calcium and sodium and
most of the filtered load is reclaimed in the thick ascending
limb of the loop of Henle.  Thus one would expect that factors
which regulate magnesium reabsorption should act within this
important segment.  No single hormone or agent appears to

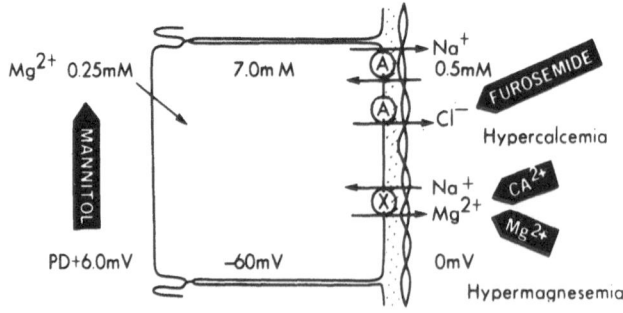

Fig. 3.  Factors which affect magnesium transport within the
         thick ascending limb of the loop of Henle.

regulate magnesium reabsorption sufficiently to account for
urinary changes; rather it appears to be a number of
intracellular and extracellular factors acting in concert to
effect day to day magnesium homeostasis.

ACKNOWLEDGEMENTS

Much of this work was supported by research grants from the
Medical Research Council of Canada.  The authors acknowledge the
contributions of Drs. Norman Wong and Shane Carney and the
excellent technical assistance of Mrs. Monique Julita, Mrs.
Sylvia Deare, Mrs. Anne Potter, Mr. Roland Blassnig, Mr. David
Ridout and Mr. Ray Dierolf.

REFERENCES

1.  Sutton, R. A. L., Quamme, G. A., and Dirks, J. H., 1979,
    Renal tubular transport of calcium, magnesium and phosphate,
    in: "Membrane Transport in Biological Membranes.  Vol. 10,"
    G. Giebisch, D. C. Tosteson and H. H. Ussing, eds.,
    Springer-Verlag, Heidelberg-New York.
2.  Morel, F., Roinel, N., and LeGrimellec, C, 1969, Electron
    probe analysis of tubular fluid composition, Nephron,
    6:350-364.
3.  LeGrimellec, C., Roinel, N., and Morel, F., 1973,
    Simultaneous Mg, Ca, P, K, Na and Cl analysis in rat tubular
    fluid.  II.  During acute Mg plasma loading, Pfluegers Arch.,
    340:197-210.
4.  Brunette, M. G., Vigneault, N. and Carriere, S.
    Micropuncture study of magnesium transport along the nephron
    in the young rat.  Am. J. Physiol., 227:891-896.
5.  De Rouffignac, C., Morel, F., Moss, N., and Roinel, N.,
    1973, Micropuncture study of water and electrolyte movements
    along the loop of Henle in Psammomys with special reference
    to magnesium, calcium and phosphorus.  Pfluegers Arch.,
    344:309-326.
6.  Quamme, G. A., Wong, N. L. M., Dirks, J. H., Roinel, N., de
    Rouffignac, C., and Morel, F., 1978, Magnesium handling in
    the dog kidney: A micropuncture study.  Pfluegers Arch.,
    377:95-99.
7.  Carney, S., Wong, N. L. M., Quamme, G. A., and Dirks, J. H.,
    1978, Renal tubular magnesium handling in the rat during
    magnesium depletion, Clin. Res., 37:4.
8.  Wen, S. F., Wong, N. L. M., and Dirks, J. H., 1971, Evidence
    for renal magnesium secretion during magnesium infusions in
    the dog, Am. J. Physiol., 220:33-38.
9.  Massry, S. G., Coburn, J. W., Chapman, L. W., and Kleeman,
    C. R., 1967, Effect of NaCl infusion on urinary $Ca^+$ and
    $Mg^+$ during reduction in their filtered load, Am. J.
    Physiol., 213:1218-1224.

10. Brunette, M. G., Wen, S. F., Evanson, R. L., and Dirks, J. H., 1969, Micropuncture study of magnesium reabsorption in the proximal tubule of the dog, Am. J. Physiol., 216:1510-1516.

11. Wong, N. L. M., Quamme, G. A., Sutton, R. A. L., and J. H. Dirks, 1978, Effect of mannitol on tubular calcium and magnesium transport, Clin. Res., 37:4.

12. Quamme, G. A. and Dirks, J. H., 1977, Microperfusion studies of magnesium transport in the proximal tubule and loop of Henle of the rat, Kidney Internat., 12:461.

13. Eknoyan, G., Suki, W. N., and Martinez-Maldonado, M., 1970, Effect of diuretics on urinary excretion of phosphate, calcium and magnesium in thyroparathyroidectomized dogs, J. Clin. Med., 76:257-266.

14. Wong, N. L.M., Quamme, G. A. and Dirks, J. H., 1979, Contrasting effects of urea and mannitol on electrolyte transport in the dog nephron, Clin. Res., 27:434.

15. Massry, S. G., Ahumada, J. J., Coburn, J. W., and Kleeman, C. R., 1970, Effect of $MgCl_2$ infusion on urinary Ca and Na during reduction in their filtered loads, Am. J. Physiol., 219:881-885.

16. Coburn, J. W., Massry, S. G., and Kleeman, C. R., 1970, The effect of calcium infusion on renal handling of magnesium with normal and reduced glomerular filtration rate, Nephron, 7:131-143.

17. Blassnig, R., and Quamme, G. A., 1978, Effect of hypercalcemia on calcium and magnesium transport along the loop of Henle and distal tubule, Clin. Res., 26:867.

18. Massry, S. G., Coburn, J. W., and Kleeman, C. R., 1969, Renal handling of magnesium in the dog, Am. J. Physiol., 216:1460-1467.

19. Burnatowska, M., Harris, C.A., Sutton, R.A.L., and Dirks, J.H., 1977, Effects of PTH and cAMP on the renal handling of calcium, magnesium and phosphate in the hamster, Am. J. Physiol., 233:514-518.

20. Sorensen, O.H., and Hindberg, I., 1972, The acute and prolonged effect of porcine calcitonin on urine electrolyte excretion in intact and parathyroidectomized rats, Acta Endocrinolgia, 70:295-307.

21. Poujoel, P., Touvay, C., Roinel, N. and de Rouffignac, C., 1978, Effets de la thyrocalcitonine sur le comportement renal du calcium, du magnesium et des phosphates, Abstracts of VII International Congress of Nephrology, Montreal.

22. Kuntziger, H., Amiel, C., Roinel, N., and Morel, F., 1974, Effects of parathyroidectomy and cyclic AMP on renal transport of phosphate, calcium and magnesium, Am. J. Physiol., 227:905-911.

23. Quamme, G.A., Carney, S., Wong, N.L.M., and Dirks, J.H., 1979, Effect of parathyroid hormone on renal calcium and magnesium reabsorption in magnesium deficient rats, Clin. Res., 27:427.

24. Chabardes, D., Imbert-Teboul, M., Clique, A., Montegut, M., and Morel, F., 1976, Distribution of calcitonin-sensitive adenylate cyclase activity along the rabbit kidney tubule, Proc. Natl. Acad. Sci., 73:3608-3612.
25. Brunette, M.G., Chabardes, D., Imbert-Teboul, M., Clique, A., Montegut, M., and Morel, F., 1979, Hormone sensitive adenylate cyclase along the nephron of genetically hypophosphatemic mice, Kidney Internat., 15:357-369.
26. Walser, M., 1969, Renal excretion of alkaline earts, in: "Mineral Metabolism, Vol. III", C.L. Comar and F. Bronner, eds., Academic Press, New York, p. 235-320.
27. Walser, M., 1971, Calcium-sodium interdependence in renal transport, in: "Renal Pharmacology". J.W. Fisher, ed., Appleton-Century-Crofts, New York, p. 21.
28. Baker, P.F., 1976, Regulation of intracellular calcium and magnesium in squid axons, Federation Proceedings, 35:2589-2596.
29. Case, G.D., VanderKooi, J.M., and Scarpa, A., 1974, Physical properties of biological membranes determined by the fluorescence of the Ca ionophore A23187, Arch. Biochem. and Biophys., 162:174-181.
30. Proverbio, F., Condiescu-Guidi, M., and Whittembury, G., 1975, Ouabian-insensitive Na stimulation of $Mg^+$-dependent APTase in kidney tissue, Biochem. Biophys. Acta., 394:281-286.

# THE INTERRELATIONSHIP BETWEEN PHOSPHATE AND MAGNESIUM METABOLISM

Shaul G. Massry and Nachman Brautbar

Division of Nephrology, Department of Medicine
USC School of Medicine
2025 Zonal Avenue
Los Angeles, California 90033

A large body of evidence exists indicating a close interrelationship between body stores of phosphate and magnesium. In our presentation we will attempt to explore the relationship between the homeostasis of these two ions and to examine the possible mechanisms underlying these interactions.

## Effect of Magnesium Depletion on Phosphate Homeostasis

It is well known that magnesium depletion is associated with phosphaturia in the rat (1-5). Smith et al (1) in 1962 and Whang and Welt (2) in 1963 reported that magnesium depletion in the rat produced marked increments in urinary phosphate excretion which occurred within the first week of feeding the animals with magnesium restricted diet (Figure 1). This phenomenon was attributed to a decrease in the proximal tubular reabsorption of phosphate (1). Indeed, Ginn and Shanbour (3) demonstrated that the phosphaturia of magnesium depletion was due to a decrease in maximum tubular reabsorptive capacity for phosphate (TmP) (Figure 2). This phosphaturia could not be due to increased activity of the parathyroid glands since it occurred in parathyroidectomized animals (3-5), and the TmP is reduced during magnesium depletion in parathyroidectomized rats (3) (Figure 3).

In the dog (6) and in humans (7,8) magnesium depletion is not associated with phosphaturia. Levi et al (6) reported that fractional excretion of phosphate was 9.5±2.1% before and 5.7±2.4% after several weeks of magnesium depletion. Muldowney et al (8) found a direct relationship between the renal clearance of phosphate and serum magnesium in patients with intestinal malabsorption with phosphate clearance being lowest in those with severe hypomagnesemia

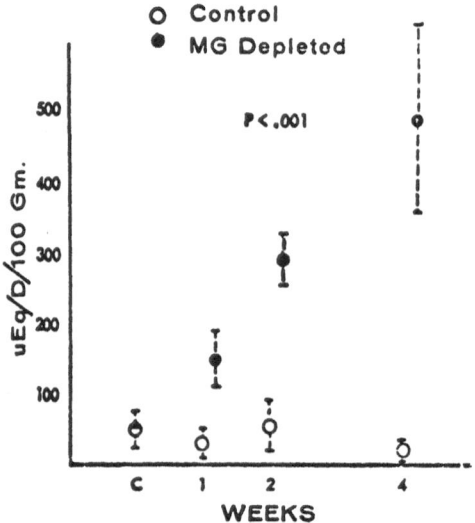

Fig 1.   Urinary phosphate excretion expressed as μEq/day/100 g body
         weight during magnesium depletion in rats.   From Smith et
         al (1).

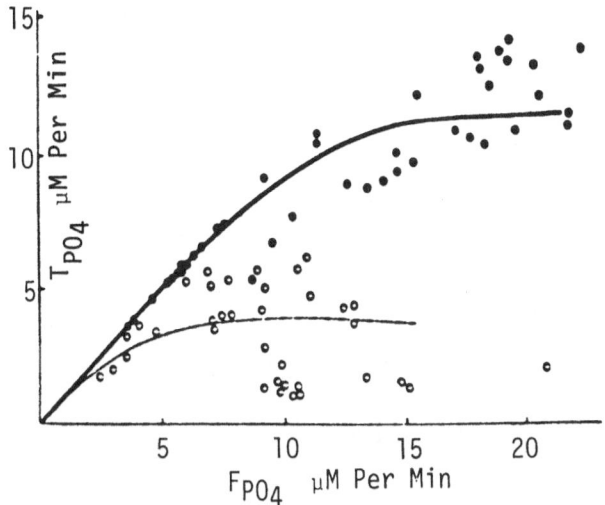

Fig 2.   Tubular phosphate reabsorption in non-parathyroidectomized
         control (●) and magnesium depleted (0) rats.  $F_{pO4}$ denotes
         filtered load of phosphate and $T_{pO4}$ indicates tubular reab-
         sorption of phosphate.   From Ginn and Shanbour (3).

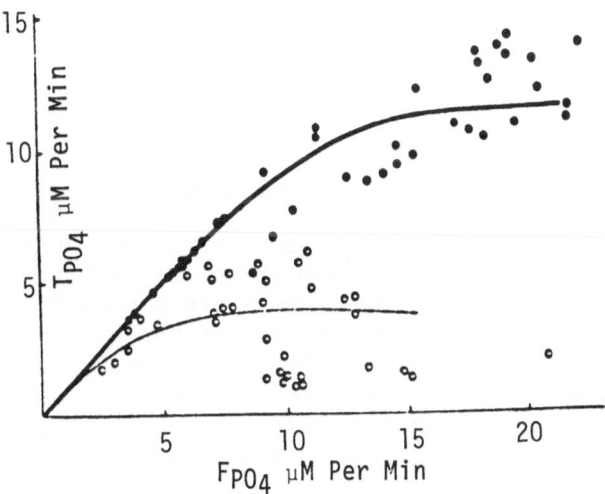

Fig 3.   Tubular phosphate reabsorption in parathyroidectomized con-
         trol (●) and magnesium depleted (0) rats.  $F_{pO4}$ denotes
         filtered load of phosphate and $T_{pO4}$ indicates tubular
         reabsorption of phosphate.   From Ginn and Shanbour (3).

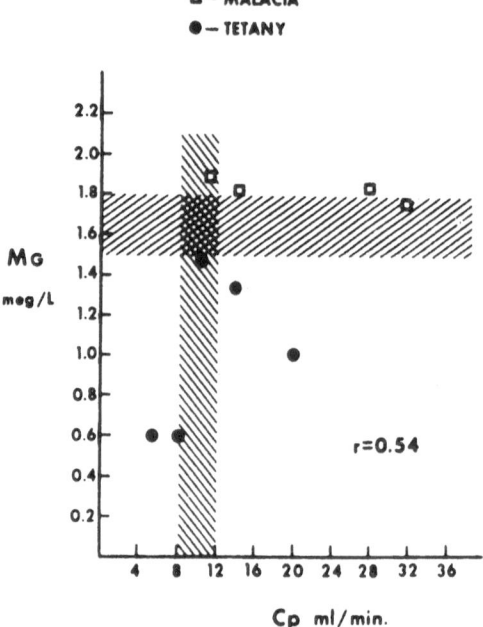

Fig 4.   Correlation between serum magnesium concentration and renal
         phosphate clearance (Cp) in nine patients with intestinal
         malabsorption.  Cross hatched areas indicate the normal
         range.  From Maldowney et al (8).


(Figure 4).  Thus, it appears that the effect of magnesium deficiency on urinary excretion of phosphate is species dependent causing phosphaturia in rats while it could be associated with reduced
urinary phosphate excretion in dogs or humans.

     The effects of parathyroid hormone (PTH) on the renal excretion
of phosphate have also been studied in animals and humans with magnesium depletion (6-9), and the results are not consistent.  Hahn,
Chase and Avioli (9) found that in the rat the increments in urinary
phosphate and in the renal production of cyclic AMP following the
administration of PTH is not affected by magnesium depletion.  In
contrast, Levi et al (5) in dogs (Figure 5) and Estep et al (7) in
humans reported that the phosphaturic response to PTH is impaired
during magnesium depletion and is restored to normal after magnesium
repletion.  Maldowney et al (8) on the other hand, could not confirm
Estep et al's observation (7) in their two magnesium depleted subjects who displayed a normal phosphaturic response to PTH,

     Magnesium depletion may also affect the concentration of serum
phosphorus.  The early studies in rats (1-3) showed that magnesium
depletion did not produce a significant fall in levels of serum
phosphorus.  However, Gitelman et al (4) and Slatopolsky et al (5)

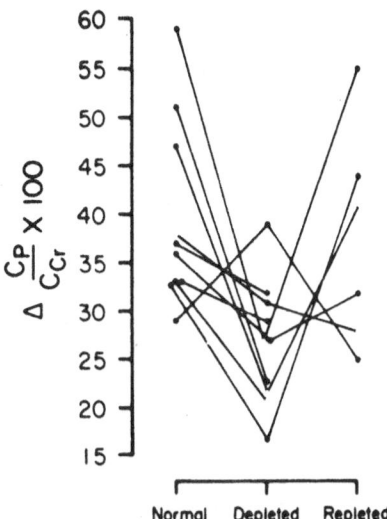

Fig 5.   The changes in the percent filtered phosphate excreted
         ($\Delta Cp/C_{cr}$ x 100) induced by infusion of parathyroid extract
         in normal animals, during the depleted state and after
         magnesium repletion.  Open circles represent the mean of
         two studies in the animals and the lines connect data in
         the same dog.  From Levi et al (6).

reported that magnesium depletion is associated with significant
hypophosphatemia in the rat.  The latter authors (5) found that
several factors may underlie the hypophosphatemia in their animals;
these include increased urinary losses of phosphate and lack of
augmentation in intestinal absorption of phosphate and mobilization
of this ion from bone.  In the dog, magnesium depletion is not associated with hypophosphatemia (6).  The effect of magnesium deficiency
in humans on the levels of serum phosphorus are variable; a fall,
a rise, or no change have been reported (10,11).  Magnesium depletion in intact or parathyroidectomized rats was associated with
increase total carcus phosphorus content (4).

## Effects of Hypermagnesemia on Phosphate Homeostasis

     Massry et 21 (12) studied the effects of acute rise in serum
magnesium produced by $MgCl_2$ infusion in normal and thyroparathyroidectomized dogs.  The elevation in the concentration of serum
magnesium was associated with a gradual and significant rise in
the levels of serum phosphorus.  This occurred whether $MgCl_2$ was
infused during the morning (Figure 6) (from 4.0±.37 to 6.8±.58 mg/dl,

p<0.01) or the afternoon (Figure 7) (from 4.9±.2 to 8.1±.58 mg/dl, p<0.01) hours and was independent of the activity of the parathyroid gland since the hyperphosphatemia developed in TPTX dogs as well (from 5.5±.37 to 7.4±.21 mg/dl, p<0.01). The mechanisms for this hyperphosphatemia are not elucidated. A rise in serum levels of phosphorus occurs also during hypercalcemia (13) and has been attributed to shifts of phosphate from soft tissues to extracellular space. It is possible that hypermagnesemia exerts a similar effect.

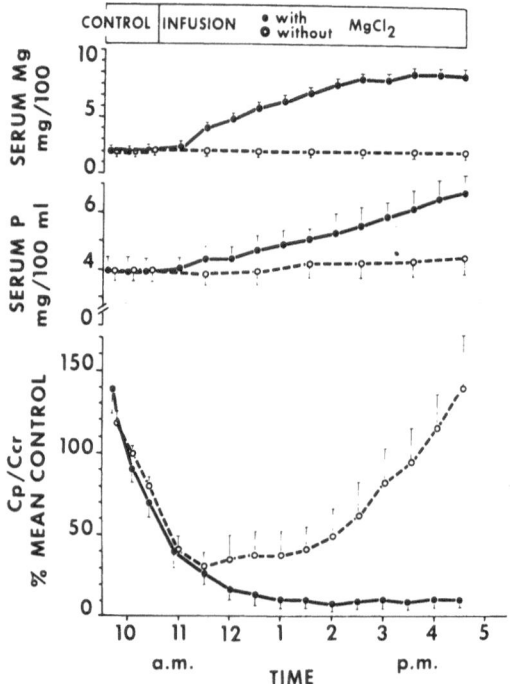

Fig 6.   MgCl infusion during morning hours. The changes in mean levels of serum magnesium (Mg) and phosphorus (P) and in fraction of filtered phosphate excreted (Cp/C$_{cr}$) in seven intact dogs with and without the infusion of MgCl$_2$. In order to reduce the variability in absolute values of Cp/C$_{cr}$ from one experiment to another, the changes in Cp/Cr are expressed as the percent of the mean of three control clearances in each individual experiment. Brackets represent ±1SE. From Massry et al (12)

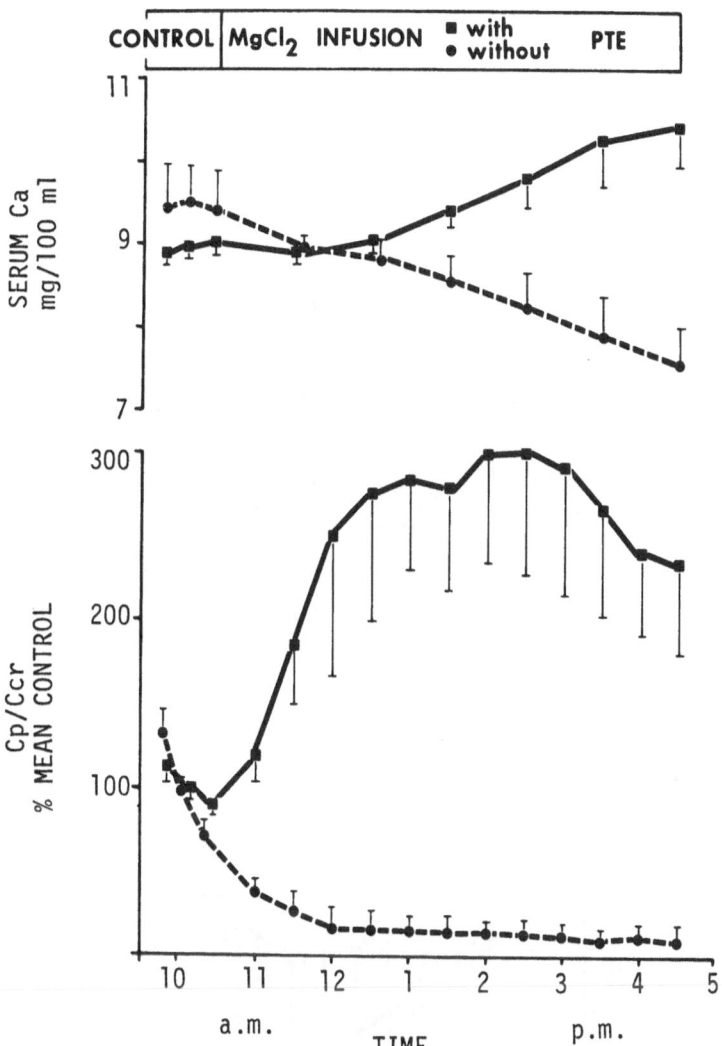

Fig 7. MgCl2 infusion during afternoon hours. The changes in mean
levels of serum magnesium (Mg), calcium (Ca) and phosphorus
(P) and in the fraction of filtered phosphate excreted
(Cp/Ccr) in four intact dogs with and without the infusion
of MgCl2. The data of Cp/Ccr are expressed as in Figure 6.
Brackets denote ±1SE. From Massry et al (12).

Despite the hyperphosphatemia, the fractional excretion of
phosphate (Cp/Ccr fell markedly during the hypermagnesemia, and
the values for Cp/Ccr were significantly lower from values observed
at the same time of the day in paired control dogs (Figure 6 and 7).

Magnesium infusion did not affect $Cp/C_{cr}$ in TPTX dogs (Figure 8).
The pattern of the fall in $Cp/C_{cr}$ during magnesium infusion resembled
that observed after hypercalcemia or following the removal of the
parathyroid glands.  The infusion of PTH to dogs receiving $MgCl_2$ produced a significant rise in $Cp/C_{cr}$ and in serum calcium levels (Figure 9).  These data indicate that the effects of hypermagnesemia on
urinary phosphate excretion are mediated through the suppression of
the activity of the parathyroid gland.  Furthermore, hypermagnesemia
does not appear to affect the phosphaturic and calcemic responses to
PTH indicating there is no end organ resistance to PTH during
hypermagnesemia.

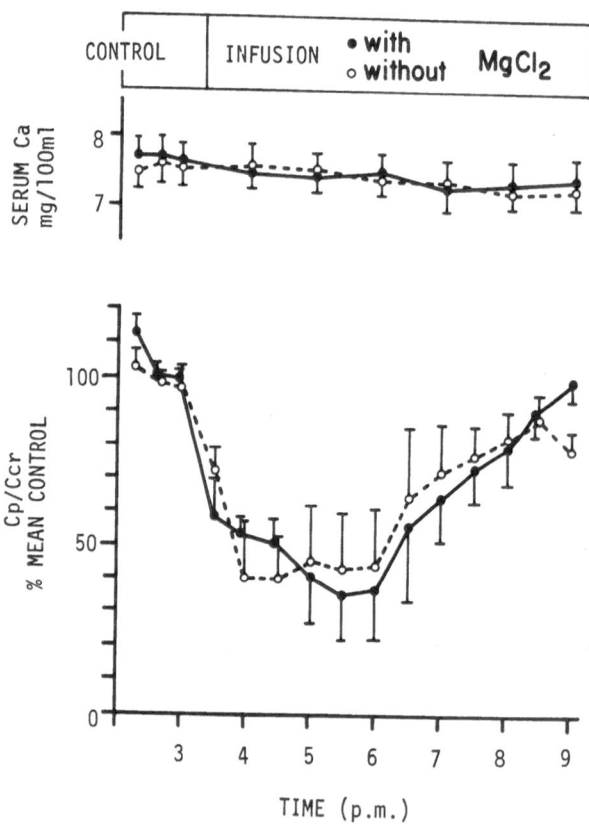

Fig 8.   The changes in mean levels of serum calcium (Ca) and in the
         changes in the fraction of filtered phosphate excreted (Cp/
         $C_{cr}$) in four thyroparathyroidectomized dogs with and without
         $MgCl_2$ infused.  The changes in $Cp/C_{cr}$ are expressed in Fig-
         ure 6.  Brackets represent ±1SE.  From Massry et al (12).

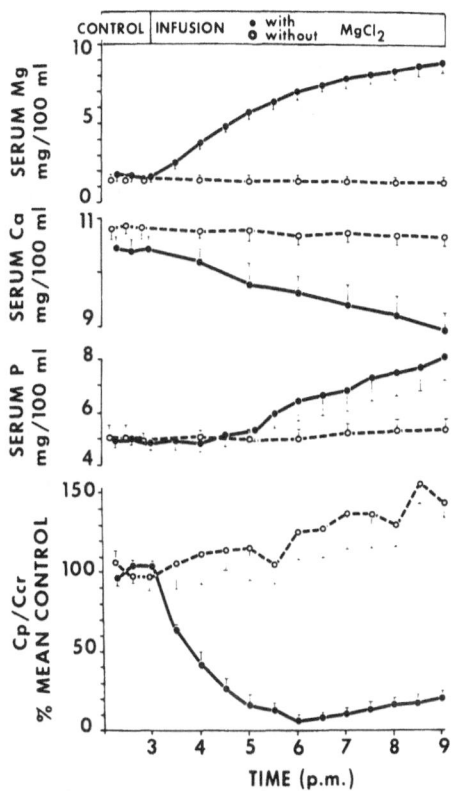

Fig 9. The mean values of serum calcium (Ca) and the changes in the fraction of filtered phosphate excreted (Cp/C$_{cr}$) in four intact dogs receiving MgCl$_2$ with and without the administration of parathyroid extract (PTE). The changes in Cp/C$_{cr}$ are expressed as in Figure 6. Brackets denote ±1SE. From Massry et al (12).

## Effects of Phosphate Depletion on Magnesium Homeostasis

Phosphate depletion affects magnesium metabolism and the magnitude of this effect is species dependent. Coburn and Massry (14) found that modest magnesuria without consistent changes in plasma magnesium may occur during phosphate depletion in adult dogs.

Similar observations were reported in man (15).  In contrast, marked
magnesuria and hypomagnesemia develops rapidly during phosphate
depletion in the rat (16-18).

We have evaluated in detail the alteration in magnesium homeostasis during phosphate depletion in the rat (17).  A significant
(p<0.01) increment in urinary magnesium from 46±2.7 to 126±24 µeq/24
hr occurred during the first day of phosphate depletion; urinary
magnesium reached a peak of 300±24 µeq/24 hr by the 3rd day and
remained high ranging between 150-300 µeq/24 hr thereafter (Figure
10).  The magnitude of the magnesuria was related to the degree of
hypophosphtemia (Figure 11) and was not affected by lowering the
calcium intake and reducing the hypercalciuria.  The concentration
of serum magnesium fell significantly (p<0.01) from 1.2±.02 to
0.79±.10 µEq/l by the first day and remained low throughout
(Figure 12).

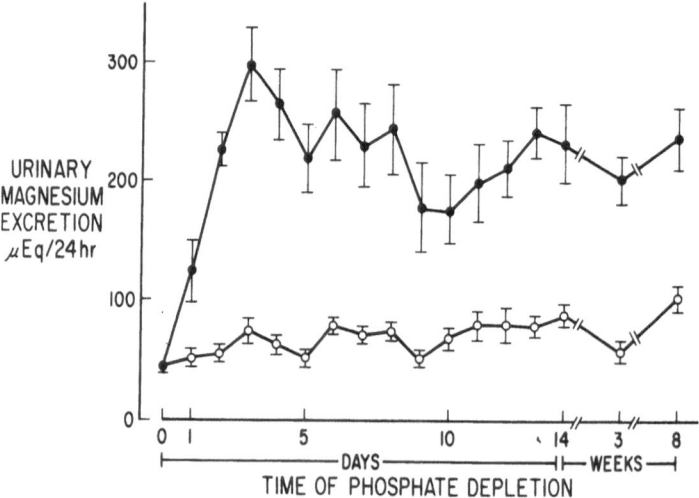

Fig 10.   The changes in urinary excretion of magnesium in rats
          with phosphate depletion (●) and in pair fed control
          animals (0).  Brackets denote ±1SE.  From Kreusser et al
          (17).

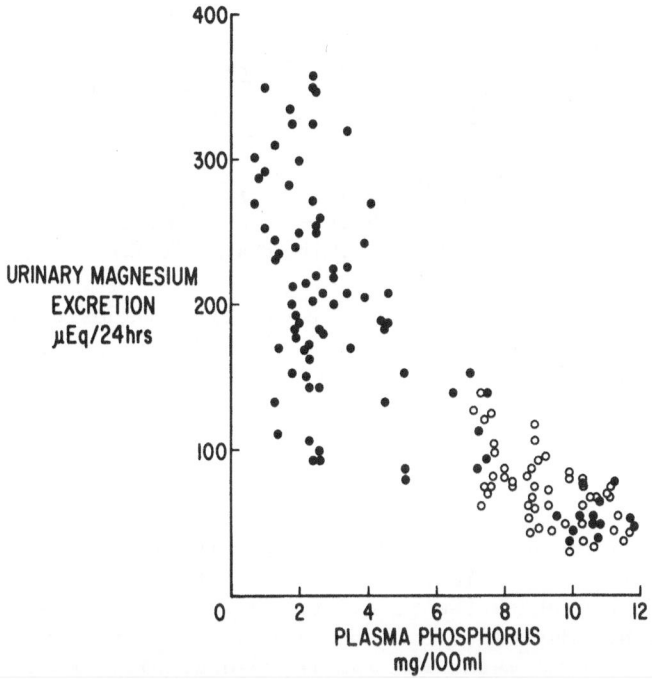

Fig 11.  The relationship between the concentration of phosphorus
in serum and urinary excretion of magnesium.  Closed
symbols denote data from rats ingesting a low dietary
phosphate and open symbols represent data from pair fed
animals.  From Kreusser et al (17).

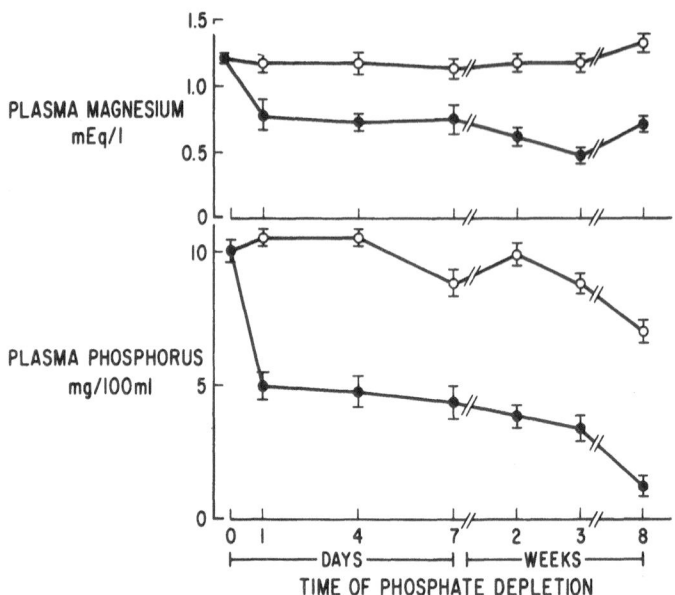

Fig 12.   Changes in the concentration of serum magnesium and phos-
          phorus in phosphate depleted (●) and pair fed rats (O).
          Brackets denote ±1SE.   From Kreusser et al (17).

Magnesium balance became negative during the first day of
phosphate depletion and remained so during the entire study.   This
occurred despite a significant increment in the fraction of ingested
magnesium absorbed which became evident by the third week of phosphate depletion.   Magnesium content of muscle, kidney and liver were
not affected but bone magnesium was reduced significantly.   The
change in bone magnesium was not due to an overall reduction in bone
mineral content because bone calcium content was not affected.
Supplementation of amgnesium in the drinking water produced a normalization of serum magnesium but did not bring about restoration
of bone magnesium despite a positive magnesium balance.   These
disturbances in magnesium metabolism were independent of the age or
weight of the animals (Figure 13).

These data indicate that phosphate depletion is associated with
a) magnesuria due to a decrease in the net renal tubular reabsorption
of magnesium with the mean source of urinary losses being bone
magnesium, b) hypomagnesemia secondary to the renal leak of magnesium, c) negative magnesium balance, and d) increase in the intestinal fractional absorption of magnesium.   The latter was not adequate
to compensate for the urinary losses of magnesium.

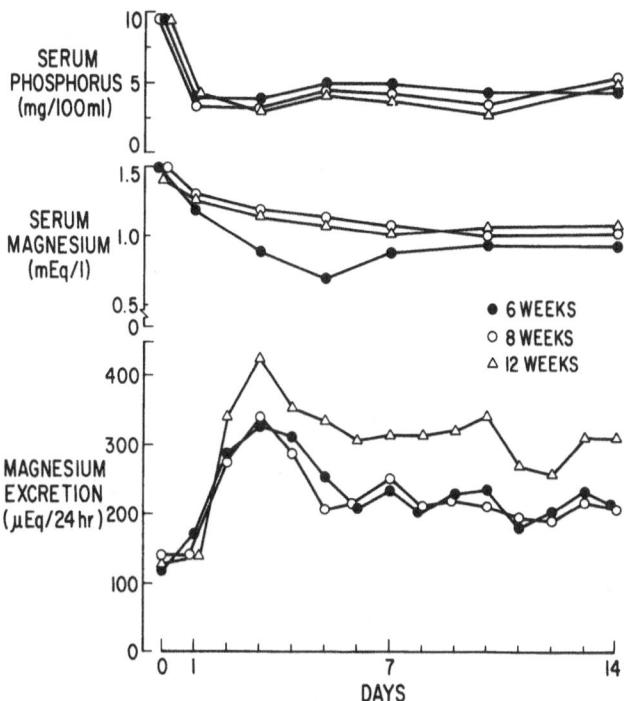

Fig 13.  Effect of low dietary phosphate on levels of serum phosphorus and magnesium and on urinary excretion of magnesium
in rats of different size and weight.  Data adapted from
Kreusser et al (17).

Similar observations were reported by Brautbar et al (18).
They demonstrated that phosphate depletion in the rat is associated
with magnesuria, negative magnesium balance and reduced bone magnesium content.  They also found that adequate dietary magnesium could
prevent the hypomagnesemia.

Several mechanisms may be responsible for the magnesuria in
phosphate depleted rats.  It is evident that a decrease in tubular
reabsorption of magnesium exists since the magnesuria develops in
the face of falling filtered loads of this ion (17).  Suppression
of the parathyroid gland activity by phosphate depletion (15,19) is
not a critical factor in the genesis of the magnesuria since the
latter occurred in phosphate depleted TPTX rats (16).  Additional
studies in our laboratory (20) have demonstrated that substantial
magnesium secretion by the kidney occurs during phosphate depletion
in the rat (Figure 14).  Thus, the magnesuria is due to decreased
tubular reabsorption and enhanced secretion of magnesium.

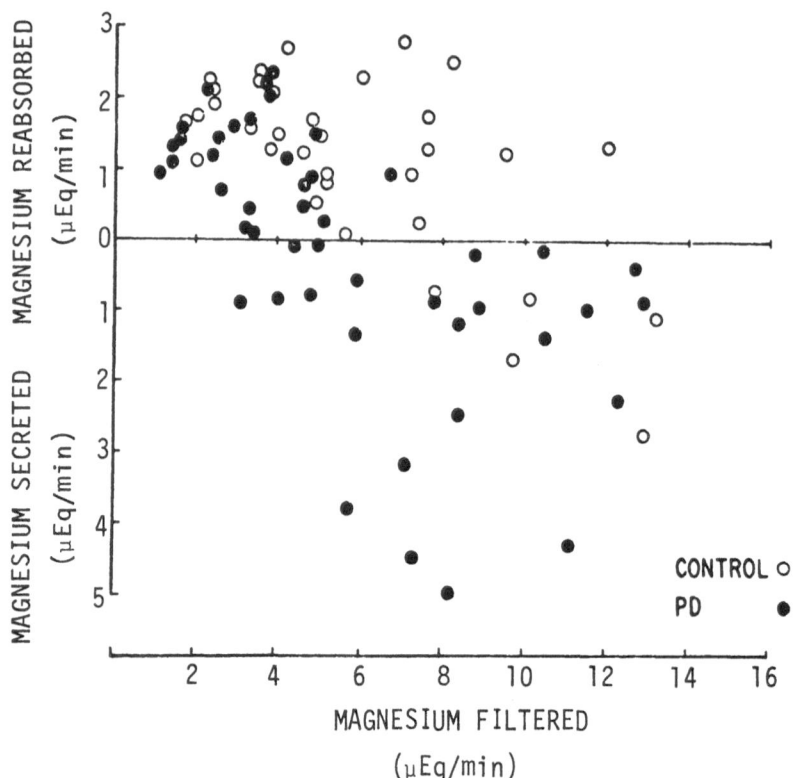

Fig 14.  The changes in the quantity of magnesium reabsorbed or
          secreted at various levels of filtered magnesium in control
          rats (O) and phosphate depleted animals (●).  Symbols below
          the zero line denote magnesium secretion.  Each data point
          is the average of two to three clearance periods obtained
          at the end of each level of magnesium infusion.  From
          Sachtjen et al (20).

     In summary:  a) it appears that the interrelationship between
phosphate and magnesium metabolism is complicated and the mechanisms
involved are not fully understood, b) the interaction between the
homeostasis of these two ions is species dependent and its full
expression is most evident in the rat, c) body depletion of either
of these ions may result in marked changes in the blood levels,
intestinal absorption, renal handling and body content of the other,
d) hypermagnesemia causes hyperphosphatemia and decreased urinary
excretion of phosphate, and e) the effects of hyperphosphatemia on
magnesium are not elucidated as yet.

REFERENCES

1.  W.O. Smith, D.J. Baxter, A. Linder and H.E. Ginn:  Effect of
magnesium depletion on renal function in the rat.  J. Lab. Clin.
Med. 59:211 (1962).

2.  R. Whang and L.G. Welt:  Observations in experimental magnesium
depletion.  J. Clin. Invest. 42:305 (1963).

3.  H.E. Ginn and L.L. Shanbour:  Phosphaturia in magnesium-defi-
cient rats.  Amer. J. Physiol. 212:1347 (1967).

4.  H.J. Gitelman, S. Kukolj, and L.G. Welt:  The influence of the
parathyroid glands on the hypercalcemia of experimental magnesium
depletion in the rat.  J. Clin. Invest. 47:118 (1968).

5.  E. Slatopolsky, J. Lewis, K. Martin, and S. Klahr:  On the
hypophosphatemia of magnesium depletion in the rat.  Proc. Amer.
Soc. Nephrol. 10:8A (1977).

6.  J. Levi, S.G. Massry, J.W. Coburn, F. Llach and C.R. Kleeman:
Hypocalcemia in magnesium-depleted dogs:  Evidence for reduced
responsiveness to parathyroid hormone and relative failure of
parathyroid gland function.  Metab. 23:323 (1974).

7.  H. Estep, W.A. Shaw, C. Waltington, R. Hobe, W. Holland and
St. G. Tucker:  Hypocalcemia due to hypomagnesemia and reversible
parathyroid hormone unresponsiveness.  J. Clin. Endocrinol. Metab.
29:842, 1969.

8.  F.P. Muldowney, T.J. McKenna, L.H. Kyle, R. Freaney, and
M. Swan:  Parathormone-like effect of magnesium replenishment in
steatorrhea.  New Eng. J. Med. 282:61 (1970).

9.  T.J. Hahn, L.R. Chase, and L.V. Avioli:  Effect of magnesium
depletion on responsiveness to parathyroid hormone in parathyroidectomized rats.  J. Clin. Invest. 51:886 (1972).

10.  M.J. Dunn and M. Walser:  Magnesium depletion in normal man.
Metab. 15:895 (1965).

11.  M.E. Shills:  Experimental human magnesium depletion.  Medicine
48:61 (1969).

12.  S.G. Massry, J.W. Coburn, and C.R. Kleeman:  Evidence for
suppression of parathyroid gland activity by hypermagnesemia.  J.
Clin. Invest. 49:1619 (1970).

13.  P.S. Chen, Jr., and W.F. Neuman:  Renal reabsorption of calcium
through its inhibition by various chemical agents.  Amer. J. Physiol.
180:632, (1955).

14.  J.W. Coburn and S.G. Massry:  Changes in serum and urinary calcium during phosphate depletion:  Studies on mechanisms.  J. Clin. Invest. 49:1073 (1970).

15.  J.H. Dominguez, R.W. Gray and J. Lemann, Jr.:  Dietary phosphate deprivation in women and men:  Effects on mineral and acid balances, parathyroid hormone and the metabolism of 25-OH-vitamin D.  J. Clin. Endocrinol and Metab. 43:1056 (1976).

16.  P. Cuisinier-Gleizes, M. Thomasset, F. Saintery-Debove, and H. Mathieu:  Phosphorus deficiency, parathyroid hormone and bone resorption in growing rats.  Calcif. Tissue Res. 20:235 (1976).

17.  W.J. Kreusser, K. Kurokawa, E. Aznar, E. Sachtjen, and S.G. Massry:  Effect of phosphate depletion on magnesium homeostasis in rats.  J. Clin. Invest. 61:573 (1978).

18.  N. Brautbar, D.B.N. Lee, J.W. Coburn and C.R. Kleeman:  Dietary magnesium in experimental phosphate depletion:  Bone and soft tissue mineral changes.  Amer. J. Physiol. 237:E152 (1979).

19.  H.C. Stoerk and W.H. Carnes:  The relation of the dietary Ca:P ratio to serum Ca and to parathyroid volume.  J. Nutr. 29:43 (1945).

20.  E. Sachtjen, W.A. Meyer and S.G. Massry:  Evidence for magnesium during phosphate depletion in the rat.  Proc. Exptl. Biol. Med. 162: 416 (1979).

# $PO_4$ TRANSPORT IN SUPERFICIAL AND JUXTAMEDULLARY NEPHRONS

# IN THE CAT:  EVIDENCE FOR NEPHRON HETEROGENEITY

Stanley Goldfarb, M.D.

Renal-Electrolyte Section, Dept. of Medicine
Hospital of the University of Pennsylvania
Philadelphia, Pennsylvania USA

Many micropuncture studies have demonstrated a difference between the delivery of $PO_4$ from late superficial distal convoluted tubules and final urinary $PO_4$ excretion.  This difference could be due to $PO_4$ transport in nephron segments beyond the late distal tubule (1) or to differing transport rates in deep nephrons (2). The latter possibility would suggest that lesser amounts of $PO_4$ delivered from deep nephrons combined with the $PO_4$ delivered from superficial nephrons and the algebraic sum is the final urinary $PO_4$ content.  To study the role of deep nephrons in $PO_4$ transport with particular reference to the quantitative contribution of deep and superficial nephrons, micropuncture and A-V extraction studies were performed in the cat kidney.  The cat is useful as a model for the study of nephron heterogeneity of transport since the superficial and juxtamedullary cortex are drained by discrete and accessible venous drainage systems (3).

## METHODS
A-V extraction studies were performed by cannulating super-ficial (surface), and deep renal veins  (3).  Standard clearance studies were performed simultaneously.  Thirty-four separate determinations were made in eleven cats.  $PO_4$, $^3H$ inulin, and Ca in blood and urine were determined as previously described (4).

Micropuncture studies were performed by sampling late proximal (n = 18) late distal (n = 24) tubules as well as simultaneous clearance studies as previously described (4).

## RESULTS
The  %FE $PO_4$ from superficial and deep nephrons as well as %FE $PO_4$ in the final urine are described in Table 1 as are the

results of segmental PO$_4$ transport in micropuncture studies.

TABLE I.        RENAL PO$_4$ HANDLING IN THE CAT

### A-V Extraction Studies

| Deep | Superficial | Final Urine |
|------|-------------|-------------|
| %FD PO$_4$ 22.35 | 42.94 [a,b] | 29.05 |
| ±2.05 | ±2.42 | ±2.01 |

### Micropuncture

| Proximal Tubule | Distal Tubule | Final Urine |
|-----------------|---------------|-------------|
| %FD PO$_4$ 66.21 | 41.63 [c] | 30.24 |
| ± 4.23 | ±3.61 | ±2.22 |

Values as mean ± SEM of % fractional delivery of PO$_4$.

a = p < .001 vs deep system
b = p < .001 vs final urine
c = p < .025 vs final urine

## DISCUSSION

These studies suggest that a qualitatively similar amount of PO$_4$ is delivered from superficial late distal convoluted tubules as from the entire population of superficial cortical nephrons in the cat. Thus, the differences in PO$_4$ delivery, observed between late distal tubules and final urine may be accounted for by a lower delivered load of PO$_4$ entering the urine from deeper nephrons. However, a direct measurement of PO$_4$ transport in deep nephrons or in the collecting duct system is necessary before these results can be definitively attributed to internephron heterogeneity.

REFERENCES
1. E. Pastoriza-Munoz, R. E. Colindres, W. E. Lassiter, and C. Lechene, Effect of parathyroid hormone on phosphate reabsorption in rat distal convolution, Am. J. Physiol. 235(4):F321 (1978).
2. J. A. Haas, T. Berndt, and F. G. Knox, Nephron heterogeneity of phosphate reabsorption, Am. J. Physiol. 234(4):F287 (1978).
3. O. I. Nissen, The function of superficial and deep areas of the cat kidney, Danish Med. Bull. 16 Suppl. III:1 (1969).
4. S. Goldfarb, G. R. Westby, M. Goldberg, Z. S. Agus, Renal tubular effects of chronic PO$_4$ depletion, J. Clin. Invest. 59:770 (1977).

# ADAPTIVE CHANGES IN RENAL CORTICAL BRUSH BORDER MEMBRANE

Thomas P. Dousa, Stephen A. Kempson and Sudhir V. Shah

Mayo Clinic and Foundation

Rochester, MN 55901, USA

## INTRODUCTORY COMMENT

The kidney plays a key role in phosphorus (P)[*] homeostasis.[1]
The amount of phosphate (Pi) excreted by the kidney depends mostly
on the extent to which Pi filtered in glomeruli is reabsorbed back
to peritubular circulation in tubules.[2] The bulk of the filtered
Pi is reabsorbed in the proximal tubule[2] and the first step in
the mechanism of Pi transport from the lumen across the proximal
tubule epithelium is a $Na^+$-dependent Pi uptake across the luminal
brush border membrane (BBM).[3,4] Studies on [32]Pi uptake by BBM
vesicles isolated from the renal cortex allows analysis of this
initial step in tubular Pi reabsorption in a variety of pathophysiologic situations, independent of immediate supply of energy from
tubular cell metabolism and independent of other factors which
could contribute to or regulate overall proximal tubular Pi reabsorption in situ.

Luminal BBM of renal proximal tubule is characterized not only
by unique transport properties, but also by a distinct structural
characteristic (numerous microvilli forming brush border) and by
the fact that it is equipped with a set of enzymes present in this
structure in a very high specific activity, so-called "BBM
enzymes."[4,5,6,7] Brush border-like arrangement of luminal mem-

---

[*] Abbreviations used in this paper: P = phosphorus; Pi = inorganic
phosphate; AlPase = alkaline phosphatase; $\gamma$-GT = gamma glutamyl
transferase; LAP = leucinaminopeptidase; PTH = parathyroid hormone
BBM = brush border membrane; LPD = low phosphorus diet; HPD =
high phosphorus diet.

brane is believed to increase the contact surface for reabsorption, but the functional significance of BBM enzymes is not known.[4,6] Nevertheless, their specific location in BBM is compatible with the possibility that these enzymes may have a role, direct or indirect, in BBM transport processes or their regulation,[6,7] including transport of Pi.[4]

One of the BBM enzymes, which deserve consideration with respect of its potential role in Pi transport is alkaline phosphatase (AlPase). AlPase is "intrinsic" BBM enzyme tightly bound to membrane structure,[8] consisting of only about 0.04% of BBM microvillus protein.[7] Melani et al[9] observed that rats fed for several days low P diet have a higher specific activity of renal AlPase but activity of other examined renal enzymes, mostly related to intermediary metabolism of glucose, remained unchanged. In our recent study we found that rats stabilized on low dietary P intake, have increased specific and total activity of AlPase in BBM fraction of renal cortex, but not in cytosol or in other membrane components of the renal cortical homogenate; activities of other tested BBM enzymes including γ-glutamyltransferase (γ-GT), leucinaminopeptidase (LAP) and maltase were not altered.[10] Likewise, activities of typical mitochondrial, lysosomal, microsomal and antiluminal membrane enzymes were not different between control rats and rats fed low P diet. From predominantly cytoplasmic enzymes, only cyclic 3',5'-AMP phosphodiesterase (but not cyclic 3',5'-GMP phosphodiesterase) was elevated in the cortex of rats fed low P diet.[10] From clearance,[11] microperfusion[12] and micropuncture[13] studies, it became obvious that renal tubular reabsorption of Pi and thus Pi conservation by the kidney is very closely adjusted to the amount of dietary P intake.

Such considerations led us to examine simultaneously BBM transport of Pi and, for comparison of D-glucose, and in the same BBM fractions specific activities of AlPase and other BBM enzymes, in response to variation in the alimentary P intake.

SUMMARY OF RESULTS

The experimental design was basically analogous in all experiments. The BBM fraction (vesicles) was prepared by the calcium precipitation method[10,14] from the kidney cortices pooled from 3-5 rats, treated simultaneously by various dietary regimen and/or with drugs.[15] The timing of experiments was synchronized in such a way that renal cortical BBM from rats maintained on several compared experimental conditions were prepared, and their properties (transport of $^{32}$P and D-[$^3$H]-glucose in fresh BBM, or BBM enzyme activities in deep-frozen aliquots of the same BBM) were studied always at the same time, with the use of the same biochemicals and assay conditions.[14,15]

We first investigated BBM transport of $^{32}$P and for comparison transport of D-[$^3$H]-glucose in rats stabilized on normal P diet, high P diet (HPD) and low P diet (LPD) for 2 weeks. Na$^+$-dependent $^{32}$P uptake by BBM vesicles in rats stabilized for 2 weeks on LPD was markedly higher in the initial "uphill" phase and at the peak of "overshoot", but was not different at late (120 min) period, when near equilibrium was achieved.[14] Conversely, $^{32}$P uptake was markedly decreased in rats fed for the same time period with HPD. On the other hand, Na$^+$-dependent D-glucose transport was not significantly altered in the three groups, but tended to be changed in the opposite direction--slightly increased in HPD and decreased in LPD rats. Na$^+$-independent uptake (NaCl replaced by KCl) of $^{32}$Pi or of D-[$^3$H]-glucose was not different between the three compared groups.[14] Out of the four tested BBM enzymes, the specific activity of AlPase was increased in BBM from LPD rats, and tended to be lower in BBM from HPD rats. Activities of LAP, $\gamma$-GT and maltase were not affected by differences in dietary P intake. AlPase activity showed a close positive correlation with Na$^+$-dependent $^{32}$P uptake in the "overshoot" phase, but correlation was not found between $^{32}$P uptake and other BBM enzyme activities.

Melani et al[9] reported that increase in renal AlPase induced by LPD could be prevented by actinomycin D and other inhibitors of protein biosynthesis. Administration of protein synthesis inhibitors to rats switched from normal P diet to LPD prevented or delayed the antiphosphaturic response.[15] Recently, we examined whether treatment with actinomycin D could prevent both the increase of BBM specific activity of Al Pase and the BBM and transport of $^{32}$P induced by feeding with LPD.[16] Indeed, the treatment of rats with actinomycin D prevented the LPD-induced increase in specific activity of AlPase in BBM, but activities of $\gamma$-GT and LAP were not influenced. Likewise the treatment with Actinomycin D prevented the increase in Na$^+$-dependent $^{32}$P uptake in BBM induced by LPD, but the D-[$^3$H]-glucose uptake was not affected.[16] The Na$^+$-dependent $^{32}$P-uptake in the "uphill phase" correlated significantly with the specific activity of AlPase in BBM, but not with $\gamma$-GT and LAP activities in the same preparation. These results indicate that within BBM both the Pi transport and AlPase are induced in parallel in response to short term LPD and suggest indirectly that these BBM adaptive changes depend on de novo protein synthesis.[16]

Alimentary intake of P is decreased not only if content of P in diet is selectively reduced, such as feeding with LPD, but also in total fasting; in the latter type of alimentary P deprivation profound antiphosphaturia, similar to that occurring in the response to LPD, was not observed. We compared the $^{32}$P and D-[$^3$H]-glucose BBM transport as well as BBM enzyme activities in P deprivation due to total withdrawal of food or due to feeding

with LPD for a period of 3 days.[17]  Even after this short time
period, as we noticed previously,[16] BBM transport of $^{32}$P was
markedly increased, and conversely, transport of D-[$^{3}$H]-glucose was
significantly decreased in BBM of rats fed LPD.  In contrast,
total fasting for the same period of time did not influence the
Na$^{+}$-dependent BBM transport of either $^{32}$P or D-[$^{3}$H]-glucose,
compared to the control rats[17] fed normal P diet.  It is of major
interest that both in rats fed LPD and in rats fasted for the
same periods to time, the AlPase in renal cortical BBM was significantly increased, but no increases in the activities of LAP,
γ-GT or maltase were observed.[18]

DISCUSSION AND COMMENTS

     While Na$^{+}$-dependent Pi transport across BBM of proximal
tubule is now recognized as an important and perhaps determining
step in transepithelial Pi reabsorption, its biochemical basis as
well as the mechanism of its regulation is not known.  Association
of changes in Na$^{+}$-dependent Pi transport with changes in activity
of AlPase at least in some experimental situations, characterized
by large differences in tubular Pi reabsorption, raises a question whether these two BBM elements may be directly or indirectly
related.

     First, it should be recalled that parallelity between Pi trans-
port and AlPase activity in BBM was not observed in all the experimental situations with altered BBM transport of Pi.  According to
a report by Murer et al,[19] the decrease in BBM transport of Pi
elicited by acute administration of high dose of parathyroid hormone (PTH) was not associated with changes in the AlPase activity.
It should be recalled, that acute thyroparathyroidectomy (TPTX)--
which removes physiologic levels of PTH, thyroid hormones and
calcitonin--did not cause change in Pi transport[20] and chronic
TPTX caused a rather small increase in Na$^{+}$-dependent BBM transport of Pi[20]; in vitro addition of PTH caused a relatively small
decrease in Pi transport in BBM.[21]  Alimentary P deprivation in
fasting elicited an increase in the AlPase activity but not in
the BBM transport of Pi.[17,18]  These comparisons suggest that
although AlPase could be a component of BBM transport system for
Pi, it may not represent a rate-limiting step in the whole
transmembrane Pi movement.

     Analysis of BBM ultrastructural organization, based mostly on
studies with use of enzyme digestion,[7,8,22,23] indicate that
AlPase is localized rather deeply inside the thickness of BBM.
This suggests that in Pi transfer from luminal surface inside the
cell, AlPase would unlikely serve as a receptor for Pi or intra-
membranous transport carrier for Pi.[23]  On the other hand, AlPase

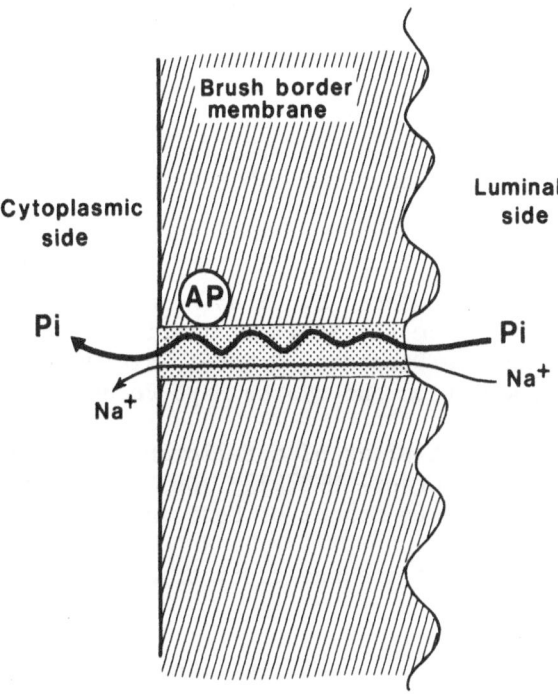

Fig. 1.    Schematic summary of the putative role of alkaline phos-
           phatase in the Pi transfer across the luminal BBM of the
           proximal tubule, assuming that the $Na^+$-dependent Pi trans-
           port is a specific process involving perhaps several
           steps.  Alkaline phosphatase (AP), which is an intrinsic
           membrane protein deeply inserted into membrane structure
           may be involved as an integral or modulatory, but not
           rate-limiting, factor in the Pi system close to the
           cytoplasmic aspect of BBM.

may be operational through its esterolytic[24] or transesterifi-
cation activity[25] on components of Pi membrane transfer which are
located close to cytoplasmic aspect of BBM (Fig. 1).

    Variations in renal BBM activity of AlPase paralleled quan-
titatively major changes in $Na^+$-dependent BBM transport of Pi,
which are associated with steadily increased or decreased renal
tubular Pi reabsorption.  This aspect may indicate that alterations of BBM AlPase play a role primarily in long-term adjust-
ments of kidney capacity to handle Pi.  On the other hand,
changes in AlPase may not be operative in acute regulation of

renal Pi transport, such as those elicited by PTH or other regulating aents which have a rapid onset of action, and effect of
which is quickly reversible.

Finally, it is still possible that observed changes in BBM
activity of AlPase which parallel those of $Na^+$-dependent Pi
transport are coincidental and that the function(s) of AlPase is
related primarily to BBM functions other than Pi reabsorption.

## ACKNOWLEDGMENTS

This research was supported by USPHS Research Grants AM-16105,
AM-21114 and AM-19715 from the National Institute of Arthritis,
Metabolism and Digestive Diseases, Grant-in-Aid MHA-36 from the
Minnesota Heart Association and by the Mayo Foundation.

S.V. Shah was the recipient of a fellowship from the Public
Health Service Training Grant AM-07013.  Dr. Shah's current
address:  Tulane University School of Medicine, New Orleans, LA.

S.A. Kempson, Ph.D. is the recipient of a Minnesota Heart
Association Fellowship.

T.P. Dousa, M.D., Ph.D. is an Established Investigator of the
American Heart Association (AHA-74182).

Mrs. Ardith Walker provided expert secretarial assistance.

## REFERENCES

1.  W. Kreusser and E. Ritz, The phosphate-depletion syndrome,
        Contr. Nephrol. 14:162 (Karger, Basel 1978).
2.  F.G. Knox, H. Osswald, G.R. Marchand, W.S. Spielman, J.A.
        Haas, T. Berndt, and S.P. Youngberg, Phosphate transport
        along the nephron, Am. J. Physiol. 233:F261 (1977).
3.  N. Hoffmann, M. Thees, and R. Kinne, Phosphate transport by
        isoated renal brush border vesicles, Pflugers Arch.
        362:147 (1976).
4.  F.G. Knox, A. Hoppe, S.A. Kempson, S.V. Shah, and T.P. Dousa,
        Cellular mechanism of phosphate transport, in "Renal
        Handling of Phosphate," S. Massry, ed., Plenum Press, NY
        (1979), in press.
5.  B. Sacktor, The brush border of the renal proximal tubule and
        the intestinal mucosa, in "Mammalian Cell Membranes,"
        G.A. Jamieson and D.M. Robinson, eds., Butterworths,
        Boston (1977), pp. 221-254.
6.  B. Sacktor, Transport in membrane vesicles from mammalian
        kidney and intestine, in "Current Topics in
        Bioenergetics," 6:39-81 (1977).

7.  A.J. Kenny and A.G. Booth, Organization of the kidney
        proximal-tubule plasma membrane, Biochem. Soc. Trans. 4:
        1011 (1976).
8.  A.G. Booth and A.J. Kenny, Identification of protein subunits
        in the kidney microvillous membrane. Biochem. Soc.
        Trans. 4:348 (1976).
9.  F. Melani, G. Ramponi, M. Farnararo, E. Cocucci, and A.
        Guerritore, Regulation by phosphate of alkaline phospha-
        tase in rat kidney, Biochim. Biophys. Acta 138:411
        (1967).
10. S.A. Kempson, J.K. Kim, T.E. Northrup, F.G. Knox, and T.P.
        Dousa, Alkaline phosphatase in adaptation to low dietary
        phosphate intake. Am. J. Physiol. (Endocrine) (1979),
        in press.
11. U. Trohler, J.-P. Bonjour, and H. Fleisch, Inorganic
        phosphate homeostasis. Renal adaptation to the dietary
        intake in intact and thyroparathyroidectomized rats. J.
        Clin. Invest. 57:264 (1976).
12. J.W. McKeown, P.C. Brazy, and V.W. Dennis, Axial heteroge-
        neity of phosphate transport along proximal convoluted
        tubules:  influence of phosphate restriction. Kidney
        Int. 14:641 (1978).
13. R.C. Muhlbauer, J.-P. Bonjour, and H. Fleisch, Tubular loca-
        lization of adaptation to dietary phosphate in rats, Am.
        J. Physiol. 233:F342 (1977).
14. S.A. Kempson and T.P. Dousa, Phosphate transport across
        renal cortical brush border membrane vesicles from rats
        stabilized on a normal, high or low phosphate diet, Life
        Sci. 24:881 (1979).
15. S.V. Shah, S.A. Kempson, T.E. Northrup, and T.P. Dousa,
        Renal adaptation of rats to low phosphate diet (LPD):
        Possible role of protein synthesis, Clin. Res. 26:42A
        (1978).
16. S.A. Kempson, S.A. Shah, and T.P. Dousa, Renal cortical
        brush border membrane (BBM) adaptation to short-term
        dietary phosphate (P) deprivation and its blockade by
        actinomycin D (Act.D), Clin. Res. 27:420A (1979).
17. S.A. Kempson, S.V. Shah, D.M. Heublein, and T.P. Dousa,
        Phosphate transport by renal cortical brush border
        membrane (BBM) vesicles:  Influence of fasting compared
        to selective depriation of dietary phosphate (P), Clin.
        Res. 27:419A (1979).
18. S.A. Kempson, S.V. Shah, and T.P. Dousa, Differential
        effects of phosphate (P) deprivation due to low P diet
        or due to starvation on renal cortical brush border
        membrane (BBM), Abstr. 12th Ann. Meeting of Amer. Soc.
        Nephrol. (1979),in press.
19. H. Murer, C. Evers, R. Stoll, and R. Kinne, The effect of
        parathyroid hormone and dietary phosphate on the sodium-
        dependent phosphate transport system located in the rat

renal brush border membrane, in: "Biochemical
Nephrology," W.G. Guder and U. Schmidt, eds., Hans
Huber, Bern (1978), pp. 455-461.

20. T.E. Northrup and T.P. Dousa, Increased transport of
    phosphate (Pi) across renal brush border membranes of
    thyroparathyroidectomized (TPTX) rats, Abstr. 61st Ann.
    Meeting of The Endocrine Society, Anaheim, CA (1979), p.
    81, Abstr. #51.

21. B. Sacktor and L. Cheng, Phosphate transport in rabbit renal
    proximal tubule membrane vesicles and its regulation,
    Fed. Proc. 38:246 (1979).

22. L. Thomas and R. Kinne, Studies on arrangement of aminopep-
    tidase and alkaline phosphatase in microvilli of iso-
    lated brush border of rat kidney, Biochem. Biophys. Acta
    255:114 (1972).

23. L. Noronha-Blob. Effects of papain on enzyme a transport
    function of isolated rabbit brush border membrane
    vesicles. Federation Procedings 38:838 (Abstr. No.
    3204) (1979).

24. W.H. Fishman, Perspectives on alkaline phosphatase isoen-
    zymes, Am. J. Med. 56:617 (1974).

25. H.N. Fernley, Mammalian alkaline phosphatases, in: "The
    Enzymes," 3rd ed., P.D. Boyer, ed., Academic Press, New
    York, vol. 4, pp. 417-445.

# MICROPUNCTURE STUDY OF DISTAL TUBULAR ACTIVATION

# OF PHOSPHATE REABSORPTION IN THE RAT

Ph. Jaeger, B. Karlmark, B. Stanton, R.G. Kirk,
T. Duplinsky and G. Giebisch

Department of Physiology
Yale University School of Medicine
333 Cedar Street, New Haven, Conn., 06510, U.S.A.

## INTRODUCTION

A considerable body of evidence suggests a reciprocal relationship between the urinary excretion rate of potassium and urinary pH[1]. In addition, attention has also been drawn to a reciprocal relationship between potassium and ammonium excretion[2,3]. The relationship between the excretion rate of urinary buffers, mainly phosphate, and potassium, is less well defined. In order to evaluate this aspect of renal tubular acidification, micropuncture studies were carried out in which the effects of acute potassium loading upon phosphate transport were investigated.

## MATERIAL AND METHODS

Male Sprague-Dawley rats (Charles River Breeding Laboratories) weighing 250 to 300 g were fed a standard rat diet (Purina laboratory chow diet #5010, phosphate content: 0.83%). Two groups of animals were used. Both received an intravenous infusion at 3 ml/hour. The control group (Na-rats) received a solution containing 135 mmol/l of NaCl, 5 mmol/l of KCl, 1 mmol/l of $NaH_2PO_4$, 1 mmol/l of $Na_2HPO_4$ and 5% mannitol; the other group (K-rats) received a similar solution in which the proportion of NaCl and KCl was reversed. $^3H$ inulin was added to these solutions in appropriate amounts to achieve counting rates in collected tubular fluid samples of several times background. Rats were anesthetized with Inactin (100 mg/kg). Details on the technical preparation of the animals in clearance and free flow

77

micropuncture experiments were similar to those previously used in this laboratory[4].

Three techniques were used to estimate phosphate (respec-tively phosphorus): (1) a spectrophotometric (phosphomolybdate) method[5] for plasma and final urine, (2) electron microprobe analysis[6], a technique also used for tubular fluid, and, (3) for urine and tubular fluid we introduced acid-base titration, a coulometric method described by Karlmark[7]. It allows deter-mination of total titratable acid (TA) in nanoliter samples. An up-to-date description of the method is given elsewhere[8]. The goal of the addition of this third technique was to test whether in experimental conditions in which phosphate is the main urinary buffer, acid-base titration is an adequate method for determin-ing inorganic phosphate. The rational is that the pKa of phos-phate is 6.8 and that the pH range used for titration extends from the actual in vivo pH of the sample (pH $\cong$ 6.5) to pH 7.4. From a practical point of view, this means that only uric acid (pKa 5.8) and creatinine (pKa 4.65) could be additional buffer specicies that could generate additional amounts of titratable acid: however, under almost all experimental conditions these buffers are not present in concentrations which could introduce a serious error. Ammonium will also not create a serious inter-ference. Firstly, because its pKa is 9.2 and secondly, because using the formaldehyde method[7], ammonium can be measured at the same time. However, as mentioned by Lemann[9] precipitation of calcium and ammonium phosphate close to the titration end point of 7.4 does create $H^+$ ions which could falsely increase TA concentration of tubular samples.

A comparison between urinary TA and inorganic phosphate excretion is shown in Figure 1: under the two experimental conditions of the present study, one mmol of chemically measured inorganic phosphate corresponds to 0.84 mmol of titrated inor-ganic phosphate; it is apparent that the amount obtained by titration is smaller than the amount obtained by spectrophoto-metry, showing that interference by uric acid and by creatinine, under normal conditions, is probably quite small. The reason why TA excretion rates are smaller than those of true inorganic phosphate is obvious, if one realizes that by stopping titration at pH 7.4, not all the phosphate present in the sample will have been titrated into its divalent form. According to the Henderson-Hasselbalch equation, an estimate may be obtained of the untitrated fraction of phosphate. For example, in our two experimental conditions, the mean urinary pH was 5.7. In this case, using the Henderson-Hasselbalch equation, one predicts a value of 80% of $PO_4$ to be titrated. This value closely ap-proaches the value of 84% which was actually obtained (see Figure 1). Although these data were obtained in final urine

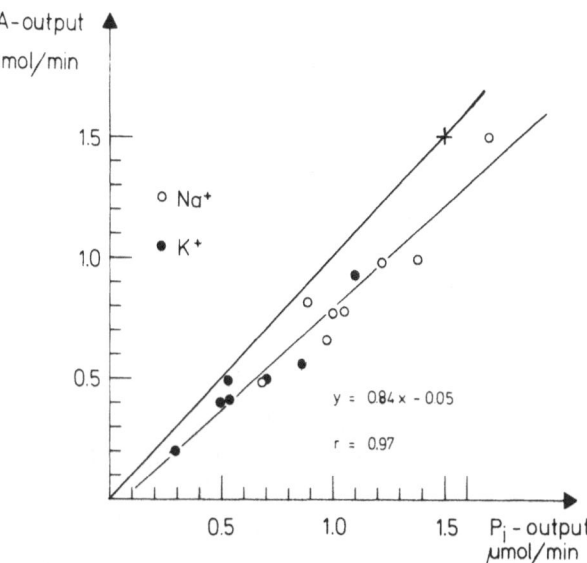

Fig. 1.    Comparison between titratable acid determination
(obtained by titration) and inorganic phosphate determination (obtained by spectrophotometry) in final
urine of 15 rats after NaCl or KCl infusion (see
above). Mean urine pH was 5.68 in the Na-group and
5.77 in the K$^+$-group.

samples it is likely that a similar close relationship between
titratable acid and phosphate also exists in tubular samples.


## RESULTS

Infusion of potassium resulted in significant elevation of
the plasma potassium level (6.87 mM ± 0.31) and a dramatic
urinary kaliuresis (Δ K excretion: + 155%). Importantly, there
were only minor changes in glomerular filtration rate, urinary
flow rate and urine pH. Nevertheless, urinary phosphate excretion significantly decreased by 45%.

Our micropuncture data clearly show that the effect of
potassium administration upon titratable acid excretion involves
the distal tubule. The following values of the slopes of phosphate concentrations (electron microprobe analysis) and of
titratable acid concentration as function of distal tubular

length (expressed as inulin TF/P concentration ratios) were, respectively:  Na-rats: 0.76 and 0.82, K rats: 0.36 and 0.26. These data indicate that acute potassium loading depresses equally both distal tubular phosphate excretion and titratable acid generation.  The similarity of those slopes in control conditions as well as after potassium loading shows that phosphate ions make up most of the titratable acid generated along the distal tubule.


## DISCUSSION

These studies add evidence to the notion that the late distal tubule of superficial nephrons is a site at which phosphate transport can be modulated[10,11].  In the present study, phosphate reabsorption was significantly augmented following potassium loading, a situation known to accentuate distal tubular potassium secretion[12]

The precise mechanism by which stimulation of potassium secretion enhances phosphate transport is not known.  Changes in intraluminal pH can be excluded since direct measurements of tubular pH in situ by means of antimony electrodes have shown no difference of pH along the distal tubule (mean control value $6.51 \pm 0.04$ (n = 21), potassium loading:  $6.52 \pm 0.06$ (n = 12). Indeed, it is known that changes in intraluminal pH may modify renal phosphate transport, probably by changing the ratio of divalent over monovalent phosphate[13,14] or, alternatively, by a direct effect of luminal pH·upon the $V_{max}$ of phosphate transport[15].  However, these luminal pH effects have been observed at the level of the proximal tubule and it should be noted that the presently distal effect can be demonstrated in the absence of luminal pH changes.

It is possible that the present effects are modulated by intracellular pH changes since it is known that alterations in potassium balance affect cellular pH[16].  Hyperkalemia may be expected to lead to intracellular alkalosis.  Indeed, studies involving changes in acid base balance have been shown to affect urinary phosphate excretion.  The results of Webb et al[17] and of Chan and Bartter[18] are consistent with the notion that intracellular alkalosis enhances overall phosphate reabsorption.  On the other hand, Ullrich and his associates have interpreted their results on proximal tubular phosphate transport to show that intracellular acidosis enhances phosphate reabsorption[19]. Clearly, more direct studies are needed in which distal tubular cell pH and phosphate transport are evaluated simultaneously.

It is also relevant to point out that hormonal factors could be involved.  For instance, the potential role of PTH depression after potassium loading has not been evaluated. Also relevant are studies by DeFronzo et al[20]: these investigators have demonstrated in man that insulin administration enhances tubular phosphate reabsorption, probably across the proximal convoluted tubule. Since hyperkalemia activates insulin release, it is possible that diminished distal phosphate delivery as a consequence of augmented proximal reabsorption limits distal tubular titratable acid formation.

In conclusion, our experiments have verified that a large fraction of distal tubular acid is formed by phosphate titration. Following activation of distal tubular potassium secretion, titratable acid generation is reduced along the distal tubule. This effect occurs without changes in distal tubular pH and is due to enhanced phosphate reabsorption.

## ACKNOWLEDGEMENTS

This work was supported by N.I.H. Grant No. AM17433-06.

## REFERENCES

1. R.W. Berliner, Renal mechanisms for potassium excretion. Harvey Lect. 55:141.
2. R.L. Tannen, Relationship of renal ammonia production and potassium homeostasis. Kidney Int. 11:453 (1977).
3. Ph. Jaeger, B. Karlmark, and G. Giebisch, Micropuncture study of relationship between $K^+$ and tubular acidification. Kidney Int. 12:562 (1977) (Abstr.).
4. J. Diezi, P. Michoud, A. Grandchamp, and G. Giebisch, Effect of nephrectomy on renal salt and water transport in the remaining kidney. Kidney Int. 10:450 (1976).
5. P.S. Chen, Jr., T.Y. Toribara, and H. Warner, Microdetermination of phosphorus. Anal. Chem. 28:11:1756 (1956).
6. Ph. Jaeger, B. Karlmark, B. Stanton, R.G. Kirk, T. Duplinsky, and G. Giebisch, Manuscript in preparation.
7. B. Karlmark, The determination of titratable acid and ammonium ions in picomole amounts. Anal. Biochem. 52:69 (1973).
8. B. Karlmark, Ph. Jaeger, and G. Giebisch, Coulometric acid-base titration in nanoliter samples with glass and antimony electrodes. A technical description. Manuscript in preparation.
9. J. Lemann, Jr., E.J. Lennon, J. Brock, A potential error in the measurement of urinary titratable acid. J. Lab. Clin. Med. 67:906 (1966).
10. C. Amiel, H. Kuntziger, S. Couette, C. Coureau, N. Bergounioux, Evidence for a parathyroid-independent

calcium modulation of phosphate transport along the
nephron. J. Clin. Invest. 57:256 (1976).

11.  L.H. Beck, M. Goldberg, Mechanism of the blunted phos-
     phaturia in saline-loaded thyroparathyroidectomized dogs.
     Kidney Int. 6:18 (1974).

12.  G. Malnic, and G. Giebisch, Micropuncture study of renal
     potassium excretion in the rat. Am. J. Physiol. 206:674
     (1964).

13.  K. Baumann, G. Rumrich, G., F. Papavassiliou, and S. Klöss,
     pH dependence of phosphate reabsorption in the proximal
     tubule of rat kidney. Pflügers Arch. 360:183 (1975).

14.  N. Bank, H. Aynedjian, and S.W. Weinstein, A microper-
     fusion study of phosphate reabsorption by the rat proximal
     renal tubule. J. Clin. Invest. 54:1040 (1974).

15.  H. Murer, Transport of phosphate by rat proximal tubular
     brush border vesicles. Presentation at the 4th International
     Workshop on Phosphate and Other Minerals, Strasbourg, 1979.

16.  S. Adler, and D.S. Fraley, Potassium and intracellular pH.
     Kidney Int. 11:433 (1977).

17.  R.K. Webb, Ph.B. Woodhall, C. Tischer, G. Glaubiger,
     F.A. Neelon, and R.R. Robinson, Relationship between
     phosphaturia and acute hypercapnia in the rat. J. Clin.
     Invest. 60:829 (1977).

18.  J.C.M. Chan, and F.C. Bartter, Effect of acidosis and
     alkalosis on calcium and phosphorus metabolism in normal
     man. Mineral and Electrolyte Metabolism 2:214 (1979)
     Abstract.

19.  K.J. Ullrich, G. Rumrich, S. Klöss, Phosphate transport
     in the proximal convolution of the rat kidney. Pflügers
     Arch. 377:33 (1978).

20.  R.A. DeFronzo, M. Goldberg, and Z. Agus, The effects of
     glucose and insulin on renal electrolyte transport.
     J. Clin. Invest. 58:83 (1976).

# THE INFLUENCE OF D-GLUCOSE ON PHOSPHATE ABSORPTION IN THE RAT PROXIMAL TUBULE

T. F. Knight, H. O. Senekjian, and E. J. Weinman

Renal Section, Department of Internal Medicine,
Veterans Administration Medical Center and
Baylor College of Medicine, Houston, Texas 77211

## INTRODUCTION

Recent microperfusion studies utilizing both in vitro and in vivo techniques have focused attention on the effects of intraluminal factors on the control of absorptive processes in the proximal tubule. Thus, D-glucose and/or alanine are responsible for the negative potential differences recorded in the proximal convoluted tubule and for at least some component of net sodium absorption.[1] Dennis and Brazy and Corman and associates have also shown that D-glucose in the tubular lumen inhibits the reabsorption of phosphate.[2,3] We have recently shown in our laboratory that D-glucose also inhibits the reabsorption of urate in the proximal convoluted tubule of the rat.[4] The mechanism of the interaction of glucose with phosphate, on the one hand and with urate on the other, appears to be quite distinct in that phloridzin mimics the inhibitory effect of glucose on urate absorption while not affecting phosphate transport. The present study was, therefore, performed to re-examine the effects of D-glucose on phosphate transport in the rat proximal tubule. In addition, the effects of flow rate and initial phosphate concentration on phosphate absorption were examined.

## METHODS

Male Sprague-Dawley rats weighing between 250-350 grams were anesthetized with nembutal (50-60 mg/kg body wt) injected intraperitoneally. A thyroparathyroidectomy was performed utilizing electrical cautery, following which the animals were prepared for micropuncture as previously described from this laboratory.[5] Two hours were allowed to elapse after parathyroidectomy before

83

experiments were started.  Fractional excretion of phosphate in all
animals was less than 2.3%, confirming adequate removal of all
parathyroid tissue.  In vivo microperfusions of proximal convoluted
tubules were performed using a Hampel microperfusion apparatus.
After each microperfusion, a latex cast of the tubule was made and
the distance between the perfusion and collection pipets was determined.  The tubular length was between 1 and 2.5 mm and all
tubules were localized to the middle third of the proximal convoluted tubule.  The perfusion solution contained sodium, 139 mM/L;
chloride, 119 mM/L; bicarbonate, 25 mM/L; potassium, 5 mM/L; and
urea, 5 mM/L.  $NaH_2PO_4$ was added to the solution to a final concentration of either 2 or 8 mM/L.  Where examined, glucose was added
in a concentration of 5.6 mM and phloridzin in a concentration of
$10^{-4}$ M.  Methoxy-$^3$H inulin and $^{32}$P-ortho-phosphate were added to
the solution in amounts sufficient to permit accurate isotope
counting.  Perfusion rate, water absorption and phosphate absorption
were determined from standard formulae and all values are expressed
as the mean ± S.E.M.  Statistical significance was determined by the
t-test for unpaired data.

RESULTS AND DISCUSSION

       As noted in Figure 1, phosphate absorption for the 2 mM phos-
phate solution increased from 6.7±0.9 pmol/min/mm at an average
perfusion rate of 8.2 nl/min to 12.3±1.4 pmol/min/mm (P<0.01) as
the perfusion rate was increased to 15.3 nl/min.  Further increases
in perfusion rate beyond this did not result in any increase in
phosphate absorption.  For all perfusions performed at rates above

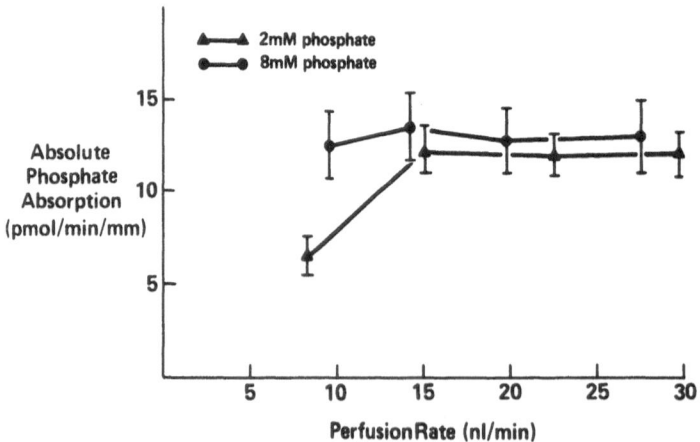

Fig. 1.    Relationship of perfusion rate and absolute phosphate ab-
           sorption for 2 concentrations of inorganic phosphate.
           Values represent mean ± S.E.M.  See text for statis-
           tics.

15 nl/min, phosphate absorption averaged 12.0±0.7 pmol/min/mm.  With
the 8 mM phosphate solution, phosphate absorption was independent of
flow rate and averaged 12.5±2.0 pmol/min/mm.  This value was not
significantly different from that obtained with the 2 mM phosphate
solution at perfusion rates in excess of 15 nl/min.  These results
clearly show a maximal rate of phosphate absorption in the thyroparathyroidectomized rat.  Once the delivery rate of phosphate exceeds this value, phosphate absorption is independent of either
perfusion rate or initial phosphate concentration.  These results
are consistent with those of Dennis et al., who found little effect
of altering delivery rate of phosphate by either increasing perfusion rate or the initial phosphate concentration on phosphate absorption in isolated perfused rabbit proximal convoluted tubules.[6]

Figure 2 shows the results for absolute phosphate absorption
when D-glucose was added to the perfusion solution.  At any rate of
perfusion, phosphate absorption was less than with the solution not
containing glucose.  This decrease was not significant, however,
until the perfusion rate exceeded 15 nl/min.  For all perfusions
above 15 nl/min, phosphate absorption averaged 6.2±0.5 pmol/min/mm
(P <0.001 compared to the non-glucose containing solution).  In Figure 3 are shown the results of studies performed with phloridzin
added to the perfusion solution.  There was no significant effect on
phosphate absorption at any rate of perfusion.  With the addition of
both D-glucose and phloridzin to the perfusion solution, shown in
Figure 4, phosphate absorption was again similar to values obtained
with the 2 mM phosphate solution.  For all perfusions over 15 nl/min,
phosphate absorption averaged 10.6±0.6 pmol/min/mm (P=NS compared to

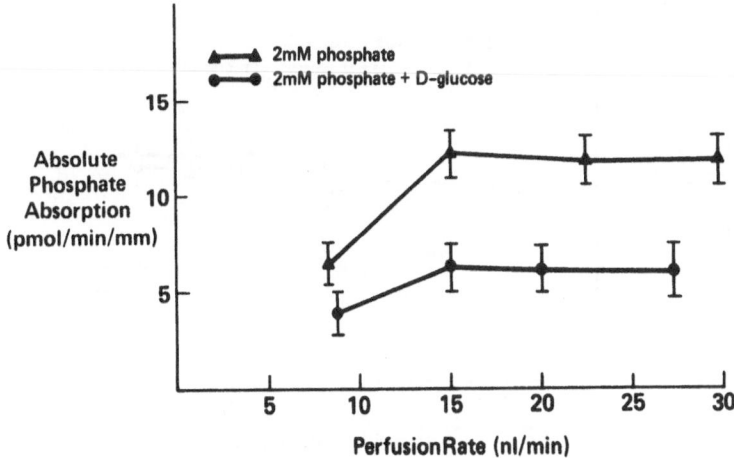

Fig. 2.   Effect of intraluminal D-glucose on absolute phosphate ab-
          sorption.  Values represent mean ± S.E.M.  See text for
          statistics.

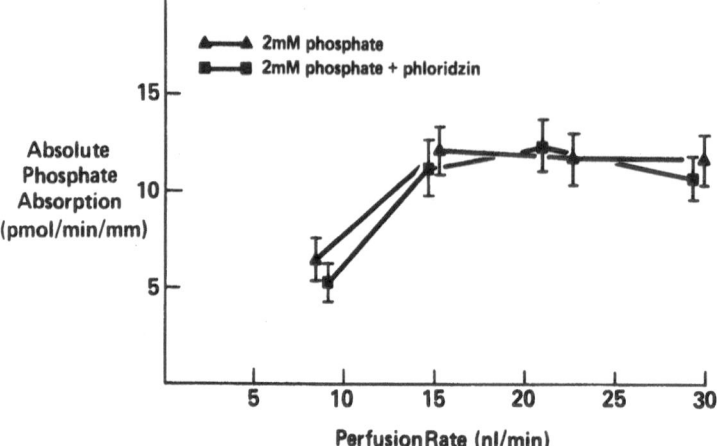

Fig. 3.   Effect of intraluminal phloridzin on absolute phosphate
          absorption.  Values represent mean ± S.E.M.  There was no
          significant effect on absolute phosphate absorption at any
          perfusion rate.

2 mM phosphate solution; P<0.001 compared to 2 mM phosphate solution
with D-glucose).  Thus, these studies, which demonstrate that the
presence of D-glucose in the lumen of the proximal convoluted
tubule inhibits phosphate absorption, confirm the studies of Dennis
and Brazy in the isolated rabbit proximal convoluted tubule.[2]  They

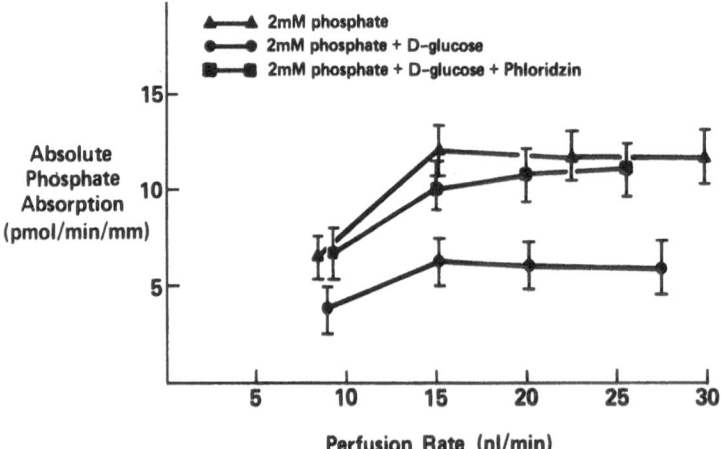

Fig. 4.   Effect of intraluminal D-glucose and phloridzin (shown in
          the middle line) on absolute phosphate absorption.  Values
          represent mean ± S.E.M.  See text for statistics.

extend the observations of Corman et al. in the rat,[3] in that they demonstrate that phloridzin inhibits the effect of glucose on phosphate transport. Thus, in the rat, as in the rabbit, the inhibitory effect of glucose on phosphate absorption is dependent on the absorption of glucose and not the result of competition for a common carrier on the brush border membrane. Corman argued convincingly that the site of this interaction in the rat was most likely the proximal convoluted tubule, and the present study shows that this is indeed the case.[3] The results reported here can be contrasted to recent findings in our laboratory that glucose inhibits urate reabsorption in the proximal convoluted tubule.[4] This glucose-urate interaction, however, appears to result from competition for a single carrier on the luminal membrane, in that phloridzin had the same effect as glucose. By contrast, it has been suggested that phosphate absorption is inhibited by glucose secondary to changes in electrical potentials due to the rheogenic nature of sodium-dependent glucose transfer across the brush border membrane.[2] The results of the present studies, in conjunction with others, suggest that glucose is an important modulator of absorptive function in the proximal convoluted tubule.

In summary, the present studies demonstrate that a tubular maximum for phosphate absorption is present in the proximal tubule of the rat. In addition, the presence of D-glucose in the solution on the luminal side of the renal tubular cells inhibits phosphate absorption. The effect of D-glucose on phosphate absorption requires the tubular absorption of D-glucose and does not appear to be due to an interaction between glucose and phosphate at the luminal surface of the renal tubular cells.

REFERENCES

1. J. P. Kokko, Proximal tubule potential difference. Dependence on glucose, $HCO_3$, and amino acids, J. Clin. Invest. 52:1362 (1973).

2. V. W. Dennis and P. C. Brazy, Sodium, phosphate, glucose, bicarbonate and alanine interactions in the isolated proximal convoluted tubule of the rabbit kidney, J. Clin. Invest. 62:387 (1978).

3. B. Corman, C. Touvay, P. Poujeol, and C. deRouffignac, Glucose mediated inhibition of phosphate reabsorption in the rat kidney, Am. J. Physiol. 235:F430 (1978), or Am. J. Physiol.: Renal Fluid Electrolyte Physiol. 4:F430 (1978).

4. T. F. Knight, H. O. Senekjian, and E. J. Weinman, Effects of intraluminal D-glucose and probenecid on urate absorption in the rat proximal tubule, Am. J. Physiol. 236:F526

(1979), or Am. J. Physiol.: Renal Fluid Electrolyte
Physiol. 5:F526 (1979).

5.  E. J. Weinman, W. N. Suki, and G. Eknoyan, The influence
    of the extracellular fluid volume on the tubular reabsorp-
    tion of uric acid, J. Clin. Invest. 55:283 (1975).

6.  V. W. Dennis, P. B. Woodhall, and R. R. Robinson, Charac-
    teristics of phosphate transport in isolated proximal
    tubule, Am. J. Physiol. 231:979 (1976).

# TUBULAR LOCALIZATION OF THE EFFECT OF 1,25-DIHYDROXY-VITAMIN D3 AND DIETARY PHOSPHATE ON THE TRANSPORT OF PHOSPHATE IN THYROPARATHYROIDECTOMIZED RATS

R. Mühlbauer, J.-P. Bonjour and H. Fleisch

Department of Pathophysiology
University of Berne
Murtenstrasse 35, 3010 Berne, Switzerland

Clearance studies in vitamin D-replete thyroparathyroid-ectomized (TPTX) rats have shown that chronic administration of 1,25-dihydroxyvitamin $D_3$ (1,25$(OH)_2D_3$, 2 x 13 pmol/day intraperitoneally for 7 days) decreased the overall tubular capacity to reabsorb inorganic phosphate (Pi) (1). In the present work, the influence of 1,25$(OH)_2D_3$ on the tubular handling of Pi was localized by random free-flow micropunctures.

TPTX Wistar rats of 180-200 g were used for this study. They were pair-fed for 7 days a diet containing 1.2 g % phosphorus and 1.1 g % calcium. 1,25$(OH)_2D_3$ in ethanol was administered twice daily at a dose of 2 x13 pmol for 7 days. The control animals received ethanol alone. At the day of the micropuncture experiment they were prepared as previously described (2). Inulin was infused to allow measurement of whole kidney clearance and functional localization of micropunctures with respect to water reabsorption (TF/P)In. Inulin in plasma, urine and tubular fluid was determined using diphenylamine after acid hydrolysis to fructose (2,3). Pi in plasma, urine and tubular fluid was determined using a molybdate malachite green reagent (2,4).

The effect of 1,25$(OH)_2D_3$ was compared to those of 1) increasing dietary P in TPTX rats, and 2) chronic removal of thyroparathyroid glands. Differences in plasma Pi concentration ([Pi]Pl.) as a result of pretreatment were corrected by acute infusion of Pi. The influence of 1,25$(OH)_2D_3$, dietary Pi and TPTX was studied at these similar [Pi] Pl. so attained.

The results show that in TPTX rats the administration
of $1,25(OH)_2D_3$ or an increase in dietary phosphorus
from 0.2 to 1.2 %, inhibits net Pi reabsorption from
glomerulus to early proximal tubule but not from early
to late accessible proximal tubule.  Along the first
portion of convoluted proximal tubules, pretreatment
with $1,25(OH)_2D_3$ and high Pi diet do not only block
completely the net reabsorption of Pi, but appear to
promote a net secretion of Pi.  Such a net entry of Pi
into the tubular lumen of early proximal convolutions
has already been reported in intact rats (2,5,6).

Removal of the thyroparathyroid glands did not alter
net Pi reabsorption along the first portion of the
proximal tubule when measured at similar filtered load
of Pi 48 h after the operation.  In these rats chronically TPTX, however, an increase in net Pi reabsorption
from mid to late accessible proximal tubule was observed.
This data showing that chronic TPTX affects the second
but not the first portion of the proximal tubule might
explain the original observation made by Amiel et al.
(7): these authors studied chronic TPTX rats at their
endogenous (significantly elevated) [Pi] Pl. and found
in these animals more Pi being delivered to the early
proximal tubule as compared to intact counterparts.
This apparently paradoxal result could be explained by
an increased filtrered load of Pi delivered to a segment (the early proximal tubule) of which the transport capacity is not influenced by chronic TPTX.

Comparison between the fraction of filtered Pi excreted
in the urine and that recovered in the distal tubule
suggested that $1,25(OH)_2D_3$ or high phosphorus diet
decreased, whereas chronic TPTX increased, the net
tubular reabsorption along the terminal nephron.  Thus
these data confirm our previous observations which
strongly suggested that the terminal nephron can be the
site of either a net secretion or a net reabsorption of
Pi (2,6).  To what extent the apparent net movement
between the end of the distal tubule and the final
urine could be due to a difference in the handling of
Pi between superficial and deep nephrons (8) remains to
be established.

In conclusion, this study indicates that $1,25(OH)_2D_3$
given to TPTX rats affects the Pi transport along the
same tubular segments as does an increase in dietary
Pi.  Along the proximal tubule the localization of the

influence of 1,25(OH)$_2$D$_3$ and dietary Pi differs
form that of chronic TPTX.  The results also suggest
that besides some portions of the proximal convoluted
tubule, more distal segments appear to respond to
1,25(OH)$_2$D$_3$, dietary Pi, and chronic thyroparathyroidectomy.

## Acknowledgements

This work has been supported by the Swiss National
Science Foundation (3.725.76), by F. Hoffmann-La Roche
& Co. AG, Basel, Switzerland, and by the Ausbildungs-
und Förderungsfonds der Arbeitsgemeinschaft für Osteo-
synthese (AO), Chur, Switzerland.  We thank Mrs. C.
Marti and R. Rubli for skilled technical assistance.

## References

1. J.-P. Bonjour, C. Preston, and H. Fleisch, Effect of
   1,25-dihydroxyvitamin D$_3$ on the renal handling of
   Pi in thyroparathyroidectomized rats. J.Clin.Invest.
   60: 1419 (1977).
2. R.C. Mühlbauer, J.-P. Bonjour, and H. Fleisch, Tubular localization of adaptation to dietary phosphate
   in rats, Am.J.Physiol. 233: F342 (1977).
3. H.E. Harrison, A modification of the diphenylamine
   method for determination of inulin, Proc.Soc.Exptl.
   Biol. Med. 49: 111 (1942).
4. H.J. Altman, E. Fürstenau, A. Gielewski, and L.
   Scholz, Photometrische Bestimmung kleiner Phosphat-
   mengen mit Malachitgrün, Z.Anal.Chem. 256: 274 (1971).
5. C. Le Grimellec, Micropuncture study along the proximal convoluted tubule. Electrolyte reabsorption in
   first convolutions. Pflügers Arch. 354: 133 (1975).
6. J.F. Boudry, U. Tröhler, M. Touabi, H. Fleisch, and
   J.-P. Bonjour, Secretion of inorganic phosphate in
   the rat nephron. Clin.Sci.Mol.Med. 48: 475 (1975).
7. C. Amiel, H. Kuntziger, and G. Richet, Micropuncture
   study of handling of phosphate by proximal and distal
   nephron in normal and parathyroidectomized rat.
   Evidence for distal reabsorption. Pflügers Arch. 317:
   93 (1970).
8. C. de Rouffignac, P$_{32}$Poujeol, and R.L. Jamison,
   Microinjections de $^{32}$P phosphate dans les segments
   grêles des néphrons juxtamedullaires: Existence d'un
   segment réabsorbant les phosphates localisé entre la
   pointe des anses et les canaux collecteurs, in:
   Abstracts VIIth International Congress of Nephrology,
   Montreal, 1978, E-14 (1978).

# NATRIURESIS AND PHOSPHATURIA DURING EXTRACELLULAR VOLUME EXPANSION, BLOOD VOLUME EXPANSION OR STIMULATION OF THE INTRA-THORACIC VOLUME RECEPTORS

H.A. Jahn, G.M. Rocha, M. Kondo, D.C. Schohn,
R.L. Schmitt

Service de Néphrologie
67005 Strasbourg Cedex France

It has been shown that extracellular fluid volume expansion (ECVE) produces natriuresis (1,2) and phosphaturia (3,4,5) due to a decrease in the renal tubular reabsorption of these ions (3,4,5,6). However the biological signals for this phenomenon are as yet not elucidated.

In a effort to examine the possible pathways involved, studies were carried out to evaluate the effects of ECVE, of preferential blood volume expansion and of an increase in the volume of the central cardiovascular compartment induced by water immersion (WI) or negative pressure breathing (NPB) on the urinary excretion of sodium and phosphate.

## METHODS

Studies were performed in 29 normal volunteers. There were 10 females and 19 males. Their age ranged between 21 and 50 years with a mean of $31 \pm 9$ years. The nature of the experiments was explained to the subjects and their consents for the participation in the studies were obtained.

In 6 subjects ECVE was produced by the infusion of normal saline at a rate of $16 \pm 3$ ml/min for 2 hours. A week later the same subjects received an infusion of modified fluid gelatine (MFG) at a rate of $16 \pm 3$ ml/min for 30 minutes then $3 \pm 3$ ml/min for the next 90 minutes. The MFG contained degraded polymerized gelatine (35 g/l), sodium and chloride (145 mEq/l), potassium (5.1 mEq/l) and calcium 12.5 mEq/l. The oncotic pressure of the MFG was 29 to 30 mm Hg, its pH 7.0 to 7.5 and relative viscosity 1.6 to 1.9. With the saline infusion, we obtained a gain in weight near 2 % of body

weight. Urine collections of 2 hour duration were obtained before,
during and after the infusions. Echocardiographic studies (7) were
performed before and during the expansion in order to determine the
sound beam diameter of the left atrium.

Twenty three individuals were subjected to WI, according to the
technique of Gauer and al. (8), for 2 hours. This procedure
produced an increase in the volume of the central cardiovascular
compartment and an increase in the diameter of the left atrium, measured on the echocardiogram (Figure 1). Urine was collected for 2 hour
periods before, during and after WI.

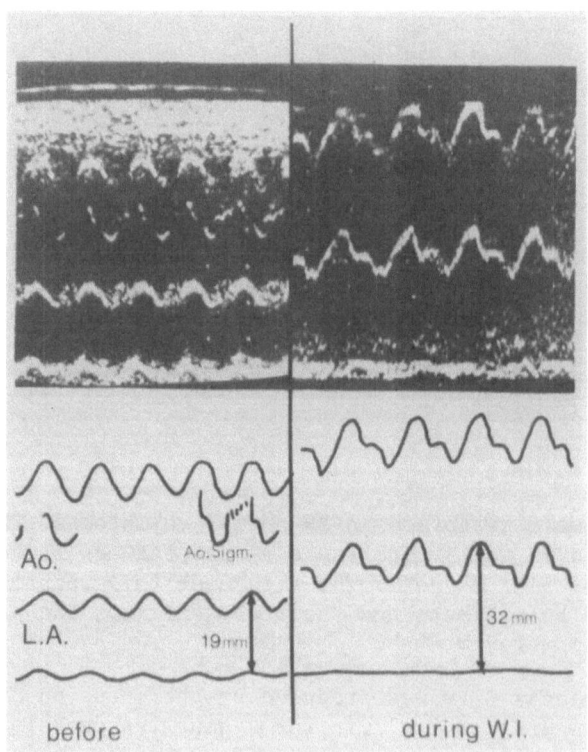

## WATER IMMERSION

Fig 1    The effect of water immersion (WI) on the echocardiogram.
         Note the increase in diameter of the left atrium from
         19 to 32 mm. Ao = aorta and LA = left atrium.

In 8 subjects stimulation of the stretch receptors of the left
atrium was produced by NPB (pressure at -6 cm $H_2O$ for 20 minutes).
Urine collections were obtained for 20 minutes periods before, during
and after the NPB. Echocardiogram was also recorded in this study.

In order to examine whether WI is associated with the production
of natriuretic and/or phosphaturic material(s), the urines collected
before, during and after WI in 10 individuals were subjected to gel
filtration and dry freezing. The effects of the resultant volume of
urine on the urinary excretion of sodium and phosphate were tested in
female Whistar rats (200 g) undergoing mild and stable saline diuresis
produced by the infusion of 0.4 % NaCl solution. After a stable u-
rinary flow was obtained, 0.5 ml of the prepared human urine was
injected intravenously into the test rats and their urines were
collected for 4 - 5 periods of 10 minutes each. The urine flow was
recorded drop by drop on a potentiometric recorder, the urinary fluid
losses replaced with 0.4 % saline infusion utilizing a computerized
servocontrol infusion pump.

The concentrations of creatinin, sodium, calcium and phosphate
in blood and urine were measured with standard techniques. Statistical
analysis were made using the Student paired sample test.

RESULTS

The effects of ECVE produced by saline infusion and of blood
volume expansion produced by MFG on pulmonary arterial pressure (PAP)
and urinary excretion of sodium and phosphate are given in Figure 2.
There were significant increments in PAP during both procedures but
the rise in PAP was greater during MFG infusion. ECVE produced a
significant ($p < 0.005$) increment in urinary sodium excretion
(from 0.097 $\pm$ 0.03 to 0.28 $\pm$ 0.08 mmol/min) and a significant
($p < 0.025$) increment in phosphaturia (from 7.59 $\pm$ 2.64 to
15.09 $\pm$ 2.72 µmol/min). The infusion of MFG also produced natriuresis
(from 0.14 $\pm$ 0.06 to 0.39 $\pm$ 0.16 mmol/min) and the percent increment
in sodium excretion (178 %) was only slightly different from that
observed during ECVE (225 %). Although MFG infusion also produced
phosphaturia (from 8.69 $\pm$ 2.44 to 11.94 $\pm$ 2.30 µmol/min), the
magnitude of the rise in phosphate excretion was smaller than that
with ECVE ($p < 0.05$). The plasma concentration of calcium during MFG
infusion (2.50 $\pm$ 0.09 mmol/1) was not significantly different from
that during saline infusion (2.27 $\pm$ 0.04 mmol/1) and therefore changes
in blood calcium and consequently in blood parathyroid hormone levels
could not account for the difference in the phosphaturia noted during
the two procedures. The echocardiogram did not show an increase in
left atrium diameter during ECVE or blood volume expansion with MFG.

The effects of WI on urinary sodium and phosphate excretion are
given in Figures 3, 4 and 5. All 23 subjects exhibited marked and
significant ($p < 0.001$) natriuresis (from 0.077 $\pm$ 0.010 to

0.22 ± 0.029 mmol/min ; Figure 3). However, the effects of WI on phosphate excretion varied among the various individuals and was dependent on the initial rate of urinary phosphate (Figure 4). The 9 subjects who started with low rate of phosphate excretion (5.4 ± 1 µmol/min) displayed significant phosphaturia during WI (from 5.4 ± 1 to 11.2 ± 1.3 µmol/min, p < 0.005). On the other hand 14 subjects in whom phosphate excretion was higher prior to WI (15 ± 2.2 µmol/min) had a decrease in urinary phosphate during WI (from 15 ± 2.2 to 8.7 ± 1 µmol/min).

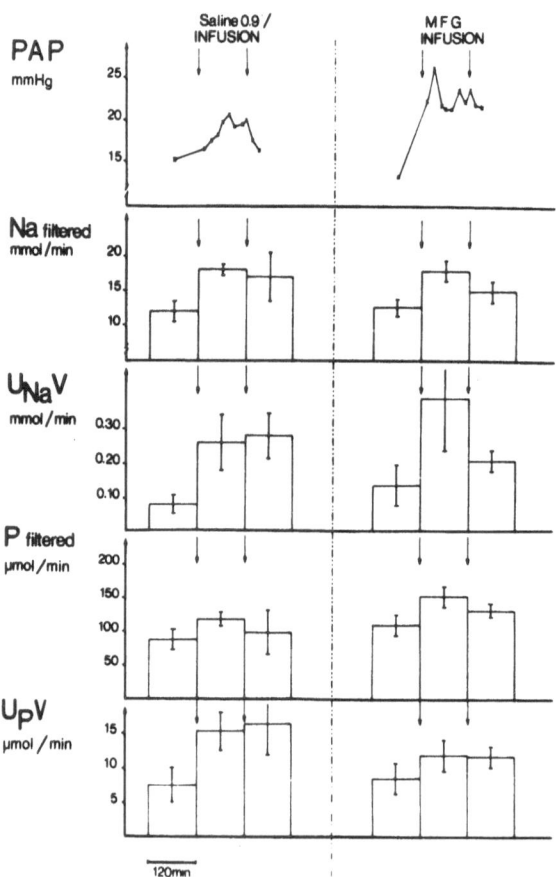

Fig 2    Effects of ECVE produced by saline infusion (left) and blood volume expansion produced by modified fluid gelatin infusion (MFG) (right) on PAP and on filtered sodium and phosphate and on their excretory rates. Each column represents the mean values with the brackets denoting standard error (SE).

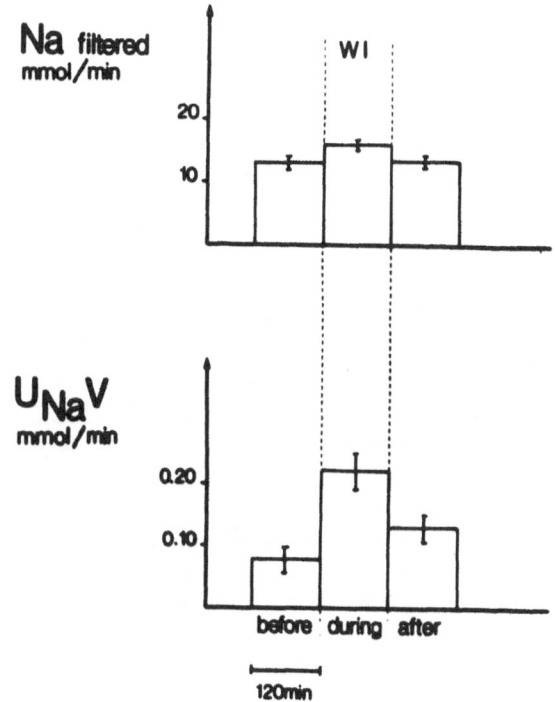

Fig 3    The effects of WI on filtered sodium and its urinary excretion. Each bar represents the mean values with brackets
denoting SE.

        Figure 5 shows a significant and inverse correlation between
the phosphate excretion before WI and the phosphate excretion during
WI. In all the subjects in whom echocardiogram was done, WI was associated with a significant increase in the diameter of the left atrium
(Figure 1).

        The effects of NPB on urinary excretion of sodium and phosphate
are shown in Figure 6. There were no significant changes in urinary
excretion of sodium. However, modest but significant phosphaturia
was noticed (+ 6 $\pm$ 2 $\mu$mol/min, p<0.001). Echocardiogram demonstrated that NPB was associated with a slight increase in the diameter of the left atrium (Figure 7).

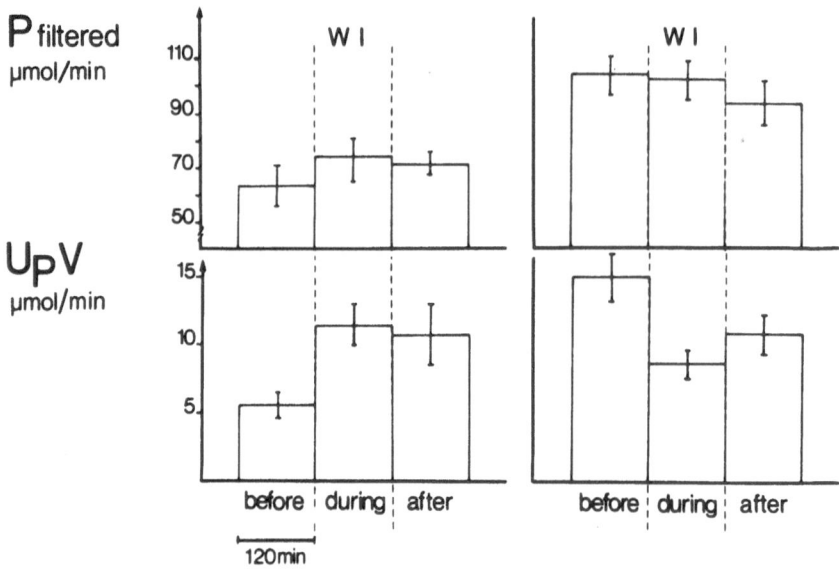

Fig 4    The effects of WI on filtered phosphate and its excretion
rates. Subjects who had initial low urinary phosphate are
shown on the left panel and those with higher initial phosphate excretion are shown on the right panel. Each column
represents the mean value with the brackets denoting SE.

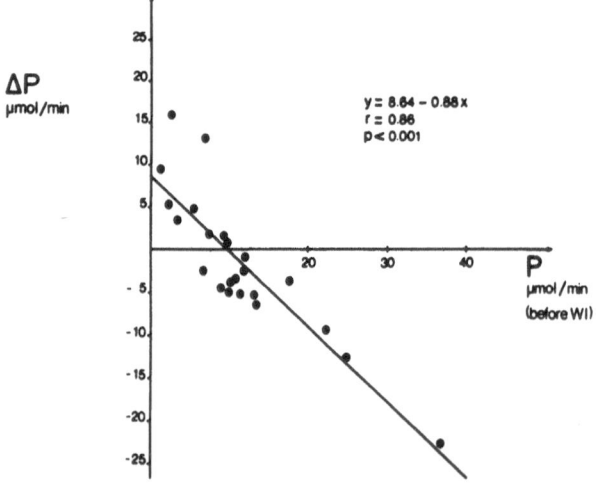

Fig 5    The relationship between initial phosphate excretion and
the change observed during WI in 23 normal subjects.

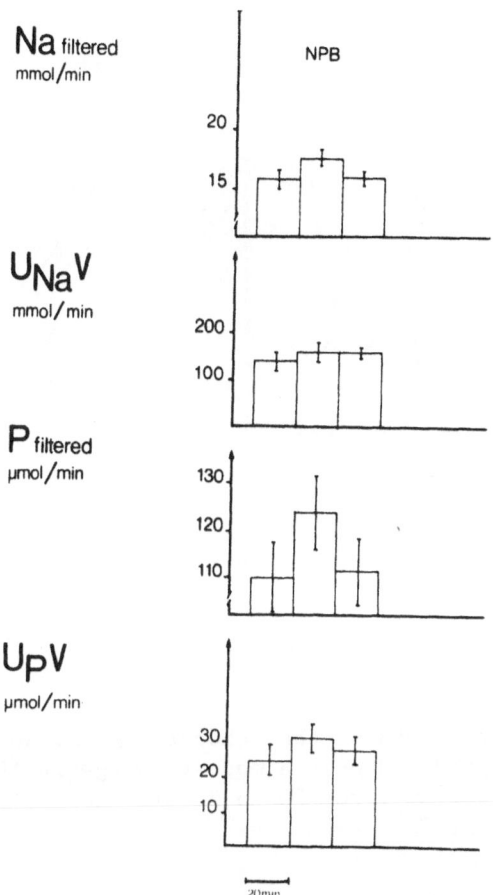

Fig 6    The effects of negative pressure breathing (NPB) on filtered
         loads of sodium and phosphate and on their excretion rates.
         Each column represents the mean value with the brackets
         denoting SE.

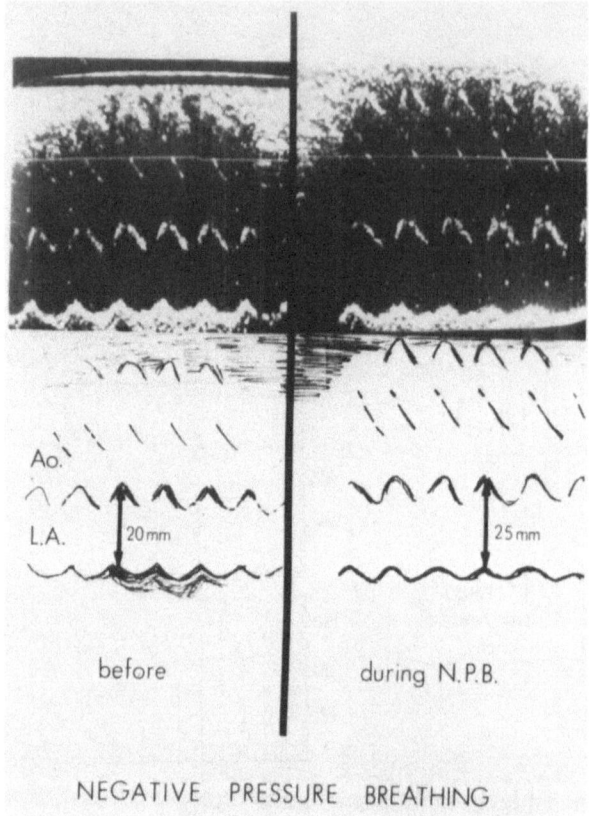

Fig 7    The effect of NPB on the echocardiogram. Note that this
         maneuvre produced only a modest change in the diameter of
         the left atrium (from 20 to 25 mm). Ao = aorta and
         LA = left atrium.


     The effects of the injection of prepared human urines collected
before, during and after WI on urine volume and urinary excretions
of creatinin, sodium and phosphate in test rats are shown in Figure 8.
Urinary excretion of creatinin did not change significantly, indicating that glomerular filtration rate was stable throughout the study.
Urine volume and urinary excretion of sodium and phosphate increased
significantly after the injection of prepared human urine obtained
after WI. It is of interest that even the urine from subjects that
did not have phosphaturia during WI produced significant phosphaturia
when injected into the rats.

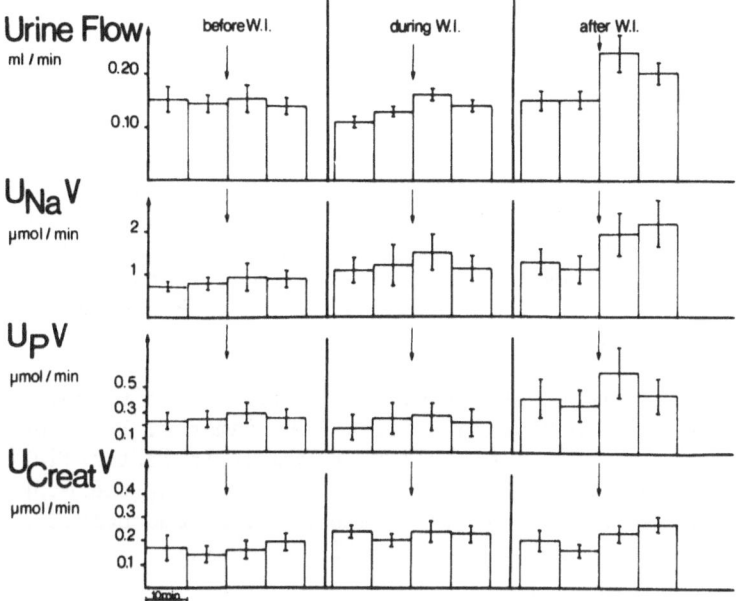

Fig 8    The effects of the intravenous injection of prepared human
urines obtained from 10 patients before, during and after
water immersion (WI) on urine flow and urinary excretion of
sodium, phosphate and creatinin in test rats. Each column
represents the mean value with the brackets denoting SE.
The first two columns in each panel represent data before
the injection of the human urine and the 3rd and 4th columns
the data after the injection of the human urine.


DISCUSSION

    The results of the present study show that ECVE with saline,
preferential blood volume expansion with MFG and WI produced comparable degrees of natriuresis but NPB failed to significantly
increase urinary sodium excretion. Since these different maneuvres
probably produce various hemodynamic changes, one may suggest that
alterations in various circulatory sites are involved in the control
of renal handling of sodium.

    Expansion of the extracellular fluid volume or blood volume
alone produced similar increments in sodium excretion despite different increments in PAP during the two procedures. This would
suggest that either the magnitude of the rise in PAP is not a critical factor for the modulation of sodium excretion or only a modest
rise in PAP is needed to reduce tubular sodium reabsorption and further increment in PAP do not produce greater natriuresis. Indeed the
work of Toor et al. (9) suggests an important role for the rise in
PAP in the control of sodium excretion.

It should be emphasized that during both ECVE and MFG infusion, there was no increase in the diameter of the left atrium as demonstrated by echocardiography. Although this observation may suggest that an alteration in the diameter of the left atrium is not an important regulatory factor in the control of sodium excretion ; the data from the studies with WI do not support such a contention. During the latter procedure, there was a marked increase in the diameter of the left atrium which was associated with marked natriuresis. It appears therefore, that the increase in urinary sodium excretion during ECVE and MFG infusion are not triggered by an increase in left atrial diameter although a change in the latter can affect the renal handling of sodium.

It is surprising that NPB did not produce significant natriuresis despite a rise in left atrial diameter. It is possible that this is related to the smaller increment in left atrial diameter than that observed during WI. One may suggest, therefore, that a finite increase in left atrial diameter is needed before an effect on renal tubular sodium reabsorption is evident.

The data of the present study are consistent with the notion that a certain degree of expansion of the extracellular volume, the vascular volume or the central compartment of the circulation stimulates baroreceptors or the receptors within or outside the cardiovascular system. This stimulation form the afferent limb of an integrated system that modulate the sodium reabsorption by the renal tubule. The efferent system through which the signals are transmitted to kidney and by which the changes in sodium reabsorption are dictated is not as yet well elucidated. Such a system may involve changes in renal hemodynamics (10,11) or the release of a humoral factor(s) (12,13,6,14,15,16,17,18,19).

Several investigators have provided data supporting the formation of a natriuretic hormone during ECVE and have suggested that at least part of the natriuresis of ECVE is due to the effect of this hormone on sodium transport by the kidney. Our results obtained during WI in humans indicate that the urine of these subjects contains a natriuretic material(s) and it is possible that such a substance is responsible for part of the sodium diuresis observed during WI. Our data and these of others suggest that the release of a possible natriuretic hormone may occur not only during ECVE but even during expansion of the central compartment of the cardiovascular system.

It has been reported by several investigators that the renal handling of sodium and phosphate are closely linked and phosphaturia occurs during natriuresis. Our results confirm in part such observations but further indicate that the renal excretion of these two ions could be dissociated. This was particularly evident during WI when the effect of this procedure on phosphate excretion was dependent on the initial excretory rate of phosphate.

It has been shown that many factors may affect the renal reabsorption of phosphate in addition to changes in sodium transport. These may include parathyroid hormone (20,21), calcitonin (22,23), growth hormone (24), state of body stores of phosphate (25), blood calcium levels (26), or state of vitamin D metabolites (27,28). Variation in these parameters may explain our findings. However, we did not evaluate these factors in our subjects and we can not, therefore, point toward any of them alone or in combination as the cause of the differences in the phosphaturic response during WI.

Our data clearly indicate that some of our subjects had strong phosphate retaining forces that overcome the phosphaturic effect of WI. These forces, therefore, are responsible for the dissociation between the renal handling of sodium and phosphate. This postulate is supported by the observation that the urine of these subjects contained a phosphaturic material since it produced significant phosphaturia when injected into rats.

REFERENCES

1. L. G. WESSON Jr, W. P. ANSLOW, L. G. RAISZ, A. A. BOLOMEY, and M. LADD, Effect of sustained expansion of extracellular fluid volume upon filtration rate, renal plasma flow and electrolyte and water excretion in the dog, Am. J. Physiol. 162:677 (1950).
2. I. H. MILLS, H. E. DE WARDENER, C. J. HAYTER, and W. F. CLAPHAM, Studies on the efferent mechanism of the sodium chloride diuresis which follows intravenous saline in the dog, Clin. Sci., 21:249 (1961).
3. S. G. MASSRY, J. W. COBURN, and C. R. KLEEMAN, The influence of extracellular volume expansion on renal phosphate reabsorption in the dog, J. Clin. Invest., 48:1237 (1969).
4. W. N. SUKI, M. MARTINEZ MALDONADO, D. ROUSE, and A. TERRY, Effect of expansion of extracellular fluid volume on renal phosphate handling, J. Clin. Invest., 48:1888 (1969).
5. T. H. STEELE, Increased urinary phosphate excretion following volume expansion in normal man. Metabolism, 19:129 (1970).
6. F. C. RECTOR Jr, G. VAN GIENSEN, F. KILL, and D. W. SELDIN, Influence of expansion of extracellular volume on tubular reabsorption of sodium independent of changes in glomerular filtration rates and aldosterone activity, J. Clin. Invest. 43:341 (1964).
7. R. GRAMIAK, P. M. SHAH, and D. H. KRAMER, Ultrasound cardiography : contrast in anatomy and function, in "Ultrasono graphia medica", ed. J. Böck - K. Ossoinig, Wiener Medizinische Akademie, WIEN, III:407 (1971).
8. C. BEHN, O. H. GAUER, K. KIRSCH, and P. ECKERT, Effects of

sustained intrathoracic vascular distension on body fluid distribution and renal excretion in man, Pflügers Arch. Klin. Chir. 313:123 (1969).

9.  M. TOOR, M. DULFANO and J. YAHINI in Hahnemann Symposium on Hypertension, Saunders (1957).

10. L. E. EARLEY, and R. M. FRIEDLER, Changes in renal blood flow and possibly the intrarenal distribution of blood during the natriuresis accompanying saline loading in the dog, J. Clin. Invest. 44:929 (1965).

11. L. E. EARLEY, and R. M. FRIEDLER, Studies on the mecanism of natriuresis accompanying increased renal blood flow and the renal response of extracellular volume expansion, J. Clin. Invest. 44:1847 (1965).

12. H. JAHN, F. STEPHAN et J. STAHL, Activité diurétique du sang et des urines de chien oedémateux, C. R. Soc. Biol., 150:1449 (1956).

13. H. JAHN, F. STEPHAN et J. STAHL, Activité antidiurétique et diurétique urinaire après saignée chez le chien normal, Arch. Sci. Physiol. 14:421 (1960).

14. E. SLATOPOLSKY, C. WEERTS, and N. S. BRICKER, Observations on the central system regulating sodium excretion in uremic man, J.Lab. and Clin. Med 68:1017 (1966).

15. H. JAHN, M. JAHN, A. HEUSSNER et J. STAHL, Mise en évidence chez l'homme et chez le chien d'un facteur diurétique et natriurétique dans le sang et les urines après l'expansion du volume extra-cellulaire, C. R. Acad. Sci. 265:1145 (1967).

16. J. E. SEALEY, J. D. KIRSHMAN, and J. H. LARAGH, Natriuretic activity in plasma and urine of salt loaded man and sheep, J. Clin. Invest. 48:2210 (1969).

17. V. M. BUCKALEW Jr, and D. B. NELSON, Natriuretic and sodium transport inhibitory activity in plasma of volume expanded dogs, Kid. Inter. 5:12 (1974).

18. H. G. KRAMER, B. GOSPODINOV, and F. KRUCK, Humorale Hemmung des epitelialen Natrium transports nach akuter Expansion des Extracellular Volumens, Klin. Mochenschr. 52:801 (1974).

19. H. C. GONICK, and L. F. SALDANHA, A natriuretic principle derived from kidney tissue of volume expanded rats, J. Clin. Invest. 56:247 ( 1975).

20. A. H. SAMIY, P. F. HIRSH, and A. G. RAMSAY, Localization of phosphaturic effect of parathyroid hormone in the nephron of the dog, Am. J. Physiol. 208:73 (1965).

21. Z. S. AGUS, L. B. GARDNER, L. H. BECK, and M. GOLDBERG, Effects of parathyroid hormone on renal tubular reabsorption of calcium, sodium and phosphate. Am. J. Physiol. 224:1143 (1973).

22. A. D. KENNY and C. A. HEISKELL, Effect of crude thyrocalcitonin on calcium and phosphorus metabolism in rats, Proc. Soc. Exp. Biol. Méd. 120:269 (1965).

23. R. J. ARDAILLOU, J. P. FILLASTRE, G. MILHAUD, R. ROUSSELET, F. DELAUNAY, and G. RICHET, Renal excretion of phosphate, calcium and sodium during and after a prolonged thy-

rocalcitonin infusion in man, Proc. Soc. Exp. Biol. Med. 131:56 (1969).

24. D. IKKOS, R. LUFT, and C. A. GEINZELL, The effect of human growth hormone in man, J. Clin. Invest. 39:1223 (1960).

25. D. D. THOMPSON, and H. H. HIATT, Effects of phosphate loading and depletion on the renal excretion and reabsorption of inorganic phosphate, J. Clin. Invest. 36:566 (1957).

26. H. H. HIATT, and D. D. THOMPSON, Some effects of intravenously administered calcium on inorganic phosphate metabolism, J. Clin. Invest. 36:573 (1957).

27. H. E. HARRISON, and H. C. HARRISON, The normal excretion of inorganic phosphate in relation to the action of vitamin D and parathyroid hormone, J. Clin. Invest. 20:47 (1941).

28. J. B. PUSCHETT, J. MORANZ, and W. S. KURNICK, Evidence of a direct action of cholecalciferol and 25-Hydroxycholecalciferol on the renal transport of phosphate, sodium and calcium, J. Clin. Invest. 51:373 (1972).

ADAPTATION OF TUBULAR PHOSPHATE TRANSPORT: RELATION
BETWEEN PHOSPHATE REQUIREMENT, AS INFLUENCED BY GROWTH,
AND SUPPLY

J. Caverzasio, J.-P. Bonjour and H. Fleisch

Department of Pathophysiology
University of Berne
Murtenstrasse 35, 3010 Berne, Switzerland

It has become more and more evident over the last few
years that parathyroid hormone (PTH) is not the only
factor controlling the renal handling of inorganic
phosphate (Pi). Indeed the tubular transport of Pi is
also regulated by a PTH-independent mechanism, which
responds to variations in the alimentary supply of Pi
(1,2,3). This specific mechanism appears to control
both the basal tubular Pi transport capacity and the
acute tubular phosphaturic response to PTH without,
however, affecting the action of the peptide hormone
on calcium reabsorption and cyclic-3',5'-AMP excretion
(4,5,6,7). This specific adaptive response to the Pi
supply has been localized by free-flow micropunctures
in intact (8) and more recently also in thyroparathyroidectomized (TPTX) rats (9) in the first portion of the
proximal tubule and probably also along the terminal
nephron. Recent studies indicate furthermore that the
change in the renal Pi transport capacity induced
by varying the intake of Pi of chronically TPTX rats
is associated with a specific alteration in the sodium-
dependent Pi transport system present in the brush
border membranes of cortical tubules (10). In a
former presentation (4) we have suggested that this
adaptive mechanism may also respond to fluctuations in
the Pi demand of the organism. This suggestion was
based on experiments showing that in growing rats a
decrease in net Pi uptake by the skeleton, as induced
by treatment with the diphosphonate EHDP, was associated
with a specific alteration in the tubular Pi transport
capacity (6). This PTH-independent alteration was

similar to that characterizing the tubular response to
an increased Pi supply (4,6,11,12).

In this report we should like to present results which
sustain further the concept that the renal tubule
adapts, in presence as well as in absence of PTH, its
Pi transport capacity to Pi requirement, as influenced
by the growth of the organism.

In a first series of experiments the renal handling of
Pi of young growing rats (2 months old) was compared to
that of adult ones (8 months old).  The tubular Pi
transport capacity was assessed by measuring the net Pi
reabsorption at several plasma Pi concentrations under
acute i.v. Pi infusion, as previously described (1,13).
The results show that the tubular capacity for net Pi
reabsorption decreased when rats become adult.  This
finding is in agreement with observations in man indicating that the tubular reabsorption of Pi is greater
in children than in adult (14).  We have then assessed
the possible role of PTH in this growth-related alteration by comparing the renal handling of Pi in young
and adult rats after thyroparathyroidectomy.  The results show that the removal of thyroparathyroid glands
did not reduce, but rather increased the difference
in the tubular Pi transport capacity observed between
young and adult rats.  The marked change in the renal
handling of Pi which occurs with age was not associated
with any apparent alteration in the glomerular filtration rate monitored per kidney weight, or in the renal
handling of calcium and sodium.  Finally the difference
in the tubular capacity to reabsorb Pi between young
and adult rats was still more pronounced when the Pi
content in the diet was reduced from 0.8 to 0.2 %.
This derives from the fact that the renal response to
Pi restriction was much greater in young growing than
in adult rats.

In a second series of experiments the influence of
hypophysectomy (HPX) and growth hormone on the renal
handling of Pi was studied in two month old rats.
Pituitary glands were removed by the parapharyngeal
approach.  Adequacy of HPX was assessed by the arrest
of growth over a period of two weeks and by direct
examination of the sphenoidal area after the renal
study.  In order to normalize the low glomerular
filtration rate consecutive to the removal of the
pituitary glands, hypophysectomized rats were supplemented with ACTH and thyroxyine.  The study of the relation between plasma concentration and net tubular re-

absorption of Pi indicated that in these conditions the overall reabsorptive capacity was reduced after HPX. Treatment with bovine growth hormone (3 x 0.15 IU/week s.c.) abolished the difference in the renal handling of Pi between hypophysectomized and intact rats. These results are in agreement with previous observations concerning the influence of growth hormone on the tubular transport of Pi (15,16). They are consistent with the concept that the renal tubule adapts its Pi transport capacity to a reduction in the growth rate, and thus to the Pi demand of the organism.

In order to assess whether or not growth hormone would play a critical role in the tubular adaptation to variations in the Pi supply, the renal response to a low P diet was studied in hypophysectomized rats. In these animals a significant augmentation in the tubular capacity to reabsorb Pi was observed during Pi restriction. However, the rise in the tubular reabsorptive capacity determined 3, 6 and 12 days after a reduction of the dietary Pi content from 1.2 to 0.2 % was less pronounced in hypophysectomized than in age-matched and pair-fed intact counteparts. A reduced Pi requirement can be expected to occur in young rats after removal of the pituitary gland (17). This could explain why the adaptive response of the tubular Pi transport system to a Pi restriction is less dramatic in hypophysectomized than in fast growing animals. Finally we have also observed that the tubular Pi adaptation to Pi restriction can take place in hypophysectomized rats after thyroparathyroidectomy.

In conclusion, the results of the present report are consistent with the existence of an adaptation of the renal Pi transport system to growth-related variations in the Pi demand. The effect of growth hormone on the renal handling of Pi could thus be indirectly mediated by the increased Pi requirement that the hormone imposes upon the organism. Finally our experiments indicate that the presence of growth hormone is not required for the occurence of the tubular adaptation to variation in the alimentary supply of inorganic phosphate.

Acknowledgements: We acknowledge the excellent technical help of Mrs. R. Faundez, I. Tschudi, C. Marti, G. Kunz, and Miss I. Ryba. This work was supported by the Swiss National Science Foundation (grant 3.725.76) and by the Ausbildungs- und Förderungsfonds der Arbeitsgemeinschaft für Osteosynthese (AO), Switzerland.

## References

1. U. Tröhler, J.-P. Bonjour, and H. Fleisch, Inorganic phosphate homeostasis. Renal adaptation to the dietary intake in intact and thyroparathyroidectomized rats, J.Clin.Invest. 57: 264 (1976).

2. T.H. Steele and H.F. DeLuca, Influence of dietary phosphorus on renal phosphate reabsorption in the parathyroidectomized rats, J.Clin.Invest. 57: 867 (1976).

3. U. Tröhler, J.-P. Bonjour, and H.- Fleisch, Renal tubular adaptation to dietary phosphorus, Nature 261: 145 (1976).

4. J.-P. Bonjour, U. Tröhler, R. Mühlbauer, C. Preston, and H. Fleisch, Is there a bone-kidney link in the homeostasis of inorganic phosphate (Pi)? in: "Phosphate Metabolism", S.G. Massry and E. Ritz, eds., Plenum, New York (1977).

5. T.H. Steele, J.L. Underwood, B.A. Stromberg, and C.A. Larmore, Renal resistance to parathyroid hormone during phosphorus deprivation. J.Clin. Invest. 58: 1461 (1976).

6. J.-P. Bonjour, U. Tröhler, C. Preston, and H. Fleisch, Parathyroid hormone and renal handling of Pi: Effect of dietary Pi and diphosphonates, Am. J.Physiol. 234: F497 (1978).

7. H.J. Gloor, J.-P. Bonjour, and H. Fleisch, Resistance to the phosphaturic and calcemic actions of parathyroid hormone during phosphate depletion. Prevention by 1,25-dihydroxyvitamin $D_3$, J.Clin. Invest. 63: 371 (1979).

8. R.C. Mühlbauer, J.-P. Bonjour, and H. Fleisch, Tubular localization of the adaptation to dietary phosphate in rats, Am.J.Physiol. 233: F342 (1977).

9. R. Mühlbauer, J.-P. Bonjour, and H. Fleisch, Tubular handling of phosphate in thyroparathyroidectomized rats treated with 1,25-dihydroxyvitamin $D_3$, Kindney Int., abstract, in press.

10. R. Stoll, R. Kinne, H. Murer, H. Fleisch, and J.-P. Bonjour, Phosphate transport by rat renal brush border membrane vesicles: Influence of dietary phosphate, thyroparathyroidectomy, and 1,25-dihydroxyvitamin $D_3$, Pflügers Arch. 380: 47 (1979).

11. J.-P. Bonjour, R. Mühlbauer, H. Fleisch, R. Stoll, H. Murer, and R. Kinne, Renal phosphate transport: Parallel changes in whole kidney, proximal tubule and brush border membrane vesicles, Kidney Int., abstract, in press.

12.  R. Stoll, H. Murer, H. Fleisch, and J.-P. Bonjour,
     Effect of diphosphonate treatment on phosphate
     transport by renal brush border vesicles, submitted.
13.  J.-P. Bonjour, C. Preston, and H. Fleisch, Effect
     of 1,25-dihydroxyvitamin $D_3$ on the renal handling
     of Pi in thyroparathyroidectomized rats, J.Clin.
     Invest. 60: 1419 (1977).
14.  J. Corvilain and M. Abramow, Growth and renal
     control of plasma phosphate, J.Clin.Endocr. 34:
     452 (1972).
15.  J. Corvilain and M. Abramow, Some effects of human
     growth hormone on renal hemodynamics and on
     tubular phosphate transport in man, J.Clin.Invest.
     41: 1230 (1962).
16.  J. Corvilain and M. Abramow, Effect of growth
     hormone on tubular transport of phosphate in normal
     and parathyroidectomized dogs, J.Clin.Invest. 43:
     1608 (1964).
17.  D.B.N. Lee, N. Brautbar, N.W. Walling, H.E.
     Carlson, C. Golvin, J.W. Coburn, and D.R. Kleeman,
     The biochemical indices of experimental phosphorus
     depletion (PD): A re-examination of their physiolo-
     gical implications, in: "Homeostasis of Phosphate
     and Other Minerals", S.G. Massry, E. Ritz and A.
     Rapado, eds., Plenum, New York (1978).

# INDIRECT EFFECT OF HYPERCAPNIA ON THE PHOSPHATURIA OF RESPIRATORY ACIDOSIS

Sung-Feng Wen

Department of Medicine, University of Wisconsin
Center for Health Sciences
Madison, WI 53792

## INTRODUCTION

The mechanism for the phosphaturia of respiratory acidosis is not well understood because there are concomitant alterations in arterial blood $pCO_2$, pH, bicarbonate and phosphate which could all affect urinary phosphate excretion[1-6].  Recently, Webb et al[1] demonstrated in the rat that alterations in the blood levels of phosphate, bicarbonate and parathyroid hormone could not entirely account for the phosphaturia of respiratory acidosis and concluded that it was the result of a direct effect of the elevated blood $pCO_2$ on renal phosphate transport.  Our present clearance and micropuncture experiments were, therefore, designed to reexamine the relationship between blood $pCO_2$ and the phosphaturia of respiratory acidosis.

## METHODS

Clearance and/or micropuncture studies were performed in 13 dogs 2 hours after thyroparathyroidectomy.  In Group I of 6 dogs, the control phase was followed by a second phase of hypercapnia induced by 20% $CO_2$ breathing and 30 - 45 minutes were allowed before the second phase collections began.  The third phase of hypocapnia was induced by hyperventilation immediately following the second phase and 10 - 15 minutes were allowed before the third phase collections were started.  In Group II of 7 dogs, clearance studies were performed with the sequence of respiratory acidosis and alkalosis reversed.

Table 1.  Clearance and Micropuncture Data in Group I

| Exptl Phase | $B_{pCO_2}$ mmHg | $B_{pH}$ | $B_{HCO_3}$ mM | GFR ml/min | $UF_{PO_4}$ mM | $FE_{PO_4}$ % | SNGFR nl/min | $FD_{PO_4}$ % |
|---|---|---|---|---|---|---|---|---|
| C | 40.6 | 7.33 | 21.1 | 32.7 | 1.99 | 6.9 | 56.5 | 45 |
| ↑CO$_2$ | 79.4** | 7.12** | 23.6* | 31.8 | 2.63** | 16.0** | 52.3 | 57** |
| ↓CO$_2$ | 21.9** | 7.53** | 17.8* | 28.0* | 2.00** | 18.3* | 46.3 | 61 |

B, blood; GFR, glomerular filtration rate; UF, plasma ultrafiltrate; FE, fractional excretion; SN, single nephron; FD, fractional
delivery in late proximal tubule; C, control; ↑CO$_2$, hypercapnia;
↓CO$_2$, hypocapnia; *P<0.05; **P<0.01 re preceding phase.

RESULTS

Clearance and proximal tubule micropuncture data in Group I
are summarized in Table 1.  Respiratory acidosis in the second phase
was associated with increases in arterial blood pCO$_2$, bicarbonate
and UF phosphate and a fall in blood pH.  There was a marked phosphaturia which was due to the reduction in fractional reabsorption
of phosphate in the proximal tubule.  When respiratory alkalosis
was induced in the third phase, the changes in blood pCO$_2$, bicarbonate and pH were reversed and UF phosphate returned to the control
level.  Despite the correction of these parameters, high fractional
delivery of phosphate in the proximal tubule and final urine
persisted.

Clearance data in Group II with reversed sequence of respiratory acidosis and alkalosis are shown in Table 2.  Hypocapnia in
the second phase led to reduction in GFR, UF phosphate and absolute
and fractional phosphate excretion.  In the third phase, however,
respiratory acidosis failed to induce significant phosphaturia
despite the reversal of acid-base parameters and restoration of
the filtered load of phosphate.

Table 2.  Clearance Data in Group II.

| Exptl Phase | $B_{pCO_2}$ mmHg | $B_{pH}$ | $B_{HCO_3}$ mM | GFR ml/min | $UF_{PO_4}$ mM | $U_{PO_4}V$ μmol/min | $FE_{PO_4}$ % |
|---|---|---|---|---|---|---|---|
| C | 41.5 | 7.34 | 21.8 | 31.8 | 1.89 | 3.26 | 5.66 |
| ↓CO$_2$ | 20.3** | 7.51** | 15.8** | 27.4* | 1.55** | 1.48* | 2.82* |
| ↑CO$_2$ | 83.2** | 7.15** | 26.8** | 24.2 | 2.25** | 2.47* | 4.44 |

$U_{PO_4}V$, absolute phosphate excretion; other abbreviations as in
Table 1; *P<0.05; **P<0.01 re preceding phase.

DISCUSSION

Our present studies demonstrated that respiratory acidosis leads to phosphaturia by inhibition of fractional phosphate reabsorption in the proximal tubule. The associated changes in arterial blood $pCO_2$, bicarbonate, pH and UF phosphate were not directly related to the phosphaturia since the phosphaturia persisted even when these parameters were corrected or reversed. Their indirect effect was also supported in Group II studies in which phosphaturia was blunted when the respiratory acidosis was preceded by respiratory alkalosis. Our results suggest the possibility that alteration in intracellular phosphate metabolism could be responsible for the phosphaturia of respiratory acidosis.

REFERENCES

1. R. K. Webb, P. B. Woodhall, C. C. Tisher, G. Glaubiger, F. A. Neelon, and R. R. Robinson, Relationship between phosphaturia and acute hypercapnia in the rat, J. Clin. Invest. 60:829 (1977).
2. M. Fulop and P. Brazeau, The phosphaturic effect of sodium bicarbonate and acetazolamide in dogs, J. Clin. Invest. 47:983 (1968).
3. N. Bank, H. S. Aynedjian, and S. W. Weinstein, A microperfusion study of phosphate reabsorption by the rat proximal renal tubule, J. Clin. Invest. 54:1040 (1974).
4. K. Baumann, G. Rumrich, F. Papavassiliou, and S. Klöss, Letters and notes: pH dependence of phosphate reabsorption in the proximal tubule of rat kidney. Pflügers Arch. 360: 183 (1975).
5. J. B. Puschett and M. Goldberg, The relationship between the renal handling of phosphate and bicarbonate in man, J. Lab. Clin. Med. 73:956 (1969).
6. A. Mercado, E. Slatopolsky, and S. Klahr, On the mechanisms responsible for the phosphaturia of bicarbonate administration, J. Clin. Invest. 56:1386 (1975).

# PHOSPHATE HANDLING BY THE REMNANT DOG KIDNEY IN THE PRESENCE AND ABSENCE OF THE CONTRALATERAL NORMAL KIDNEY

N.L.M. Wong, G.A. Quamme, J.H. Dirks, & R.A.L. Sutton

Department of Medicine, University of British Columbia

Vancouver General Hospital, 755 West 12th Avenue, Vancouver, B.C., V5Z 1M9, Canada

The fractional urinary excretion of filtered inorganic phosphate ($P_i$) increases progressively from the normal value of less than 15% up to 80% or more in advanced renal failure. The mechanisms responsible for this adaptation have been examined by several investigators. Slatopolsky et al (1) suggested that a reduction in glomerular filtration led to an increase in plasma $P_i$, which in turn decreased plasma ionised calcium concentration and stimulated increased parathyroid hormone secretion. $P_i$ retention was thus considered to be responsible for secondary hyperparathyrodism, which in turn decreased tubular $P_i$ reabsorption and tended to correct or minimise the rise in the plasma $P_i$ concentration. Recently Bricker et al (2) have suggested that there is an increased responsiveness to the phosphaturic effect of PTH in renal failure, and that this may contribute to phosphate homeostasis in this circumstance. By contrast, Swenson et al (3) reported that PTH was not required for phosphate homeostasis in renal failure in the dog. In a recent micropuncture study in the rat, Bank et al (4) concluded that, in this species in renal failure, the proximal tubule has a greatly enhanced intrinsic capacity for $P_i$ reabsorption which is unmasked by parathyroidectomy, but is normally suppressed by the secondary hyperparathyroidism of renal failure.

The present micropuncture studies in the dog were undertaken to examine further the mechanisms responsible for the high fractional urinary $P_i$ excretion in renal failure. These studies, like those of Swenson et al (3), suggest that PTH may not be resposible for this phenomenon in the dog, but rather that tubular $P_i$ reabsorption may be inhibited as a result of $P_i$ retention or hyperphosphatemia by mechanisms independent of PTH.

METHODS

The experiments were performed in mongrel dogs weighing 8 – 16 Kg. A 'remnant' left kidney was produced at a preliminary operation by ligating about 80% of the main renal artery branches as previously described (5). Two groups of dogs with such a remnant left kidney were then studied in micropuncture experiments. One group of seven dogs was studied 2 weeks after production of the remnant kidney, while the normal kidney was still in situ. These animals (Stage II) were not azotemic. The second group of ten dogs underwent a right nephrectomy after the creation of the left remnant kidney, and were studied by micro-puncture 1 week later, at which time they were azotemic. The dogs were allowed free access to food and water prior to study; no attempt was made to control food intake in either group.

All dogs were thyroparathyroidectomised (TPTX) on the day of the micropuncture study. Anaesthesia was maintained and 2 hours later, standard 3-phase clearance and micropuncture experiments were performed on the left (remnant) kidney. All experiments comprised a first, hydropenic phase (Phase 1), followed by volume expansion with 5% body weight of Ringer's solution containing 3 mEq/l calcium. Urinary losses were replaced with additional Ringer's solution (Phase 2). In the final phase 3, purified bovine PTH (Inolex Pharmaceutical Division, Park Forest South, Illinois, 331 units/mg.) was given i.v. in an initial dose of 60 units, followed by an infusion of 60 units/hour. Urine was collected from both ureters in Stage II. Micropuncture and analytical methods were as previously described from this laboratory (6); tubule fluid samples were collected from late proximal and random distal tubules and were analysed for phosphorus as well as other elements with the electron microprobe.

RESULTS

The Stage III animals were azotemic (mean BUN 62 mg/100 ml, plasma creatinine 4.9mg/100 ml) whereas the Stage II dogs had normal BUN and creatinine levels (13 and 1.2 mg/100 ml respectively). Mean inulin clearance was 9 ml/min in Stage III, while in Stage II the mean for the normal right kidney was 41 ml/min and for the remnant left kidney 7 ml/min. Hematocrit and plasma $UF_{Ca}$ (2.9 mEq/l in Stage III and 3.0 mEq/l in Stage II) were not significantly different in the two groups, whereas plasma $P_i$ concentration was higher in Stage III than in Stage II animals (5.8 $\pm$0.5 mg/100 ml vs 4.4 $\pm$0.4 mg/100 ml, p <0.05).

## TABLE 1

### CLEARANCE DATA

| Phase | Stage II 1 | 2 | 3 | Stage III 1 | 2 | 3 |
|---|---|---|---|---|---|---|
| **RIGHT KIDNEY** | | | | | | |
| GFR  ml/min | 41+5 | 39+6 | 35+3* | | | |
| $FE_{Na}$  % | 3+6 | 6+1* | 7+1 | | | |
| $FE_{Pi}$  % | 10+4 | 16+6 | 56+15* | | | |
| **LEFT KIDNEY** | | | | | | |
| GFR  ml/min | 7+1 | 7+1 | 7+1 | 9+2 | 9+2 | 9+2 |
| $FE_{Na}$  % | 2+0.4 | 9+3* | 8+1 | 7+1 | 15+4* | 10+2 |
| $FE_{Pi}$  % | 6+2 | 16+5* | 45+8* | 48+9 | 51+10 | 68+7* |

FE = fractional urinary excretion of the filtered load of sodium
or phosphate.    *$p < 0.05$ compared with previous phase

Table 1 summarises the Na and $P_i$ clearance data from the
3-phase experiments in both groups of dogs.  In Stage II,
fractional urinary excretions (FE) of sodium and $P_i$ were similar
in the normal and remnant kidneys.  In hydropenia (phase 1)
$FE_{Pi}$ was 6% in the remnant kidney and 10% in the normal
kidney, and this increased to 16% in phase 2 in both kidneys and
to 46 and 56% respectively after PTH (phase 3).  By contrast in
the Stage III kidney, $FE_{Pi}$ was much higher in all phases,
increasing from 48% in hydropenia to 51% after volume expansion
(ns) to 68% after PTH ($p < 0.05$).

## TABLE 2

### MICROPUNCTURE DATA

| | Proximal Tubule $TF/P_{In}$ | $TF/UF_{Pi}$ | Distal Tubule $TF/P_{In}$ | $TF/UF_{Pi}$ |
|---|---|---|---|---|
| Stage II-Phase 1 | 1.57+0.05 | 0.65+0.04 | 5.2+0.5 | 0.45+0.08 |
| -Phase 2 | 1.41+0.06* | 0.75+0.03* | 3.1+0.2* | 0.45+0.05 |
| -Phase 3 | 1.31+0.05* | 0.95+0.03* | 3.0+0.1 | 0.99+0.08* |
| Stage III-Phase 1 | 1.34+0.03† | 1.08+0.05† | 3.7+0.4† | 1.92+0.14† |
| -Phase 2 | 1.21+0.04* | 1.22+0.10* | 2.9+0.2* | 1.55+0.14* |
| -Phase 3 | 1.20+0.04 | 1.23+0.14 | 3.3+0.3* | 2.62+0.33* |

*$p < 0.05$ compared with previous phase
†$p < 0.05$ compared with Stage II

Table 2 summarises the micropuncture data from the remnant kidney in Stage II and Stage III dogs.  Fig. 1, which is derived from the micropuncture data in table 2, shows the fraction of filtered $P_i$ remaining at the various nephron sites in each group.

In Stage II, a significant increase in delivery of $P_i$ to proximal and distal tubule and final urine is observed after volume expansion, and a further increase after PTH.  In Stage III proximal $P_i$ reabsorption is markedly inhibited in phase 1, being only 22% of filtered load.  This is a result both of a decrease in fractional water reabsorption compared with Stage II ($TF/P_{inulin}$ 1.34 compared with 1.57, p <0.05) and of a high $TF/UF_{Pi}$ ratio (1.08 compared with 0.65, p <0.05).

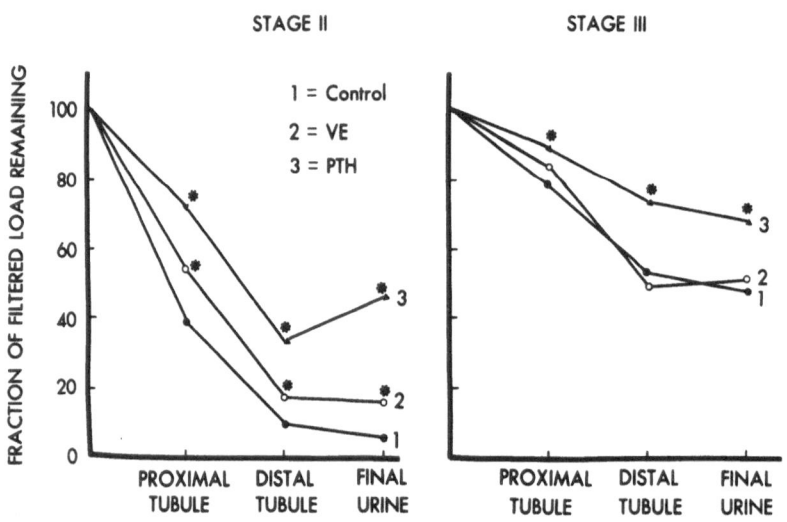

PHOSPHATE HANDLING  BY REMNANT KIDNEY

* significantly different from previous phase  p <0.05

Fig. 1. Fraction of filtered $P_i$ remaining at successive nephron sites  in the 3 phases in the Stage II (left panel) and Stage III (right panel) remnant kidney.  * Indicates a significant difference (p <0.05) from previous phase.

Likewise, $P_i$ reabsorption is inhibited in the 'loop segment' (which includes the pars recta). Despite the greater $P_i$ delivery to this segment, both fractional and absolute $P_i$ reabsorption are much reduced compared with Stage II. Volume expansion in Stage III did not significantly alter fractional phosphate delivery to proximal or distal tubules or to the final urine. PTH, however, significantly increased fractional $P_i$ delivery to each of these sites; Fig. 1 suggests that the effect of PTH to inhibit $P_i$ reabsorption may have been mediated both before and beyond the late superficial proximal micropuncture site.

DISCUSSION

     Clearly there is a major inhibition of tubular $P_i$ reabsorption in Stage III (azotemia) compared with the Stage II dogs. All animals had undergone total thyroparathyroidectomy at least 2 hours prior to the commencement of these clearance and micropuncture studies. It is therefore unlikely that the difference between the two groups is attributable to differences in parathyroid function; the half life of biologically active PTH is such that it would not be expected to be present in signif- icant quantities in these animals. However, PTH levels were not determined during these experiments; furthermore PTH levels were probably higher in Stage III than Stage II prior to TPTX since these animals were azotemic. It is possible, therefore, that a somewhat greater residual PTH effect could have been present in the renal tubules of the Stage III than in those of the Stage II dogs. The demonstration of similar increments in $P_i$ excretion with similar doses of exogenous PTH (phase 3) in Stage II and Stage III dogs, however, further suggests that the differences in baseline $P_i$ reabsorption (phase 1) were not due to a major residual PTH effect in Stage III.

     Volume expansion is a well documented cause of inhibition of tubular $P_i$ reabsorption. It is possible that Stage III dogs were more volume expanded than Stage II dogs in phase 1. However, even after 5% volume expansion (phase 2) in Stage II dogs, which increased $FE_{Na}$ to 9%, $FE_{Pi}$ was only 16% compared with 48% in the non-expanded Stage III animals (phase 1), in which $FE_{Na}$ was 7%. Thus it seems unlikely that volume expansion was responsible for the major inhibition of $P_i$ reabsorption in the azotemic, Stage III dogs.

     Plasma ionised calcium concentration may influence tubular $P_i$ reabsorption. A decrease in calcium concentration may cause a decrease in tubular $P_i$ reabsorption (7, 8). However, the mean plasma ultrafilterable calcium concentration was not significantly different in Stage II and Stage III animals, and it therefore seems unlikely that calcium concentration could be responsible for the major differences observed in tubular $P_i$ reabsorption.

Both dietary $P_i$ (9, 10) and plasma $P_i$ concentration have been shown to have a noteworthy effect on renal $P_i$ handling which is independent of PTH. A high $P_i$ diet causes a reduction in tubular reabsorptive capacity for $P_i$ at any given plasma $P_i$ concentration or filtered $P_i$ load (9). In the present experiments plasma $P_i$ was higher in the Stage III than in the Stage II animals (5.8 vs 4.4 mg/100 ml, p <0.05). It seems likely that the $P_i$ retention may itself have influenced tubular $P_i$ handling, independently of PTH, in the Stage III animals. The mechanism of this effect of dietary $P_i$ upon tubular $P_i$ reabsorption has not been clarified, though Bonjour et al (11) have presented evidence suggesting that $1,25(OH)_2$ vitamin $D_3$ is required for the adaptation to a high $P_i$ diet in the rat. A deficiency of $1,25(OH)_2D_3$, such as would be expected in severe renal failure, might therefore interfere with this adaptation of tubular phosphate handling to phosphate retention.

That the alteration in tubular $P_i$ handling in the Stage III dogs may be the result of a PTH independent effect of $P_i$ retention or hyperphosphatemia is further suggested by the striking similarities between the present micropuncture data from Stage II and Stage III remnant kidneys, and data presented at the previous phosphate workshop (12) at which we showed that $P_i$ infusion in the TPTX dog, causing elevation of plasma $P_i$ from 4.15 mg/100 ml to 6.62 mg/100 ml, resulted in an increase in proximal non-reabsorbed $P_i$ from 44 to 85%, in distal non-reabsorbed $P_i$ from 6 to 54%, and in $FE_{pi}$ from 3 to 62%. The latter changes in tubular $P_i$ handling in response to $P_i$ infusion are strikingly smilar to those in the remnant kidney in response to azotemia.

CONCLUSION

Comparison of segmental $P_i$ handling in the remnant kidney in the presence (Stage II) and in the absence (Stage III) of the contralateral normal kidney reveals a noteworthy inhibition of $P_i$ reabsorption in the proximal tubule and loop segment (including pars recta) in the azotemic (Stage III) dogs. This inhibition appears to be independent of PTH, and is not attributable to differences in volume expansion or in plasma calcium levels. The azotemic dogs were significantly hyperphosphatemic, and it seems likely that this hyper-phosphatemia, or the associated $P_i$ retention of azotemia, may have caused the inhibition of $P_i$ reabsorption by mechanisms independent of PTH.  These may be similar or identical to the as yet undefined PTH-independent mechanisms which mediate changes in tubular $P_i$ reabsorptive capacity in response to antecendent dietary $P_i$ intake.  If, as others have suggested (13), such mechanisms do contribute to altered tubular $P_i$ handling in renal failure, they may be mediated via changes in intracellular $P_i$ or organic phosphate concentrations.  Furthermore, such mechanisms would make experiments employing proportional reduction of dietary $P_i$ intake during the development of renal failure very difficult to interpret, since $P_i$ retention during the evolution of the renal failure, even if modest, might itself alter renal $P_i$ handling independently of PTH, and might also influence the phosphaturic response to PTH.

REFERENCES

1.  E. Slatopolsky, S. Caglar, L. Gradowska, J. Canterbury, E.,
    E. Reiss, & N.S. Bricker, On the pathogenesis of hyper-
    parathyroidism in chronic experimental renal insufficiency
    in the dog.  J. Clin. Invest. 50:492 (1971).
2.  N.S. Bricker, L.G. Fine, M. Kaplan, M. Epstein,
    J.J. Bourgoignie, & A. Light, "Magnification phenomenon"
    in chronic renal disease.  New Eng. J. Med. 299:1287
    (1978).
3.  R.S. Swenson, J.R. Weisinger, J.L. Ruggeri, & G.M. Reaven,
    Evidence that parathyroid hormone is not required for
    phosphate homeostasis in renal failure.  Metabolism
    24:199 (1975).
4.  N. Bank, W-S. Su & H.S. Aynedjian, A micropuncture study of
    renal phosphate transport in rats with chronic renal
    failure and secondary hyperarathyroidism.  J. Clin.
    Invest.61:884, (1978).
5.  S-W. Wen, N.L.M. Wong, R.L. Evanson, E.A. Lockhart, &
    J.H. Dirks, Micropuncture studies of sodium transport in
    the remnant kidney of the dog.  J. Clin. Invest. 52:386
    (1973).
6.  B.R. Edwards, P.G. Baer, R.A.L. Sutton, & J.H. Dirks, Micro-
    puncture study of diuretic effects on sodium and calcium
    reabsorption in the dog nephron.  J. Clin. Invest. 52:2418
    (1973).
7.  C. Amiel, H. Kuntziger, S. Couette, C. Coureau, &
    N. Bergounioux, Evidence for a parathyroid hormone
    independent calcium modulation of phosphate transport
    along the nephron.  J. Clin. Invest. 57:256, 1976.
8.  F. Lang, H. Oberleithner, R. Greger, & P. Deetjen, Factors
    involved in the altered phosphate reabsorption during
    phosphate loading in thyroparathyroidectomized rats.  Adv.
    Exp. Med. & Biol. 103:81 (1978).

9.  U. Tröhler, J-P. Bonjour & H. Fleisch, Inorganic Phosphate
    homeostasis.  Renal adaptation to the dietary intake in
    intact and thyroparathyroidectomized rats.  J.Clin. Invest
    Invest. 157:264, (1976).

10. T.H. Steele & H.F. DeLuca, Influence of dietary phosphorus
    on renal phosphate reabsorption in the parathyroidect-
    omized rat.  J. Clin. Invest. 57:867, (1976)

11. J-P. Bonjour, C. Preston & H. Fleisch, Effect of 1,25-
    dihydroxyvitamin $D_3$ on the renal handling of $P_i$ in
    thyroparathyroidectomized rats.  J. Clin. Invest. 60:1419
    (1977).

12. R.A.L. Sutton, G.A. Quamme, T. O'Callaghan, N.L.M. Wong &
    J.H. Dirks, Renal tubular phosphate reabsorption in the
    phosphate depleted dog.  Adv. Exp. Med. & Biol. 103:405
    (1978).

13. A.M. Parfitt & B. Frame, Phosphate loading and depletion in
    vitamin D treated hypoparathyroidism.  In (eds.)
    L. Avioli, Ph. Bordier, H. Fleisch, S. Massry, &
    E. Slatopolsky. Phosphate Metabolism Kidney and Bone,
    p. 179, 1975. Armour Montagu Cy, Paris.

# PHOSPHATE TRANSPORT IN THE RABBIT CORTICAL

# COLLECTING TUBULE

Zalman S. Agus and G. Reza Shareghi

Renal Section, Dept. of Medicine
University of Pennsylvania School of Medicine
Philadelphia, Pennsylvania U.S.A.

The presence and mode of phosphate transport beyond the late distal convoluted tubule remains controversial. Micropuncture studies in the parathyroidectomized rat have been for the most part suggestive of a difference between phosphate delivery to the late distal tubule in superficial nephrons and that appearing in the final urine (1,2). This difference may be accounted for in one of two ways. First, there may be differences in the phosphate reabsorptive capacity of superficial and deeper nephron populations (3). Thus, increased phosphate reabsorption by more proximal segments of deep nephrons would reduce delivery to the late distal tubule of those nephrons and the mixture of these two populations would result in a urinary value lower than that obtained in the superficial distal tubule. Alternatively, phosphate reabsorption could continue in segments of the nephron beyond the late distal convoluted tubule.

## METHODS

In order to evaluate the role of distal segments directly, we utilized the technique of isolated tubule perfusion. Segments of the light portion of the collecting duct were dissected from the cortex and outer medulla of the rabbit kidney and perfused with artificial solutions in an isotonic bath. Net phosphate transport was measured using electron probe microanalysis and the effects of transepithelial potential difference, phosphate concentration and parathyroid hormone (1 U/ml) were evaluated.

## RESULTS

Perfusion of isolated cortical collecting tubules with isotonic perfusate and bath and an identical phosphate concentration of

125

4 mg/dl in both fluids resulted in net reabsorption of phosphate at a rate of 0.34±0.09 pmol/mm/min with a transepithelial potential difference of -17.8±2.3 millivolts, lumen negative. There was sodium and chloride reabsorption, net potassium secretion and no detectable net transport of either calcium or magnesium.

There was a linear relationship between net transport and PD as follows, $y = 0.20x + 0.01$, $r = 0.87$, $p < .01$.

Similarly, there was a significant linear relationship between net phosphate reabsorption and the concentration gradient for phosphate between lumen and bath (Table 1) such that increasing the difference between lumen and bath phosphate concentration from -8.0 mg/dl to +8.0 mg/dl was associated with a step-wise increase in net phosphate reabsorption.

Table 1.  Effects of Phosphate Concentration Gradient

| Perfusate/Bath PO$_4$ Concentration mg/dl | Net Phosphate Transport pmol/mm/min |
|---|---|
| 8/0 | 0.95 |
| 8/4 | 0.77 |
| 4/8 | 0.14 |
| 0/8 | -0.18 |

Addition of PTH to the bath had no detectable effect upon net phosphate transport.

### DISCUSSION AND CONCLUSIONS

These studies indicate that there is a reabsorptive capacity for phosphate in the cortical collecting tubule of the rabbit. Transport in this segment appears to be determined by passive forces such as concentration gradient and transepithelial potential difference. Phosphate transport is not influenced by large concentrations of PTH compatible with previous studies indicating the absence of detectable PTH sensitive adenylate cyclase activity in this segment (4).

REFERENCES

1.  C. Amiel, H. Kuntziger and G. Richet, Micropuncture study of handling of phosphate by proximal and distal nephron in normal and parathyroidectomized rats. Evidence for distal reabsorption, Pflueg. Arch. 317:93 (1970).

2.  E. Pastoriza-Munoz, R.E. Colindres, W.E. Lassiter and C. Lechene, Effect of parathyroid hormone on phosphate reabsorption in rat distal convlutions. Amer. J. Physiol. 235:F321 (1978).

3.  J.A. Haas, T. Berndt and F.G. Knox, Nephron heterogeneity of
    phosphate reabsorption.  Amer. J. Physiol. 234:F287 (1978).

4.  D. Chabardes, M. Imbert, A. Clique, M. Montegut and F. Morel,
    PTH sensitive adenyl cyclase activity in different segments
    of the rabbit nephron.  Pflueg. Arch. 354:229 (1975).

# ADDITIVITY OF THE PHOSPHATURIC ACTION OF PARATHYRIN AND CALCITONIN IN THE RAT KIDNEY [*]

H.Oberleithner, F.Lang, R.Greger and H.Sporer

Physiologisches Institut, Universität Innsbruck
Fritz-Pregl-Str. 3
A-6020 Innsbruck   Austria

Several investigations performed in man as well as in different animal species have been carried out to define the effects of parathyrin and calcitonin on renal phosphate transport.

In the majority of the studies the hormones were given intravenously leading to systemic effects due to the fact that they act at various sites such as bone, gut and kidney.

For example, when calcitonin is administered to nonparathyroidectomized animals phosphaturia occurs. The observed phosphaturic action, however, may be due to increased secretion of parathyrin in response to calcitonin-induced hypocalcaemia (2,6,9) rather than due to direct renal response to calcitonin.

Even if influences of endogenous hormone secretion are excluded by thyroparathyroidectomy, systemic infusion of the hormones alters plasma concentration of both calcium and phosphate, which in turn could influence renal transport of phosphate (1,4,5,7,11).

The present study was designed to evaluate renal effects of calcitonin and parathyrin. In order to avoid systemic effects of the hormones microinfusions of single nephrons were performed and the hormones were applied directly (superfused) to the microinfused nephron surface. The hormonal amounts, used for superfusion are too minute to exert any systemic effects.

---

[*]This study has been supported by the Legerlotz-Stiftung

Studies were carried out in 35 male Munich Wistar rats (Ivanovas,
Kisslegg, GFR) weighing 250 g. The animals were fed a standard
altromin chow and had free access to tap water. The animals were
anaesthetized with Inactin (120 mg/kg B.W., i.p., Byk Gulden,
Konstanz, GFR) and placed on an electrically heated table to maintain body temperature at 37°C. Following tracheostomy, thyroparathyroidectomy was performed (8) and the right femoral artery can-
nulated. A bladder catheter served for sampling urine of the contralateral kidney, whereas the ipsilateral urine was collected by
an uretheral catheter.

All animals were infused with a Ringer solution at a rate of 0.2
ml/min·kg B.W. Systemic infusion started 120 min before the first
tubule was microinfused and was continued throughout the whole
experiment.

Microinfusion and simultaneous superfusion were performed as
follows (Fig. 1):

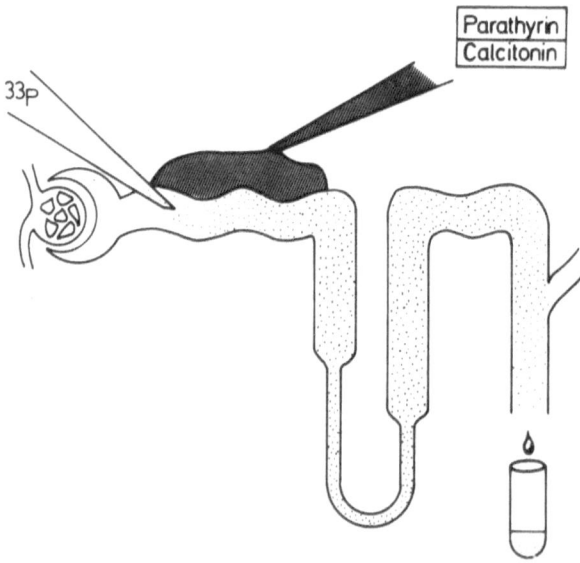

Fig. 1. Microinfusion and simultaneous superfusion in proximal
        tubules of thyroparathyroidectomized rats.

A sharpened glass pipette (tip diameter 12 μm), mounted on a microinfusion pump (10) was inserted in an early loop of a proximal
tubular segment. Isotonic saline containing $^{33}$P phosphate (4
mmol/l, specific activity 100 mCi/mol, New England Nuclear, Boston, Mass.) and $^{3}$H inulin (120 mg/l, specific activity 400 mCi/g,
Amersham, Radiochemical centre, Buckinghamshire, GB) was microinfused continuously for 42 min at a rate of 5 nl/min. This low
flow rate ensures a minimum interference with normal intratubular
hydrodynamics of the unblockes proximal tubules (3).

The $^{3}$H and $^{33}$P activities in the urine were measured by liquid
scintillation counting. Fractional reabsorption of $^{33}$P phosphate
was calculated from $^{33}$P recovery as described elsewhere (8).

The superfused solutions were delivered from another glass pipette to the area of the microinfused tubule after a control period
of 18 min. The superfusate (NaCl 150 mmol/l, 5 μl) contained
either parathyrin (0.1 IU synthetic bovine parathyrin, Beckman
Instruments, Wien) or calcitonin (5 ng, salmon calcitonin, Sandoz
AG, Basel, CH) and covered the area of the microinfused tubule
for 24 min.

Data are expressed as mean values ± standard error of the mean
(SEM). Statistical significance of difference was evaluated by
paired students' t-test. $p < 0.05$ indicates "significantly different".

Superfusion of either hormone, calcitonin and parathyrin leads to
a decrease of phosphate reabsorption within minutes (Fig. 2).

After a 24 min superfusion period fractional phosphate reabsorption is decreased for about 15% related to the 6 min value at the
beginning of microinfusion. Since in time controls no change of
phosphate reabsorption is apparent (Fig. 2, dotted line), altered
phosphate reabsorption during hormonal superfusion has to be due
to action of parathyrin and calcitonin.

In further experiments supramaximal doses of parathyrin (15 IU/h)
were infused systemically and simultaneously calcitonin was
superfused on the microinfused tubule. The results are shown in
Fig. 3.

Again, within minutes phosphate reabsorption decreases. Is parathyrin superfused, no change of phosphate reabsorption occurs indicating that the parathyrin-sensitive system is activated maxi-
mally in these animals. On the other hand, when parathyrin is su-

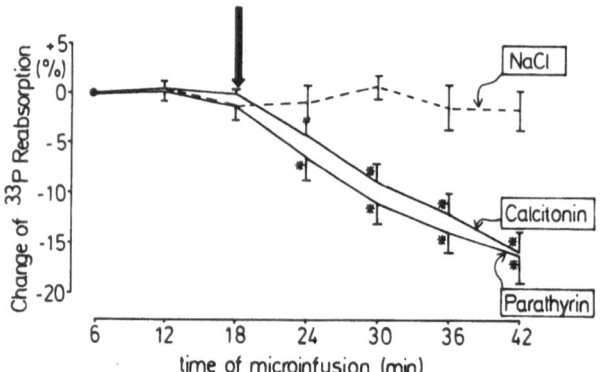

Fig 2.  Superfusion of the solvent (NaCl), parathyrin and calci-
        tonin.  Change of fractional 33p-phosphate reabsorption in
        percent - related to the 6 min value - is plotted versus
        time of continuous microinfusion.  Superfusions were
        started 18 min after commencement of microinfusion.

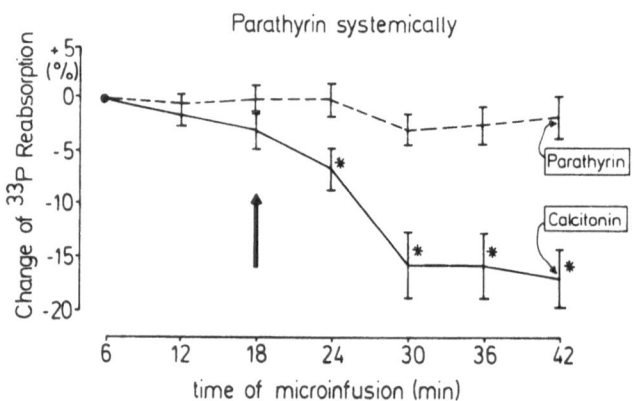

Fig 3.  Effect of local parathyrin and calcitonin in thyropara-
        thyroidectomized rats receiving systemic infusion of
        parathyrin.

perfused in calcitonin loaded animals (3 µg/h) a similar decline
of phosphate reabsorption can be demonstrated whereas superfusion
of calcitonin has no additional effect (Fig. 4):

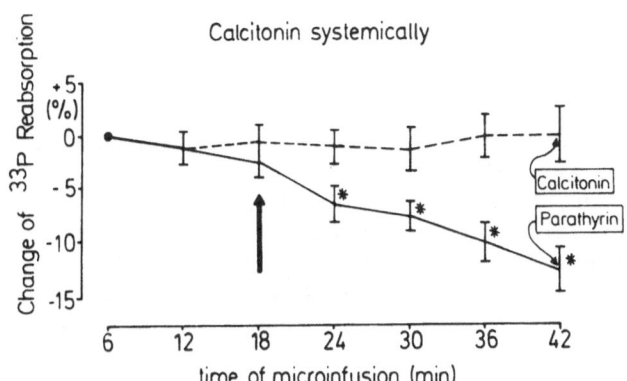

Fig. 4. Effect of local parathyrin and calcitonin in thyroparathyroidectomized rats receiving systemic infusion of
calcitonin.

From these results we conclude that
1. Both parathyrin as well as calcitonin exert a direct phosphaturic effect in the rat kidney and
2. the actions of the two hormones are additive.

References
1.  Amiel, C., Kuntzinger, H., Couette, S., Coureau, C., Bergounioux, N.: Evidence for a parathyroid hormone-independent
calcium modulation of phosphate transport along the nephron.
J. Clin. Invest. 57, 256-263 (1976)
2.  Grubb, S.A., Markham, T.C., Talmage, R.V.: Effect of Salmon
Calcitonin Infusion on Plasma Concentrations of Recently Administered 45Ca. Calcif. Tiss. Res. 24, 201-208 (1977)
3.  Lang, F., Greger, R., Lechene, C., Knox, F.G.: Micropuncture
Techniques. In: Methods in Pharmac., Vol. 4B. Ed.: Manuel
Martinez-Maldonado, Plen. Publ. Corp., New York (1978)

4.  Le Grimellec, C., Roinel, N., Morel, F.: Simultaneous Mg, Ca,
    P, K, and Cl analysis in rat tubular fluid. III. During acute
    Ca plasma loading. Pflügers Arch. 346, 171–188 (1974)
5.  Le Grimellec, C., Roinel, N., Morel, F.: Simultaneous Mg, Ca,
    P, K, and Cl analysis in rat tubular fluid. IV. During acute
    phosphate plasma loading. Pflügers Arch. 346, 186–204 (1974)
6.  Nielsen, S.P., Buchanan-Lee, B., Matthews, E.W., Moseley, J.
    M. and Williams, C.C.: Acute effects of synthetic procine cal-
    citonin on the renal excretion of magnesium, inorganic phos-
    phate, sodium and potassium. In: J. Endocrinol., 51, 455
    (1971)
7.  Oberleithner, H., Greger, R., and Lang, F.: Role of calcium
    in the decline of phosphate reabsorption during phosphate
    loading in acutely thyroparathyroidectomized rats: Pflügers
    Arch. 374, 249–254 (1978)
8.  Oberleithner, H., Lang, F., Greger, R., and Sporer, H.: In-
    fluence of calcium and ionophore 23187 on tubular phosphate
    reabsorption. Pflügers Arch. 379, 37–41 (1979)
9.  Pak, C.Y.C., Ruskin, B., and Caspen, A.: Renal effects of
    porcine thyrocalcitonin in the dog. In: Endocrinol. 87, 262
    (1970)
10. Sonnenberg, H., Deetjen, P.: Methode zur Durchströmung ein-
    zelner Nephronabschnitte. Pflügers Arch. Ges. Physiol. 278,
    669–674 (1964)
11. Ullrich, K.J., Rumrich, G., Klöss, S.: Phosphate transport
    in the proximal convolution of the rat kidney. Pflügers Arch.
    375, 97–103 (1978)

THE EFFECT OF BICARBONATE ON ANION REABSORPTION ALONG THE DOG

NEPHRON.

Norman L. M. Wong
Gary A. Quamme
John H. Dirks

Department of Medicine and
G. F. Strong Laboratory for Medical Research
University of British Columbia
Vancouver, Canada

Alkalosis, either of metabolic or respiratory origin, alters urinary phosphate excretion in man (1,2), dogs (3-5) and rats (6-10). Thus alkalinization of the urine with infusions of sodium bicarbonate decreases renal tubular phosphate reabsorption. A number of indirect factors have been used to explain the resultant phosphaturia following bicarbonate infusion, including volume expansion, enhanced filtered load, hypocalcemia, and endogenous release of parathyroid hormone (PTH). Alternatively, a direct action of $HCO_3^-$ on tubular phosphate could explain the resultant phosphaturia. This could arise from intraluminal alkalinization with an increase in the $HPO_4^=/H_2PO_4^-$ ratio. Bank et al (6) have shown by in vivo microperfusion studies that $H_2PO_4^-$ is transported more readily by the rat proximal tubule than $HPO_4^=$. These findings however are at variance with findings of Ullrich and colleagues (7,10) suggesting that it is the divalent form which is preferentially reabsorbed. Furthermore, Ullrich et al (10) have demonstrated that intracellular alkalosis in addition to luminal acidosis inhibits transtubular phosphate transport. The interaction of $HCO_3^-$ with phosphate has been most extensively examined in the rat (6-10). In this species, $HCO_3^-$ is preferentially reabsorbed relative to other anions in the early proximal tubule, resulting in large transtubular $HCO_3^-$, chloride and phosphate gradients in the later segments. Phosphate reabsorption, although avid in the early proximal convoluted tubule, is markedly slower (average half-times for acidification were some five times faster compared to phosphate reabsorption (8)) than changes in tubular pH and so its effect on proximal tubular acidification is of minor importance (8). However, changes in $HCO_3^-$ reabsorption, i.e. $H^+$ secretion may significantly affect phosphate reabsorption. Thus evidence from the rat suggests $HCO_3^-$ infusions directly affect phosphate reabsorption (9) through changes in intraluminal or intracellular pH (10,11). These conclusions, however, have been disputed in the dog (5) in which PTH has been postulated to form the major link between phosphate and $HCO_3^-$ reabsorption. Sodium bicarbonate infusion would decrease ionized calcium resulting in PTH release and the observed phosphaturia. Micropuncture studies to date suggest a different mechanism of $HCO_3^-$ reabsorption in the dog. The proximal $HCO_3^-$ concentration in the dog has been reported to fall only slightly (12,13) or not at all (14,15) in contrast to the rat. These species differences may account for the discrepancies reported in the literature and reflect different mechanisms of bicarbonate-phosphate interaction in the proximal convoluted tubule of the dog.

The present experiments were designed to investigate the effect of graded bicarbonate infusions on proximal phosphate reabsorption in the dog. Care was taken to minimize the effects of volume expansion, plasma calcium, circulating parathyroid hormone and filtered phosphate load. The results indicate that bicarbonate directly inhibits phosphate reabsorption in the proximal tubule of the dog similar to reports with the rat (9,10) and indicates the importance of intraluminal and intracellular pH on phosphate reabsorption.

METHODS

Three phase clearance and recollection micropuncture experiments were carried out in eight mongrel dogs. Thyroparathyroidectomy (TPTX) was performed on the morning of the study and two hours were allowed to elapse after TPTX before starting the experiments. An initial phase of volume expansion (3% body weight) with modified Ringer's solution containing 25 meq/l $NaHCO_3$ was administered during which several late proximal and distal tubules were identified and sampled. This was then followed by an intravenous infusion of modified Ringer's containing 90 meq/l $NaHCO_3$ until 3% of the body weight had been given. Tubular fluid was then sampled from previously punctured sites. In the final phase the animals received 3% body weight of 150 meq/l of $NaHCO_3$ Ringer's. $CaCl_2$ was infused throughout the three phases to maintain plasma calcium at control levels.

The micropuncture and analytical methods were as previously described from this laboratory; tubule fluid was analysed for phosphorus, sodium, and chloride with an electron microprobe by a

technique described by Morel and colleagues (16,17). Tubule
fluid bicarbonate was measured using the picapnotherm method of
Vurek (18).

RESULTS

The plasma and clearance data are presented in Table 1.
Since the clearance data from both the left and right kidney were
the same, only those from the left are reported. Plasma
$HCO_3^-$ concentration rose stepwise with graded sodium
bicarbonate infusion. This was accompanied by significant
increases in $PCO_2$ and plasma phosphate concentration with a
significant decrease in plasma chloride. Figure 1 illustrates
the changes in fractional phosphate and $HCO_3^-$ excretion.
Fractional $HCO_3^-$ excretion rose proportional to enhanced
$HCO_3^-$ load whereas fractional phosphate rose markedly despite
no change in filtered phosphate. The increase in anion excretion
was accompanied by an increase in urinary sodium and a fall in
chloride excretion. The mean proximal and distal micropuncture
data are shown in Tables 2 and 3. Following bicarbonate infusion
there was a progressive rise in mean proximal TF/P $HCO_3$ and
TF/P Pi ratios while the mean TF/P inulin ratio was unaltered in
all three phases. Figure 2 demonstrates the fraction of
delivered $HCO_3^-$ and phosphate remaining at the late proximal
sampling site at the three plasma $HCO_3^-$ concentration levels.

Table 1.  Graded Bicarbonate – Clearance Data.

|  | ECVE | Modest $HCO_3$ | High $HCO_3$ |
|---|---|---|---|
| P $HCO_3$, mEq/l | 22+1 | 33+1* | 48+1* |
| P $CO_2$, mmHg | 37+8 | 41+4* | 47+6* |
| C In, ml/min | 23+2 | 20+2* | 15+2* |
| P Na, mEq/l | 149+1 | 151+2 | 150+2 |
| P Pi, mg % | 5.3+0.5 | 5.7+0.5* | 5.6+0.3 |
| P Cl, mEq/l | 113+1 | 107+2* | 91+2* |
| FE $H_2O$, % | 13+2 | 21+2* | 29+2* |
| FE Na, % | 7+1 | 12+1* | 19+2* |
| FE $HCO_3$, % | 9+2 | 29+4* | 52+4* |
| FE Pi, % | 2+1 | 9+3* | 16+4* |
| FE Cl, % | 8+1 | 11+2* | 11+2 |

ECVE represents 3% extracellular volume expansion with
modified Ringer's.
*$p < 0.01$ compared with previous phase.

Table 2.   Graded Bicarbonate − Mean Proximal Micropuncture Data.

|            | ECVE | Modest HCO$_3$ | High HCO$_3$ |
|------------|------|----------------|--------------|
| TF/P In    | 1.45+0.01 | 1.48+0.10 | 1.50+0.10 |
| TF/P CO$_2$ | 0.81+0.02 | 0.84+0.02 | 0.93+0.03* |
| TF/P Cl    | 1.05+0.01 | 1.01+0.03* | 0.99+0.02* |
| TF/P Pi    | 0.67+0.02 | 0.80+0.10* | 0.93+0.10* |
| TF/P Na    | 0.97+0.03 | 0.97+0.02 | 0.97+0.03 |

ECVE represents 3% extracellular volume expansion with modified Ringer's.
*p<0.01 compared with previous phase

Table 3.   Graded Bicarbonate − Mean Distal Micropuncture Data.

|            | ECVE | Modest HCO$_3$ | High HCO$_3$ |
|------------|------|----------------|--------------|
| TF/P In    | 3.61+0.19 | 2.89+0.18* | 2.28+0.13* |
| TF/P CO$_2$ | 0.39+0.04 | 0.73+0.05* | 1.01+0.06* |
| TF/P Cl    | 0.46+0.07 | 0.57+0.06* | 0.42+0.05* |
| TF/P Pi    | 0.17+0.04 | 0.46+0.07* | 0.62+0.07* |
| TF/P Na    | 0.33+0.03 | 0.53+0.05* | 0.61+0.03* |

ECVE represents 3% extracellular volume expansion with modified Ringer's.
*p<0.01 compared with previous phase

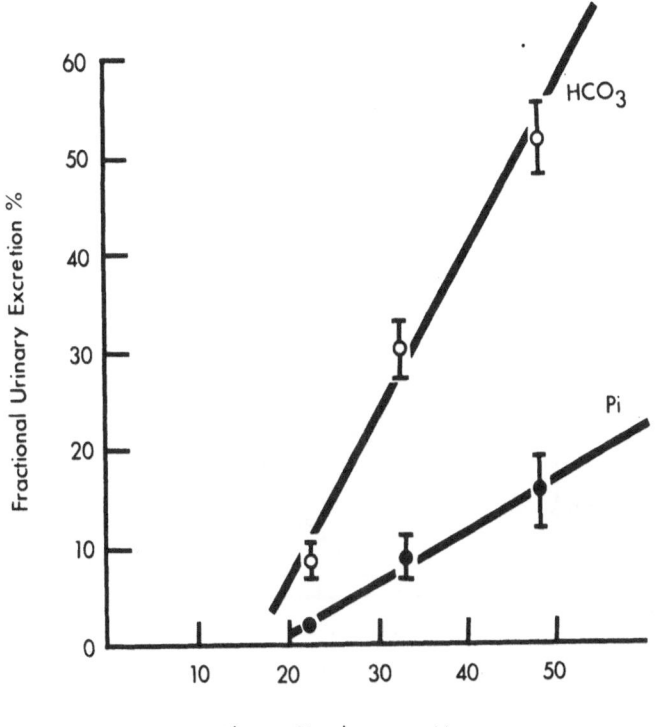

Figure 1. Effect of bicarbonate infusion on urinary bicarbonate and phosphate excretion.

Fractional phosphate reabsorption was inhibited to a greater extent than $HCO_3^-$ for each plasma concentration. Absolute tubular fluid chloride concentration fell as a function of intraluminal $HCO_3^-$ concentration. This was in part due to a fall in plasma chloride concentration and in part due to inhibition of fractional $HCO_3^-$ reabsorption (Fig. 2). Absolute $HCO_3^-$ reabsorption increased as a function of load, however fractional reabsorption fell, resulting in the observed fall in proximal chloride concentration. Distal tubule TF/P inulin fell and TF/P $HCO_3$ rose progressively whereas TF/P chloride remained constant in the second phase and fell with high luminal $HCO_3^-$. TF/UF Pi rose from 0.17 progressively to 0.62 in the final phase. This was accompanied by a significant increase in TF/P Na. The fraction of the delivered phosphate load remaining increased from 0.05 to 0.27 in the final $HCO_3^-$

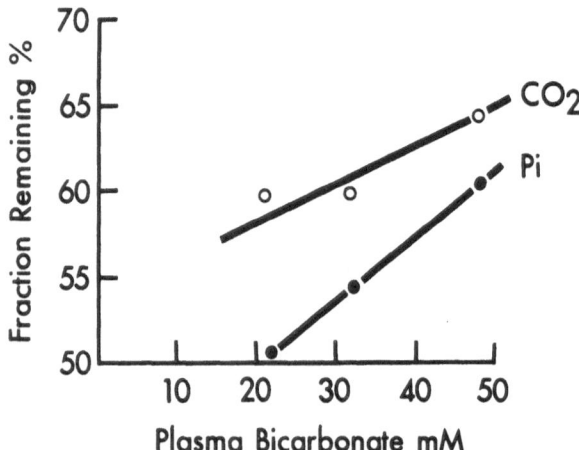

Figure 2. Effect of bicarbonate infusion on the fraction of filtered bicarbonate and phosphate remaining at the late proximal tubule.

loading phase. Fractional $HCO_3^-$ remaining increased by a greater extent from 0.11 to 0.44, suggesting a relatively greater distal effect of alkalosis on $HCO_3^-$ compared to phosphate reabsorption.

DISCUSSION

The object of the present studies was to investigate the interrelationship of renal bicarbonate and phosphate reabsorption in the dog. It has been assumed that since the TF/P bicarbonate ratio in the dog does not fall significantly, the reabsorptive activity for bicarbonate is less compared with the rat (19,20). This may reflect different acidification mechanisms and a different interaction with phosphate.

The data from the present studies indicate the dog proximal tubule handles $HCO_3^-$ in a manner similar to rats (21-23). This is at distinct variance with all previously reported micropuncture studies in the dog (12-15). Thus a TF/P $HCO_3^-$ ratio of 0.81 was observed at TF/P inulin ratio of 1.45 in volume-expanded dogs. This was supported by a TF/P Cl ratio of 1.05 for these tubular fluid samples, demonstrating a preferential reabsorption of $HCO_3^-$ similar to that observed in rats. Moreover, graded bicarbonate infusion resulted in a modest elevation of intraluminal $HCO_3^-$ with parallel but reciprocal changes in chloride concentration. More importantly, $HCO_3^-$ infusion resulted in stepwise increases in luminal phosphate concentration independent of proximal sodium reabsorption. This produced proportional stepwise changes in urinary phosphate excretion as distal sodium and phosphate reabsorption increased only modestly with the increased deliveries. Variables which could indirectly influence phosphate were carefully controlled. The experiments were done on TPTX dogs to avoid alterations in circulating PTH and calcitonin which may lead to a phosphaturia. The dogs were initially volume expanded with Ringer's comparable to that observed during bicarbonate infusion to minimize volume expansion effects. In addition, serum calcium was maintained within control levels by addition of $CaCl_2$ to the Ringer's maintenance infusion. Finally, an attempt was made to control plasma P $CO_2$ to avoid influences on phosphate reabsorption (11). However, it is possible that this mechanism played some role at the tubular level (9) and more importantly at the intracellular level (10) as the plasma $PCO_2$ increased modestly albeit significantly in the present experiments.

Our data are consistent with the view that $HCO_3^-$ has a direct effect on phosphate reabsorption in the dog. Furthermore, these studies demonstrate the proximal tubule is the major site of inhibition of phosphate reabsorption during sodium bicarbonate infusion in TPTX dogs. The direct mechanisms are not evident from the present experiments but as in the rat intracellular and intraluminal pH must be considered (10), for indirect mechanisms including volume expansion, calcium and PTH are not adequate to explain the inhibition of phosphate reabsorption by bicarbonate infusions.

ACKNOWLEDGEMENTS

The authors gratefully acknowledge the expert technical assistance of Mr. Edward Mak, Mr. Ray Dierolf, Mr. David Ridout, Mrs. Sylvia Deare, and Mrs. Monique Julita, and the superb typing expertise of Mrs. Pat Pinder.

This study was supported by grants from the Medical Research Council of Canada to Dr. J. H. Dirks (MT-1915, MA-5431) and the

British Columbia Health Care Research Foundation to Drs. G. A. Quamme and N. L. M. Wong.

REFERENCES

1.  Mostellar, M. E., and Tuttle, E. P., Jr., 1964, Effects of alkalosis on plasma concentration and urinary excretion of inorganic phosphate in man, J. Clin. Invest., 43:138-149.
2.  Puschett, J. B., and Goldberg, M., 1969, The relationship between the renal handling of phosphate and bicarbonate in man, J. Lab. Clin. Med., 73:956-969.
3.  Malvin, R. L., and Lotspeich, W. D., 1956, Relation between tubular transport of inorganic phosphate and bicarbonate in the dog, Am. J. Physiol., 187:51-56.
4.  Fulop, M., and Brazeau, P., 1968, The phosphaturic effect of sodium bicarbonate and acetazolamide in dogs, J. Clin. Invest., 47:983-991.
5.  Mercado, A., Slatopolsky, E., and Klahr, S., 1975, On the mechanisms responsible for the phosphaturia of bicarbonate administration, J. Clin. Invest., 56:1386-1395.
6.  Bank, N., Aynedjian, H. S., and Weinstein, S. W., 1974, A microperfusion study of phosphate reabsorption by the rat proximal tubule. Effect of parathyroid hormone, J. Clin. Invest., 54:1040-1048.
7.  Baumann, K., Rumrich, G., Papvassiliou, F., and Kloss, S., 1975, pH-dependence of phosphate reabsorption in the proximal tubule of rat kidney, Pfluegers Arch., 360:183-187.
8.  Cassola, A. C., and Malnic, G., 1977, Phosphate transfer and tubular pH during renal stopped flow microperfusion experiments in the rat, Pfluegers Arch., 367:249-255.
9.  Zilenovski, A. M., Kuroda, S., Bhat, S., Bank, D. E., and Bank, N., 1979, Effect of sodium bicarbonate on phosphate excretion in acute and chronic PTX rats, Am. J. Physiol., 236:184-191.
10. Ullrich, K. J., Rumrich, G., and Kloss, S., 1978, Phosphate transport in the proximal convolution of the rat kidney. III. Effect of extracellular and intracellular pH, Pfluegers Arch., 377:33-42.
11. Webb, R. K., Woodhall, P. B., Tisher, C.C., Glaubiger, G., Neelon, F. A., and Robinson, R.R., 1977, Relationship between phosphaturia and acute hypercapnia in the rat, J. Clin. Invest., 60:829-837.
12. Clapp, J. R., Watson, J. R., and Berliner, R. W., 1963, Osmolality, bicarbonate concentration and water reabsorption in proximal tubule of the dog nephron, Am. J. Physiol., 205:273-280.
13. Bernstein, B. A., and Clapp, J. R., 1968, Micropuncture study of bicarbonate reabsorption by the dog nephron, Am. J. Physiol., 214:251-257.

14.  Puschett, J. B., and Zurbach, P., 1976, Acute effects of parathyroid hormone on proximal bicarbonate transport in the dog, Kidney Inter., 9:501–510.

15.  Puschett, J. B., Sylk, D., and Teredesai, P. R., 1978, Uncoupling of proximal sodium bicarbonate from sodium phosphate transport by bumetanide, Am. J. Physiol., 235:403–408.

16.  Morel, F., and Roinel, N., 1969, Application de la microsonde electronique a l'analyse elementaire quantitative d'echantillons liquides d'un volume inferieur a $10^{-9}$l, J. Chim. Phys., 66:1084–1091.

17.  Morel, F., Roinel, N., and LeGrimellec, C., 1969, Electron probe analysis of tubular fluid composition, Nephron, 6:350–364.

18.  Vurek, G. G., Warnock, D. G., and Coisey, R., 1975, Measurement of picomole units of carbon dioxide by calorimetry, Anal. Chem., 47:765–769.

19.  Rector, F. C., Jr., 1976, Renal acidification and ammonia production in: "The Kidney", Vol. I, Chap. 9, W. B. Saunders Co.

20.  Seldin, D. W., 1976, Metabolic alkalosis in: "The Kidney", Vol. I, Chap. 17, W. B. Saunders Co.

21.  Rector, F. C., Jr., Carter, N. W., and Seldin, D. W., 1965, The mechanism of bicarbonate reabsorption in the proximal and distal tubules of the kidney, J. Clin. Invest., 44:278–290.

22.  Vieira, F. L., and Malnic, G, 1968, Hydrogen ion secretion by rat renal cortical tubules as studied by an antimony microelectrode, Am. J. Physiol., 214:710–718.

23.  Levine, D. Z., Nash, L. A., Chan, T., and Dubrovskis, A. H. E., 1976, Proximal bicarbonate reabsorption during Ringer and albumin infusions in the rat, J. Clin. Invest., 57:1490–1497.

THE PHOSPHATURIC ACTION OF PTH IN THE STEADY STATE IN PATIENTS

WITH NORMAL AND IMPAIRED RENAL FUNCTION

M. Kleerekoper,[1] C. Cruz,[2] R.S. Bernstein,[1] N.W. Levin,[2]
C.C. Foreback,[3] and A.M. Parfitt[1]

Bone and Mineral Research Laboratory,[1] Division of
Nephrology,[2] Department of Clinical Chemistry[3]
Henry Ford Hospital, Detroit, Michigan  48202

INTRODUCTION

The phosphaturic action of parathyroid hormone (PTH) is mediated via stimulation of adenylate cyclase at the basal pole of the
cells of the proximal convoluted tubules, with a resultant increased
synthesis of 3', 5' adenosine monophosphate (c'AMP).[1] Some of the
newly formed c'AMP enters the circulation but most passes into the
cell.  Together with increased entry of calcium, this decreases entry
of phosphate into the luminal pole of the cell.[2] We have examined
the steady-state relationship between serum immunoreactive PTH (iPTH)
and renal production of c'AMP (nephrogenous c'AMP or Nc'AMP) in subjects with varying levels of parathyroid function and normal renal
function and in patients with chronic renal failure.  We have also
examined the steady-state relationship between these two independent
indices of PTH secretion and the tubular maximum reabsorption of
phosphate/unit of GF (TMP/GFR) as an index of phosphaturic action
of PTH.

MATERIALS AND METHODS

i)    Experimental Subjects

Normal controls.  Thirty-eight subjects had normal serum calcium, serum inorganic phosphate (Pi) and endogenous creatinine
clearance (Ccr), of whom 22 were normal volunteers on no medication
at the time of the study and 16 were patients with a variety of disorders, in whom no abnormality in calcium homeostasis could be demonstrated clinically, biochemically, or radiographically.

Post-surgical hypoparathyroidism (PTX). Thirteen patients had a history of thyroid or parathyroid surgery followed by hypocalcemia for a period of at least 4 weeks and had normal renal function without other demonstrable cause of hypocalcemia. All were untreated (and hypocalcemic) at the time of the study.

Primary hyperparathyroidism (PHPT). Of 88 patients with normal renal function 50 had surgical confirmation and 38 had persistent hypercalcemia (>2 determinations) without other cause of hypercalcemia after adequate clinical, biochemical and radiographic evaluation.

Chronic renal failure (CRF). Forty-seven patients had stable chronic renal failure (Ccr <70 ml/min/1.73m$^2$) and had not been treated with peritoneal or hemodialysis. They were not grouped according to etiology, but in none was this attributed to acute or chronic hypercalcemia. They were on a variety of medications at the time of study, but none had been taking either phosphate binding agents, calcium supplements or any form of vitamin D.

## ii)  Study Protocol

All subjects underwent an identical study protocol. Beginning at 2100 the previous night the subjects fasted but were encouraged to drink water ad lib. At 0730 an oral water load of 8 fl.oz. every 30 minutes was begun and continued throughout the study. The subjects voided at 0755 and again at 0800 and the urine was discarded. All urine passed between 0800 and 1000 was collected and stored at 4°C. At 0900 a venous blood sample was obtained; a portion was collected into chilled tubes containing 10.5mg EDTA, centrifuged at 4°C, and the serum stored at -20°C until used.

## iii)  Analytical Methods

a)  Pi and creatinine in serum and urine were analyzed on the day of collection by standard autoanalyzer techniques.

b)  Serum iPTH. The immunoassay used was essentially as previously described,[3] using a guinea pig anti-bovine PTH antiserum (GP 14) (a gift from Dr. John Haddad) which recognizes predominantly the carboxyl-terminal portion of the PTH molecule.

c)  Cyclic AMP in plasma and urine was assayed within 7 days of specimen collection by competitive protein binding using the method of Tovey et al,[4] without prior extraction.

## iv)  Calculation of Results and Statistical Analyses

a) <u>Nephrogenous cyclic AMP (Nc'AMP)</u>. Nc'AMP production expressed as nmol/dl glomerular filtrate, was calculated as the difference between the total urine c'AMP in the 2-hour collection period
and the filtered load of c'AMP where the filtered load was in turn
calculated as the product of the plasma c'AMP and the endogenous
creatinine clearance.  The calculated value is equivalent to
tubular secreted c'AMP/unit of GF, and is given by:

$$P_{c'AMP} - U_{c'AMP}/Ccr$$

b) <u>Tubular maximum reabsorption of phosphate (TmP)</u>.  TmP
expressed as mg/dl glomerular filtrate was calculated as described
by Bijvoet et al.[5]


RESULTS

a)   <u>Patients with Normal Renal Function</u>

There was a direct linear relationship between serum iPTH and
Nc'AMP (Figure 1).  The relationships between iPTH and TmP/GFR
(Figure 2) and Nc'AMP and TmP/GFR (Figure 3) were non-linear; they
could be described by an exponential equation (Figure 2) or a hyper-
bolic equation (Figure 3) with equal statistical validity.  In
patients with PHPT considered separately the relationships between
iPTH and TmP/GFR and between Nc'AMP and TmP/GFR were linear but
the correlation was not as good.

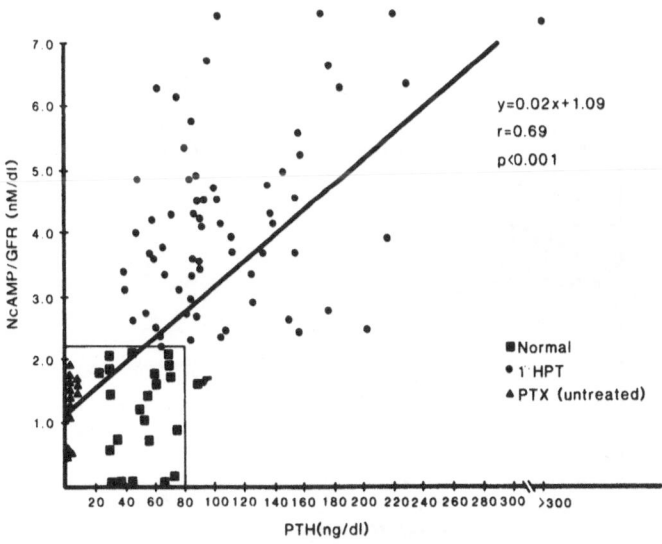

Fig. 1.   Relationship between iPTH and Nc'AMP in normal subjects
(■), and patients with surgical hypoparathyroidism (▲)
and primary hyperparathyroidism (●).

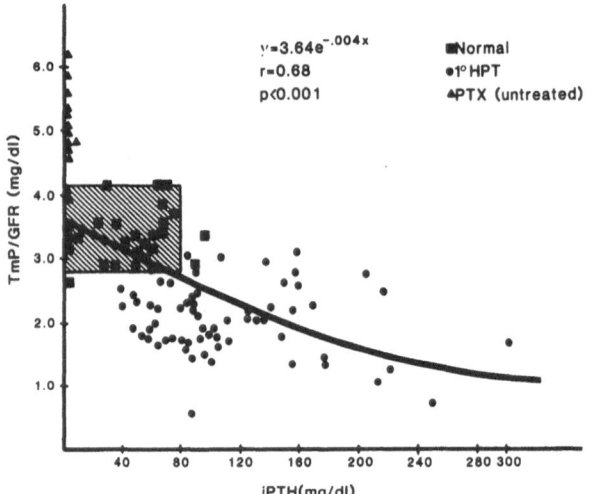

Fig. 2.   Relationship between iPTH and TmP in patients with normal
          renal function.  Symbols are the same as in Figure 1.


b)    Patients with Impaired Renal Function

        None of the three measurements of parathyroid function, alone
or in combination (Figure 4, Table 1) was able to distinguish between PHPT and hyperparathyroidism secondary to CRF.  Serum iPTH and
Nc'AMP increased linearly as endogenous creatinine clearance de-

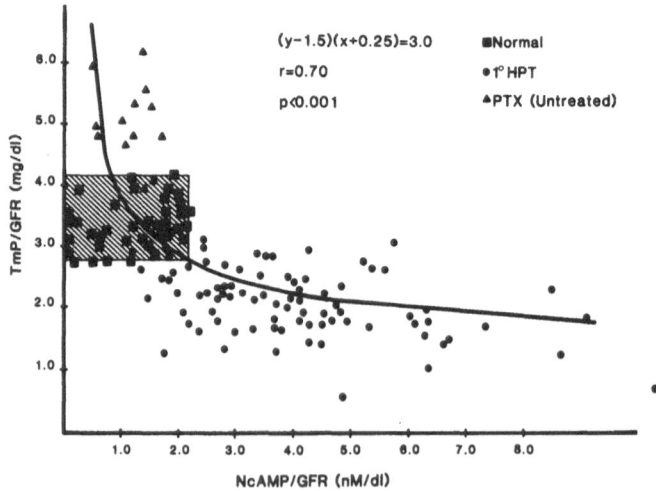

Fig. 3.   Relationship between Nc'AMP and TmP in patients with normal
          renal function.  Symbols are the same as in Figure 1.

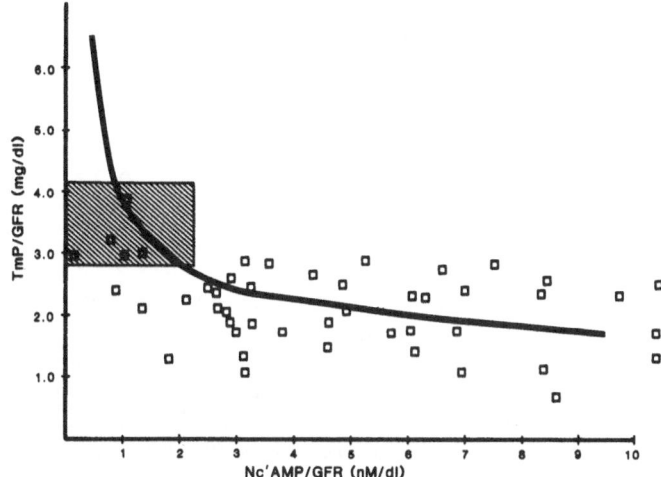

Fig. 4. Relationship between Nc'AMP and TmP in patients with chronic renal failure. Regression line is for patients with normal renal function as in Figure 3.

clined (Table 2) but no relationship could be demonstrated between TmP/GFR and creatinine clearance. Nevertheless, there was a significant relationship between fasting serum Pi and Ccr (Figure 5).

The three curves in Figure 5 are theoretical curves that predict serum Pi according to the formula:

$$\text{Serum Pi} = \frac{\text{UPi}}{\text{GFR}} + \frac{\text{TmP}}{\text{GFR}}$$

The upper curve assumes constant values for UPi and TmP/GFR equal to the mean values obtained in the 38 control subjects. The middle curve assumes a constant, reduced UPi equal to the mean UPi obtained

Table 1. Comparison of statistical relationships between the three independently measured indices of parathyroid function (iPTH, Nc'AMP and TmP) in patients with primary hyperparathyroidism (PHPT) and chronic renal failure (CRF). There was no significant difference between the slope of the regression nor the intercept for the three pairs of data.

|  |  | y = | r = | p < |
|---|---|---|---|---|
| PTH vs Nc'AMP | PHPT | 2.30 + 0.016x | 0.49 | 0.001 |
|  | CRF | 2.84 + 0.015x | 0.42 | 0.01 |
| PTH vs TmP | PHPT | 2.38 - 0.003x | -0.30 | 0.01 |
|  | CRF | 2.42 - 0.002x | -0.23 | NS |
| Nc'AMP vs TmP | PHPT | 2.59 - 0.13x | -0.45 | 0.001 |
|  | CRF | 2.45 - 0.071x | -0.31 | 0.05 |

Table 2.   Relationship between indices of parathyroid function and
           creatinine clearance in patients with chronic renal failure

|              | y =          | r =    | p <    |
|--------------|--------------|--------|--------|
| Nc'AMP vs Ccr | 7.25 - 0.09x | -0.59 | 0.001 |
| TmP vs Ccr    | 1.96 + 0.6x  | 0.17  | NS    |
| PTH vs Ccr    | 211 - 2.65x  | -0.57 | 0.001 |

in the 47 patients with CRF, with the same value for TmP/GFR as in
the controls.  The lower curve assumes constant values for both UPi
and TmP/GFR equal to the mean values obtained in the patients with
CRF.  For all curves GFR was the only variable.  The relationship
between these theoretical curves and the individual data points
indicates a reduction in both excreted load and threshold for
phosphate excretion in CRF.

    Hyperphosphatemia was not present in the fasting state in the
18 patients with CRF in whom Ccr was >30 ml/min/1.73m$^2$, and in 9 of
these patients the serum Pi was <3.0 mg/dl.  In Table 3 the 47 patients with CRF are arbitrarily divided into two groups on the basis
of the residual renal function.  With progression from mild (Ccr >
30 ml/min/1.73m$^2$) to severe (Ccr <30 ml/min/1.73m$^2$) renal failure,
there was also progression of hyperparathyroidism, as assessed by
iPTH and Nc'AMP.  TmP/GFR was significantly lower than normal in
both groups, but was not significantly different between the groups.
As a result of the fall in TmP/GFR patients with mild CRF had hypophosphatemia; the progression to hyperphosphatemia in severe CRF
was delayed by reduction in the excreted load of phosphate, but not
by any further reduction in TmP/GFR.


DISCUSSION

    Using graded doses of exogenous PTH, Kaminsky et al[6] demonstra-
ted that the maximum phosphaturic action of PTH was achieved at much
lower doses than the maximum production of renal cyclic AMP.  They
proposed that  the effect of PTH on phosphate transport was rate
limited at a point beyond production of cyclic AMP.  Similar observations were made by Walker et al,[7] who also demonstrated apparent
rate limitation of the cyclic AMP response at higher doses of
exogenous PTH.

    Our data, obtained in the steady state in man, are in complete
agreement with these acute infusion experiments and we can summarize
the relationships between PTH, cyclic AMP production, and inhibition
of phosphate reabsorption as follows:  If Nc'AMP production accurately reflects the interaction between PTH and its renal receptors then
it is not possible to saturate these receptors by endogenous PTH in

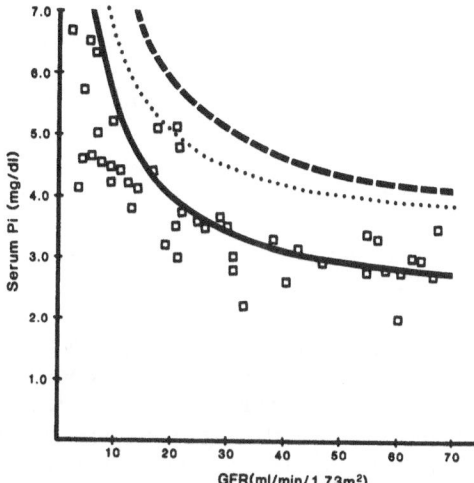

Fig. 5.   Effect of GFR on serum phosphate in chronic renal failure
(CRF).  Comparison of observed values with relationships
predicted from: Mean TmP/GFR and mean $U_pV$/GFR in normal subjects (upper curved line), mean TmP/GFR in normal subjects
and mean $U_pV$/GFR in patients with CRF (middle curved line)
and mean TmP/GFR and mean $U_pV$/GFR in patients with CRF
(lower curved line).

either primary hyperparathyroidism (Figure 1, Table 1), or in hyperparathyroidism secondary to chronic renal failure (Table 1).  On the
other hand, if the inhibition of phosphate reabsorption (reduction
in TmP) reflects the end-organ response to stimulation by the hormone, this response is rate limited at a point distal to hormone-
receptor interaction (Figures 2, 3).  A similar rate limited end-
organ response at a point beyond c'AMP production was demonstrated
for c'AMP mediated stimulation of adrenal steroidogenesis.[8]

Table 3.   Comparison of biochemical data in mild and severe renal
failure where mild renal failure has been arbitrarily defined as Ccr between 30 and 70 ml/min/1.73m²

| Group (N) | | Mild CRF (19) | Severe CRF (29) | Normal (38) |
|---|---|---|---|---|
| Serum Ca | (mg/dl) | 9.7 ± 0.6 | 8.7 ± 1.20 | 9.6 ± 0.4 |
| Serum Pi | (mg/dl) | 2.9 ± 0.4 | 4.7 ± 1.2 | 3.3 ± 0.4 |
| C.Cr. | (ml/min/1.73m²) | 50 ± 13 | 13 ± 8 | 120 ± 39 |
| Serum iPTH* | (ng/dl) | 92 ± 69 | 204 ± 87 | 45 ± 29 |
| Nc'AMP/GFR† | (nM/dl) | 2.59 ± 1.46 | 6.29 ± 2.98 | 1.15 ± 0.74 |
| TMP/GFR § | (mg/dl) | 2.19 ± 0.59 | 2.06 ± 0.79 | 3.34 ± 0.34 |

Normal ranges:   * 0-80; † 0-2.20; § 2.78-4.15

Of particular interest was the finding that the phosphaturic response (fall in TmP/GFR) was maximal with only small increments of iPTH and Nc'AMP above the normal range. This is in keeping with the clinical observation that reduction in serum Pi concentration is a poor index of the severity of primary hyperparathyroidism, in contrast to the rise in serum calcium concentration that relates very well to the severity of the disease.[3] There is evidently a major component of renal phosphate transport which is independent of PTH.

The failure to find a progressive decline in TmP/GFR as renal function deteriorates (Figure 4, Table 2) despite the progressive increase in iPTH and Nc'AMP supports the hypothesis that small increments in PTH secretion produce maximal phosphaturic response to the hormone. Provided that both TmP and nephrogenous c'AMP are expressed per unit of creatinine clearance, the relationships between iPTH, Nc'AMP, and TmP/GFR are evidently the same in patients with stable chronic renal failure as in patients with normal renal function, although obviously this cannot be true with extremes of renal failure when urine production is negligible.

Hyperparathyroidism develops early in the course of renal failure and becomes progressively worse as renal function declines. From the limited number of patients included in this study, it is difficult to determine the level of renal impairment at which biochemical evidence of hyperparathyroidism is first seen but 4 out of our 6 patients with an endogenous creatinine clearance between 60 and 70 ml/min/1.73m$^2$ had an elevated Nc'AMP and a subnormal TmP. The etiology of the secondary hyperparathyroidism in uremia has been controversial for some time. The "trade-off" hypothesis[9] postulates phosphate retention in early renal failure as the initiating event for the development of hyperparathyroidism. This is supported by good experimental data in the dog[10] but phosphate retention has never been documented in early renal failure in man. In fact, as shown in our studies (Figure 5, Table 3) and previously reported by several other groups, phosphate retention is not seen until the creatinine clearance is below 20-30 ml/min/1.73m$^2$ [11] and in early renal failure mild hypophosphatemia is seen.[12] This suggests that the initiation of secondary hyperparathyroidism is due to factors outside the kidney, possibly skeletal resistance to the calcium homeostatic action of PTH.[13]

The reduction in the TmP/GFR seen in our patients with early renal failure is greater than is required to maintain normophosphatemia and so must be at least partly due to factors other than the need to maintain phosphate homeostasis. The absence of phosphate retention and the appropriateness of the phosphaturic response to increased PTH strongly suggests that phosphate retention only modestly contributes to the initiation of the secondary hyperparathyroidism. In addition, since the phosphaturic response to PTH is maximal early in the course of hyperparathyroidism (primary or secondary) progression of hyperparathyroidism between mild and severe renal failure cannot make a significant further contribution to the maintenance of phosphate homeostasis in uremia. The plot of serum Pi concentration against creatinine clearance obtained in our patients (Figure 5) is very similar to the theoretical curve one would obtain if one mathematically determined serum Pi under conditions of a fixed reduced TmP/GFR and varying GFR,[11] with a modest reduction in phosphate load because of poor intake and impaired intestinal absorption.

## CONCLUSIONS

1)    In normal subjects and in patients with surgical hypoparathyroidism and primary hyperparathyroidism there is a linear relationship between PTH and Nc'AMP in the fasting state, and a curvilinear relationship between TmP/GFR and PTH and between TmP/GFR and Nc'AMP.

2)    Only a small increase in iPTH and Nc'AMP is needed to lower the high TmP/GFR of hypoparathyroidism to normal, but large further increases in iPTH and Nc'AMP had little further effect on TmP/GFR.

3)    The relationships between these variables are essentially the same in the secondary hyperparathyroidism of chronic renal failure as in primary hyperparathyroidism.

4)    The reduction in TmP/GFR in early renal failure is greater than is required to maintain normophosphatemia and so must be due to factors other than the need to preserve phosphate homeostasis; it does not fall further in severe renal failure.

5)    Phosphate retention does not occur in early renal failure and so cannot contribute to the initiation of secondary hyperparathyroidism.

6)    With the transition from mild to severe renal failure, the already low TmP/GFR, together with a reduction in excreted load of phosphate, postpones the onset of hyperphosphatemia, but the further progression of hyperparathyroidism makes no significant further contribution to the maintenance of phosphate homeostasis.

## REFERENCES

1.  L. J. Shlatz, I. L. Schwartz, E. Kinne-Saffran, and R. Kinne, Distribution of parathyroid hormone-stimulated adenylate cyclase in plasma membranes of cells of the kidney cortex, J. Membrane Biol. 24:131 (1975).

2.  A. M. Parfitt and M. Kleerekoper, The divalent ion homeostatic system: Physiology and metabolism of calcium, phosphorus, magnesium and bone, in: "Clinical Disorders of Fluid and

Electrolyte Metabolism, 3rd Edition," M. Maxwell and C. R. Kleeman, eds. (in press)

3. M. Kleerekoper, J. P. Ingham, J. P. McCarthy, and S. Posen, Parathyroid hormone assay in primary hyperparathyroidism: Experiences with a radioimmunoassay based on commercially available reagents, Clin. Chem. 20:369 (1974).

4. K. C. Tovey, K. G. Oldham, and J. A. M. Whelan. A simple direct assay for cyclic AMP in plasma and other biological samples using an improved competitive protein binding technique, Clin. Chim. Acta 56:221 (1974).

5. O. L. M. Bijvoet and J. Van Der Sluys Veer, The interpretation of laboratory tests on bone disease, Clin. Endocrinol. Metab. 1:217 (1972).

6. N. I. Kaminsky, A. E. Broadus, J. G. Hardman, D. J. Jones, Jr., J. H. Ball, E. W. Sutherland, and G. W. Liddle, Effects of parathyroid hormone on plasma and urinary adenosine 3', 5'-monophosphate in man, J. Clin. Invest. 49:2387 (1970).

7. D. A. Walker, S. J. Davies, K. Siddle, and J. S. Woodhead, Control of renal tubular phosphate reabsorption by parathyroid hormone in man, Clin. Sci. Mol. Med. 53:431 (1977).

8. D. G. Grahame-Smith, R. W. Butcher, R. L. Ney, and E. W. Sutherland, Adenosine 3', 5'-monophosphate as the intracellular mediator of the action of adrenocorticotropic hormone on the adrenal cortex, J. Biol. Chem. 242:5535 (1967).

9. N. W. Bricker, E. Slatopolsky, E. Reiss, and L. V. Avioli, Calcium, phosphorus and bone in renal disease and transplantation, Arch. Intern. Med. 123:543 (1969).

10. E. Slatopolsky, S. Caglar, J. P. Pennel, D. D. Taggart, J. M. Canterbury, E. Reiss, and N. S. Bricker, On the pathogenesis of hyperparathyroidism in chronic experimental renal insufficiency in the dog, J. Clin. Invest. 50:492 (1971).

11. O. L. M. Bijvoet, Kidney function in calcium and phosphate metabolism, in "Metabolic Bone Disease, Vol. I," L. V. Avioli and S. M. Krane, eds., Academic Press, New York (1977).

12. T. Friis, S. Hahnemann, and E. Weeke, Serum calcium and serum phosphorus in uremia during administration of sodium phytate and aluminium hydroxide, Acta Med. Scand. 183:497 (1968).

13. A. M. Parfitt, The actions of parathyroid hormone on bone. Relation to bone remodelling and turnover, calcium homeostasis and metabolic bone disease. IV. The state of the bones in uremic hyperparathyroidism. The mechanisms of skeletal resistance to PTH in renal failure and pseudohypoparathyroidism and the role of PTH in osteoporosis, osteopetrosis and osteofluorosis, Metabolism 25:1157 (1976).

# MECHANISM OF THE PHOSPHATURIA DUE TO CHLOROTHIAZIDE

Jules B. Puschett, J. Winaver, and P. Teredesai

Renal-Electrolyte Division, University and VA Hospitals, University of Arkansas for Medical Sciences and Allegheny General Hospital and the University of Pittsburgh School of Medicine, Pittsburgh, Pennsylvania

There appears to be general agreement with regard to the characteristic effects of the thiazide diuretics on sodium and calcium excretion. However, the action of these drugs on phosphate excretion remains a controversial matter. Thus, some investigators find that a significant phosphaturia results when the thiazides are administered both in the presence of normal parathyroid function as well as following removal of the parathyroid glands.[1,2] Others report either no phosphaturia or only a minimal increase in excretion in either circumstance.[3,4] The studies to be reported here were undertaken to identify and evaluate those factors which determine the pattern of phosphate excretion following the acute administration of chlorothiazide (CTZ). Accordingly, acute clearance studies were performed both in intact and chronically thyroparathyroidectomized (TPTX) dogs. In our earlier studies, we compared the effects of the drug on phosphate excretion in intact dogs with those in a group of animals in which parathyroid ablation had been accomplished at least 48 hours previously. We found that the intact animals could be divided into two groups: those with an initial low rate of phosphate excretion responded to CTZ with a phosphaturia. On the other hand, in animals with baseline phosphate excretion greater than approximately 15% of filtered load, the drug did not alter phosphate excretion in any consistent manner. In TPTX dogs, CTZ appeared to result in a consistent phosphaturia, greatly resembling that obtained in the intact dogs with low baseline phosphate excretion.

It is well recognized that urinary pH and/or bicarbonate content are usually altered in the same direction as urinary phosphate excretion.[5,6] Indeed, a causal relationship has been suggested for this phenomenon.[6] Furthermore, CTZ has been determined to increase urinary pH and is considered to act in the proximal nephron by virtue of an ability to inhibit carbonic anhydrase.[7] We therefore attempted to determine the actions of CTZ on urinary phosphate excretion when the drug was superimposed during three maneuvers which alter urinary phosphate excretion by differing mechanisms: volume expansion with saline, acetazolamide (ACTZ) and sodium bicarbonate loading. Preliminary studies have provided the following observations:

The expansion of TPTX dogs by 10% of body weight with saline resulted in increases in urinary pH and bicarbonate as well as phosphate excretion. Addition of CTZ produced a further rise in all three parameters. These data therefore suggest that CTZ alters phosphate excretion by mechanisms which differ from those mediating the saline expansion effect. An additional possibility is that the drug acts at a different nephron site than does saline expansion.

Bicarbonate loading, like saline expansion, augmented urinary bicarbonate and phosphate excretion and alkalinized the urine as did saline expansion. However, contrary to the previous studies, while the superimposition of CTZ resulted in a continued rise in bicarbonate excretion, neither urinary pH nor phosphate excretion increased. Thus, CTZ dissociated the actions of pH from those of bicarbonate on phosphate excretion.

As was the case with bicarbonate loading, ACTZ caused a marked rise in urinary pH and in both bicarbonate and phosphate excretion. When CTZ was then added, there was no further increase in phosphate excretion. Bicarbonate excretion showed no consistent rise and urinary pH actually fell. Thus, CTZ was incapable of augmenting phosphate excretion when the proximal impairment of phosphate reabsorption had already been accomplished by carbonic anhydrase inhibition.

In summary, CTZ caused a phosphaturia when baseline phosphate excretion was not already high. Furthermore, when the influence of PTH is withdrawn, the excretion of phosphate appears to be largely affected by changes in urinary pH.

REFERENCES

1.  G. Eknoyan, W. N. Suki, and M. Martinez-Maldonado, Effect of diuretics on urinary excretion of phosphate, calcium, and magnesium in thyroparathyroidectomized dogs, J Lab Clin Med 76:257 (1970).
2.  S. R. Steinmuller and J. B. Puschett, Effect of metolazone in man:comparison with chlorothiazide, Kidney International 1:169 (1972).

3.  R. J. Smith, R. M. Friedler, and J. W. Coburn, The effect of chlorothiazide on renal handling of phosphate, International Workshop on Phosphate Metabolism Kidney and Bone, L. Avioli, P. Bordier, H. Fleisch, S. Massry, and E. Slatopolsky, eds., p. 291 (1975).

4.  P. C. Fernandez and J. B. Puschett, Proximal tubular actions of metolazone and chlorothiazide, Am J Physiol 225:954 (1973).

5.  M. Fulop and P. Brazeau, The phosphaturic effect of sodium bicarbonate and acetazolamide in dogs, J Clin Invest 47:983 (1968).

6.  J. B. Puschett and M. Goldberg, The relationship between the renal handling of phosphate and bicarbonate in man, J Lab Clin Med 73:956 (1969).

7.  J. B. Puschett and M. Goldberg, The acute effects of furosemide on acid and electrolyte excretion in man, J Lab Clin Med 71:666 (1968).

# EFFECT OF UNILATERAL NEPHRECTOMY AND ITS ACCOMPANYING HEMODYNAMIC CHANGES ON CALCIUM AND PHOSPHATE EXCRETION IN THE DOG

Juan C. Ayus and Garabed Eknoyan

Renal Section, Department of Medicine
Baylor College of Medicine
Houston, Texas 77030

Acute unilateral nephrectomy (AUN) results in a prompt increase in electrolyte excretion by the controlateral kidney in the dog (1). Humphreys and Ayus have shown that this increased electrolyte excretion by the remaining kidney consists mainly of $Na^+$ and $K^+$ and is accompanied by striking systemic hemodynamic changes (2). The latter consists of a drop in cardiac output; an increase in diastolic pressure and total peripheral resistance; but a constant glomerular filtration rate. These findings resemble those observed following closure of a systemic arteriovenous fistula (3, 4). Of particular interest in this regard is the fact that when an artificial arteriovenous fistula is created at the time of uninephrectomy, all of the changes seen following AUN are abolished only to reappear again when the fistula is closed. Thus, it is evident that AUN induces hemodynamic changes resembling those seen following closure of a systemic arteriovenous fistula and that the observed increase in electrolyte excretion following AUN is not the result of the removal of the kidney itself, but rather secondary to the hemodynamic changes induced by the AUN.

Since the increased excretion of monovalent cation (Na+K) by the remaining kidney after AUN was accompanied by a significant rise of phosphate excretion (2), the possibility that the parathyroid hormone might be playing a role in these changes was entertained. The present study was designed to investigate the changes in calcium and phosphate excretion following AUN and to determine the role of PTH on them.

MATERIALS AND METHODS

Experiments were carried out in 33 mongrel dogs of either sex and weighing between 16 and 27 kg. Anesthesia was induced with intravenous sodium pentobarbital (30 mg/kg) and ventilation maintained via a cuffed endotracheal tube attached to a Harvard respirator. The kidneys were approached through subcostal flank incision and catheters placed in each renal vein and ureter. Following a loading dose, all animals received a maintenance solution of isotonic saline via a foreleg vein at 0.5 ml/min containing sufficient inulin and sodium p-aminohippurate to achieve plasma concentrations of 25 and 1 mg/dl respectively. All animals received a 5 mg intramuscular injection of desoxy-corticosterone acetate in oil prior to initiation of the experiments. Three groups of animals were studied.

GROUP I: Ten dogs served as controls. After concluding preparatory renal surgery as described above, urine and blood collections for clearance measurements were commenced for a period of 120 minutes, following which a left subcostal incision was made, the kidney exposed and gently manipulated. Collections were then continued for an additional 4 hours.

GROUP II: In this group 10 dogs were studied. After a control period of 60-120 minutes in which clearance determinations were done, complete left surgical nephrectomy was performed by doubly ligating and severing the renal artery and vein, and removing the kidney. The maintenance infusion was then slowed in half and observations repeated starting 60 minutes after the nephrectomy for an additional 2 hours.

GROUP III: In this group of 13 dogs total thyroparathyroidectomy (TPTX) was performed 24 hours before study. On the day of experiment after a control period of 60-120 minutes in which clearance determinations were obtained, complete left surgical nephrectomy was performed as on Group II and clearance collections obtained in the same sequences following the uninephrectomy.

Clearance periods were 20 or 25 minutes in length, five such periods were averaged to yield a single value for each experimental period. Arterial and renal venous blood samples were obtained at the midpoints of every period. Blood samples were immediately placed in chilled, heparinized tubes, centrifuged in the cold, and frozen until later analysis. GFR was calculated from the clearance of inulin, renal blood flow (RBF) from the clearance and extraction of p-aminohippurate and the arterial hematocrit. Fractional excretion (FE) of $PO_4$ was calculated from $C_{PO_4}/C$ inulin X 100; $FE_{Na}$ from $C_{NA}/C$ inulin X 100;

## TABLE I

### EFFECT OF ACUTE UNILATERAL NEPHRECTOMY ON GFR AND ELECTROLYTE EXCRETION BY THE REMAINING KIDNEY

**Group II - AUN in Intact Dogs (n=10)**

| | GFR ml/min | | $U_{Na+K}V$ µEq/min | | $U_{PO_4}V$ µmol/min | | $U_{Ca}V$ µmol/min | |
|---|---|---|---|---|---|---|---|---|
| | C | E | C | E | C | E | C | E |
| m | 33.5 | 33.8 | 66.1 | 123.2 | 6.4 | 23.7 | 0.50 | 0.40 |
| ±SE | ±1.8 | ±1.5 | ±2.2 | ±3.2 | ±5.0 | ±4.6 | ±0.13 | ±0.13 |
| P | N.S. | | <0.001 | | <0.001 | | N.S. | |

**Group III - AUN in TPTX Dogs (n=13)**

| | GFR ml/min | | $U_{Na+K}V$ µEq/min | | $U_{PO_4}V$ µmol/min | | $U_{Ca}V$ µmol/min | |
|---|---|---|---|---|---|---|---|---|
| | C | E | C | E | C | E | C | E |
| m | 43.2 | 54.4 | 38.2 | 82.3 | 4.1 | 12.6 | 0.15 | 0.12 |
| ±SE | ±3.3 | ±4.7 | ±6.4 | ±10.8 | ±1.2 | ±2.4 | ±0.04 | ±0.03 |
| P | <0.01 | | <0.001 | | <0.001 | | N.S. | |

*Values are means ± SE of measurements before (C) and after (E) acute unilateral nephrectomy in Groups II and III.

P = level of significance using Student's T test for paired data.

N.S. = not significant.

and $FE_K$ from $C_K$/Cinulin X 100.  Values are the means ± 1 SE.  The
statistical significance of the difference between periods was
assured using two methods.  In the proper case  in which two observations were compared, Students' T test for paired observations was used.  In the proper  case. in which more than two observations were performed, analyses of the variance was used.

RESULTS

Serial observations over the 6-hour duration of the experiment in the control sham operated dogs showed no change in glomerular filtration rate, renal blood flow or Na+K excretion.
However, phosphate excretion rose significantly from 8.4±1.1 to
15.7±1.4 µmol/min (p <0.05) from Period 1 (0-2 hours) to Period
2 (2-4 hours) but remained constant thereafter up to the sixth
hour termination of collections.

The effects of AUN in the intact dogs is presented in Table
I.  AUN resulted in a significant increase in the excretion of
Na+K and phosphate, but no change in calcium excretion.  These
changes occurred without significant alterations in GFR and RBF.

The results of AUN in dogs parathyroidectomized 24 hours
prior to study are also shown in Table I.  As in the intact animals, AUN produced a significant increase in the excretion of
Na+K and of phosphate; but calcium excretion again remained unchanged.  However, in contrast to the intact animals, there was
a significant increase in GFR from 43.2±3.3 to 54.4±4.7 ml/min
(p <0.01) after AUN in TPTX animals.  RBF also showed an increase from 214.0±26.1 to 261.0±34.5 ml/min after AUN but this
increase was not statistically significant.

Table II shows the fractional excretion of Na, K and $PO_4$ in
Group II and III animals.  Despite the fact that GFR and RBF increased after AUN in the TPTX dogs (Group III), no difference in
the fractional excretions of Na, K and $PO_4$ was present between
the two groups.

Table III depicts the serum calcium and phosphate in Group
II and III animals.  No change in either of these values was observed after AUN.

DISCUSSION

The results of the present study confirm the previous observation that AUN induces changes in electrolyte excretion (1,
2).  In the present study, the increased excretion of Na+K is
shown to be accompanied by a significant increase of phosphate

## TABLE II

### EFFECT OF ACUTE UNILATERAL NEPHRECTOMY ON FRACTIONAL EXCRETION OF ELECTROLYTES BY THE REMAINING KIDNEY

#### Group II - AUN in Intact Dogs (n=10)

|  | FE Na% | | FE K% | | FE PO$_4$% | |
|---|---|---|---|---|---|---|
|  | C | E | C | E | C | E |
| m | .60 | .90 | 25.0 | 46.0 | 11.0 | 34.0 |
| ±SE | ±.14 | ±.20 | ±4.3 | ±5.2 | ±2.0 | ±1.9 |
| P | <.05 | | <0.001 | | <0.001 | |

#### Group III - AUN in TPTX Dogs (n=13)

|  | FE Na% | | FE K% | | FE PO$_4$% | |
|---|---|---|---|---|---|---|
|  | C | E | C | E | C | E |
| m | .22 | .51 | 13.0 | 24.0 | 5.0 | 13.0 |
| ±SE | ±.06 | ±.10 | ±.94 | ±2.2 | ±1.6 | ±2.3 |
| P | <.005 | | <0.001 | | <0.001 | |

Symbols and abbreviations same as Table I.

excretion in both the intact and the thyroparathyroidectomized dogs. Thus, the phosphaturia induced by AUN must be independent of parathormone. Since an increase in phosphate excretion was also seen in the sham operated group, the changes in the experimental groups might be attributed to time variation (5, 6). However, the increased excretion of phosphate in the sham group was present during the collection period between the 2nd and the 4th hours, with no further increase after that. In the two experimental groups, collections after AUN extended beyond the fourth hour of the initiation of the experiment, thus making the possibility that the observed changes in phosphate excretion in the experimental groups were due to temporal spontaneous variation most unlikely.

## TABLE III

### EFFECT OF ACUTE UNILATERAL NEPHRECTOMY ON

### SERUM CALCIUM AND PHOSPHORUS

#### Group II - AUN in Intact Dogs  (n=10)

|       | $CA_{mmol/l}$ | | $PO_{4mmol/l}$ | |
|-------|------|------|------|------|
|       | C | E | C | E |
| m     | 2.4 | 2.3 | 1.6 | 1.9 |
| ±SE   | ±.17 | ±.19 | ±.2 | ±1.2 |
| P     | N.S. | | N.S. | |

#### Group III - AUN in TPTX Dogs (n=13)

|       | C | E | C | E |
|-------|------|------|------|------|
| m     | 1.7 | 1.6 | 1.6 | 1.8 |
| ±SE   | ±.12 | ±.10 | ±.07 | ±.1 |
| P     | N.S. | | N.S. | |

Symbols and abbreviations same as Table I.

Calcium excretion on the other hand did not increase after AUN, neither in the intact animals nor in the TPTX group. A direct relationship between the excretion of sodium and calcium has been shown to be present under various types of diuretic conditions (7). Since these earlier reports, however, several exceptions demonstrating a dissociation of sodium from calcium excretion have been reported (8, 9). The results of the present study demonstrating a dissociation of the excretion of sodium from that of calcium following AUN, provides evidence for yet another experimental model in which the excretion of $Na^+$ and of $Ca^+$ are not directly related.

Our previous studies of the AUN model showed that creating an artificial arteriovenous fistula at the time of AUN not only prevented the excretion of Na+K but that of phosphate as well (2). The suggestion was then made that these changes were mediated by a hemodynamic signal located in the vascular bed. Since bilateral cervical vagotomy failed to abolish the increased electrolyte excretion after uninephrectomy; the conclusion was drawn that intrathoracic receptors could not be responsible for initiating these changes (10). More recent observations, utilizing bilateral carotid denervation, indicate that the carotid baroreceptors are most likely the afferent pathway mediating the observed changes (11).

Since the increased electrolyte excretion following AUN, occurs in the absence of changes in renal hemodynamics and is also present in the absence of PTH as well as maximal doses of desoxycorticosterone, the possibility of a direct tubular effect of the efferent mechanism must be considered. The site within the tubule where this effect must be exerting itself cannot be determined from the present studies. Certainly the increase in phosphate excretion would suggest inhibition of proximal tubular reabsorption. If this were indeed the case, the failure to observe an accompanying calciuresis must be attributed to the presence of a component of tubular calcium reabsorption situated beyond the proximal tubule which is not inhibited by AUN and is independent of PTH. The more correct definition and tubular localization of this effect must await clarification by more direct studies.

## ACKNOWLEDGEMENTS

The authors wish to gratefully acknowledge the most able technical assistance of Geraldine B. Tasby and the secretarial assistance and manuscript preparation of Charlia Due.

## REFERENCES

1.  Coe, F. L., Suki, W. N., Kurtzman, N. A., Rector, F. C. Jr.

and Seldin, D. W.:  The mechanism of natriuresis immediately following unilateral nephrectomy.  CLIN. RES. 16: 380, 1968 (Abstr.).

2.  Humphreys, M. H. and Ayus, J. C.:  Role of hemodynamic changes in the increased cation excretion after acute unilateral nephrectomy in the anesthetized dog.  J. CLIN. INVEST. 61: 590, 1978.

3.  Epstein, F. H., Shadle, O. W., Ferguson, T. B. and McDowell, M. E.:  Cardiac output and intracardiac pressures in patients with arteriovenous fistulas.  J. CLIN. INVEST. 32: 543, 1953.

4.  Epstein, F. H., Post, R. S. and McDowell, M. E.:  The effect of an arteriovenous fistula on renal hemodynamics and electrolyte excretion.  J. CLIN. INVEST. 32: 233, 1953.

5.  Massry, S. G., Coburn, J. W. and Kleeman, C. R.:  Evidence for suppression of parathyroid gland by hypermagnesemia. J. CLIN. INVEST. 49: 1619, 1970.

6.  Hartenbower, D. L., Friedler, R. M., Coburn, J. W. and Massry, S. G.:  Spontaneous variation in electrolyte excretion in the dog.  CLIN. RES. 21: 283, 1973 (Abstr.).

7.  Walser, M.:  Ion association.  VII.  Dependence of calciuresis on natriuresis during sulfate infusion.  AMER. J. PHYSIOL. 201: 769, 1961.

8.  Suki, W. N., Hull, A. R., Rector, F. C. Jr. and Seldin, D. W.: Mechanism of the effect of thiazide diuretics on calcium and uric acid.  CLIN. RES. 15: 78, 1967 (Abstr.).

9.  Suki, W. N., Schwettmann, R. S., Rector, F. C. Jr. and Seldin, D. W.:  Effect of chronic mineralocorticoid administration on calcium excretion in the rat.  AMER. J. PHYSIOL. 215: 71, 1968.

10.  Humphreys, M. H., Ayus, J. C. and Stanton, J. C.:  Role of the vagus in the hemodynamic changes following acute unilateral nephrectomy (AUN).  KIDNEY INT. 12: 561, 1977 (Abstr.).

11.  Ayus, J. C. and Humphreys, M. H.:  On the mechanism of hemodynamic changes caused by acute unilateral nephrectomy (AUN) in the dog.  KIDNEY INT. 14: 748, 1978 (Abstr.).

EFFECT OF METABOLIC ACIDOSIS AND ALKALOSIS ON THE RENAL RESPONSE

TO PARATHYROID HORMONE INFUSION IN NORMAL MAN

James C.M. Chan, M.D. and Frederick C. Bartter, M.D.

From the Section on Seteroid and Mineral Metabolism,
National Heart Lung and Blood Institute, National
Institutes of Health, Bethesda, Maryland.  Dr. Chan
is now in the Department of Pediatrics, Medical College
of Virginia, Richmond, Va., and Dr. Bartter, VA Hospital-
University of Texas, San Antonio, Texas.

ABSTRACT

Six normal volunteers were observed for 24 days on a constant
metabolic diet in a study designed to test the hypothesis that the
action of parathyroid hormone may be altered by renal acidosis.

Parathyroid extract (PTE 200 units) was administered intravenously with 4 subsequent urine collections at 30-minute intervals
on the fifth day of each 5-day balance period in a protocol where
"steady state" (a) metabolic acidosis (blood total $CO_2$ of 20±2
mEq/l) was achieved with ammonium chloride (200 mEq/$m^2$/day) and (b)
metabolic alkalosis (total $CO_2$ of 30±2 mEq/l) by substitution of

---

*Abbreviations:   parathyroid extract (PTE), parathyroid hormone (PTH)
blood total carbon dioxide concentration (total
$CO_2$), sodium bicarbonate ($NaHCO_3$).

200 mEq NaHCO$_3$ for the 200 mEq of dietary sodium chloride. The acidotic and alkalotic states were produced twice in each subject.

In response to PTE infusion, the maximal calcium clearances were 12.8±4.4, 35.2±21.6 and 15.5±7.2 ml/min during the control, acidosis and alkalosis periods, respectively. Similarly, the maximal phosphorus clearances were 91.9±7.2, 166.7±62.2 and 73.5±17.7 ml/min for the control, acidosis and alkalotic periods, respectively.

The data, therefore, show that in normal man: (1) metabolic acidosis alters the effect of PTE on calcium (p<0.05) and phosphorus (p<0.02) clearances and (2) metabolic alkalosis does not affect such clearances. The results support the contention that metabolic acidosis significantly alters the effect of PTH on the kidneys.

INTRODUCTION

Diverse abnormalities of calcium metabolism have been reported in patients with acute and chronic acidosis: in the kidney with hypercalciuria [1-4], hypocitraturia [5,6], nephrocalcinosis and at the bone surface with loss of calcium carbonate [9,19]. In addition, metabolic acidosis is thought to stimulate parathyroid hormone (PTH) secretion resulting in further bone resorption and negative calcium balance [11,12]. However, it has been recently demonstrated that positive hydrogen ion and negative calcium balances are seen without changes in PTH concentrations. [13,14] The present study is, therefore, designed to test the hypothesis that acidosis may enhance the actions of PTH on the renal clearances of calcium and phosphorus. In addition, a more complete characterization of the renal response to PTH infusion under conditions of acidosis and alkalosis will be examined here.

MATERIAL AND METHODS

All studies were performed in the Clinical Center of the National Institutes of Health with the informed consent of the normal volunteers and the approval of the Research Committee of the National Heart, Lung and Blood Institute.

Four men and two women, aged 21 to 26 years were studied for 29 days on a constant metabolic diet containing 209 mEq/day of sodium as 200 mEq of sodium chloride supplement and 9 mEq of dietary sodium, 900 mg/day of calcium and 1,000 mg/day of phosphorus, and 60 mEq/day of potassium. After four days of control observations, the daily fluid intake in the form of distilled water was held constant.

Two hundred units of parathyroid extract (Eli Lilly and Co.,

Indianapolis) were administered intravenously on the morning of the fifth day of each 5-day balance period in a protocol in which "steady-state" (a) metabolic acidosis was achieved with ammonium chloride (200 mEq/m$^2$/day) given in gelatin-coated (not enteric coated) capsules and (b) metabolic alkalosis by substitution of 200 mEq of sodium bicarbonate for the 200 mEq of sodium chloride supplement. The 5-day acidotic and 5-day alkalotic states were produced sequentially, and each was repeated once in each subject.

Two hours prior to the PTE infusions, 20 ml/kg of distilled water were administered orally; 30-minute aliquots of urine were then collected. The urine output was replaced over the subsequent 30 minutes with an equal volume of distilled water to ensure a good urine output. Two pre-infusion and 4 post-infusion urine collections were obtained and analyzed for calcium, phosphorus and creatinine. Blood was obtained through a heparin lock every 30 minutes (corresponding to the mid-point of each 30-minute collection) and aliquots of serum were analyzed for calcium, phosphorus, creatinine and carbon dioxide by methods previously described.(13)

In addition, blood was obtained on the fourth and fifth day of each study period and analyzed for total carbon dioxide to demontrate the steady-state of acid-base balance.


RESULTS

A steady-state metabolic acidosis (plasma $CO_2$ content 20$\pm$2 mEq/l) was achieved in each subject by the fourth and fifth day with the daily intake of 200 mEq/m$^2$ of ammonium chloride. Similarly, a steady-state metabolic alkalosis (plasma $CO_2$ content, 30$\pm$2 mEq/l) was achieved in each subject by the fourth and fifth day, by substitution of 200 mEq NaHCO$_3$ for the 200 mEq of supplemental NaCl. These states of acidosis and alkalosis were produced twice in each subject. The body weight did not change significantly in any subject during the entire study after the initial 4 days of observation.

Table 1 summarizes the results of the PTE infusions. In normal


Table 1: Maximal renal response to parathyroid extract infusion

| Study Period | Calcium Clearance ml/min | Phosphorus Clearance ml/min |
|---|---|---|
| Control | 12.8 ± 4.4 | 91.9 ± 7.2 |
| Acidosis | 35.2 ± 21.6 | 166.7 ± 62.2 |
| Alkalosis | 15.5 ± 7.2 | 73.5 ± 17.7 |

subjects: (1) metabolic acidosis greatly alters the effect of
PTE on calcium ($p<0.05$) and phosphorus ($p<0.02$) clearances and
(2) metabolic alkalosis does not affect such clearances.


DISCUSSION

It has been repeatedly demonstrated that PTH concentrations in
the blood change little during metabolic acidosis as compared to
control states [14,15]. Thus it has been frequently held that the
acceleration of net bone resorption [14] during acidosis is not
the result of increased PTH action on the bone. The result of the
present study tends to suggest that during acidosis, PTE results in
a significantly greater renal response of calcium ($p<0.05$) and
phosphorus ($p<0.02$) clearances than it does in control studies. It
seems reasonable to conclude that acidosis strongly alters the
action of PTE on the renal tubule.

It is well established that metabolic acidosis can produce
hypercalciuria [16,17], but aside from its association with sodium
excretion [18] the exact mechanism of the hypercalciuria is unknown. [19] It is interesting to speculate that the hypercalciuria
may be related to altered sensitivity of the renal tubule to PTH
in the presence of metabolic acidosis. [20,21]

It is also clearly shown in the present study that metabolic
alkalosis is achieved without body weight changes by substitution
of equal amounts of sodium bicarbonate for sodium chloride, and
that metabolic alkalosis in contrast to metabolic acidosis, does
not have any influence on the renal response to PTH.


REFERENCES

1.  Simpson, D.P.: Control of hydrogen ion homeostasis and renal
       acidosis. Medicine 50: 503, 1971.
2.  Pak, C.Y.C., Ohata M, Lawrence EC, and Synder W: The hyper-
       calciurias:causes, parathyroid functions and diagnostic
       criteria. J Clin Invest 54: 387, 1974.
3.  Albright, F., Henneman P., Benedict, P.H., and Forbes, A.P.:
       Idiopathic hypercalciuria. J Clin Endocrinol Metab 13:
       860, 1953.
4.  Nordin, B.E.C., Peacock, M., and Marshall, D.H.: Calcium
       excretion and hypercalciuria. In "Urolithiasis Research".
       H. Fleisch, W.G. Robertson, C.H. Smith, W. Vahlensiech (Eds)
       Plenum Press, NY, 1976, pp 101-115.
5.  Dedmon, R.E., and Wrong, O.: The excretion of organic anion in
       renal tubular acidosis with particular reference to citrate.
       Clin Sci 22: 19, 1962.

6.  Norman, M.E., Feldman, N.I., Cohn, R.M., Roth, K.S., and McCurdy, D.I.C.:  Urinary citrate excretion in the diagnosis of distal renal tubular acidosis.  J Pediatr 92: 394, 1978.

7.  Pak, C.Y.C.: "Calcium urolithiasis:  Pathogenesis, diagnosis and management." Plenum Medical Book Co. NY 1978, p  162.

8.  Chan, J.C.M.:  Renal electrolyte and mineral disorders in children.  Curr Probl Pediatr 8: 1, 1978.

9.  Lemann, J. Jr., Litzow, J.R. and Lennon, E.J.:  The effects of chronic acid loads in normal man:  Further evidence for the participation of bone mineral in the defense against chronic metabolic acidosis.  J Clin Invest 45:  1608, 1966.

10. Kaye, M., Fruch, A.J., and Silverman, M.:  A study of vertebral bone powder from patients with chronic renal failure.  J Clin Invest 49:  442, 1970.

11. Chu, H.I., Liu, S.H., Yu, T.F., Hsu, H.C., Cheng, T.Y., and Chao, H.C.:  Calcium and phosphorus metabolism in osteomalacia.  X. Further studies in vitamin D action, early sign of depletion and effect of mineral doses.  J Clin Invest 19:  349, 1940.

12. Gray, S.P., Morris, J.E.W., and Brooks, C.J.:  Renal handling of calcium, magnesium, inorganic phosphate and hydrogen ions during prolonged exposure to elevated carbon dioxide concentration.  Clin Sci Molecular Med 45:  751, 1973.

13. Chan, J.C.M.:  Acid-base, calcium, potassium and aldosterone metabolism in renal tubular acidosis.  Nephron 23: 152, 1979.

14. Weber, H.P., Gray, R.W., Dominquez, J.H., and Lemann J. Jr.: The lack of effect of chronic metabolic acidosis on 25-OH-Vitamin D metabolism and serum parathyroid hormone in humans.  J Clin Endocrinol Metab 43: 1047, 1976.

15. Coe, F.L., Firpo, J.J., Hollandsworth, D.L., Segil, L., Canterbury, J.M. and Reiss, E.M.:  Effect of acute and chronic metabolic acidosis on serum immunoreactive parathyroid hormone in man.  Kidney Int 8:  262, 1975.

16. Walzer, M:  The separate effects of hyperparathyroidism, hypercalciuria of malignancy, renal failure and acidosis on the state of calcium, phosphate and other ions in plasma.  J Clin Invest 41:  1454, 1962.

17. Reidenberg, M.M.:  Mechanisms of hypercalciuria in acidosis. Clin Res 15:  328, 1967.

18. Wills, M.R., Gill, J.R., Jr., and Bartter, F.C.:  The interrelationships of calcium and sodium excretions.  Clin Sci (Oxford) 37: 621, 1969.

19. Walzer, M.:  Divalent cations:  physicochemical state in glomerular filtrate and urine and renal excretion.  Chapter 18 in Orloff, J. and Berliner, R.W. (eds): "Handbook of Physiology, Section 8:  Renal Physiology." Williams & Wilkins Co. Baltimore, 1973, p 521.

20. Chan, J.C.M. and Bartter, F.C.:  Effect of metabolic acidosis and alkalosis on the renal response to parathyroid hormone infusion in normal man.  Kidney Int 14:  637, 1978 (abstract).

21.  Batlle, D., Hays, S., Arruda, J.A.L, and Kurtzman, N.A.:
     Parathyroid hormone (PTH) dependent hypercalciuria in metabolic
     acidosis (MA).  Clin Res 27:  362 (A), 1979. (abstract).

## ACKNOWLEDGEMENT

The authors wish to thank the nursing, dietary and technical
staff of the Clinical Center, N.I.H. for expert patient care and
balance collections and Mrs. Cindy Alawar for secretarial support.

# PHOSPHATE HOMEOSTASIS
# IN HEALTH AND DISEASE

PHOSPHATE METABOLIC CONTROL OF POTASSIUM MOVEMENT -

ITS EFFECT ON OSMOTIC PRESSURE OF THE CELL

Samuel P. Bessman, M.D. and Nandita Pal, Ph.D.

University of Southern California
School of Medicine
Los Angeles, CA  90033

Certain features of intracellular inorganic ion metabolism must be considered in any discussion of extracellular phosphate metabolism.  This report will present our concepts in three areas: the potassium and phosphate shifts related to glucose uptake and insulin stimulation, the osmotic effects of energy metabolism, and some changes in cerebral intracellular ions caused by various hyperosmolar states.

It is well known that potassium moves into the cell under the influence of insulin and that this effect is reversed even while the insulin and glucose continue to be administered.  Figure 1. It is apparent that insulin does not "drive potassium into the cell" for the second half of Fig. 1 would give just as good evidence that insulin drives potassium out of cells as the first half gives to support the conventional view.  In fact, insulin probably has no effect on net potassium movement at all, certainly not at the order of magnitude of millimoles.  The same transitory change in phosphate occurs as is seen in potassium.  Indeed, this was seen long ago.  It was known long before the potassium fall was reported (1).  The thesis which we wish to propose is that all movements of potassium in the milliequivalent range are passively related to glycolysis or esterification of organic phosphate or increases or decreases in negative ions (organic acids) within the cell.

Let us look at Figure 2 to see the passive role of potassium and phosphate in the uptake of glucose by the cell.  The first step after glucose enters the cell is phosphorylation of glucose, catalyzed by hexokinase.  This produces a mole of glucose-6-phosphate with two negative charges in equilibrium with two potassium

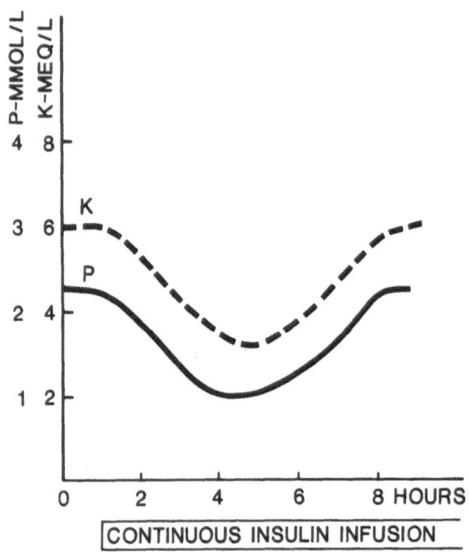

Figure 1.   Effect of Insulin on Serum Potassium and Phosphate

ions.  The ADP undergoes oxidative phosphorylation using inorganic
phosphate, $K_2HPO_4$.  A second molecule of $K_2HPO_4$ is required to re-
phosphorylate the ADP formed when phosphate is added to fructose 6
to make fructose 1,6 diphosphate, $K_4$.  Two more $K_2HPO_4$ molecules
are required to form the two moles of 1,3 diphosphoglyceric acid
$(P_4K_8)$.  Thus to reach maximum phosphorylation in the glycolytic
process a mole of glucose must bind the equivalent of four moles of
$K_2HPO_4$.  To move 1.80 grams of glucose (about maximum hourly usage
per kilo) into the 1,3 diphosphoglycerate step would require 40
millimoles per kilo of $K_2HPO_4$ including eighty milliequivalents of
potassium.  In fact Fig. 1 shows that about 1 meq of K enters the

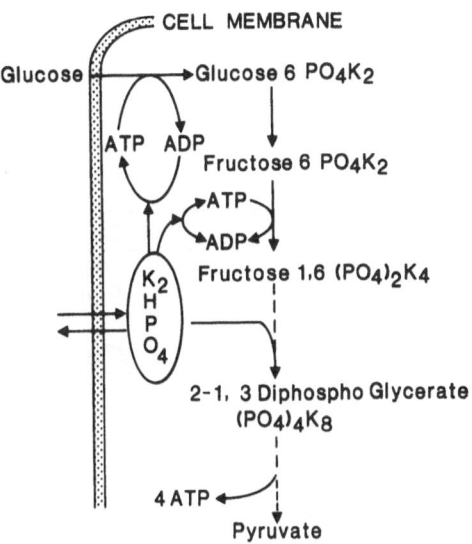

Figure 2

cell during the period of maximum fall of serum K.    This would be equivalent to 0.5 meq of phosphate.    These shifts represent only about 1.25% of the theoretical (Fig. 2) requirement of $K_2HPO_4$ to permit optimal metabolism.    Where then lies the discrepancy?

    Fig. 2 shows that in the metabolic steps from 1,3 diphospho-glycerate to pyruvate the potassium phosphate groups are trans-ferred to ADP to make ATP.    This is where most of the rephosphory-lation of ATP used at the hexokinase and phosphofructokinase steps occurs.    These phosphate movements recycle intracellular phosphate. Why does potassium enter the cell at all?   We must turn to the chemistry of the "transitional state" to explain the transitory drop seen in serum potassium and phosphate.    (Figure 3 shows what I call the "tunnel theory").

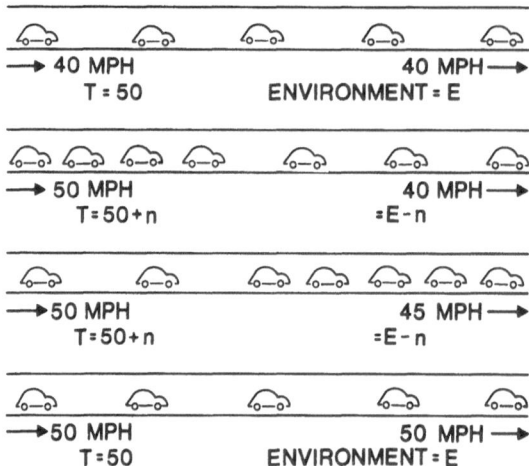

Figure 3

Let us assume there is a tunnel 5000 feet long through which
cars are traveling at 40 miles per hour. They maintain the legal
spacing distance of 100 feet, so there are fifty cars (T) present
in the tunnel. Let the number of cars in the environment of the
tunnel be E. Now comes rush hour and it is necessary to pass cars
through the tunnel at a greater rate, say 50 miles per hour. The
policeman at the proximal end of the tunnel waves the cars in faster, permitting them to tailgate until the new rate of entry is
50 miles per hour. But some cars are still leaving the tunnel at
40 mph. There is a little "clot" of extra cars (N cars) in the
tunnel for a short time until the speed of all cars is 50 mph,
when they enter at 100 ft. intervals again, but at the faster rate.
During this transitional period there are (T+N) cars in the tunnel
and E-N cars in the environment. After the transition the extra
"clot" of cars has reentered the environment and there are again
T cars in the tunnel and E cars in the environment. Although the
rate of movement is faster the number of cars present in the tunnel is the same as at the lower rate of movement. Only in the
transition period is there a net displacement from tunnel to environment or back. This is the basis for the transitory changes

TABLE I

THE EFFECT OF INSULIN ON INTRACELLULAR PHOSPHATE COMPOUNDS OF ISOLATED
RAT DIAPHRAGM INCUBATED IN THE PRESENCE OF GLUCOSE (nm/mg protein)

| Incubation time (min) | Insulin | CP | Intra-Cellular $P_i$ | DHAP | F6P | G6P | PGA | PEP | FDP | ADP | ATP |
|---|---|---|---|---|---|---|---|---|---|---|---|
| 0.5 | – | 52.7 | 48.1 | 0.38 | 0.25 | 1.25 | 0.25 | 0.17 | 0.37 | 4.40 | 21.4 |
|     | + | 54.1 | 48.2 | 0.42 | 0.32 | 1.38 | 0.29 | 0.19 | 0.33 | 4.55 | 22.7 |
| 1   | – | 41.8 | 42.0 |      | 0.30 | 1.14 | 0.29 | 0.17 | 0.29 | 4.01 | 21.7 |
|     | + | 43.2 | 42.0 |      | 0.29 | 1.17 | 0.33 | 0.19 | 0.31 | 3.61 | 22.1 |
| 2   | – | 54.7 | 51.4 | 0.23 | 0.26 | 0.93 | 0.29 | 0.14 | 0.25 | 4.71 | 20.9 |
|     | + | 57.0 | 55.3 | 0.33 | 0.31 | 1.29 | 0.34 | 0.18 | 0.33 | 4.75 | 21.2 |
| 5   | – | 51.7 | 39.0 |      |      | 0.75 | 0.37 | 0.25 | 0.33 | 4.45 | 21.7 |
|     | + | 53.6 | 41.0 |      |      | 0.83 | 0.37 | 0.25 | 0.30 | 4.53 | 21.3 |
| 14  | – | 36.4 | 63.4 | 0.32 | 0.28 | 1.11 | 0.35 | 0.34 | 0.40 | 4.33 | 22.3 |
|     | + | 39.6 | 60.2 | 0.29 | 0.31 | 1.31 | 0.39 | 0.36 | 0.36 | 4.80 | 21.0 |

of serum potassium and phosphate, caused by insulin glucose administration in fructose  feeding.  Table I shows the changes with
time in concentration of organic phosphates when insulin was added
to rat diaphragm in vitro.  The maximum changes in total intracellular organic phosphate concentration seem trivial after insulin, amounting to about 1 milliequivalent per liter, but this is
enough to account for the entire drop in extracellular potassium.

A 1 milliequivalent change in intracellular potassium is impossible to measure accurately, but radioactive measurements, e.g.,
from Ken Zieller's group, are essentially in agreement with this
analysis.  There are about 100 meq of organic phosphates in the
cell - about equal to extracellular chloride concentration.  A
change in these organic phosphates within the cell must be balanced by equal and opposite net change in the extracellular fluid.
Since there is twice as much intracellular as extracellular fluid
a 1 milliequivalent change intracellularly causes an opposite 2
milliequivalent change in the extracellular fluid.  The organic
phosphates cannot leave or enter the cell.  $K_2HPO_4$ is the only
movable form of phosphate and it is freely diffusable.  It is therefore clear that what appears to be a trivial change in intracellular fluid total phosphate produces a major change in the extracellular potassium and phosphate concentrations.

A second general consideration relates to the effect of
changes in cellular organic phosphate as they can affect the osmotic pressure of the cell.  The magnitude of the actual osmotic pressure is generally not appreciated.  The osmotic pressure of an
isotonic solution is 5,000 millimeters of mercury, equivalent to
about 200 feet of water.  In physiological terms this means that
each milliosmole exerts a pressure of about 17 mm of mercury
($\frac{5000}{300}$).  Putting it another way we can say that a differential of
one milliosmole between extracellular and intracellular fluid will
cause water to move into the cell with a pressure of 17 mm of
mercury.  In the case of the brain which is in an inelastic space
a differential of about 10 millimoles between plasma and brain
tissue will cause water to move into the brain cells causing the
brain cells to swell into the vascular space at 170 mm pressure,
effectively obliterating it.  This is irreversible because the
only way the swelling could be reduced is by equilibration via
the vascular spaces.  This is why it is extremely important to
alter the osmolarity very slowly in hyperosmolar states.  A ten
milliosmolar change in intracellular fluid is rather easily attained simply by alterations in ATP and creatine phosphate.

Let us refer to Figure 4.  ATP is composed of a nucleotide
triphosphate with four negative charges which equilibrate with
four intracellular potassium ions, making a total of 5 milliosmoles per millimole of ATP.  With cellular activity ATP breaks

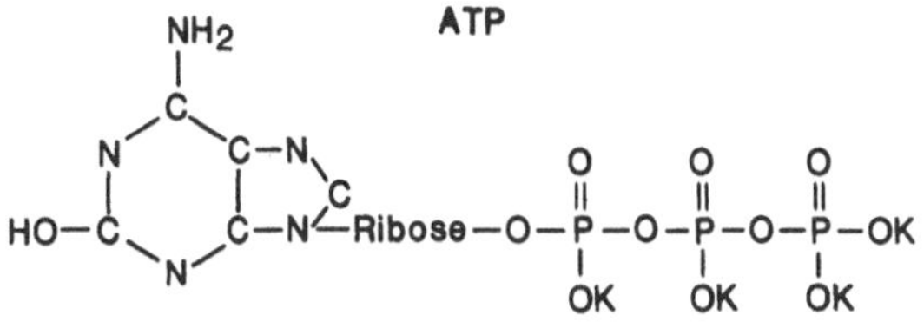

OSMOTIC EFFECTS OF NUCLEOTIDE HYDROLYSIS

|  | Negative Ion | $H\overline{P}O_4$ | $\overset{+}{K}$ | Total Osmoles |
|---|---|---|---|---|
| ATP | 1 | — | 4 | 5 |
| ADP + P | 1 | 1 | 5 | 7 |
| AMP + 2P | 1 | 2 | 6 | 9 |

Figure 4

down to a mole of ADP with three negative charges, a phosphate ion with two negative charges, a proton which exchanges with extracellular potassium, and the four potassium ions originally with ATP. The total milliosmoles is now seven. Conversion of ADP to AMP (which immediately goes to inosinic acid) causes the formation of another phosphate ion, and entrance into the cell of another potassium ion in exchange for a proton. This further increases the total osmoles derived from the original ATP to nine. The total ATP of normal resting muscle is approximately ten millimoles per liter and of brain is about 5 millimoles. The complete breakdown of ATP, e.g. from anoxia would furnish forty extra milliosmoles in a muscle and 20 in brain. This is enough to account for the irreversible death of brain after even short periods of anoxia. This is compounded by the fact that breakdown of creatine phosphate furnishes an additional ten to fifteen milliosmoles.

This brings us to the third problem - the "idiogenic" osmoles seen in hyperosmolar states. In general the organic phosphate compounds of brain have not been considered by any of the investigators of osmotic changes. Recent estimates of phosphate were done by methods which convert all of the ATP and creatine phosphate to

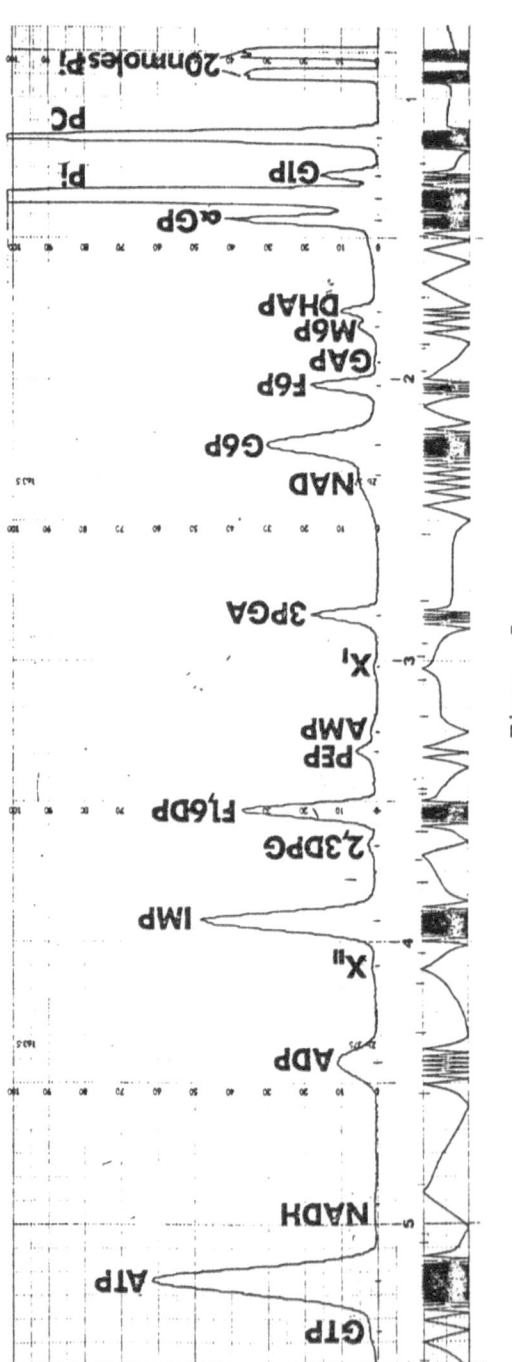

Figure 5

inorganic phosphate, AMP and creatine.  This effectively prevents
any insight into the actual osmotic state of the organic phosphate
since every molecule of phosphate is counted as if it existed as a
free milliosmole even though the bulk of phosphate in the cell is
tied up as ATP (about 40%) and creatine phosphate (20%).

A second fact which has not been considered is the osmotic
contribution of chloride ion.  Dr. Nandita Pal in our laboratory
has demonstrated that the sodium and chloride "spaces" are not
equal and in general the sodium space is much smaller than the
chloride space particularly in hyperchloremia.

Table II shows the data on mice subjected to hyperglycemia
and hyperchloremia.  In order to study the organic phosphate which
comprises at least two thirds of the negative charges of the cell
we have utilized an automatic apparatus constructed in our laboratory which permits us to measure twelve or more of the organic
phosphate compounds in highest concentration in small bits of
tissue.  Figure 5 taken from a chapter to appear shortly shows
the organic phosphates of a piece of muscle tissue.

Swiss Webster mice weighing 35-40 g were used.  In one group
of experiments the mice were given i.p. injections of 1 ml of 4M
NaCl/100 g or 4 ml of 2 M glucose/100 g.  Control mice were given
1 ml of normal saline.  Animals were killed 60 minutes after the
injection.  In another group of experiments the mice were made
diabetic with a single injection of streptozotocin (100 mg/Kg) and
used two weeks later.  These mice were either given 16 units of
insulin or 1.5 ml of 25% glucose over a period of 120 minutes and
killed at 180 minutes.  The mice were killed by a beam of micro-
waves focused on the head for 3 seconds from a 1.5 Kilowatt mi-
crowave oven.  The head was bisected in a vertical sagittal plane
and the brain removed from the right half of the cranium, weighed
and immediately homogenized in ice-cold 10% TCA.  The neutralized
TCA filtrates were analyzed for phosphorylated intermediates by
placing aliquots corresponding to 40 mg wet wt. of tissue on the
columns of the automated phosphate analyzer (2).
The left half of the brain was weighed and dried in an oven at
108° C for 2 hours.  Sodium and potassium were determined by
Perkin-Elmer atomic absorption spectrophotometer using nitric acid
(0.75N) digests.  Chloride was assayed in the same digest using a
Buchler-Cotlove chloridometer.  The plasma electrolytes were assayed using O-tolouidine (3).

The intracellular fluid (ICF) values were based on the sodium
space.  The ICF values based on the chloride space were smaller
hence it was assumed that some chloride may have moved intracel-
luarly.  The calculation of amino acid nitrogen (AAN) and lactate
was based on the data of Chan and Fishman (4).

TABLE II

ACUTE HYPEROSMOLALITY IN MICE

| mmole/Kg $H_2O$ | Control | 4 M NaCl | 2 M Glucose |
|---|---|---|---|
| **Brain** | | | |
| $H_2O$ (%) | 80.7±0.57 (7) | 78.9±1.2 (4) | 74.0±0.61 (7) |
| Organic P | 15.6±0.89 (7) | 17.5±4.6 (4) | 15.4±1.5 (7) |
| Pi | 17.0±1.09 (7) | 32.0±3.4 (4) | 32.0±1.7 (7) |
| $K^+$ | 158 ±2.5 (7) | 224 ±6.8 (4) | 211 ±4.0 (7) |
| Total P + $K^+$ plus AAN, $\bar{L}$ A and cellular Cl | 191 214 | 274 334 | 258 311 |
| **Plasma** | | | |
| $Na^+$ | 138 ±4.5 (7) | 179 ±5.1 (4) | 171 ±6.6 (7) |
| $K^+$ | 4.03±0.01 (7) | 5.1±0.5 (4) | 5.7±0.23 (7) |
| $Cl^-$ | 98 ±0.01 (7) | 171 ±10.1 (4) | 124 ±6.3 (7) |
| Glucose | 5.8±0.34 (7) | 5.8±0.24 (4) | 33.4±2.0 (7) |
| $Na^+ + Cl^- +$ Glucose | 241 | 355 | 328 |

Table III shows that the major osmolar changes in diabetic mice injected with glucose or insulin are related to the phosphate compounds and potassium. In the control animal the total brain phosphate is about 33 milliosmolar but in the diabetic animals it ranged from 50 to 63 milliosmolar, an increment of 18 to 30 milliosmoles. If we assume two potassiums equilibrated with each phosphate this should account for an increment of 36 to 70 potassium ions. The potassium increments are from 58 to 88, and parallel the phosphate changes. There is an excess increment of potassium over phosphate of 22 to 28 milliequivalents, rather uniformly in all diabetic animals.

TABLE III

CHANGES IN DIABETIC MICE

| mmole/Kg $H_2O$ | Control | Diabetic | Diabetic + Insulin | Diabetic + 25% Glucose |
|---|---|---|---|---|
| **Brain** | | | | |
| $H_2O$ (%) | 80.7 ± 0.57 (7) | 78.5 ± 0.77 (8) | 79.1 ± 0.20 (11) | 76.0 ± 0.77 (4) |
| Organic P | 15.6 ± 0.89 (7) | 40.0 ± 2.55 (8) | 22.8 ± 1.9 (11) | 22.5 ± 2.9 (4) |
| Pi | 17.0 ± 1.09 (7) | 23.0 ± 0.35 (8) | 28.7 ± 1.1 (11) | 36.7 ± 3.6 (4) |
| $K^+$ | 158 ± 2.5 (7) | 216 ± 3.1 (8) | 197 ± 3.3 (11) | 206 ± 7.3 (4) |
| Total P + $K^+$ | 191 | 279 | 249 | 265 |
| **Plasma** | | | | |
| $Na^+$ | 138 ± 4.5 (7) | 134 ± 2.0 (8) | 128 ± 3.1 (8) | 129 ± 6.0 (4) |
| $K^+$ | 4.03 ± 0.01 (7) | 4.65 ± 0.32 (8) | 4.69 ± 0.27 (8) | 4.79 ± 0.16 (4) |
| $Cl^-$ | 98 ± 0.01 (7) | 87 ± 0.01 (8) | 99 ± 3.6 (8) | 83 ± 1.8 (4) |
| Glucose | 5.8 ± 0.34 (7) | 22.8 ± 2.26 (8) | 4.6 ± 1.2 (8) | 68.6 ± 10.0 (4) |
| $Na^+$ + $Cl^-$ + Glucose | 241 | 244 | 232 | 281 |

In the case of non-diabetic mice rendered hyperosmolar by intraperitoneal administration of 2 molar glucose or 4 M sodium chloride we find that major osmotic adjustment occurs through changes in intracellular phosphates of about 18 millimoles in both cases. This accounts only for an increment of 36 meq of potassium about half of the actual increment of potassium seen. The difference is apparently made up by intracellular chloride, lactate and amino acids, with chloride being predominant.

A further cause for osmotic changes was noted by A.V. Hill who observed that osmotic changes occurring with muscle contraction could only be accounted for by assuming that a large portion of nucleotides were tightly bound to protein at rest and released by exercise or anoxia, which caused increases in osmotic pressure much greater than could be accounted for.

It is quite clear that until we account for the inorganic and organic phosphate changes, the chloride movement into cells and the binding of nucleotides, it is premature to postulate "idiogenic" osmoles.

Reference:

1.  Quantitative Clinical Chemistry. Interpretations Vol. I, Peters and Van Slyke, 2nd Edition. Williams & Wilkins, Baltimore, MD., 1946

2.  D.P. Bessman, P.J. Geiger, T.C. Lu., and E.R.B. McCabe, Separations and automated analysis of phosphorylated metabolic intermediates, Ann. Biochem. 59:533-546 (1974).

3.  K.M. Dubowski, An O-toluidine method for body-fluid glucose determination, Clin. Chem. 8:215-235 (1962).

4.  R.A. Fishman, M. Reiner, and P.H. Chan, Metabolic changes associated with iso-osmotic regulation in brain cortex slices, J. Neuro. Chem. 28:1061-1067 (1977).

# PHOSPHATE AND ACID-BASE HOMEOSTASIS

Neil A. Kurtzman, M.D.  and Jose A.L. Arruda, M.D.

Departments of Medicine and Physiology
University of Illinois Medical Center
Chicago, Illinois 60612

Both because of its properties as a buffer and its function as a major intracellular anion, phosphate plays a pivotal role in the maintenance of acid-base homeostasis.  This review is concerned with the impact of phosphate on three interrelated aspects of acid-base physiology and pathophysiology.  These are the role of phosphate as a urinary buffer, its relationship to the formation of urinary carbon dioxide tension, and the effects of phosphate depletion on urinary acidification.

## PHOSPHATE AS A URINARY BUFFER

While phosphate is a minor extracellular buffer, under ordinary circumstances it is the single most important urinary buffer (1).  As can be seen fom the following reaction divalent and monovalent phosphate constitute a buffer pair with a pK of 6.8.

$$H^+ + HPO_4^= \xrightleftharpoons[\qquad]{pK\ 6.8} H_2PO_4^-$$

Since the pH of urine is commonly close to the pK of the phosphate buffer pair, it functions as an ideal urinary buffer.  The secretion of protons by the nephron titrates the basic form of phosphate to its acidic form.  The excretion of this buffered acid represents the vast majority of urinary titratable acid.

It is thus apparent that even in the presence of an intact renal acidifying apparatus, urinary acid excretion will be diminished if sufficient phosphate is not delivered to the distal nephron.  Table I lists some of the pathophysiologic states associated with increased distal phosphate delivery.  It is

TABLE I

Decreased Distal $PO_4$ Delivery

1. Hypophosphatemic States

   a. Alcoholics given carbohydrate

   b. Glucose and insulin
      -hyperalimentation
      -treated diabetic ketoacidosis

   c. Respiratory alkalosis

   d. $Al(OH)_3$

   e. Malabsorption

   f. ↓ dietary $PO_4$ intake

2. Renal

   a. Hypoparathyroidism

   b. ↓ effective arterial
      blood volume

   c. Obstructive uropathy

obvious that any hypophosphatemic state will be associated with
decreased delivery of phosphate to the distal nephron owing to
the decrease in filtered load resulting from hypophosphatemia.
Hypophosphatemia may result either from the shift of phosphate
from extracellular to intracellular fluid, or as the result of a
decrease in dietary phosphate intake or the inability to absorb
phosphate across the GI tract.  States associated with high
levels of available insulin or with primary hyperventilation are
examples of the former, while administration of phosphate binders,
malabsorption, and decreased dietary phosphate intake are examples of the latter (2).

     In the presence of normal or even increased concentrations
of phosphate in the blood, decreased distal delivery of phosphate
may result from a variety of renal mechanisms.  These mechanisms
are seen in patients with hypoparathyroidism, a contraction of
effective arterial blood volume, and in subjects with obstructive
uropathy.  The impact of a decrease in titratable acid excretion
owing to decreased distal delivery of phosphate will depend upon
the integrity of the urinary acidifying apparatus and the state
of extrarenal buffering.  Since phosphate depletion has a considerable influence on these processes, the exact state of acid-base
function in any individual instance will depend upon the specific
circumstances which resulted in the decrease in titratable acid
excretion.  These events will be discussed below in the section
on phosphate depletion.

PHOSPHATE AND URINARY $pCO_2$

During the past few years there has been a considerable
increase in the interest in the use of urinary carbon dioxide
tension as an index of distal nephron acidifying capacity.  While
there is still some controversy concerning the precise definition
of the factors which control the generation of a urinary carbon
dioxide tension which exceeds that of plasma (3-5), there is
complete agreement concerning the role of phosphate in this
process.  In a highly alkaline urine (pH greater than 7.8)
normal subjects exhibit a carbon dioxide tension in their urine
which exceeds that of blood by about 30 mmHg.  This carbon dioxide (U-B) gradient is the result of two general processes.  The
first is acidification of the urine, while the second results
from concentration of the urine (3-5).  Concentration of the
urine, by increasing bicarbonate concentration, increases the
generation of $CO_2$.  Acidification of the urine likewise generates
$CO_2$.  Both these processes are illustrated below.

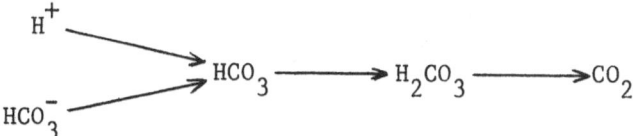

The use of the U-B $pCO_2$ gradients as an index of distal
acidification is predicated on the assumption that the $CO_2$
generated in the urine is the result of hydrogen ion secretion

DISTAL NEPHRON

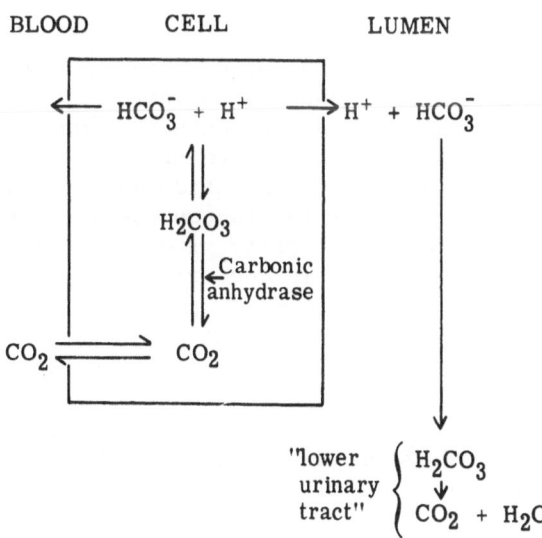

Fig 1: Relationship of $H^+$ secretion to urinary $CO_2$ formation

(Fig 1). If one corrects for the urinary bicarbonate concentration, then the U-B $pCO_2$ gradient in the urine will reflect the
integrity of the acidifying apparatus. Since the pK for the
phosphate buffer system is 6.8, in a highly alkaline urine
almost all phosphate present in the urine will be in its basic
form. This form of phosphate, since it is a base, cannot donate
a hydrogen which in turn would react with urinary bicarbonate to
form $CO_2$. For phosphate to play a role in the generation of
urinary carbon dioxide it must be in a form in which it is capable of donating a proton. In other words, phosphate will play a
role in the generation of a high U-B $pCO_2$ gradient when protons
secreted by a distal nephron can react with a basic form of
phosphate (see below) to form its acidic form.

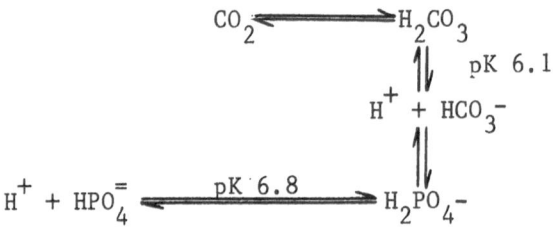

This acid phosphate will, in the lower urinary tract, release
hydrogen ions which in turn, by combining with bicarbonate, will
generate $CO_2$. Thus it is apparent that while phosphate will not
play a role in the generation of carbon dioxide in an alkaline
urine, in a urine which has a pH close to the pK of phosphate,
urinary phosphate concentration will play a crucial role in the
generation of carbon dioxide. If the urinary pH is very much
lower than 6.8 phosphate will be in its acid form, but there will
be no bicarbonate available to titrate to $CO_2$.

Under circumstances where the urinary pH is close to the pK
of phosphate, the ability to generate an increased U-B $pCO_2$
gradient is totally dependent on the concentration of urinary
phosphate (3). The relationship between urinary carbon dioxide
tension and urinary phosphate concentration is linear; i.e., the
higher the phosphate the higher the carbon dioxide tension.
Thus, when one evaluates the integrity of distal acidification by
measuring the U-B $pCO_2$ gradient in the urine of subjects which
have a pH of around 6.8, one must make certain that there is
adequate phosphate in the urine. Normal subjects with low urinary phosphate concentrations will not raise the U-B $pCO_2$ gradient even though the distal acidifying apparatus is totally intact.

In general, disorders of distal renal tubular acidification
can be grouped into two broad classifications (1,5). In one, the
failure of acidification is the result of a defect in hydrogen
ion secretion. The other type of defective distal acidification
results from a defect in urinary acid excretion which is associa-

ted with an intact capacity to secrete protons. Examples of such
defective acidification (Table II) include increased back diffusion of acid (amphotericin-induced renal tubular acidosis), an
inability to maintain a negative intraluminal potential difference in the distal nephron (lithium-induced renal tubular acidosis), a decrease in intraluminal potential difference secondary
to increased tubular permeability to chloride (chloride shunt
acidosis), and enhanced chloride for bicarbonate exchange (no
known example).

TABLE II

Distal renal tubular acidosis

A. Secretory

    1. Abnormal response of U-B $pCO_2$ to $PO_4$ (or Tris)

    2. Abnormal response to $Na_2SO_4$. Examples:

       a. classical dRTA

       b. urinary tract obstruction

B. Non-Secretory

    1. Normal response of U-B $pCO_2$ to $PO_4$ (or Tris)

    2. Normal response to $Na_2SO_4$. Examples:

       a. gradient - amphotericin

       b. PD dependent - lithium

       c. increased permeability to Cl; Cl shunt acidosis

       d. enhanced $HCO_3$-Cl exchange; no known example


    Secretory distal renal tubular acidosis may be distinguished
from renal tubular acidosis associated with normal hydrogen ion
secretory capacity (non-secretory renal tubular acidosis) by a
number of maneuvers (5). One such maneuver includes the administration of phosphate under conditions where the urinary pH is
close to the pK of the phosphate buffer system. In subjects with
impaired proton secretion, the administration of phosphate under
this circumstance will not elicit the normal increase in urinary
carbon dioxide tension associated with an increase in urinary
phosphate concentration. Patients with non-secretory renal
tubular acidosis will respond to phosphate in a normal fashion,
i.e., phosphate administration will result in the expected increase in urinary carbon dioxide tension. This increase will
result since proton secretion is intact, and since secreted
proton is buffered in the tubule, and thus trapped there, by the
phosphate. The formation of acid phosphate will provide the
source of protons necessary for $CO_2$ generation in the post-

papillary urine.  Thus the administration of phosphate to patients
known to have defective distal acidification will distinguish
secretory from non-secretory types of renal tubular acidosis.

PHOSPHATE                          TABLE III

PO$_4$ Depletion and Acid-Base Homeostasis

1. Gold et al (7)

   a. HCO$_3$ wastage in dogs

   b. Proximal RTA

2. Emmett et al (8)

   a. HCO$_3$ wastage in rats

   b. Mild metabolic acidosis

   c. Enhanced extrarenal buffering

3. Kurtz and Hsu (9)

   a. No HCO$_3$ wastage

   b. No metabolic acidosis

   c. Impaired urinary acidification
      after NH$_4$Cl

4. Julka et al (10)

   a. No HCO$_3$ wastage

   b. No metabolic acidosis

   c. Impaired urinary acidification
      after NH$_4$Cl

   d. ↓ NH$_4^+$ excretion

   e. Enhanced extrarenal buffering

   f. Normal U-B pCO$_2$ gradient

PHOSPHATE DEPLETION AND ACID-BASE HOMEOSTASIS (Table III)

     Deficiency of phosphate, as has been mentioned above,
decreases urinary acid excretion by removing the substrate for
titratable acid formation in urine (6).  In addition to this
mechanism it has become quite clear, in recent years, that phosphate depletion also impairs the acidifying apparatus.  Gold and
colleagues (7) demonstrated that dogs which were phosphate depleted developed metabolic acidosis.  The degree of metabolic acidosis was linearly correlated to the plasma phosphate concentration.
The greater the degree of phosphate depletion and hypophosphatemia

the greater the degree of metabolic acidosis. These workers
showed that the phosphate depleted animals had a major defect in
bicarbonate reclamation. In other words, these animals had
proximal renal tubular acidosis. Since the intracellular pH of
skeletal muscle in these animals was greatly increased during
phosphate depletion it was hypothesized that the defect in proximal acidification resulted from an elevation of intracellular pH
of the proximal tubule.

Emmett and coworkers (8) studied urinary acidification in
the phosphate depleted rat. They demonstrated bicarbonate wastage in their animals. An effort was not made in this study to
distinguish between defective proximal or distal acidification,
so the site of impaired acidification responsible for the bicarbonate leak cannot be ascertained. The animals studied had mild
metabolic acidosis. The moderate degree of this metabolic acidosis was attributed to enhanced extrarenal buffering capacity in
phosphate depleted animals. Enhanced extrarenal buffering capacity would counteract the tendency of decreased renal acid
excretion to cause acidemia. When phosphate depleted animals
were nephrectomized, plasma concentration and pH remained at
significantly higher values than were seen in normal animals that
were nephrectomized and similarly studied. An effect of phosphate depletion to enhance bone buffering was suggested from
additional studies which showed that colchicine, an agent which
inhibits bone resorption, resulted in a marked fall in plasma
bicarbonate concentration in phosphate depleted animals.

Kurtz and Hsu (9), in a recent study of phosphate depleted
rats, failed to demonstrate bicarbonate wastage and also did not
observe metabolic acidosis. They did, however, note that phosphate depleted rats failed to lower urinary pH appropriately
during ammonium chloride induced metabolic acidosis.

In a study just completed in our laboratory, we observed
that phosphate depleted rats did not develop metabolic acidosis
or bicarbonate wastage (10). Bicarbonate reclamation during
bicarbonate loading was the same as that seen in control animals.
We noted, as did Kurtz and Hsu (9), that the ability to acidify
the urine following ammonium chloride administration was impaired
by phosphate depletion. In addition, we noted that animals
phosphate depleted for 60 days had a marked decrease in urinary
ammonium excretion. The combination of decreased urinary acid
excretion secondary to decreased ammonium excretion and the
decrease in titratable acid excretion, owing to the phosphate
depletion, resulted in a major decline in net acid excretion.
Despite this major defect in urinary acidification, the animals
did not have metabolic acidosis. This failure to develop metabolic acidosis was doubtless the result of enhanced extrarenal
buffering capacity as suggested by Emmett and coworkers (8).

This was demonstrated by the administration of hydrochloric acid
to normal animals and to phosphate depleted animals. This procedure resulted in a greatly attenuated fall in blood pH and
bicarbonate concentration in the phosphate depleted animals as
compared to the normal controls.

Additional studies suggested that the defect in urinary
acidification observed in phosphate depletion was of the non-
secretory type. This conclusion was reached because of the
response of urinary $pCO_2$ to bicarbonate loading and buffer administration. During bicarbonate loading phosphate depleted animals
had a urinary $pCO_2$ tension which was equal to that of control
animals. Since phosphate depleted animals were the subject of
this investigation, phosphate could not be administered to test
the integrity of the acidifying apparatus; in its place Tris
buffer was infused. The response of urinary carbon dioxide
tension to Tris buffer administration is the same as that to
phosphate administration. Following this maneuver urine carbon
dioxide tension increased to the same degree in the phosphate
depleted animals as it did in the control animals. The most
likely explanation for the impaired acidifying capacity of phosphate depleted animals is that phosphate depletion results in
intracellular alkalosis (Fig 2). Intracellular alkalosis markedly
decreases the capacity to secrete protons even though the proton
secretory pump itself is uninvolved. The integrity of this pump

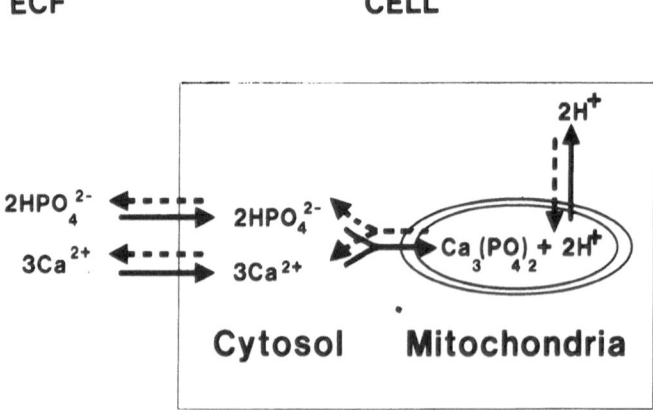

Fig 2:  Mechanism whereby phosphate depletion decreases cytosolic
        $H^+$ concentration.

is demonstrated by a normal response of urinary carbon dioxide
tension to buffer administration.  It is possible that under
extreme degrees of phosphate depletion the energy requirements of
the pump will not be met and proton secretion will be impaired by
this mechanism as well.

It seems likely that both proximal and distal acidification
may be impaired by phosphate depletion (Table IV).  The site in

TABLE IV

Response to $PO_4$ Depletion.

1. Impaired proximal $HCO_3$ reabsorption

2. Impaired distal acidification

   a. ↓ $PO_4$ delivery

   b. ↓ $NH_3$ excretion/production

   c. ↓ pH gradient

3. Enhanced extrarenal buffering capacity

the nephron and the degree of deficient acidification will vary
according to the species studied and to the degree of phosphate
depletion induced.  Depending upon these variables, one may see
impaired proximal bicarbonate reabsorption which will manifest
itself as proximal renal tubular acidosis.  Under other circumstances, impaired distal acidification may predominate as the
result of at least three effects attributable to phosphate depletion.  The first is a decrease of phosphate delivery to the
distal nephron which results in decreased titratable acid formation.  The second is that phosphate depletion appears to retard
the kidney's ability to form and excrete ammonium (10,11).  In
this regard additional studies which directly measure ammonium
production are required before such a conclusion can be reached
with finality.  The third way that phosphate depletion can impair
distal acidification is by reducing the capacity to generate a
maximum pH gradient between the blood and the lumen of the distal
nephron.  The expression of the derangement in urinary acidification induced by phosphate depletion will be attenuated to the
degree that extrarenal buffering capacity is enhanced by phosphate depletion.  The factors responsible for this enhanced
extrarenal buffering response and the exact nature of its mechanism are still to be elucidated.

REFERENCES

1.  Arruda JAL and Kurtzman NA: Metabolic acidosis and alkalo-
    sis.  Clin Nephrol 7:201-215, 1977.

2.  Massry SG and Coburn JW: Divalent ions and the kidney.  In Pathophysiology of the Kidney (Kurtzman NA and Martinez-Maldonado M, eds); Charles C. Thomas, Springfield, 1977.

3.  Arruda JAL, Nascimento L, Kumar SK and Kurtzman NA: Factors influencing the formation of urinary carbon dioxide tension. Kidney Internat 11:307-317, 1977.

4.  Arruda JAL, Nascimento L, Mehta PK, Rademacher DR, Sehy JT, Westenfelder C and Kurtzman NA: The critical importance of urinary concentrating ability in the generation of urinary carbon dioxide tension.  J Clin Invest 60:922-935, 1977.

5.  Kurtzman NA and Arruda JA: Physiologic significance of urinary carbon dioxide tension.  Min Elect Metab 1:241-246, 1978.

6.  Massry SG: Effect of phosphate depletion on renal function and metabolism.  Proc VIIth Internat Cong Neph 7:625-633, 1978.

7.  Gold SW, Massry SG, Arieff AI and Coburn JW: Renal bicarbonate wasting during phosphate depletion.  A possible cause of altered acid-base homeostasis in hyperparathyroidism.  J Clin Invest 52:2556-2565, 1973.

8.  Emmett M. Goldfarb S, Agus ZS and Narins RC: The pathophysiology of acid-base changes in chronically phosphate depleted rats.  Bone-Kidney interactions.  J Clin Invest 59:291-298, 1977.

9.  Kurtz TW and Hsu CH: Impaired distal nephron acidification in chronically phosphate depleted rats.  Pflüg Arch 337:229-234, 1978.

10. Julka NK, Sabatini S, Arruda JAL and Kurtzman NA: Distal acidification defect (AD) induced by phosphate depletion. Clin Res 26:691A, 1978.

11. Kohaut EC, Klish WJ, Beachler CW and Hill LL: Reduced renal acid excretion in malnutrition: A result of phosphate depletion.  Amer J Clin Nutr 30:861-867, 1977.

# PHOSPHATE, CALCIUM AND LIPID METABOLISM

Eberhard Ritz, Claus-Christian Heuck,
Ricardo Boland

Department Internal Medicine and
Max-Planck-Institut Heidelberg, Germany

There exists a rather extensive literature on possible interrelations between calcium and phosphate metabolism on the one hand and lipid metabolism on the
other hand. Unfortunately, much of the information is da-
ted or contradictory and few of the interrelationships
have been clarified with respect to the underlying mechanism. For the purpose of this discussion, table 1 provides a conceptual framework of how various aspects of
Ca and phosphate homeostasis may act on different reactions in lipid metabolism.

Table 1

Schema of possible interactions between calcium or
phosphate  and lipid metabolism

| Ca or Pi | may act directly | lipolysis |
|---|---|---|
| (extra- and/or | or indirectly | lipoprotein synthesis |
| intracellular), | (e.g.via insulin) | or catabolism |
| intestinal Ca, | on: | |
| vitamin D | | |
| PTH | | |

Historically, much interest in this area has been
generated by the association of water hardness and cardiovascular disease. In several countries it was found
that the highest death rates from various forms of cardiovascular mortality are observed in areas with soft
drinking water (1,2,3).

Table 2

Mean death rates per 1oo.ooo (1958-64) from cardiovascular disease at ages 45-64 years related to water Ca

| Water Ca<br>(p.p.m.) | Males | Females |
|---|---|---|
| < 1o | 751 | 355 |
| 1o - 39 | 721 | 33o |
| 4o - 69 | 636 | 3o6 |
| 7o - 99 | 633 | 281 |
| > 1oo | 546 | 248 |

After Shaper, Clayton and Morris (ref. 3)

Anatomical studies failed to show a higher preva-
lence of extensive atheroma and more severe stenosis of
the coronary arteries in hard as opposed to soft water
areas (3). In epidemiological studies, differences of
heart rate and casual diastolic pressure were observed
between hard and soft water areas, but less consistent
differences between such areas were found for serum cholesterol. Consequently, it is far from settled whether
the effect of water hardness is mediated by changes in
lipid metabolism. Furthermore, since drinking water Ca
content is correlated with water acidity and water trace
metal content, it may well be that water Ca is only an
index of some other underlying pathogenic factor.

A suggestive correlation between vitamin D consumption and myocardial infarction (4) was not confirmed in
a more recent prospective study, in which no correlation
between serum 25(OH)D levels and incidence of myocardial
infarction could be observed (5).

In adipocytes, both lipolysis, i.e. liberation of
fatty acids from triacylglycerol of adipocytes, and lipoprotein lipase activity, i.e. cleavage of free fatty
acids from circulating lipoproteins, may be modulated
by Ca. At least under some conditions, lipolysis is accompanied by cellular uptake of Ca (6,7,8). Furthermore,
in rat adipocytes, hormonal activation of lipolysis by
isoproterenol and thyrotrophin, but not the lipolytic
activity of glucagon and secretin, is reduced in the absence of external Ca (9). The activity of lipoprotein
lipase, isolated from pig adipose tissue (1o), was dependent on Ca concentration. Whether this plays any significant role in vivo remains undecided.

Dietary Ca supplements cause a decrease in serum
cholesterol and serum triglycerides in man (11) and in
rats (12). Ca acts by increasing fecal bile acids and fecal free fatty acids (13) and by a redistribution of lipids between the blood and tissue pools. As shown in
table 2, ingestion of 2 g of supplemental dietary Ca
carbonate over a period of one year by lo hyperlipemic
subjects caused a 25% decrease in serum cholesterol and
a striking decrease in serum triglycerides despite no
change in body weight (14). Short term infusion of rather
small amounts of Ca, in contrast to oral Ca, failed to
affect serum cholesterol and ß-lipoproteins (15).

Table 3

Effect of long term administration of supplemental dietary Ca (2 g) on serum cholesterol (mg/dl)

| before | after |
|---|---|
| 316 | 274 |
| 435 | 272 |
| 525 | 36o |
| 393 | 293 |
| 3o7 | 27o |
| 372 | 269 |
| 247 | 2o6 |
| 244 | 224 |
| 276 | 187 |
| 375 | 326 |

| | | |
|---|---|---|
| mean + SD | 349 | 262 |
| | + 28,3 | + 16,6 |

After Bierenbaum et al., LIPIDS, 7, 2o2, 1972 (ref.14)

Apart from Ca, vitamin D is known to influence
serum lipid concentrations. In 1932, Pfleiderer (16)
observed that the development of atherosclerosis was
stimulated by the combined administration of vitamin D
and cholesterol. Other investigators observed that vitamin D intensified the degree and increased the rate
of development of hypercholesterolemia in rabbits on a
cholesterol diet (17) or in rats subjected to a variety
of dietary and endocrine manoeuvres (18). It is also of
note that in children with idiopathic hypercalcemia, a
state of hypersensitivity to vitamin D, a rise in total
cholesterol and free cholesterol with no change of cholesterol esters is consistently observed (19). In humans,
under carefully controlled conditions of dietary intake,

vitamin D in supraphysiological doses was found to reversibly raise serum cholesterol (19,2o) without change
in serum triglycerides.

Table 4

The effects of vitamin $D_3$ upon serum cholesterol (mg/dl)
in human adults (after Fleischmann et al.; ref. 2o)

| Subject | preexperi-<br>mental | after 21 days<br>5o.ooo IU daily | after 21 days<br>recovery |
|---------|--------------------|--------------------------------|-------------------------|
| 1 | 244 | 285 | 264 |
| 2 | 334 | 365 | 328 |
| 3 | 212 | 234 | 21o |
| 4 | 165 | 189 | 186 |
| 5 | 28o | 3o5 | 297 |
| 6 | 168 | 199 | 163 |
| 7 | 259 | 295 | 243 |
| 8 | 17o | 171 | 157 |

Fleischmann et al. (2o) proposed that the effect
of vitamin D was mediated by changes in intestinal Ca
transport. In a pilot study in ricketic rats, we found
a significant acute fall in serum triglycerides and a
suggestive but not significant rise in serum cholesterol
upon acute repletion with vitamin D or $1,25(OH)_2D$ (see
table 5).

Table 5

Effects of acute repletion with vitamin $D_3$ and $1,25(OH)_2D$
on serum lipids in ricketic rats

|  | triglycerides<br>mmol/L | cholesterol<br>mmol/L |
|---|-----------------------|----------------------|
| ricketic<br>(n = 9) | 1.76<br>$\pm$ o.42 | 2.94<br>$\pm$ o.36 |
| ricketic + $D_3$<br>(n = 12) | 1.12*<br>$\pm$ o.272 | 3.39<br>$\pm$ o.54 |
| ricketic + $1,25(OH)_2D$<br>(n = 12) | o.844*<br>$\pm$ o.257 | 3.17<br>$\pm$ o.55 |

Rats fed from weanling with rachitogenic diet (Altromin
1o17) were given 1o ug $D_3$ 72 and 48 h or 15 ng $1,25(OH)_2$
$D_3$ 72, 48 and 24 h before death. Animals had free access
to food and deionised water. Values are $\bar{x} \pm$ SD (* p o.o2)

This result suggests that an effect of vitamin D on intestinal Ca cannot entirely explain the vitamin D induced changes in serum lipids and that other effects, perhaps indirectly mediated by PTH (see below) have to be taken into account. Other possibilities include changes in serum Ca, Pi, insulin etc. It has also been stated, but apparently not reported in detail, that addition of vitamin D to liver homogenates stimulates cholesterol synthesis (21).

Parathyroid hormone has well defined effects on lipid metabolism. The stimulatory effect of PTH on adipose tissue lipase has been noted both in animals (22,23) and in man (24). Sinha et al. (24) observed increased glycerol release by human adipose fat tissue in vitro and increased serum FFA upon infusion of supraphysiological doses of PTH both in normal subjects and in individuals with pseudohypoparathyroidism. Furthermore, Kather and Simon (25) found a stimulatory effect of the synthetic aminoterminal 1,34 PTH fragment on the basal and GMP(PNP) liganded adenylate cyclase of human fat cell ghosts. This effect was additive to that of epinephrine. It is of note that apart from catecholamines, and with the possible exception of some gastrointestinal hormones, PTH is the only hormone known to activate adipose tissue lipase of adult humans (26). In other species, glucagon, ACTH, thyrotropin and other hormones have also been shown to activate lipolysis. The physiological role, if any, of PTH stimulated lipolysis is unknown, but it is remarkable that Hallberg and Werner (27) when studying the effect of a bolus injection of PTE in fasted dogs, saw an increase in serum glycerol and serum FFA prior to, and with lower doses even in the absence of, a change in serum Ca.

No published information is available on possible effects of PTH on de novo fatty acid synthesis and lipoprotein synthesis in the liver. Moxley et al. (28) demonstrated a PTH sensitive adenylate cyclase on hepatocytes which would clearly make such actions conceivable. Heuck and Ritz (29) found no effect of parathyroidectomy on HMG-CoA-reductase, the rate limiting enzyme in the hepatic synthesis of cholesterol.

Several authors round carbohydrate intolerance and hyperinsulinemia in primary hyperparathyroidism and proposed a role of PTH in insulin secretion or glucose catabolism. Such PTH mediated changes in insulin secretion might conceivably alter hepatic synthesis and peripheral

catabolism of lipoproteins. However, studies of Harter et al. (3o) convincingly document that PTH is not a direct insulin antagonist and has no apparent effect on either glucose- or tolbutamide stimulated insulin release. In contrast, hypophosphatemia augments glucose stimulated and hypercalcemia increases tolbutamide stimulated insulin release.
No information is available on possible effects of PTH on lipoprotein catabolism, apart from a preliminary report (29) that parathyroidectomy fails to affect the rate of catabolism of infused lipid emulsions (Intralipid R) in rats.

If the known effects of PTH on adipose tissue lipolysis were of overriding importance, one would anticipate that serum triglycerides are elevated in hyperparathyroidism as the result of increased delivery of FFA to hepatocytes. This expectation is apparently born out by an old observation of Paloyan (31). PTX caused a significant fall of serum cholesterol and administration of PTE a significant increase of both serum cholesterol and total serum lipids. However, at the dose level used, one cannot with certainty exclude nephrocalcinosis and this raises the possibility of uremic hyperlipemia. Ljunghall et al. (32) found type IV hyperlipoproteinemia in large proportion of patients with primary hyperparathyroidism. Postoperatively, peak insulin levels and insulin index had decreased and serum lipids normalized without change of adipose tissue lipoprotein lipase. It was suggested that exaggerated insulin response stimulated the synthesis of VLDL in the liver to a degree that was not compensated for by an increase in adipose tissue lipoprotein lipase.

Other authors, however, contrary to what one might anticipate, found low cholesterol (33,34) and triglyceride (34) levels in patients with primary hyperparathyroidism. Both cholesterol and triglycerides rose after surgical removal of parathyroid adenoma despite no change of body weight or serum $T_4$ levels (33,34).

In summary, in experimental and clinical hyperparathyroidism, data on changes of serum lipids and their response to withdrawal of PTH excess, are contradictory and difficult to interpret. This might well indicate that the changes observed in hyperparathyroid patients result not only from the known stimulatory effect of PTH on adipose tissue lipolysis, but are also dependent on secondary changes of Ca and Pi concentrations, insulin secretion or vitamin D metabolism.

Taking up some old observations by Cantin (35),
Massry recently proposed (3() that secondary hyperparathyroidism may contribute to hyperlipoproteinemia in
uremic subjects. This notion finds some support in the
experiments of Heuck et al. (37) who compared parathyroid
intact and parathyroidectomized rats with experimental
uremia (two stage subtotal nephrectomy  with irradiation
of renal parenchyma). In rats with this model of uremia,
the adenylate cyclase of fat cell ghosts of epididymal
fat was activated in a normal fashion by PTH (38). Consequently, in vivo lipolysis should have been stimulated
by increased endogenous PTH levels, although this was not
directly measured. As shown in table 6, fasting serum
cholesterol levels were higher in parathyroid intact
uremic as compared with parathyroid intact sham operated
pairfed control animals. However, the increment in serum
cholesterol was significantly smaller in nephrectomized
animals without parathyroids. Basically  the same behaviour could be observed for fasting serum triglycerides
and serum phospholipids.

Table 6

Influence of parathyroid status on serum cholesterol
levels in uremic rats (after Heuck et al.; ref.37)

|  | cholesterol mmol/L | triglycerides mmol/L |
|---|---|---|
| CO | 1.13 $\pm$ o.2o | o.77 $\pm$ o.23 |
| NX | 2.4 $\pm$ o.845 | o.944 $\pm$ o.156 |
| PTX | 1.18 $\pm$ o.375 | o.5o4 $\pm$ o.133 |
| PTX-NX | 1.78 $\pm$ o.473 | o.78 $\pm$ o.225 |

Values $\bar{x}$ + SD (n = lo per group); CO pair fed, sham op
controls; PTX parathyroidectomy; NX nephrectomy; duration of the experiment 2o days.

This study indicates that the presence of parathyroid glands plays some permissive role for the magnitude
of hyperlipemia in renal failure. Serum lipids in uremic
animals without parathyroids were still higher than in
control animals with parathyroids. The rise of lipids
in the absence of parathyroids shows that factors other
than PTH are responsible for the primary defect which

underlies uremic hyperlipoproteinemia.
Several lines of evidence suggest that the effect of
secondary hyperparathyroidism is not due to the associated changes of serum Ca and Pi. Normocalcemia was achieved in some PTX animals by high Ca diet. After nephrectomy, serum cholesterol, triglycerides and phospholipids
rose to an equal extent in PTX uremic animals irrespective of hypo- or normocalcemia.

Additional experiments (29,37, Heuck and Ritz, in
preparation) suggest that lipoprotein catabolism, as
evaluated by the clearance of infused exogenous lipid
emulsions (Intralipid R) was markedly diminished in uremic animals irrespective of the presence or absence of
parathyroids. This finding suggests, but does not prove,
that PTH affects lipoprotein synthesis rather than lipoprotein catabolism.

Such indirect evidence leads one to conclude that
PTH affects serum lipids in experimental uremia by modulating hepatic synthesis of lipoproteins. However, several investigators found diminished hepatic synthesis
of lipoproteins both in uremic animals (38-4o) and in
uremic man (41) despite secondary hyperparathyroidism.
This apparent contradiction can be resolved, however, by
the findings of Sanfelippo et al. (41) that diet induced
changes in hepatic triglyceride synthesis caused parallel changes in serum triglyceride levels although the absolute rate of hepatic synthesis remained lower than in
normals. Consequently, it is conceivable that by raising
delivery of FFA to the liver, PTH increases lipoprotein
synthesis in uremic individuals in such a way that the
latter, although lower than normal, becomes more inappro-
priate for the prevailing rate of lipoprotein catabolism.

It is unknown to what extent this concept which is
based on experimental studies does also apply to the situation in humans. DeMoor et al. (31) found no change of
serum lipids after PTX in patients with renal secondary
hyperparathyroidism as opposed to patients with primary
hyperparathyroidism. One group (42) reported even an inverse relation between  PTH and serum triglycerides.
Therefore, the role of secondary hyperparathyroidism on
hyperlipemia of uremic patients clearly requires further
studies.

SUMMARY

Ca and Pi interact with lipid metabolism in several
different ways. The enzymes of lipolysis and lipogenesis

are sensitive to Ca. Ca and Pi concentrations affect insulin secretion and insulin action. Raising intestinal
Ca lowers serum cholesterol and triglycerides presumably
by sequestration of cholesterol and bile acids. Administration of vitamin D or increased sensitivity to vitamin D raise serum cholesterol levels. PTH acts primarily
by activating adipose tissue lipase. Increased FFA delivery to the liver should increase hepatic lipoprotein
synthesis. Experimental data in secondary hyperparathyroidism of renal insufficiency are consistent with this
notion. Clinical observations in primary or renal secondary hyperparathyroidism, however, are not explicable by
this simple schema.

References

1. J.N. Morris, M.D. Crawford, J.A. Heady, Hardness of
   local water supplies and mortality from cardiovascular disease in county boroughs of England and Wales
   Lancet i, 860 (1961)
2. T.W. Anderson, W.H. Le Riche, J.S. Mac Kay, Sudden
   death and ischemic heart disease – correlations with
   hardness of local water supply, New Engl.J.Med.280:
   805 (1969)
3. A.G. Shaper, D.G. Clayton, J.N. Morris, Hard and soft
   water in relation to the incidence of cardiovascular
   disease, in: "Atherosclerosis III", G. Schettler,
   A. Weizel, eds., Springer, Berlin (1974) p 715
4. V. Lindén, Vitamin D and myocardial infarction, Brit.
   Med.J. 3:647 (1974)
5. V. Torstein, T. Kenneth, D.S. Thelle, O.H. Førde,
   Tromsø Heart Study: Vitamin D metabolism and myocardial interaction, Brit.Med.J. 2:176 (1979)
6. S. Werner, K. Hall, H. Löw, Similar effects of calcitonin, insulin and somatomedin on lipolysis and uptake of calcium and glucose in rat adipose tissue
   in vitro, Horm.Metab.Res. 6:319 (1974)
7. S. Akgün, D. Rudman, Relationship between mobilisation of free fatty acids from adipose tissue, and
   the concentrations of calcium in the extracellular
   fluid and in the tissue, Endocrinology 84:926 (1969)
8. S. Werner, H. Löw, Adenylate cyclase activity in rat
   adipocyte plasma membranes after adrenalectomy and
   administration of cortisone acetate – effects of
   calcium ions and hormonal stimulation, Horm.Metab.
   Res. 6:365 (1974)
9. R.J. Schimmel, The influence of extracellular calcium
   ion on hormone activated lipolysis, Biochim.Biophys.
   Acta 326:272 (1973)

10. A. Bensandoun, C. Ehnholm, D. Steinberg, W.V. Brown, Purification and characterisation of lipoprotein lipase from pig adipose tissue, J.Biol.Chem. 249: 222o (1974)

11. H. Yacowitz, H.I. Fleischman, M.L. Bierenbaum, Effect of oral calcium upon serum lipids in man, Brit.Med. J. 1:1352 (1965)

12. A.I. Fleischman, H. Yacowitz, T. Hayton, M.L. Bierenbaum, Effects of dietary calcium upon lipid metabolism in mature male rats fed beef tallow, J.Nutr. 38:255 (1966)

13. A.I. Fleischman, H. Yacowitz, T. Hayton, M.L. Bierenbaum, Long-term studies on the hypolipemic effect of dietary calcium in mature male rats fed cocoa butter, J.Nutr.91:151 (1967)

14. M.L. Bierenbaum, A.I. Fleischman, R.I. Raichelson, Long-term human studies on the lipid effects of oral calcium, Lipids 7:2o2 (1972)

15. E. Maibach, Die Beeinflussung des Gesamtcholesterins der beta-Lipoproteide und Gesamtlipide des Serums durch orale und parenterale Calciumzufuhr, Schweiz. Med.Wschr. 97:418 (1967)

16. E. Pfleiderer, Tierexperimentelle Untersuchungen über Arteriosklerose unter besonderer Berücksichtigung der Kranzarteriensklerose, Virchows Arch.Path.Anat. 284:154 (1932)

17. C.D. De Langen, W.F. Donath, Vitamin D, sclerosis of the arteries and the danger of feeding extra vitamin D to older people with a view on the development of different forms of arteriosclerosis, Acta Med.Scand. 156:317 (1956)

18. Lee Cheng-Chun, R.G. Herrmann, Effects of vitamin D sucrose, corn oil and endocrines on tissue cholesterol in rats, Circulation Res. 7:354 (1959)

19. J.O. Forfar, S.L. Tompsett, W. Forshall, Biochemical studies in idiopathic hypercalcemia of infancy, Arch.Dis.Childh. 34:525 (1959)

20. A.I. Fleischman, M.L. Bierenbaum, R. Raichelson, T. Hayton, P. Watson, Vitamin D and hypercholesterolemia in adult humans, in: "Atherosclerosis" (Proc. 2nd Intern.Symp.), R.J. Jones, ed., Springer, Berlin (197o) p 468

21. M.Dempsey, Discussion, in: "Atherosclerosis" (Proc. 2nd Intern.Symp.), R.J. Jones, ed., Springer, Berlin (197o) p 485

22. S. Werner, H. Löw, Stimulation of lipolysis and calcium accumulation by parathyroid hormone in rat adipose tissue in vitro after adrenalectomy and administration of high doses of cortisone acetate, Horm.Metab.Res. 5:292 (1973)

23. L. Gozariu, K. Forster, J.D. Faulhaber, H. Minne,
    R. Ziegler, Parathyroid hormone and calcitonin:
    Influences upon lipolysis of human adipose tissue,
    Horm.Metab.Res. 6:243 (1974)
24. T.K. Sinha, P. Thajchayapong, S.F. Queener, D.O. Allen,
    N.H. Bell, On the lipolytic action of parathyroid
    hormone in man, Metabolism 25:251 (1976)
25. H. Kather, B. Simon, Adenylate cyclase of human fat
    cell ghosts, stimulation of enzyme activity by pa-
    rathyroid hormone, J.Clin.Invest. 59:73o (1977)
26. H. Kather, B. Simon, Human fat cell adenylate cyclase:
    Responsiveness towards catecholamines, peptide hor-
    mones and prostaglandins, in: "Lipoprotein Metabo-
    lism and Endocrine Regulation", L.W. Hessel, H.M.J.
    Kraus, eds., Elsevier, Amsterdam (1979) p 189
27. D. Hallberg, S. Werner, Circulatory and lipolytic
    effects of parathyroid hormone, Horm.Metab.Res.
    9:424 (1977)
28. M.A. Moxley, N.H. Bell, R.S. Wagle, D.O. Allen,J.
    Ashmore, Parathyroid hormone stimulation of glu-
    cose and urea production in isolated liver cells,
    Am.J.Physiol. 227:1o58 (1974)
29. C.C. Heuck, E. Ritz, Does parathyroid hormone play
    a role in lipid metabolism?, Contrib.Nephrol. (in
    press)
30. H.R. Harter, J.V. Santiago, W.E. Rutherford, E. Sla-
    topolsky, S. Klahr, The relative roles of calcium,
    phosphorous and parathyroid hormone in glucose and
    tolbutamide mediated insulin release, J.Clin.In-
    vest. 58:359 (1976)
31. E. Paloyan, J. Kolar, J. Castles, D. Paloyan, V. Har-
    per, The role of parathyroid hormone in lipid me-
    tabolism, Fed.Proc. 22:676 (1963)
32. S. Ljunghall, H. Lithell, L. Wide, Hyperlipoprotein-
    emia type IV and hyperinsulinemia in primary hyper-
    parathyroidism. Effect of parathyroidectomy, Acta
    Endocr. (Kopenhagen) (in press)
33. P. De Moor, G. Creyttens, R. Bouillon, J.V. Joossens,
    Results obtained in 75 patients operated upon for
    hyperparathyroidism: low cholesterol levels in
    overt primary hyperparathyroidism, Ann.Endocr.
    34:616 (1973)
34. T. Christenson, K. Einarson, Serum lipids before and
    after parathyroidectomy in patients with primary
    hyperparathyroidism, Clin.Chim.Acta 78:411 (1977)
35. M. Cantin, Kidney, parathyroid and lipemia, Lab.
    Invest. 14:1691 (1965)

36. S.G. Massry, Is parathyroid hormone an uremic toxin? Nephron 19:125 (1977)

37. C.C. Heuck, W. Kreusser, O. Mehls, E. Ritz, Die Rolle von PTH bei der urämischen Hyperlipämie, Verh.Dtsch. Ges.Inn.Med. 85 (1979) (in press)

38. H. Kather, H.C. Heuck, W. Tschöpe, E. Ritz, B. Simon, Unchanged hormone sensitivity of rat fat cell adenylate cyclase in uremia, Clin.Nephrol.8:324 (1977)

39. J.D. Bagdade, E. Yee, D.E. Wilson, E. Shafrir, Hyperlipidemia in renal failure: Studies of plasma lipoproteins, hepatic triglyceride production and tissue lipoprotein lipase in a chronical uremic rat model, J.Lab.Clin.Med. 91:176 (1978)

40. C.C. Heuck, M. Liersch, E. Ritz, K. Stegmeier, A. Wirth, O. Mehls, Hyperlipoproteinemia in experimental chronic renal insufficiency in the rat, Kidney International 14:142 (1978)

41. M.L. Sanfelippo, R.S. Swenson, G.M. Reaven, Reduction of plasma triglycerides by diet in subjects with chronic real failure, Kidney International II:54 (1977)

42. J.D. Brunzell, A.P. Goldberg, Hormonal regulation of human adipose tissue lipoprotein lipase, in: "Atherosclerosis IV", G. Schettler et al.,eds., Springer, Berlin (1977) p 336

# PROTECTIVE EFFECT OF PHOSPHATE RESTRICTION ON RENAL FUNCTION

Allen C. Alfrey, Malcolm Karlinsky, Lewis Haut

V.A. Medical Center and University of Colorado Medical
School, Division of Nephrology, Denver, CO 80220
U.S.A.

Somewhere between 50 and 75 persons per every 1,000,000 population develop end-stage renal disease annually.  In view of the
extreme expense and in general unsatisfactory response to treatment
it would seem highly desirable to prevent rather than treat end -
stage kidney disease.  It is a well recognized fact that renal
calcium-phosphate deposits resulting from a number of clinical
conditions including sarcoidosis, milk alkali syndrome, hyperparathyroidism and vitamin D intoxication can incite an inflammatory and fibrotic response which may ultimately result in total
loss of renal function (1-4).  Since renal parenchymal calcification is also a common finding in human end-stage kidneys (5-8)
irrespective of the primary renal disease it is possible that this
promotes further damage to the diseased kidney.  It is apparent
that renal calcification could have major clinical implications.

When a critical level of renal functional deterioration has
occurred from a variety of different renal diseases, there is
almost invariable progression to total loss of renal function.
Ahlmén (9) found that the median time for renal impairment to
progress to end-stage disease after the plasma creatinine had increased to 5 mg/dl was 6 months in patients with diabetic nephropathy, 10 months in patients with glomerulonephritis and 14
months in patients with non-obstructive pyelonephritis.  Renal
parenchymal calcification could be a late common pathogenic mechanism which accelerates the rate of functional deterioration.

A number of studies have been performed to determine if calcification accelerates renal functional deterioration in the dam-
aged or diseased kidney.  It has been known for a number of years

that if a critical mass of renal tissue is removed, in a variety
of species, proteinuria and progressive deterioration of renal
function will develop in the animal, which will eventually die in
uremia (10-13). A number of different mechanisms for the progressive deterioration of renal function have been implicated. It has
been known for years that high protein intake is especially injurious to the kidney when renal mass is reduced (14-19). It was
thought that excretion of end products of protein metabolism constituted the injurious mechanism (14-16). However, it seems
equally as possible that with increasing protein intake that certain inorganics, especially phosphorus, would also be increased and
in turn could be the toxin since most studies have not attempted
to keep inorganic constituents of the diet constant. White and
Grollman suggested that autoimmune mechanisms were responsible for
the changes in the renal remnant and showed immunosuppression prevented hypertension (20). However, in their model the animals had
neither proteinuria nor glomerular disease. Koletsky and Goodsitt
suggested that the progressive renal disease resulted from hypertension (21). However Purkerson et al (22) found that treatment
of hypertension did not prevent the disease process nor did the
presence of hypertension necessarily lead to progressive glomerular
disease. These latter authors suggested that the glomerulopathy
resulted from increased capillary permeability and showed that
heparin reduced the severity of renal failure, lowered the blood
pressure and decreased the proportion of abnormal glomeruli, however had no effect on the immunofluorescence pattern or proteinuria (22).

To test the possibility that phosphorus restriction, possibly
by preventing calcification, could prevent renal failure in this
model the remnant kidney was established in 38 Sprague-Dawley rats
(23). Twelve rats were placed on a low phosphorus diet (0.05%),
(ICN Pharmaceuticals Inc., Cleveland, OH) 6-weeks prior to induction of uremia and continued on this diet throughout the remainder of the study. The remaining 26 animals served as controls
and were fed regular rat chow. The course of the disease was
markedly different in the two groups. By the 56th day plasma
creatinine was significantly higher in the control group as compared to the low P group (Fig. 1). This difference persisted
throughout the remainder of the study. By the 105th day 19 of the
26 regular P group had died whereas only 2 of the 12 P-restricted
animals had died (p < .001). At the 168th day the study was terminated and the nine surviving P-restricted animals were killed.
All normal P animals had died prior to this time (p < .001).
Kidney calcium content was significantly less in the P-restricted
animals (13 ± 1) as compared to the non-restricted animals (260 ±
5) (p < .001) (Fig. 2). In the non-restricted animals calcium was
deposited in the cortical tubular cells, tubular basement membrane
and interstitium. In addition there was a severe fibrotic and

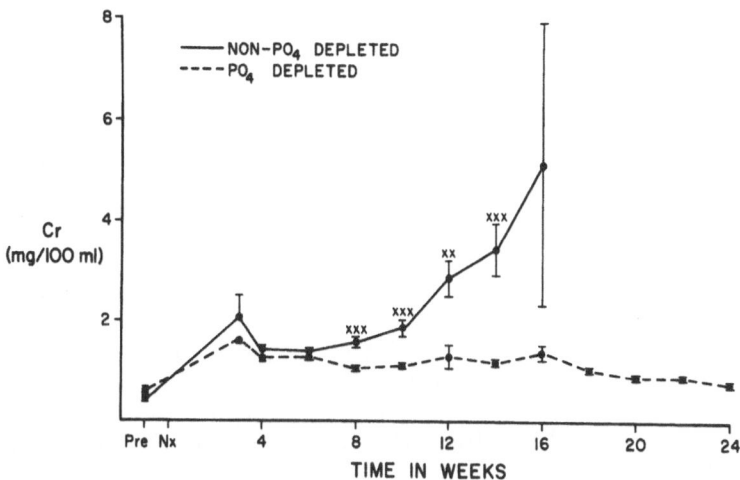

Fig. 1.  Serial plasma creatinine levels over the 168 day study.

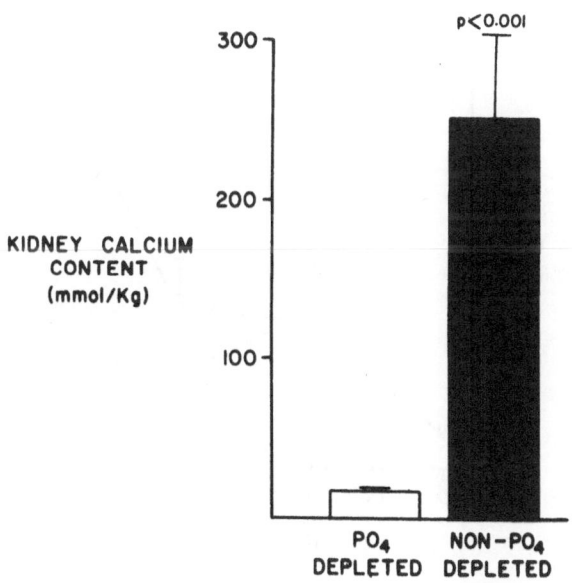

Fig. 2.  Kidney Ca concentrations in both groups of rats.

and inflammatory reaction in the remnant kidney.  In contrast the remnant kidney from the P-restricted animals was normal in appearance.  This study shows that P-restriction instituted prior to renal failure is protective in the remnant kidney model.

However, for this form of therapy to be applicable to humans it would also have to be effective after renal failure had already occurred.  To examine this possibility the remnant kidney model was established in 30 Sprague-Dawley rats.  For the first 30 days following establishment of the remnant kidney the animals were maintained on a regular diet.  At this time they were randomized into two groups of 15 animals each.  One group was fed a P-restricted diet (0.05%) where the other was given an identical diet with P added to give it a P content similar to a normal diet (0.5%).

During the study period 10 of the 15 animals in the phosphate supplemented group died and all had progressive functional deterioration (Fig. 3).  In contrast there were no deaths in the P-restricted group, renal function improved and renal histology returned to normal (Fig. 3).  In addition proteinuria also significantly improved. (Fig. 4).

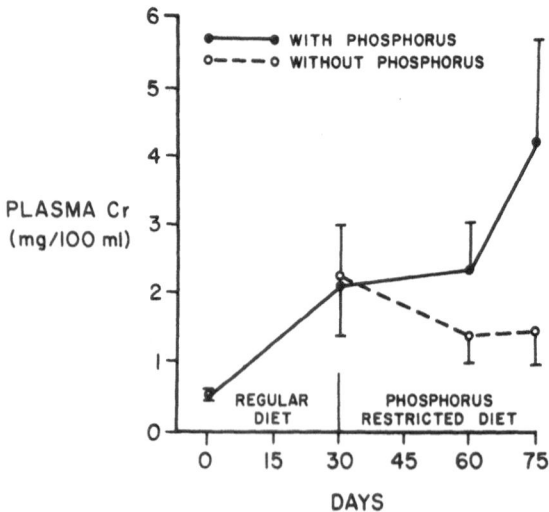

Fig. 3.   Plasma creatinine levels before nephrectomy, 30 days following nephrectomy when animals were placed on P-restriction and at 50 and 75 days.  Both of the latter values are significantly different in the two groups (p < .01).

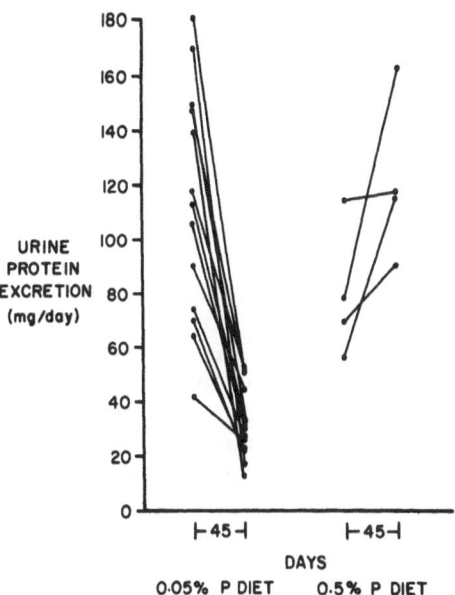

Fig. 4.  Urinary protein excretion at 30 days following nephrec-
         tomy and after 45 days on low P diet.  Urinary protein
         fell significantly in P-restricted animals (p < .01)
         whereas in the four remaining non-restricted animals it
         was actually higher on the last determination.

These studies clearly show that the destruction of the remnant
kidney is somehow mediated through phosphorus and that phosphorus
restriction prevents functional deterioration and glomerular
disease.

Stronger evidence that phosphorus restriction might have relevance to human disease has been shown in studies in our laboratory
using an animal model which closely resembles human disease (24).
The model we have employed is chronic glomerulonephritis induced
by antiglomerular basement membrane antibodies.  Anti-rat glomerular
basement membrane antibodies have been produced in rabbits by injecting them with purified rat glomerular basement membrane twice
monthly over the past year.

Over the past few decades this disease has been extensively
studied in regards to histological features and proteinuria (25-
28).  However little data are available in regards to the course

of functional deterioration (29-31). It has been felt that the disease has two phases (32-33). The first phase is the heterologous phase directly a result of the antiglomerular basement membrane antibody which results in the early induction of proteinuria. The second phase has been termed the autologous phase which results from the rat forming antibodies to the rabbit gamma globulin which is fixed to the basement membrane. This phase causes progressive proteinuria and histological abnormalities (32,33). In order to intensify the autologous phase of the disease 5-days prior to injecting uninephrectomized rats with antiglomerular basement membrane antibodies the rats were given purified rabbit gamma globulin in complete Freund's adjuvant. From a functional standpoint the disease would appear to have a tri-phasic course. Initially plasma creatinine increases in the first 7 to 21 days. It then falls and plateaus close to control values for an additional 35-45 days. At around 65 days plasma creatinine values begin to increase and the majority of animals die from uremia before 100 days. Phosphorus restriction markedly alters the course of this disease. In this study 11 animals were placed on a phosphorus restricted diet 30 days after receiving the nephrotoxic serum. Thirteen animals received the identical nephrotoxic serum and diet but had phosphorus (4 parts sodium phosphate to 1 part sodium biphosphate) added to give the diet a normal phosphorus level (0.5%). To insure that sodium was not another variable animals on the phosphorus restricted diet were given NaCl to equal the amount of sodium given with the phosphate addition to the other group. At 30 days prior to phosphate restriction, the 24-hour urine protein was 297 ± 34 mg/day in the P-restricted group as compared to 306 ± 45 mg/day (p=NS) in the non-restricted group (normal less than 20 mg/day). Following 40-days of phosphorus restriction 24-hour urinary protein was 261 ± 65 mg/24-hrs in the restricted group vs 360 ± 20 mg/24-hrs in the non-restricted group (p=NS). Even though urinary protein was somewhat less in the phosphate restricted group it was still markedly increased above normal supporting the continuing presence of glomerular disease.

As far as functionally the first two phases of the disease were identical in the two groups. However phosphate restriction totally prevented the third phase of the disease. Whereas, 12 of the 13 animals died of uremia in the non-restricted group, only 3 of the 11 animals in the P-restricted group died with only one being uremic at time of death (p < .01). This study was terminated at 146 days with the remaining animals killed. The final plasma creatinine value was 0.9 ± .1 mg/100 ml in the P-restricted group vs 3.0 ± .5 mg/100 ml in the non-restricted group (p < .001). Kidney calcium concentration was increased in all animals on a normal P diet, whereas animals on the P-restricted diet had kidney calcium concentration within the normal range.

There is additional evidence in man which also suggests that calcification of a diseased kidney may accelerate its rate of destruction. First, Walser et al (34) have shown that patients with renal disease on nutritional therapy and low phosphorus diet had stabilization or improvement of renal function. These authors attributed this finding to the prevention of renal parenchymal calcification.

Secondly, the calcium concentration is almost invariable increased in human end-stage kidney. In analyzing 59 human end-stage kidneys calcium concentration was increased above control kidneys + 2 SD in all but 2 kidneys studied (Fig. 5). Not only is calcium concentration increased to levels similar to that present in the models of experimental renal disease the calcium is also deposited in a similar manner. The calcium is largely present in cortical tubular cells, tubular basement membranes and the interstitium of the kidney.

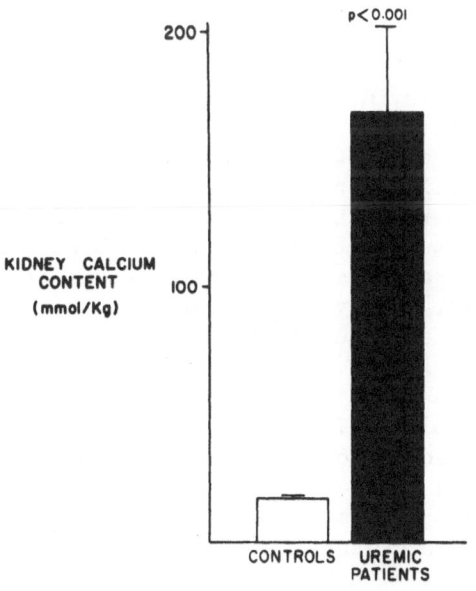

Fig. 5.   Ca concentration in human end-stage kidneys as compared to human control kidneys.

Although prevention of calcification seems the most likely reason for the protective effect of P-restriction this effect could also be mediated by suppressing PTH levels or by ameliorating some direct toxic effect of phosphorus.

In view of the expense and in general unsatisfactory response to treatment it would be highly desirable to prevent rather than treat end-stage kidney disease. The finding that P-restriction is effective in both immunologic and non-immunologic experimental renal disease gives increasing promise that this form of therapy may prove useful in retarding functional deterioration in humans with chronic renal failure.

References

1.   Britton, D.C., Thompson, M.H., Johnston, I.D.A., Fleming, L.B.: Renal function following parathyroid surgery in primary hyper-parathyroidism.  Lancet 2:74, 1971.
2.   Hecht, A., Gershberg, H., St Paul, H.:  Primary hyperpara-thyroidism: Laboratory and clinical data in 73 cases.  JAMA 233:519, 1975.
3.   Hossain, M.:  Vitamin-D intoxication during treatment of hypo-parathyroidism.  Lancet 1:1149, 1970.
4.   Burnett, C.H., Commons, R.R., Albright, F., Howard, J.E.: Hypercalcemia without hypercalciuria or hypophosphatemia, cal-cinosis and renal insufficiency: a syndrome following prolonged intake of milk and alkali.  N Engl J Med 240:787, 1949.
5.   Pollak, V.E., Schneider, A.F., Freund, G., Kark, R.M.:  Chronic renal disease with secondary hyperparathyroidism.  Arch Intern Med 103:200, 1959.
6.   Katz, A.I., Hampers, C.L., Wilson, R.E., Bernstein, D.S., Wachman, A., Merrill, J.P.:  The place of subtotal parathyroid-ectomy in the management of patients with chronic renal failure. Trans Am Soc Artif Intern Organs 14:376, 1968.
7.   Katz, A.I., Hampers, C.L., Merrill, J.P.:  Secondary hyperpara-thyroidism and renal osteodystrophy in chronic renal failure: analysis of 195 patients, with observations on the effects of chronic dialysis, kidney transplantation and subtotal para-thyroidectomy.  Medicine 48:333, 1969.
8.   Kuzela, D.C., Huffer, W.E., Conger, J.D., Winter, S.D., Hammond, W.S.:  Soft tissue calcification in chronic dialysis patients. Am J Pathol 86:403, 1977.
9.   Ahlmén, J.:  Incidence of chronic renal insufficiency.  Acta Med Scand [Suppl] 582:1, 1975.
10.  Morrison, A.B.:  Experimentally induced chronic renal insuf-ficiency in the rat.  Lab Invest 11:321, 1962.
11.  Chanutin, A., Ferris, E.B., Jr.:  Experimental renal insuf-fiency produced by partial nephrectomy.  Arch Intern Med 49: 767, 1932.
12.  Anderson, H.C.:  The relation of blood pressure to the amount of renal tissue.  J Exp Med 39:707, 1924.

13. Purkerson, M.L., Hoffsten, P.E., Lkahr, S.:  Pathogenesis of the glomerulopathy associated with renal infarction in rats. Kidney Int 9:407, 1976.

14. Koletsky, S.:  Role of salt and renal mass in experimental hypertension.  Arch Pathol 68:21, 1959.

15. Lalich, J.J., Faith, G.C., Harding, G.E.:  Protein overload nephropathy: in rats subjected to unilateral nephrectomy. Arch Pathol 89:548, 1970.

16. Lalich, J.J., Allen, J.R.:  Protein overload nephropathy in rats with unilateral nephrectomy: II. Ultrastructural study. Arch Pathol 91:372, 1971.

17. Striker, G.E., Nagle, R.B., Kohnen, P.W., Smuckler, A.: Response to unilateral nephrectomy in old rats.  Arch Pathol 87:439, 1969.

18. Inglis, J.A., Halliday, J.W.:  Renal damage after subtotal nephrectomy.  Pathology 1:177, 1969.

19. Lalich, J.J., Burkholder, P.M., Paik, W.C.W.:  Protein overload nephropathy in rats with unilateral nephrectomy.  Arch Pathol 99:72, 1975.

20. White, F.N., Grollman, A.:  Autoimmune factors associated with injection of the kidney.  Nephron 1:93, 1964.

21. Koletsky, S., Goodsitt, A.M.:  Natural history and pathogenesis of renal ablation hypertension.  Arch Pathol 69:654, 1960.

22. Purkerson, M.L., Hoffsten, P.E., Klahr, S.:  Pathogenesis of the glomerulopathy associated with renal infarction in rats. Kidney Int 9:407, 1976.

23. Ibels, L.S., Alfrey, A.C., Haut, L., Huffer, W.E.:  Preservation of function in experimental renal disease by dietary restriction of phosphate.  N Engl J Med 298:122, 1978.

24. Haut, L., Karlinsky, M.L., Buddington, B., Schrier, N., Alfrey, A.C.:  Prevention of functional deterioration in experimental glomerulonephritis (GN).  Clin Res (in press).

25. Masugi, M.:  Über das Wesen der spezifischen Veränderungen der Niere und Leber durch das Nephrotoxin bzw. das Hepatotoxin. Beitr Pathol Anat Allgem Pathol 91:82, 1933.

26. Vassalli, P., McCluskey, R.T.:  The pathogenic role of fibrin deposition in immunologically induced glomerulonephritis. Ann NY Acad Sci 116:1052, 1964.

27. Vassalli, P., McCluskey, R.T.:  The pathogenic role of the coagulation process in rabbit Masugi nephritis.  Am J Pathol 45:653, 1964.

28. Cochrane, C.G., Weigle, W.O.:  The cutaneous reaction to soluble antigen-antibody complexes; a comparison with the Arthus phenomenon.  J Exptl Med 108:591, 1958.

29. Smadel, J.E.:  Experimental nephritis in rats induced by injection of anti-kidney serum. III. Pathological studies of the acute and chronic disease. J Exptl Med 65:541, 1937.

30. Smadel, J.E., Farr, L.E.:  Experimental nephritis in rats induced by injection of anti-kidney serum. II. Clinical and functional studies.  J Exptl Med 65:527, 1937.

31.  Crosson, J.T., Lubowitz, H., Mazumdar, D.C., Weisser, F., Lang, S., Rolf, D., Germuth, F.G.:  The production of experimental glomerulonephritis in the rat.  Arch Pathol 98: 344, 1974.
32.  Kay, C.F.:  The mechanism by which experimental nephritis is produced in rabbits injected with nephrotic duck serum.  J Exptl Med 72:559, 1940.
33.  Kay, C.F.:  The mechanism of a form of glomerulonephritis. Nephrotoxic nephritis in rabbits.  Am J Med Sci 204:483, 1942.
34.  Collier, U.V., Mitch, W., Walser, M.:  The effect of spontaneous or induced lowering of plasma Ca X P product on progression of chronic renal failure (CRF).  Clin Res 26:564A, 1978.

# PHARMACOLOGY OF DISODIUM (3-AMINO-1-HYDROXYPROPYLIDENE)-1,1-BISPHOSPHONATE

Pieter H. Reitsma, Olav L.M. Bijvoet, W.B. Frijlink,
F.J.F.E. Vismans and F.J.M. van Breukelen

Clinical Investigation Unit, Dept. of
Clinical Endocrinology and Metabolism
University Hospital, Leiden
The Netherlands

## INTRODUCTION

Various bisphosphonates retard the growth and dissolution of hydroxyapatite crystals in vitro[1,2]. Growth and remodeling of bone is associated with the transition of mineral between solution and crystalline phases. The possible actions of bisphosphonates on bone metabolism have been studied in many biological systems, and this has led to the recognition of a number of pharmacological effects. The most marked of these were the appearance of unmineralized bone and cartilage, and inhibition of the resorption of bone and cartilage[3]. Inhibitory effects on the formation of matrix and longitudinal growth of bone were also noted, but received less attention[4,5].

It is still unclear whether these biological effects reflect a physicochemical or a cellular action of the compounds. Inhibition of mineralization is conventially explained by physicochemical interaction with crystal surfaces; inhibition of osteoclasts could then be secondary to that, or due to a specific metabolic action (as, for instance, alteration of the glycolytic process[6,7]). That the osteomalacia represents toxic effects on bone forming cells with the production of faulty matrix and inhibition of resorption reflects a physicochemical action, as not been considered.

Most biological and clinical studies of bisphosphonates have been carried out with 1-hydroxyethylidene-1,1-biphosphonate (EHDP), a compound with reproducible effects on mineralization and resorption of bone. The doses affecting mineralization and resorption overlap and these effects cannot be easily dissociated. However, animal studies using dichloromethylidene-1,1-biphosphonate ($Cl_2MDP$)

and another bisphosphonate, (3-amino-1-hydroxypropylidene)-1,1-bi-
phosphonate (APD), have shown that doses affecting bone resorption
may be very different from those affecting mineralization[4],[5],[6].
Cl$_2$MDP has no effect on mineralization at all, while APD only affects
it at much higher doses than those inhibiting resorption.

As bone resorption is always more sensitive to APD than to the
other compounds[6], we have studied APD both in animal and in man.
The interrelation between various pharmacological effects was
observed by comparing sequential observations during treatment.
In particular, the mineralization process, bone formation and resorption, and the secondary effects on mineral homeostasis and bone
balance were examined.

METHODS

Animal Studies

Male albino Wistar rats, 180-190 g, were used. They were
treated with APD by daily subcutaneous injections. Accumulation of
unmineralized bone was assessed after six days treatment with doses
ranging from 16-160 mol APD.kg$^{-1}$.day$^{-1}$. The distal metaphysis from
both femora and the proximal metaphysis from both tibiae were removed
and cleaned of adherent tissue, cartilage, and bone marrow. The
metaphyses from one hind leg were dried, weighed, and ashed at 600°C;
the ash was weighed and dissolved in 1 N HCl for the determination
of calcium. The contralateral metaphyses were dried, weighed, and
hydrolysed in 6 N HCl at 125°C for the measurement of hydroxyproline.
Ca/Hydroxyproline ratio was calculated by dividing μmol Ca per mg
dry weight of bone in one set of bone samples by μmol hydroxyproline
in the other set of bone samples.

The effect of APD on bone formation and bone resorption were
measured at a dose of 1.6 mol.kg$^{-1}$.day$^{-1}$ of APD. Changes in bone
formation were followed by measuring alkaline phosphatase activity
in metaphyseal bone at various intervals. All metaphyses of an
animal, isolated as described above, were pooled and homogenized,
and the alkaline phosphatase activity measured. Metabolic balance
studies were performed to measure hydroxyproline excretion, and Ca-
balance. Urine was collected daily while faeces were collected
over four day periods.

For histological observations both humeri were removed from
the rats used for the study of mineralization and alkaline phosphatase activity. Undecalcified sections were obtained by the method
of te Velde et al[8].

Clinical Studies

The clinical studies concerned patients with one of three dif-

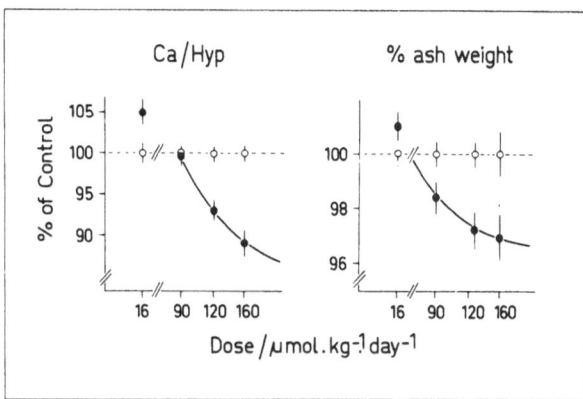

Fig. 1. Effect of APD
on bone mineralization
in rats. Results repre-
sent ± SEM for 6 rats.

ferent diseases, Paget's disease, osteolytic bone disease and osteoporosis, reflecting abnormal bone turnover, abnormal
mineral homeostasis and abnormal bone mass respectively. Details
of the patients with Paget's disease[9] and the patients with osteolytic bone disease[10] have been given previously. The method used
in the osteoporosis group were similar but maintainance doses were
3-6 μmol.kg body weight $^{-1}$.day $^{-1}$.

RESULTS AND DISCUSSION

It is clear from fig. 1 that both parameters of bone mineralization
in rats, % ash weight and Ca/hydroxyproline ratio, diminished at
doses  80  mol.kg$^{-1}$.day$^{-1}$ for 6 days, indicating an accumulation
of osteoid tissue. This was confirmed by histological examination
of the humerus, which showed, at these doses, wide osteoid seams
and broadening of the hypertrophic zone of the growth plate.
Similar results have been obtained with EHDP [4,5]. Further studies
of the effect on bone resorption and bone formation in rats were
done at a dose of 1.6 μmol.kg  .day  , which did not interfere
with bone and cartilage mineralization.

Figures 2,3 and 4 show the sequential changes in various
parameters of bone metabolism and Ca-homeostasis in rats, patients
with Paget's disease, and patients with cryptogenic osteoporosis
after start of treatment with APD. Bone resorption, measured as
urinary hydroxyproline excretion, was always inhibited with striking speed. Bone formation, measured as alkaline phosphatase activity ( in bone in the rats, and in serum in the patients ) was
reduced more slowly. In the patients with Paget's disease alkaline
phosphatase at first remained constant and in the osteoporotic
group there was even a small initial increase.

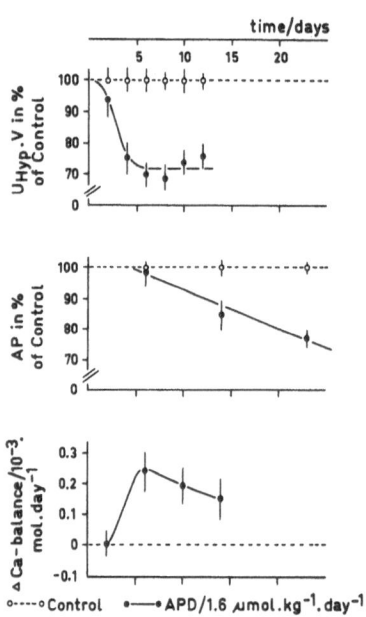

Fig. 2. Changes in urinary hydroxyproline excretion, bone AP activity, and
Ca-balance in rats during treatment
with APD. Results represent means
± SEM of rats.

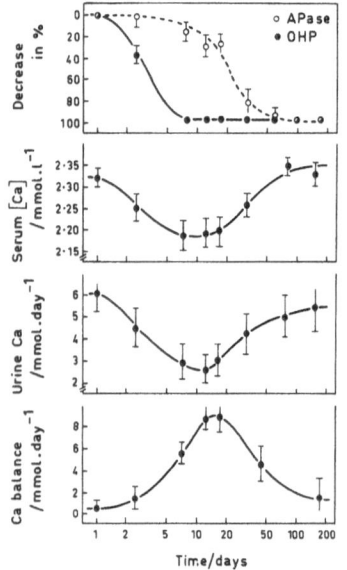

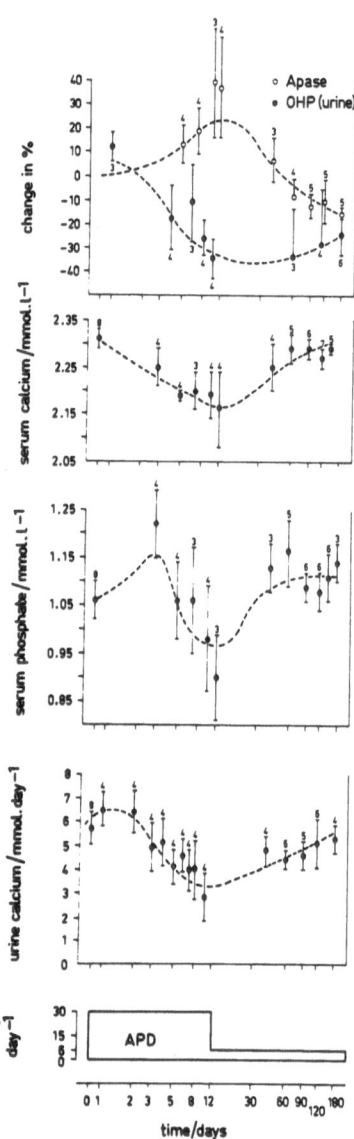

Fig. 2. Changes in various parameters
of Ca- and bone metabolism in patients
with osteoporosis during treatment with
APD. Numbers indicate number of patients.
Results represent means ± SEM.

Fig. 4. Changes in various parameters
of Ca- and bone metabolism in patients
with Paget's disease during treatment
with APD. Observations were made in 6
patients, but balances at 45 days were
calculated for 2 patients only. Results
represent means ± SEM (from ref. 9).

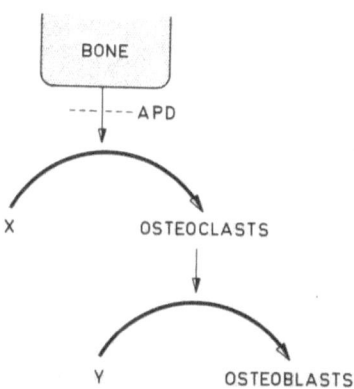

Fig. 5. Schematic representation of effects of APD on bone cells. APD blocks permissive action of bone mineral on osteoclast activation and function. Since osteoclasts have a role in new formation of osteoblasts, reduction of osteoblasts is a secondary effect.

The rapidity of the effect on hydroxyproline excretion suggests an immediate blockade of osteoclast function by APD, and the decrease of osteoclast numbers which was observed in the patients with Paget's disease[9] suggests reduced activation of new osteoclasts. The subsequent lowering of bone formation may have been due to a direct effect of APD on osteoblasts, but it is more probably the result of a normal homeostatic mechanism that maintains equilibrium between formation and resorption in many disease states, including Paget's disease[11]. If this second explanation is correct, the time needed by alkaline phosphatase to reach a new plateau represents the active life-span of the osteoblasts. Fig. 5 summarizes our interpretation of the effects of APD on bone resorption and bone formation. It shows that APD interferes with the resorption process, which in its turn affects bone formation.

There are two possible mechanisms by which APD inhibits bone resorption. There may be specific metabolic actions on osteoclasts, or alternatively, a change in the surface of bone so that its recognition by osteoclasts is blocked. If the effect on osteoclasts is due to a physicochemical action of APD on bone surface it is surprising that osteomalacia is only seen at relatively high doses. This discrepancy would be explained if the osteomalacia was not merely due to inhibited crystal growth but to altered properties of the matrix, caused by a toxic effect on bone and cartilage forming cells. In favour of this hypothesis are the observations that the formation of new matrix has been found to be inhibited by EHDP, and even by $Cl_2MDP$, resulting in impaired longitudinal growth of rat bone[4,5] and that the matrix has indeed altered biochemical properties[12]. Furthermore the recovery from EHDP induced osteomalacia in rats taken a very long time[13], indicating that

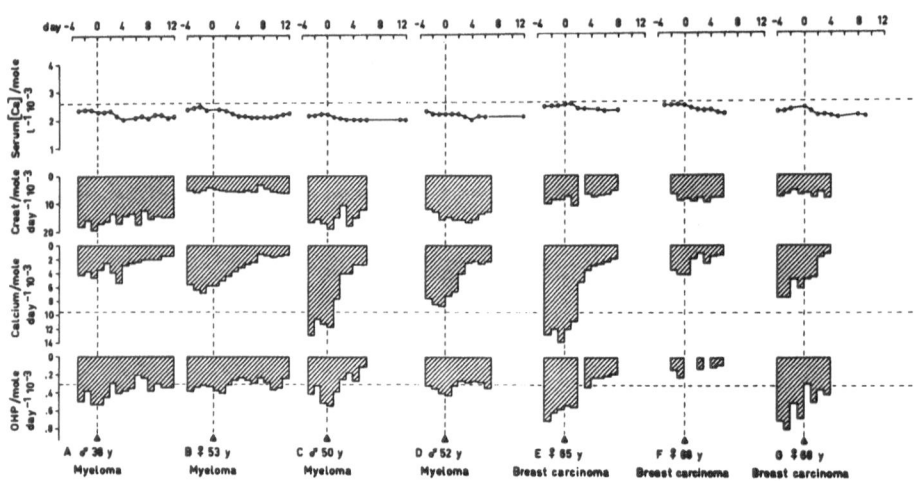

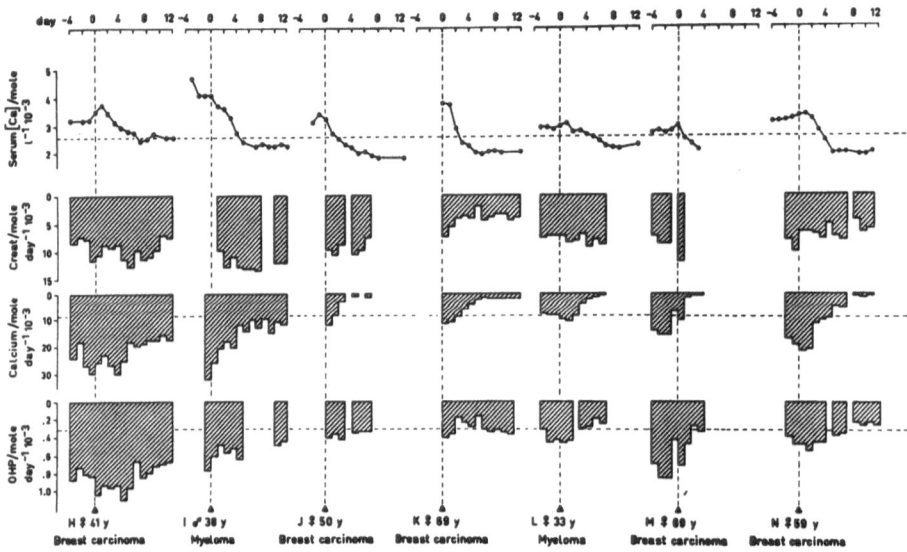

Fig. 6. Changes in serum-calcium and in
excretion-rates of creatinine, calcium,
and hydroxyproline during administration
of APD to patients with or without hypercalcaemia and with secondary osteolytic
lesions due to breast carcinoma or myeloma (from ref. 10).

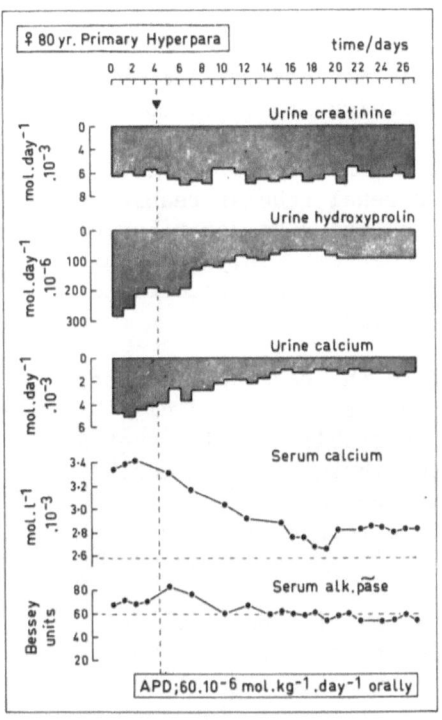

Fig. 7. Changes in various parameters of Ca- and bone metabolism in a patient with primary hyperparathyreoidism during treatment with APD.

the matrix is not suitable to calcify. We therefore suggest that phosphonate induced osteomalacia is due to a toxic effect on bone cells, and that the inhibition of resorption is due to a physicochemical action.

Fig. 8. Changes in Ca-balance in 8 patients with osteoporosis after 6 months treatment with APD.

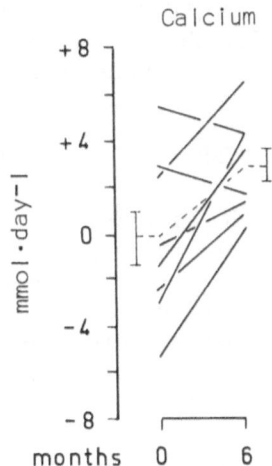

Secondary to the transient dissociation of bone resorption and formation were changes of calcium homeostasis and bone balance. The unbalanced turnover leads in man to transient hypocalcaemia and normalization of the hypercalcaemia of osteolytic bone disease (figs. 3,4,6). In hyperparathyreoidism we observed some lowering of serum calcium, but stabilization often occurred at an increased level, set by increased renal tubular reabsorption of calcium (fig.7). This illustrates the dual contribution of bone and kidney to serum calcium homeostasis. Only hypercalcaemia due directly to increased osteolysis can be expected to respond to agents that block bone resorption.

Calcium balance was positive in both the rats and patients with Paget's disease up to the moment that the equilibrium between formation and resorption was re-established. In Paget's disease calcium balance was back in equilibrium after 6 months (fig. 3). This observation stresses the need of sequential, long-term studies when the treatment of osteoporosis is considered.

The osteoporotic patients showed an initial positive calcium balance (not shown) as observed in Paget's disease. We expected calcium balance to return to zero after 6 months treatment, but this was evidently not the case (fig. 8). This may have been due to the low dose of APD used. The effect of APD on bone resorption is dose-dependent, and it is possible that a slight inhibition of osteoclast function does not produce a proportional decrease of bone formation. This subject is now under investigation.

ACKNOWLEDGEMENTS

This work was partly supported by the Foundation for Medical Research (FUNGO) which is subsidised by the Netherlands Organisation for the Advancement of Pure Research (Z.W.O.). APD was donated by Henkel KGaA, Düsseldorf.

REFERENCES

1.  M. D. Francis, The inhibition of calcium hydroxyapatite growth by polyphosphonates and polyphosphates, Calc. Tiss. Res., 3:151 (1969).
2.  H. Fleisch, R. G. G. Russell and M. D. Francis, Diphosphonates inhibit hydroxyapatite dissolution in vitro and bone resorption in tissue culture and in vivo, Science, 165:1262 (1969).
3.  H. Fleisch, R. G. G. Russell, S. Bisaz and J. P. Bonjour, The effects of pyrophosphate and diphosphonates on calcium

metabolism, in:"Hard Tissue growth, repair and reminera-
lization," Ciba Foundation Symposium 11, Associated Scientific
Publishers, Amsterdam (1973).

4.  R. Schenk, W. A. Merz, R. Mühlbauer, R. G. G. Russell and
H. Fleisch, Effect of ethane-1-hydroxy-1,1-bisphosphonate
(EHDP) and dichloromethylene diphosphonate (Cl$_2$MDP) on
calcification and resorption of cartilage and bone in the
tibial epiphysis and metaphysis of rats, Calc. Tiss. Res.,
11:196 (1973).

5.  S. C. Miller, and W. S. S. Jee, The comparitive effects of
dichloromethylene diphosphonate (Cl$_2$MDP) and ethane-1-
hydroxy-1,1-diphosphonate (EHDP) on growth and modelling
of the rat tibia, Calc. Tiss. Res., 23:207 (1977).

6.  H. H. P. J. Lemkes, P. H. Reitsma, W. B. Frijlink, H. Ver-
linden-Ooms, O. L. M. Bijvoet, A new diphosphonate:
dissociation between effects on cells and mineral in rats
and a preliminary trial in Paget's disease, in:
"Homeostasis of phosphate and other minerals," S. G.
Massry, E. Ritz and A. Rapado, eds., Plenum Publishing
Corporation, New York (1978).

7.  D. K. Fast, R. Felix, C. Dowse, W. F. Neuman and H. Fleisch,
The effects of diphosphonates on the growth and glycolysis
of connective-tissue cells in culture, Biochem. J. 172:97
(1978).

8.  J. te Velde, R. Burckhardt, K. Kleiverda, L. Leenheers-
Binnendijk, W. Sommerveld, Methyl-metacrylate as an
embedding medium in histopathology, Histopathology I:319
(1977).

9.  W. B. Frijlink, O. L. M. Bijvoet, J. te Velde, G. Heynen,
Treatment of Paget's disease with (3-amino-1-hydroxypro-
pylidene)-1,1-bisphosphonate (APD), Lancet,i:799 (1979).

10. F. J. M. van Breukelen, O. L. M. Bijvoet, A. T. van Oosterom,
Inhibition of osteolytic bone lesions by (3-amino-1-
hydroxypropylidene)-1,1-bisphosphonate (APD), Lancet,
i:803 (1979).

11. W. H. Harris, R. P. Heaney, Skeletal renewal and metabolic
bone disease, New Engl. J. Med., 280:253 (1969).

12. A. Larsson and S. E. Larsson, Light microscopic and ultrastructural observations on short-term effects of ethylene-
1-hydroxy-1,1-diphosphonate (EHDP) on rat tibia epiphysis,
Acta Path. Microbiol. Scand. Sect. A, 84:17 (1976).

13. W. R. King, M. D. Francis, W. R. Michael, Effect of disodium
ethane-1-hydroxy-1,1-diphosphonate on bone formation,
Clin. Orthop., 78:251 (1971).

EFFECT OF PHOSPHATE ON THE ARGININE-INDUCED INSULIN RELEASE BY THE

ISOLATED PERFUSED RAT PANCREAS

J.E. Campillo, A.S. Luyckx and P.J. Lefebvre

Division of Diabetes, Institute of Medicine
University of Liege -B-
4020 Liège, BELGIUM

SUMMARY

The isolated perfused rat pancreas was used to investigate the effect of extracellular phosphate on the arginine-induced insulin release. In the absence of any metabolic substrate, the insulin response to arginine was monophasic. In the absence of phosphate in the medium, the insulin release was unaffected until the 15th minute of the stimulation period, but was significantly augmented from that time onward. In the presence of oleic acid in the perfusate, the insulin response to arginine was also monophasic but occurred earlier than in controls. In this condition, phosphate omission resulted in an increase of the insulin response to arginine from the 3rd minute of the stimulatory period onward. In the presence of glucose 5.5 mM in the medium the insulin response to arginine was biphasic and was not affected by extracellular phosphate omission.

INTRODUCTION

Increasing evidence suggests that phosphate anions could play an important role in the mechanism of insulin secretion by the stimulated pancreatic beta cell. Several reports have shown that stimulation with insulin secretagogues may trigger a rapid, transient efflux of $^{32}P$ from prelabelled pancreatic islets, the so-called "phosphate flush" (1-8). It has been suggested that this phosphate flush may reflect one of the earlier components in the sequence of events that constitutes the stimulus-secretion coupling in the beta cell. Furthermore, in the isolated perfused rat pancreas and in the isolated islets from ob/ob mice, it has been shown that extracellular phosphate could be involved in the modulation of the insulin response to arginine or glucose (9-11).

229

This work aimed at further investigating the effect of extra-cellular phosphate ($H_2PO_4^-$) on the arginine-induced insulin release by the isolated perfused rat pancreas.

MATERIAL AND METHODS

Overnight fasted male Wistar rats (200-250 g) were used in all experiments. Techniques for isolation and perfusion of the rat pan-creas have been previously described (12). The pancreas was perfused using an Ambec Perfusion Unit (Boulder, Colorado) at a constant flow rate of 2.0 ml/min. The perfusate was a modified Krebs-Henseleit bicarbonate buffer containing NaCl 120 mM, KCl 4.0 mM, MgSO$_4$ 0.7 mM, CaCl$_2$ 1.0 mM, NaHCO$_3$ 25 mM, with or without 1.2 mM KH$_2$PO$_4$ for each experimental condition. In the absence of phosphate, an equivalent amount of KCl was added to avoid differences in the potassium con-centration. The perfusate was supplemented with 2 g/100 ml bovine albumin (Armour) and 2.5 g/100 ml dextran (M.W. 70,000 Poviet). In some experiments, glucose 5.5 mM (Merck) and oleic acid 1.5 mM (Merck) were added to the perfusion medium. The medium containing oleic acid was prepared as previously described (13). The medium was continuously gassed with O$_2$ and CO$_2$ (95:5).

In all experiments the pancreas was perfused from the beginning of the experiments with basal medium and this for 40 min before exposure to arginine. Arginine (L-arginine HCl, Fluka) was dissolved in the perfusate and infused into the circuit immediately above the pancrease through a side-arm perfusion pump working at a flow rate of 0.1 ml/min. The arginine reached in the perfusate a final con-centration of 10 mM. The stimulation period lasted 30 min. and was followed by a 20 min post stimulation period.

Perfusion samples (2 ml) were collected into chilled tubes con-taining 1000 U Trasylol (Bayer) and immediately frozen for storage at -20° C until assayed. Insulin (immunoreactive insulin, IRI) was measured by a double antibody procedure (14) with rat insulin as standard (Novo Industri, A.S., Copenhagen). Insulin secretion rates were calculated by multiplying the concentration in the respective samples by the flow rate and expressed as ng/min. Total release during the stimulation period was obtained by planimetry of the indi-vidual perfusion profiles. All results are expressed as mean ± stan-dard error of the mean (SEM). Statistical evaluation was performed using the Student t-test.

RESULTS

Figure 1 shows the insulin response to 10 mM arginine in the presence or in the absence of 1.2 mM phosphate ($H_2PO_4^-$) in the medium. These experiments were carried out in the absence of any metabolic substrate in the perfusion medium during the 40 minute pre-stimulation period. Both in the presence and in the absence of

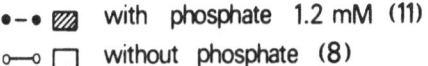

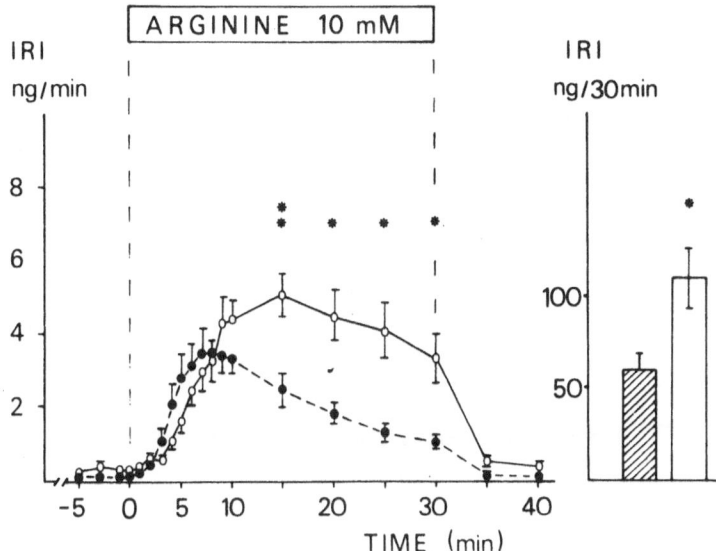

Figure 1: Insulin (IRI) response to arginine with complete medium and $H_2PO_4^-$ free medium. These experiments were performed in the absence of any metabolic substrate in the medium. The number of perfusions are indicated in parentheses. Results are given as mean ± SEM. Statistical comparison corresponds to $p < 0.05$, $p < 0.01$.

phosphate, arginine elicited a quantitatively modest monophasic insulin response. At 1.2 mM phosphate, the arginine-induced insulin release was characterized by a progressive increase in the insulin secretion rate to attain a maximum between the 6th and the 10th minute of the stimulatory period. A prompt return to the basal levels was observed when the arginine insulin was interrupted. In the absence of phosphate, the insulin release in response to arginine was identical to that obtained in the presence of phosphate until the 10th minute of the stimulatory period, but was significantly augmented from that time onward. The total amount of insulin released in response to the 30 minute arginine infusion was 60.01±8.9 ng/30 min in the presence versus 110.8±16.9 ng/30 min in the absence of phosphate ($p < 0.02$).

Figure 2 shows the insulin response to arginine in the presence
or in the absence of 1.2 mM phosphate when the perfusion medium contained 1.5 mmol/l oleic acid from the beginning of the experiment.
Both in the presence and in the absence of phosphate, the arginine-
induced insulin release was monophasic, but the insulin response
occurred significantly earlier than in the corresponding experiments
carried out in the absence of oleic acid (see Figure 1).  In the
absence of phosphate, the insulin secretion rate was significantly
augmented from the 4th minute of the stimulatory period onward.  The
total amount of insulin release in response to the 30 minute arginine
infusion was 58.5±8.2 ng/30 min in the presence versus 148.2±22.9
ng/30 min in the absence of phosphate (p< 0.005).

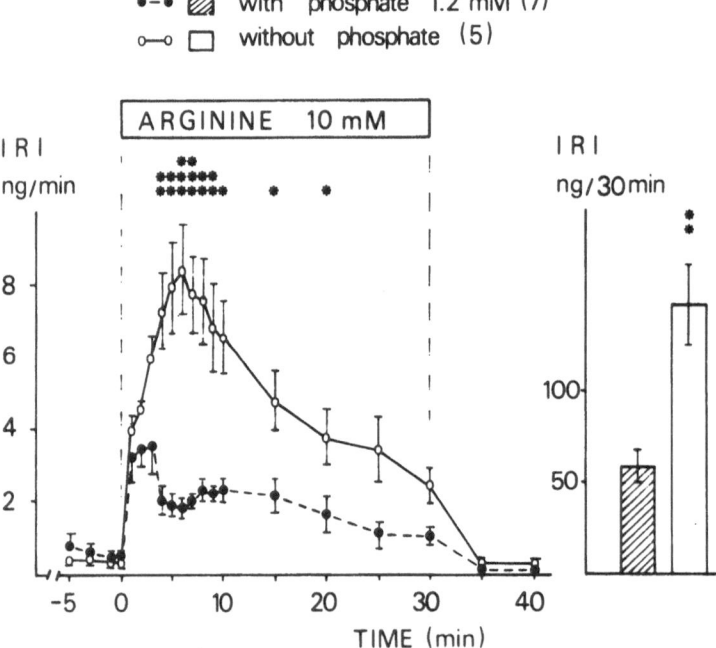

<u>Figure 2</u>:  Insulin (IRI) response to arginine with complete medium
and H₂PO₄⁻ free medium.  These experiments were performed in the
presence of oleic acid 1.5 mM in the perfusate.  The number of
perfusions is indicated in parentheses.  Results are given as
mean  SEM.  Statistical comparison corresponds to p< 0.05, p< 0.01
and p< 0.001.

Figure 3 shows the insulin response to arginine in the presence
or in the absence of 1.2 mM phosphate when the perfusion medium contained 5.5 mmol/l glucose from the beginning of the experiment.  Both
in the presence and in the absence of phosphate, the arginine-induced
insulin release was biphasic.  In comparison with the previous experiments carried out in the absence of glucose in the perfusing
medium, the insulin secretion rate was markedly increased.  No
differences were found in the total amounts of insulin released in
response to arginine both with 1.2 mM phosphate (401.8±63.9 ng/30
min) or without phosphate (447.7±99.9 ng/30 min) in the medium.

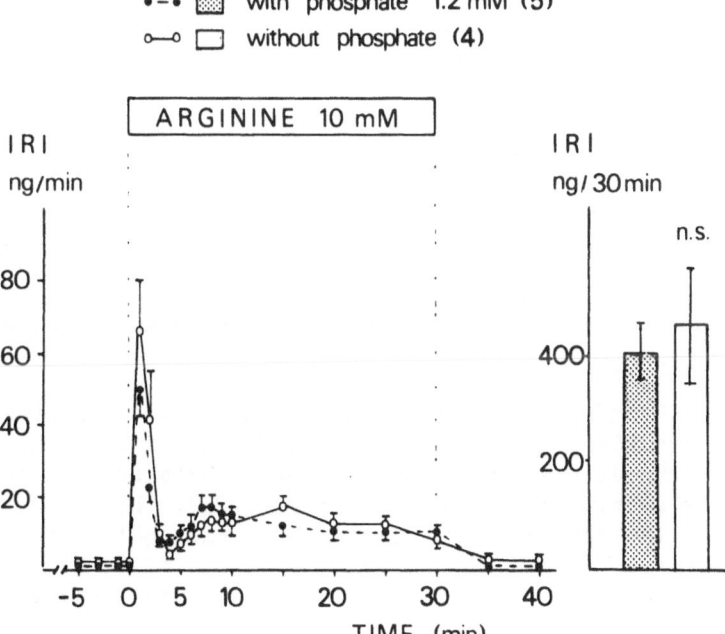

Figure 3:  Insulin (IRI) in response to arginine with complete medium
and $H_2PO_4^-$ free medium.  These experiments were performed in the
presence of glucose 5.5 mM in the perfusate.  The number of perfusions is indicated in parentheses.  Results are given as mean ± SEM.
N.S. corresponds to "not statistically significant".

DISCUSSION

The present results demonstrate that, in the isolated perfused rat pancreas, omission of extracellular phosphate ($H_2PO_4^-$) from the perfusion medium significantly enhances the insulin response to 10 mM arginine both in the absence of glucose in the perfusate or in the presence of 1.5 mM oleic acid. These results are in contrast with previous reports showing that extracellular phosphate omission severely reduced the insulin response to 16.7 mM glucose by the isolated perfused rat pancreas (11), and they are in agreement with some data obtained from beta-cell rich pancreatic islets incubated in vitro (10). On the other hand, it has been reported that experimental phosphate depletion in humans increased by 30% the plasma insulin response to intravenous glucose (15).

The mechanism(s) whereby phosphate influences insulin secretion remains to be elucidated. First, an interrelationship between phosphate and calcium in affecting insulin secretion represents an attractive hypothesis. As in various secretory cells, a rise in the concentration of cytosolic free calcium is involved in the stimulus-secretion coupling in the beta cell (16,17,18) and alterations in the rates of calcium fluxes across the plasma membrane and into or out of intracellular organelles are known to regulate cytosolic calcium concentration. In fact, in pancreatic beta cells, the mitochondria represent the major sites of calcium accumulation as they contain high concentration of exchangeable calcium and provide a far larger area for calcium transport than any other organelle (19-20). Since phosphate constitutes a permeant anion for the calcium uptake by the mitochondria in beta cells (21), extracellular phosphate variations could affect their cytosolic calcium concentration. In this way, variations in the phosphate concentrations in the medium could affect calcium movements and the so-called "calcium activity" in beta cells as in several other cells and tissues (22, 23,24).

Second, changes in the extracellular phosphate concentration could interfere with the increased turnover rate of high energy phosphate intermediates that occur in concert with several other events in the secretory sequence of insulin (25). Furthermore variations in the extracellular phosphate levels could interfere with the formation of phosphoenolpyruvate, a metabolic intermediate which reduces calcium uptake by an islet subcellular fraction (21).

Third, it has been demonstrated that in the endocrine pancreas as in other glands, specific stimulation causes an immediate increase in the rate of synthesis of the acidic phospholipids, especially phosphatidylinositol (2). Phosphate omission from the medium could interfere at this level and result in a modification of the secretory response to specific stimuli.

Finally it is well documented that insulin secretion is an energy requiring process (26) and phosphate omission could affect the ATP turnover and depress mitochondrial respiration as shown in other experimental systems (27). Moreover, phosphate omission could also reduce ATP as a substrate for adenylate cyclase and thereby cyclic AMP generation, a key step in various conditions of insulin secretion, as recently reviewed (28).

Thus, depending upon the experimental conditions, phosphate omission may lead to an enhancement of insulin secretion as is the case with arginine (through an increase in cytosolic free calcium ?) or to a decreased insulin response as is the case when a high glucose concentration (11) constitutes the stimulus (other mechanisms considered above).

ACKNOWLEDGMENTS

The authors wish to thank Mrs. M. Marchand for her technical assistance. This work was supported in part by the Fonds National de la Recherche Scientifique of Belgium. Dr. A.S. Luyckx is Maître de Recherches du F.N.R.S. (Belgium). Dr. J.E. Campillo is a visiting scientist whose permanent address is Departamento de Fisiologia y Bioquimica, Faculdad de Medicina, Universidad de Granada, Granada, Spain.

REFERENCES

1.  Freinkel, N., El Younsi, C., Bonnar, J., Dawson, R.M.C.: A new index of secretory stimulation in pancreatic islets. Trans. Assoc. Am. Physicians 87:306-314, 1974.
2.  Freinkel, N., E. Younsi, C., Bonnar, J., Dawson, R.M.C.: Rapid transient efflux of phosphate ions from pancreatic islets as an early action of insulin secretagogues. J. Clin. Invest. 54: 1179-1189, 1974.
3.  Pierce, M., Freinkel, N.: Anomeric specificity for the rapid transient efflux of phosphate ions from pancreatic islets during secretory stimulation with glucose. Biochem. Biophys. Res. Commun. 63:870-874, 1975.
4.  Bukowiecki, L., Freinkel, N.: Relationship between efflux of ionic calcium and phosphorus during excitation of pancreatic islets with glucose. Biochim. Biophys. Acta 436:190-198, 1976.
5.  Pierce, M., Bukowiecki, L., Asplund, K., Freinkel, N.: ($^{32}$P)- Orthophosphate efflux from pancreatic islets: Graded response to glucose stimulation. Horm. Metab. Res. 8:358-361, 1976.
6.  Freinkel, N., El Younsi, C., Dawson, R.M.C.: Insulin release and ion efflux from the rat pancreatic islets induced by L-leucine and its nonmetabolizable analogue 2-amino bicyclo (2,2,1) heptane-2-carboxylic acid (BCH). Proc. Natl. Acad. Sci. USA 73:3403-3407, 1976.
7.  Asplund, K., Freinkel, N.: Phosphate metabolism and glucose initiated efflux of phosphate ions in islets of fetal pancreas.

Diabetes 27:611-619, 1978.

8.  Freinkel, N., Pedley, K.C., Wooding, P., Dawson, R.M.C.:
    Localization of inorganic phosphate in the pancreatic B-cell
    and its loss on glucose stimulation. Science 201:1124-1126,
    1978.

9.  Campillo, J.E., Luyckx, A.S., Torres, M.D., Lefebvre, P.J.:
    Effect of phosphate omission on arginine-induced insulin and
    glucagon release by the isolated perfused rat pancreas. FEBS
    Letters 84:141-143, 1977.

10. Anderson, T.: Phosphate-induced modifications of $^{45}$Ca fluxes
    and secretory activity in pancreatic B-cells. Diabetologia 15:
    215, 1978 (abstract).

11. Campillo, J.E., Castillo, M., Rodriguez, E., Osorio, C.:
    Effect of phosphate on the insulin response to glucose in the
    isolated perfused rat pancreas. Diabetologia 15:223, 1978
    (abstract).

12. Campillo, J.E., Luyckx, A.S., Torres, M.D., Lefebvre, P.J.:
    Effect of various concentrations of calcium on arginine-
    induced insulin and glucagon release in vitro. Rev. Esp.
    Physiol. 34:191-198, 1978.

13. Campillo, J.E., Luyckx, A.S., Torres, M.D., Lefebvre, P.J.:
    Effect of oleic acid on insulin secretion by the isolated
    perfused rat pancreas. Diabetologia 16:267-273, 1979.

14. Hales, C.N., Randle, P.J.: Immunoassay of insulin with
    insulin-antibody precipitate. Biochem. J. 88:137-146, 1963.

15. Marshall, W.P., Banasiak, M.F., Kalkhoff, R.K.: Effects of
    phosphate deprivation on carbohydrate metabolism. Horm.
    Metab. Res. 10:369-373, 1978.

16. Rasmussen, H., Goodman, D.B.P.: Relationship between calcium
    and cyclic nucleotides in cell activation. Physiol. Rev. 57:
    421-509, 1977.

17. Malaisse, W.J., Brisson, G.R., Baird, L.E.: Stimulus
    secretion coupling of glucose induced insulin release.
    X. Effect of glucose on $^{45}$Ca efflux from perfused islets.
    Am. J. Physiol. 224:389-394, 1973.

18. Matthews, E.K.: Calcium and stimulus-secretion coupling in
    pancreatic islet cells. In Calcium transport in contraction
    and secretion, ed. by E. Carafoli, F. Clementi, W. Drabikowsky
    and A. Margreth. Amsterdam, North-Holland, 1975, p. 283-295.

19. Howell, S.L., Tyhurst, M.: Barium accumulation in rat
    pancreatic B-cells. J. Cell. Sci. 22:445-465, 1976.

20. Dean, P.M.: Ultrastructural morphometry of the pancreatic
    B-cells. Diabetologia 9:115-119, 1973.

21. Sugden, M.C., Ashcroft, S.J.H.: Effects of phosphoenolpyruvate,
    other glycolytic intermediats and methylxanthines on calcium
    uptake by a mitochondrial fraction from rat pancreatic islets.
    Diabetologia 15:173-180, 1978.

22. Borle, A.S.: Calcium metabolism at the cellular level.
    Fed. Proc. 32:1944-1950, 1973.

23.  Martin, B.R., Clausen, T., Glieman, J.:  Relationship between the exchange of calcium and phosphate in the isolated fat-cells.  Biochem. J. 152:121-129, 1975.
24.  Severson, D.L., Denton, R.M., Bridges, B.J., Randle, P.J.: Exchangeable and total calcium pools in mitochondria of rat epididymal fat-pads and isolated fat cells.  Biochem. J. 154:209-223, 1976.
25.  Malaisse, W.J., Hutton, J.C., Kawazu, S., Herchuelz, A., Valverde, I., Sener, A.:  The stimulus-secretion coupling of glucose-induced insulin release.  XXXV.  The links between metabolic and cationic events.  Diabetologia 16:325-330, 1979.
26.  Ashcroft, S.J.H., Weerasinghe, L.C.C., Randle, P.J.:  Inter-relationship of islet metabolism, adenosine triphosphate content and insulin release.  Biochem. J. 132:223-231, 1973.
27.  Seldin, D.W., Emmett, M.:  Effect of phosphate depletion on organ function.  Fourth International Workshop on Phosphate and Other Minerals.  Miner. Elect. Metab. 2:267, 1979 (abstract).
28.  Sharp, G.W.G.:  The adenylate cyclase cyclic AMP system in islets of Langerhans and its role in the control of insulin release.  Diabetologia 16:287-296, 1979.

RESPONSE OF RED CELL PHOSPHATE TO ACUTE AND CHRONIC CHANGES IN

PLASMA PHOSPHATE IN MAN

C.J. Preston, A. Challa, J.E. Phillips, S.E. Foden,
D.L. Douglas, R.G.G. Russell

Department of Human Metabolism & Clinical Biochemistry,
University of Sheffield Medical School, Beech Hill
Road, Sheffield, S10 2RX, U.K.

INTRODUCTION

Inorganic phosphate (Pi) is known to participate in many bio-chemical reactions and is a regulator in several metabolic path-ways (1). In the red blood cell the structural integrity of the membrane is dependent on metabolic energy derived from glycolysis to produce ATP (2). Pi plays a major role in the red blood cell in regulating the concentrations of ATP and 2,3-diphospho-glycerate (3). In spite of the increasing knowledge about phosphate depletion syndromes, there is still a debate about the mechanisms of phosphate transport across cell membranes and about factors which control its extracellular and intracellular concentrations.

We have developed a specific method, adapted from that of Hall (4), for measuring Pi in red blood cells. We have measured the intra- and extracellular concentrations of Pi in vitro, and in a variety of disease states associated with altered phosphate levels.

METHODS

Venous blood samples were withdrawn from normal subjects and patients after an overnight fast. The samples were collected onto ice and assayed for Pi as follows.

A 2 ml sample of whole blood (WB) and of plasma (Pl) were deproteinised by precipitation with 4 mls of ice-cold 1.0 M

perchloric acid and spun at 3,000 x g for 15 mins.  3 mls of the
supernatant was neutralised with 0.5 mls of 4.0 M potassium
hydroxide to prevent hydrolysis of organic phosphates.  1 ml of
acid ammonium molybdate (prepared as 6.7 ml 5% ammonium molybdate,
plus 2.0 ml Conc. HCl plus 1.3 ml Dist. $H_2O$) was added to 1 ml of
the neutralised extract and the resulting phosphomolybdate
complex extracted into 2 ml isobutanol:  petroleum ether (4:1) by
shaking.  To 1 ml of the organic (Upper) layer was added 5 ml
ethyl alcohol and 50 µl of a stannous chloride solution (4% (w/v)
$SnCl_2$ in 0.5 M HCl).  The blue product formed was measured
spectrophotometrically at 725 nm.  The haematocrit was measured
on a separate whole blood sample.

The red blood cell Pi concentration was calculated from the
following equation:

$$RBC\ Pi = \frac{100\ WB.Pi - (100 - x)\ Pl.Pi}{x}$$

where x is the haematocrit, WBPi is the Pi content of whole
blood and Pl.Pi that of plasma.

In vitro incubations were performed as follows:-

An aliquot of whole blood was diluted to 50 per cent of its
haematocrit value with a solution containing Isotonic Sodium
chloride and phosphate at a concentration exactly matching the
plasma concentration.  20µCi of $^{32}P$ labelled Pi was added.  The
cells were incubated at 37°C in a shaking water bath and gassed
with 5% $CO_2$/95% $O_2$.  Aliquots were taken out at various times and
assayed for intra- and extracellular Pi as above.  $^{32}P$ was
counted in aliquots of the perchloric acid supernatant, and in
the organic and aqueous layers of the assay by the Cerenkow
method.  Nucleotide levels in red blood cells were measured using
high pressure liquid chromatography.

RESULTS

The standard curve for this method was linear up to Pi concentrations of 3 mM in the starting sample.  Addition of
phosphate-containing organic compounds (ATP, hexose  phosphates,
etc.) which may be present in human blood did not interfere with
the method.  When $^{32}PPi$ was added to the assay there were no
detectable counts in the isobutanol layer, which illustrates the
great selectivity of the extraction method for Pi.  Results from
17 normal subjects showed a coefficient of variation for the
assay of 4%.  Platelets and white cells did not contribute
significantly to the measured Pi values.  There was a direct

correlation between intra- and extracellular Pi concentrations in patients with a variety of diseases associated with a wide range of plasma phosphate values.  The intracellular:extracellular ratio of Pi in red cells was the same in each of these disease states as that found in normal subjects (Fig.1).

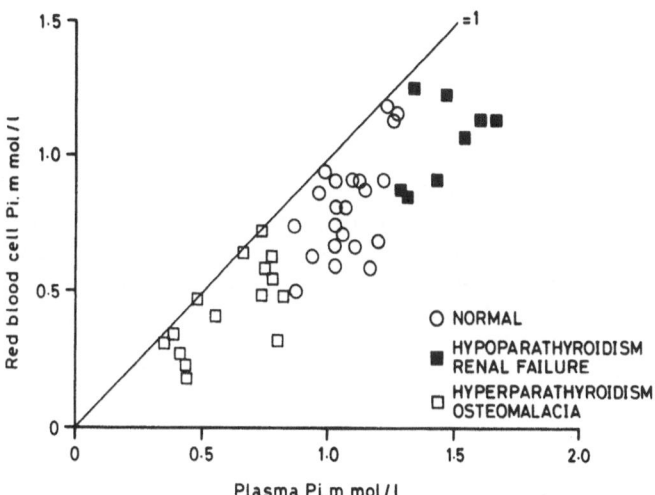

Fig.1.  Comparison of normal subjects and patients with high or low plasma phosphates.  Normal Subjects:  Ratio 0.65-0.99 (mean ± 1 S.E.M. 0.83 ± 0.02)

Patients with Paget's disease treated with the diphosphonate, ethane-1-hydroxy-1, 1-diphosphonate (EHDP) show an elevated level of plasma phosphate after two weeks of treatment. This rise is due to an increase in the reabsorptive capacity of the kidney for phosphate (Tmp/GFR) (5).  They show a normal intracellular to extracellular Pi ratio before treatment but after 2-4 weeks treatment the Pi ratio fell below the original value (Fig.2).

This was however due entirely to the rise in plasma phosphate and there was no detectable change in the red blood cell Pi.

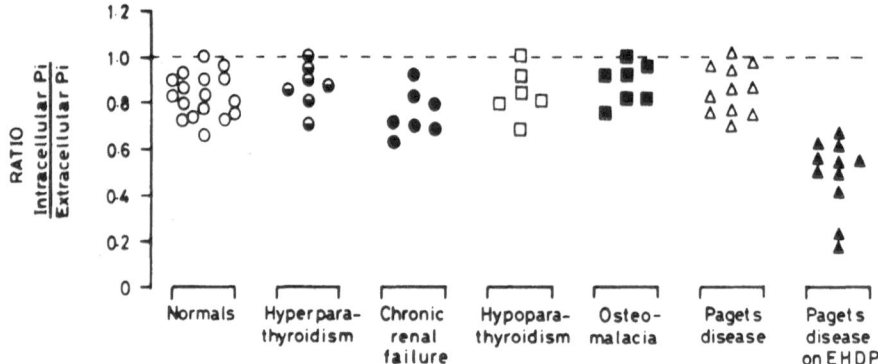

Fig. 2.    Intracellular:extracellular ratio of Pi in red blood
           cells in various disease states (see Fig.1)  Note the
           influence of EHDP on the Pi ratio in the red blood cell.
           The dose of EHDP was 80µmol/Kg/day.   Off EHDP, the Pi
           ratio was 0.70-0.99 (mean ±1 S.E.M. 0.83 ± 0.02).   On
           EHDP the ratio was 0.18-0.65 (mean ± 1 S.E.M. 0.49 ±
           0.05)


        There was also a fall in the Pi ratio   (Fig.3) in Paget's
patients treated with dichloro methylene diphosphonate ($Cl_2MDP$).
In this case both the plasma Pi and the red blood cell Pi fell
to account for the lowered ratio, but the changes did not persist
beyond the first month of treatment.

        During haemodialysis of patients with chronic renal failure
there was a fall in Pi in both plasma and red blood cells, but
the Pi ratio was unaltered.   However when haemodialysis stopped,
the plasma phosphate returned to baseline values more rapidly
than the red cell Pi.   Thus, the Pi ratio remained low for
several hours after dialysis. (Fig.4)

        Oral glucose given to two normal subjects caused a lowering
of plasma Pi but conversely a rise in the red blood cell Pi, so
that the Pi ratio rapidly approached 1.0. (Fig.5).

        Red blood cells from a normal subject incubated in vitro
with 1mM Iodoacetate to block glycolysis showed a rapid rise in
the Pi ratio during the first 30 min of incubation.   The Pi ratio
thereafter remained at 1.0, whereas the ratio remained normal
(below 1.0) in the control cells incubated without iodoacetate.

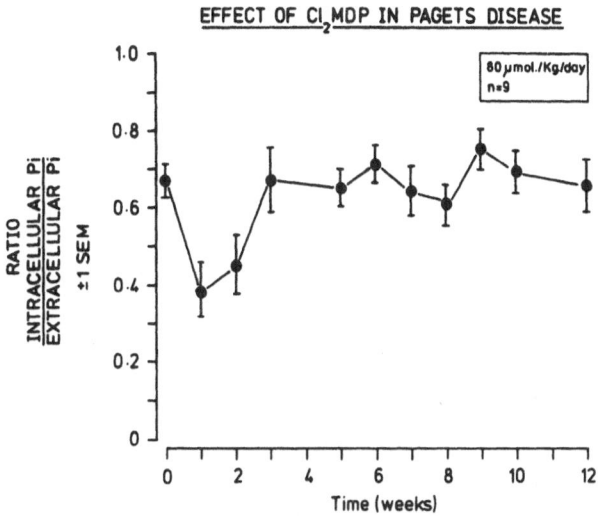

Fig. 3.    Effect of Cl$_2$MDP on the Pi ratio (mean ± 1 S.E.M)


Incorporation of $^{32}$P into red blood cells either as counts per minute or in the organic phosphate pool in the cells treated with 1 mM Iodoacetate showed a reduction when compared to control cells.

The pattern of red blood cell nucleotide changes was followed during incubation with Iodoacetate (Fig.8).  The results showed a rapid fall in ATP levels followed by a cascading effect on other nucleotides with a steady rise in hypoxanthine production.  Nucleotide levels in control cells showed no significant change during the incubation period.


SUMMARY

The measurement of Pi in red blood cells and plasma by this method is both highly selective and sensitive for Pi.  Normal subjects and several groups of patients in which plasma phosphate is altered exhibit a Pi ratio that is less than unity.  This method gives somewhat higher values for the ratio than the method of Tenenhouse & Scriver (6) which involved more manipulations of the red cells in vitro. Whether this ratio can be entirely accounted for as a diffusion equilibrium of Pi across the red cells determined by the electrochemical gradient and available intracellular water space is uncertain.  Even if this is the case,

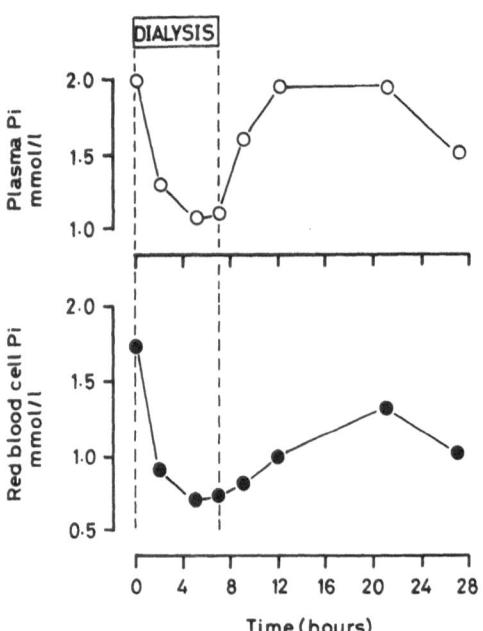

Fig. 4.   Effect of haemodialysis on plasma and red blood cell Pi
          in chronic renal failure.
          Pi ratio during dialysis (mean $\pm$ 1 S.E.M.) 0.77 $\pm$ 0.04
          Pi ratio after dialysis 0-2 hours 0.46
                                   2-4 hours 0.47
                                   4-14 hours 0.66
                                   14-21 hours 0.73

it is unclear why this normal ratio is lowered during EHDP
therapy, with the red cell failing to show the appropriate
response to the rise in plasma phosphate.   $Cl_2MDP$ produces a
similar effect on the ratio, but in the face of a lowered plasma
Pi during the first two weeks of treatment.

The Pi ratio can be shifted from its normal value during
glucose administration when it increases, and after haemodialysis
when it falls.

The response of the red blood cell to iodoacetate indicates
that the maintenance of the normal intra- to extracellular ratio
depends upon the integrity of metabolism.   Since the ratio
approaches 1 as ATP is dissipated, this may indicate that the

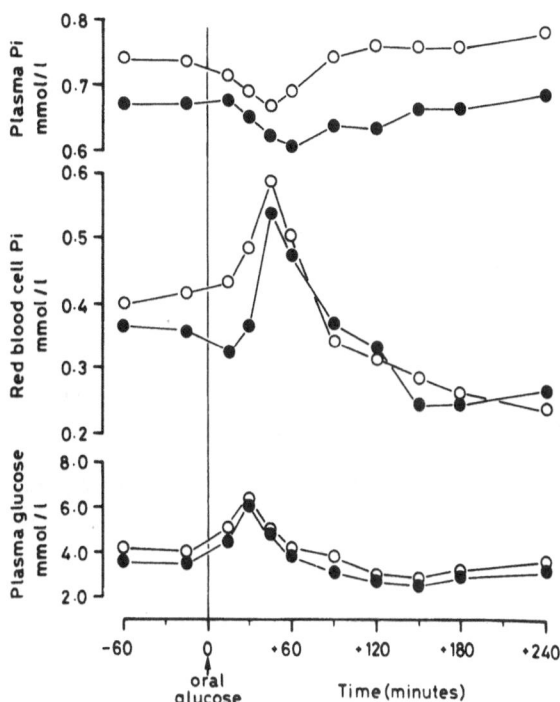

Fig. 5.   Effect of glucose on plasma and red blood cell Pi in
          two normal subjects.   The subjects received an oral
          glucose load of 50 g after an overnight fast.

available intracellular fluid volume is a higher proportion of
the total red cell volume than claimed in previous work (6).

These results suggest that the red blood cell is able to
preferentially alter its Pi content under conditions of altered
Pi metabolism and the distribution of Pi across the red cell
membrane does not appear to depend simply upon an equilibrium
determined by diffusion.

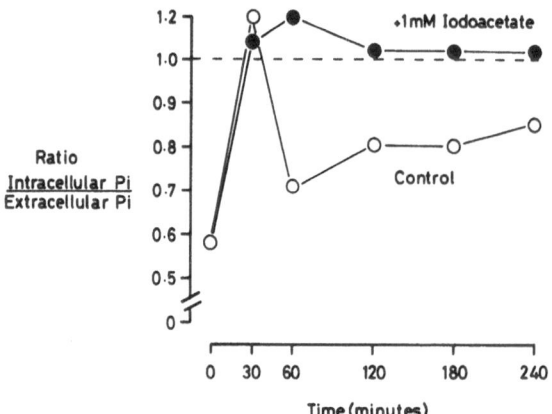

Fig. 6.   <u>In vitro</u> effect of incubation with 1 mM Iodoacetate on
          the Pi ratio in a normal subject.

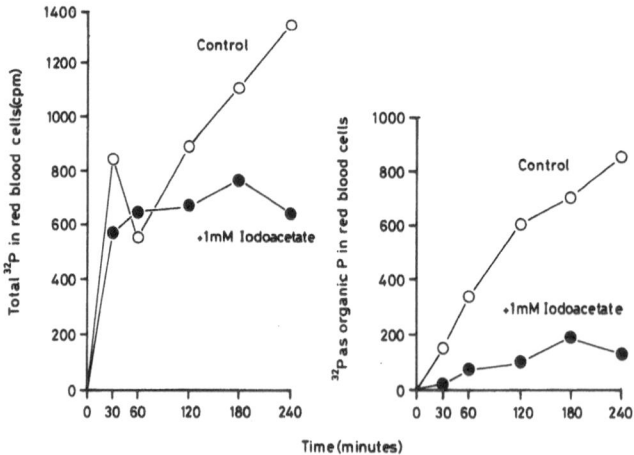

Fig.      Effect of Iodoacetate on incorporation of $^{32}$P into red
          blood cells.

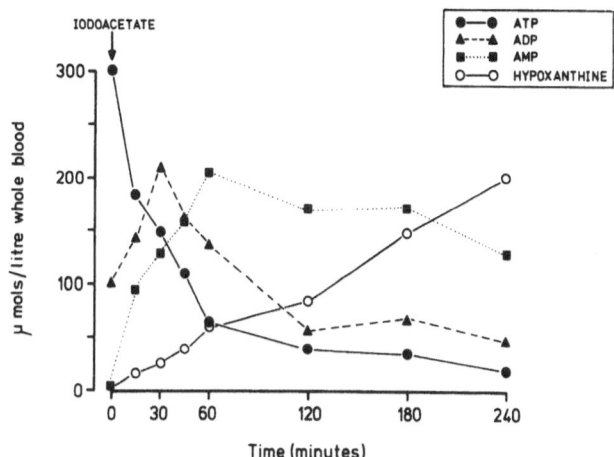

Fig. 8.  Nucleotide patterns during treatment with Iodoacetate
         (1 mM)

REFERENCES

1.  E.A. Newsholme and C. Start.  Regulation in Metabolism
        John Wiley London (1973).
2.  H.S. Jacob and T. Amsden.  Acute hemolytic anaemia and
        rigid red cells in hypophosphatemia.  New England
        Journal of Medicine.  285:1446-1450, (1971).
3.  S.I. Travis, H.I. Sugarmann and R.L. Ruberg.  Alter-
        ations of red cell glycolytic intermediates and
        oxygen transport as a consequence of hypophos-
        phatemia in patients receiving intravenous
        hyperalimentation.  New England Journal of Medicine.
        283: 763-768, (1971).
4.  R.J. Hall.  An improved method for the micro determin-
        ation of inorganic phosphate in small volumes of
        biological fluids.  Journal of Medical Laboratory
        Technology.  20 No. 2. 97-103, (1963).
5.  R.J. Walton, R.G.G. Russell and R. Smith.  Changes in
        the renal and extrarenal handling of phosphate
        induced by Disodium Etidronate (EHDP) in man.
        Clinical Science and Molecular Medicine.
        49:  45-56, (1975).

6.   H.S. Tenenhouse and C.R. Scriver.  Orthophosphate
     transport in the erythrocyte of normal subjects and
     patients with X-linked hypophosphatemia.  The
     Journal of Clinical Investigation.  55: 644-654,
     (1975).

CHRONIC HYPOPHOSPHATEMIA IN KIDNEY TRANSPLANTED CHILDREN AND YOUNG

ADULTS

Michèle Garabédian, Caroline Silve, David Lévy, Agnès
Bourdeau, André Ulmann, Michel Broyer, and Sonia Balsan

CNRS ER 126, INSERM U.30, and INSERM U.90
Hôpital des Enfants-Malades, Paris, France

INTRODUCTION

Different mechanisms have been suggested to account for the
frequently observed hypophosphatemia after renal transplantation.
One may propose, along this line, the persistence of a pretrans-
plant hyperparathyroidism[1,2], the post-transplant administration
of oral hydroxide antacids[3], the post-transplant steroid therapy[4]
a deficiency in vitamin D active metabolites[4,5], a tubular dysfunction[6], or an abnormality in intestinal phosphate absorption[7].
In an attempt to analyse the respective importance of these factors, serial measurements of biochemical and radioimmunological
parameters have been performed in the twelve subjects transplanted
during the year 1976 in the Department of Pediatric Nephrology
(Pr. M. Broyer) and considered as successful kidney transplantation.

SUBJECTS AND METHODS

Children and young adults had been selected among the 1976
allograft recipients on the basis of a satisfactory renal function throughout the investigation period. The arbitrary minimum
required level for creatinine clearance was equal to or over
50 ml/min/1.73 m2. The subject ages ranged from 9 to 20 years at
the time of transplantation (January-December 1976). All patients
had been on chronic hemodialysis for 7 to 36 months before this
time. The sources of the kidneys used for transplantation were
from cadaveric donors. HL-A identities between grafts and recipients
were 2 to 4. The warm and cold ischaemia-times of the graft varied
respectively from 1 to 5 minutes and from 2 to 26 hours.

The investigation period started at the 6th month and lasted up to the 30th-36th month following renal transplantation. This period had been deliberately chosen because of fluctuations in renal function and steroid therapy commonly observed in the early stage of the post-transplantation.

During the study period, all patients received immunosuppressive treatment (azathioprine 3 mg/kg/d, prednisone 0.2-0.5 mg/kg/d), 25-(OH) vitamin $D_3$ (15-35 µg/d), antihypertensive drugs and diuretics. Their total daily intake of phosphorus and calcium ranged respectively from 550 to 2300 mg and 400 to 2500 mg. None of them received hydroxide antacids, but all received oral aluminum phosphate antacids. One acute rejection episode occured in 4 patients. It was controlled by increasing the prednisone dosage, and by infusions of hydrocortisone.

Plasma calcium, phosphorus, creatinine, alkaline phosphatases, total protein and bicarbonates concentrations, urinary calcium phosphorus, creatinine concentrations were measured regularly one to three times monthly. Serum 25-(OH)D[8], 1,25-(OH)$_2$D[9] concentrations were measured as well as iPTH concentrations on blood samples taken from the 20th to the 36th month. The serum PTH assay utilized a carboxy-terminal antiserum. All PTH values were expressed as equivalents of purified bovine PTH. The lower limit of detection was 0.2 ng/ml. Normal values in this assay are 0.65 ng/ml or less. Urine was examined at regular intervals for the presence of reducing sugars and for detection of amino-aciduria.

RESULTS

Twenty months after kidney transplantation, 4 out of the 12 subjects had been found hypophosphatemic over periods of 5 to 14 months (i.e. phosphorus plasma concentrations lower than 1.12 mmol/1 up to the age of 12 years and lower than 1.05 mmol/1 in older subjects). At that time, comparison between normo and hypophosphatemic subjects showed that mean plasma phosphorus concentrations and mean tubular reabsorptions of phosphorus measured over the 14 month-period were significantly lower in the group of hypophosphatemic patients (Table I). As for the other parameters shown on Table I, and although the differences were not statistically significant, mean plasma calcium and creatinine concentrations were found higher and mean creatinine clearances lower in the hypophosphatemic than in the normophosphatemic group.

Extension of the investigation period to the 30th-36th month after kidney transplantation was associated with an increased number of hypophosphatemic subjects from 4 to 7. During the last 10-16 months of the study, all the seven hypophosphatemic subjects had lower renal tubular phosphate reabsorption. Six of them had

Table I. Biochemical parameters in hypo and normophosphatemic sub-
          jects measured from the 6th to the 20th month after renal
          transplantation.

|  | Normophosphatemic (8) | Hypophosphatemic (4) |
|---|---|---|
| Plasma phosphate concentration (mmol/1) | 1.23 ± 0.05* | 1.02 ± 0.07* <br> p < 0.05 |
| Plasma calcium concentration (mmol/1) | 2.52 ± 0.001 | 2.60 ± 0.001 <br> n.s |
| Plasma creatinine concentration (μmol/1) | 84.8 ± 6.2 | 105.2 ± 11.5 <br> n.s |
| Creatinine clearance (ml/min/1.73 m2) | 110 ± 13 | 85 ± 13 <br> n.s |
| Tubular reabsorption of phosphorus | 85.4 ± 1.8 | 65.1 ± 5.9 <br> p < 0.01 |

*For each parameter, the mean of all data obtained during the 14
 month period was first calculated for each subject. Values shown
 on this table are the mean ± S.D. of the previous individual means.
 Numbers in brackets are the number of subject studied in each
 group. Significant differences between the two groups are noted.
 n.s = not significant.

also higher plasma creatinine concentrations and lower creatinine
clearances when compared to 1) values found in the 5 normophosphatemic subjects ; 2) values found during the first 14 month period
in the three children who had been considered normophosphatemic
during the first 20 months after renal transplantation and hypophosphatemic for the following 10-16 months.

    Analysis of all data obtained from the 6th to the 30-36th
month after transplantation in the 12 subjects showed a positive
correlation between plasma phosphate concentrations and tubular
phosphate reabsorptions (p < 0.001), a positive correlation between
plasma phosphate concentrations and creatinine clearances (p < 0.02)
and a negative correlation between plasma phosphate and plasma

Table II. Plasma vitamin D metabolites and iPTH concentrations 20
          to 36 months after successful kidney transplantation.

|  | Normophosphatemic subjects (5) | Hypophosphatemic subjects (7) |
|---|---|---|
| 25-(OH)D ng/ml | 18.7 + 4.2 | 20.2 + 5.4 |
| 1,25-(OH)$_2$D pg/ml | 176 + 18 | 126 + 11 |
| iPTH ng/ml | 0.17 + 0.02 | 0.29 + 0.05 |

creatinine concentrations (p < 0.001). A less significant negative
correlation was also found between plasma phosphate and calcium
concentrations (p < 0.05).

Immunoreactive parathyroid hormone and vitamin D metabolites
plasma concentrations could not be measured before the 20th month
after transplantation. After this time, measurements of these
parameters were done two to four times for each subject at one to
eight month intervals. No significant difference  between the two
groups of hypo and normophosphatemic patients could be found when
comparing their mean plasma 25-(OH)D, or iPTH concentrations
(Table II). The difference in mean plasma 1,25-(OH)$_2$D concentration, lower in the hypophosphatemic group, was at the limit of
statistical significance (p < 0.05). All the plasma iPTH levels
assayed were found within the normal range as well in the hypophosphatemic as in the normophosphatemic patients.

No difference could be found between hypo and normophosphatemic children as for calcium urinary excretion, plasma alkaline
phosphatase activity, plasma bicarbonate  concentrations. Neither
amino-aciduria nor glycosuria have been detected in the urine of
the twelve subjects during the 24-30 month study. Daily phosphorus,
calcium, vitamin D intake were similar in both groups as well as
steroid and other immunosuppressive therapy, and aluminum phosphate antacid administration. No difference could be found either
when comparing the age, type of primary kidney disease, duration
of hemodialysis before renal transplantation, warm and cold

ischaemia times of the allograft, histocompatibility between cadaveric donors and young recipients.

COMMENTS

     In the present group of 12 successfully kidney transplanted
children and young adults and during the period of investigation
(6th to 30-36th month after transplantation), hypophosphatemia has
been observed in 7 subjects. The first point to be noted is that
hypophosphatemia was moderate and seemed clinically well tolerated.
This hypophosphatemia was closely correlated to a tubular phosphate
leak as previously described[3,6]. No secondary hyperparathyroidism,
no multiple tubular dysfunction and no difference in immunosuppressive therapy could account for the observed association of hypophosphatemia and renal phosphate leak. The coexistent finding of a
phosphate metabolism disorder with a slight decrease in glomerular
filtration rate has been frequent in the present investigation.
This situation could be analogous to that observed in the early
stage of renal failure[5]. At this stage, hypophosphatemia and hypocalcemia have been attributed to a relative deficit in $1,25-(OH)_2D$
synthesis in spite of the fact that some patients with renal failure at an early stage have normal circulating levels of this metabolite[10]. Similarly, in the kidney transplanted young children
with hypophosphatemia $1,25-(OH)_2D$ circulating levels, although not
markedly decreased in terms of absolute values, may have been inadequate considering the hypophosphatemic state of these patients.
However, one major difference with the observations in non-trans-
planted patients is the absence of hypocalcemia. One would have to
assume therefore that in these renal transplanted hypophosphatemic
subjects, the relative deficiency in $1,25-(OH)_2D$ synthesis would
be associated with a decrease in the activity of this metabolite
relating more on phosphate than on calcium metabolism. Similar
hypothesis has been drawn from the findings of an higher calcium
than phosphate intestinal absorption after renal transplantation[7].

     A last point to be emphasized is that even while none of the
above mentioned  factors may be decisive for the appearance of
hypophosphatemia after renal transplantation, their presence may
aggravate the phosphate metabolism disorder.

REFERENCES

1.  M. Kleerekoper, L.S. Ibels, J.P. Ingham, S.W. Mc Carthy, J.F.
        Mahony, J.H. Stewart, and S. Posen, Hyperparathyroidism
        after renal transplantation, British Medical Journal,
        3 : 680 (1975).
2.  P.G. Pletka, T.B. Strom, C.L. Hampers, H. Griffiths, R.E.
        Wilson, D.S. Bernstein, L.M. Sherwood, and J.P. Merrill,

   Secondary hyperparathyroidism in human kidney transplant
   recipients, Nephron, 17 : 371 (1976).
3. G.B. Schwartz, D.S. David, R.R. Riggio, P.D. Saville, J.C.
   Whitsell, K.H. Stenzel, and A.L. Rubin, Hypercalcemia after
   renal transplantation, Am. J. Med. 49 : 42 (1970).
4. R.G. Klein, S.B. Arnaud, J.C. Gallagher, H.F. DeLuca, and
   B.L. Riggs, Intestinal calcium absorption in exogenous
   hypercorticism. Role of 25-(OH)D and corticosteroid dose,
   J. Clin. Invest. 60 : 253 (1977).
5. N. Brautbar, and C.R. Kleeman, Disordered divalent ion metabolism in kidney disease : Comments on pathogenesis and
   treatment, in Advances in nephrology, volume 8, M.H. Maxwell,
   ed., Year Medical Book Publishers (1979).
6. J.F. Moorhead, M.R. Wills, K.Y. Ahmed, R.A. Baillod, Z. Varghese
   and G.L.V. Tatler, Hypophosphataemic osteomalacia after
   cadaveric renal transplantation, Lancet, 1 : 694 (1974).
7. K. Farrington, Z. Varghese, S.P. Newman, K.Y. Ahmed, O.N.
   Fernando, and J.F. Moorhead, Dissociation of absorptions of
   calcium and phosphate after successful cadaveric renal transplantation, British Medical Journal, 1 : 712 (1979).
8. M.A. Preece, J.L.H. O'Riordan, D.E.M. Lawson, and E. Kodicek,
   A competitive protein-binding assay for 25-hydroxycholecal-
   ciferol and 25-hydroxyergocalciferol in serum. Clin, Chim.
   Acta, 54 : 235 (1974).
9. J.A. Eisman, A.J. Hamstra, B.E. Kream, and H.F. DeLuca, 1,25-
   dihydroxyvitamin D in biological fluids : A simplified and
   sensitive assay, Science, 193 : 1021 (1976).
10. M.R. Haussler  and T.A. Mc Cain, Circulating 1,25-dihydroxy-
   vitamin D in health and disease, Clin. Res. 26 : 128A (1978).

# PATHOGENESIS OF HYPOPHOSPHATEMIA IN KIDNEY

# NECROGRAFT RECIPIENTS: A CONTROLLED TRIAL

K. Ølgaard, S. Madsen, Bi. Lund, Bj. Lund
& O.H. Sørensen

Nephrological Dept. P, Rigshospitalet, Medical
Dept. E, Frederiksberg Hospital, Dept. of
Orthopedic Surg., Hillerød Hospital and Medical
Dept. F, Herlev Hospital, Denmark

## INTRODUCTION

Disordered mineral metabolism in renal transplant
patients has attracted increasing attention in recent
years. Improved analytical methods for determination of
parathyroid hormone (PTH) and development of assays for
various vitamin D metabolites have greatly improved the
possibility of studying the pathogenesis of hypophosphatemia in kidney transplanted patients.

A high incidence of hypophosphatemia has been reported in long-term survivors after renal transplantation
(1, 2). This condition has mostly been attributed to a
renal phosphate leak and/or to an altered tubular sensitivity to PTH (2, 3).

Numerous factors can affect the renal handling of
phosphate, but it has been shown (4) that the levels of
circulating PTH has a key role in this respect. Vitamin
D may modulate the renal handling of phosphate, but the
net effect of the vitamin has been a matter of controversy. An increasing effect of various vitamin D metabolites on the tubular reabsorption of phosphate has been
proposed (5), while others have failed to demonstrate a
PTH-independent tubular effect of vitamin D (6).

Direct measurement of the biologically active vitamin D, 1.25-dihydroxyvitamin $D_3$ ($1.25(OH)_2D_3$) has shown
that most uremic patients after a successful renal transplantation achieve an increase and in many cases almost
normalization of the previously severely reduced levels
of $1.25(OH)D_3$. Therefore it should be considered whether

hypophosphatemia after kidney transplantation could be attributed to maintenance of reduced levels of $1.25(OH)_2$ $D_3$.
     In the present study, designed as a controlled trial, biochemical and clinical features were examined in normo- and hypophosphatemic kidney transplanted patients in order to elucidate the pathogenesis of hypophosphatemia after transplantation.

MATERIAL AND METHODS

     Twenty long-term survivors after kidney transplantation were investigated. Ten patients had persistent hypophosphatemia (serum phosphate below 0.78 mmol/l) and 10 patients were normophosphatemic (serum phosphate 0.78-1.48 mmol/l). The two groups were comparable as regards age, sex, duration of the previous uremic state, time after grafting, glomerular filtration rate and immunosuppressive treatment (Table I).

Table I.    Clinical data of 10 hypo- and 10 normophosphatemic kidney transplanted patients.(mean and range)

| Necrograft recipients | Serum-P mmol/l | No | Sex | Age | Mo. post transpl. | Y. of uremia | GFR ml/min | Prednisone mg/day |
|---|---|---|---|---|---|---|---|---|
| Hypophosphatemia | o.61 (o.48-o.75) | 1o | 3F, 7M | 41 (21-56) | 21 (2-118) | 4 (2-1o) | 62 (35-89) | 21 (o-3o) |
| Normophosphatemia | o.97 (o.8o-1.17) | 1o | 4F, 6M | 42 (27-54) | 27 (5-12o) | 4 (2-12) | 64 (4o-91) | 16 (o-27.5) |

     Blood samples were drawn after an overnight fast. The following parameters were measured: serum total and ionized ($Ca^{++}$) calcium, phosphate, magnesium, alkaline phosphatase, standard bicarbonate, immunoreactive PTH (i-PTH), 25-hydroxyvitamin $D_3$ ($25(OH)D_3$) and 1.25-di-hydroxyvitamin $D_3$ ($1.25(OH)_2D_3$). Finally the daily urinary excretion of calcium and phosphate was measured and the cold and warm ischaemia-times of the grafts determined. $Ca^{++}$ was measured by the Orion SS-20 (7); i-PTH by a radioimmunoassay primarily detecting the carboxy-terminal part of the PTH molecule (8); $25(OH)D_3$ by a competitive protein-binding assay (9) and $1.25(OH)_2D_3$ was measured by competitive protein-binding using rachi-

tic chick intestinal cytosol binding protein (10). The
renal handling of phosphate was expressed as the ratio
between the maximal tubular reabsorption of phosphate
and the glomerular filtration rate. This TmP/GFR index
was calculated according to the method of Walton and
Bijvoet (11).

RESULTS

Due to the selection of the patients serum phosphate
was significantly lower in the hypophosphatemic than in
the normophosphatemic patients. Furthermore the TmP/GFR
was significantly reduced in the hypophosphatemic patients (Table II). The i-PTH concentrations were signi-
cantly higher in the hypophosphatemic than in the normophosphatemic patients, while no significant differences
were found between the two groups as regards $Ca^{++}$,25(OH)
$D_3$, 1.25(OH)$_2D_3$ or any of the other measured parameters.
In particular no difference in the warm and cold ischaemia-times of the grafts existed between the two groups.

Table II.    Main results in the hypo- and
             normophosphatemic kidney trans-
             planted patients. Mean $\pm$ SD.
             *p < 0.05,**p < 0.001, n.s. not
             significant.

| | S-P mmol/l | U-P mmol/day | TmP/GFR µmol/ml | $Ca^{++}$ mmol/l | i-PTH pmol Eqv/l | 25-(OH)$D_3$ ng/ml | 1.25(OH)$_2D_3$ pg/ml |
|---|---|---|---|---|---|---|---|
| Hypophosphatemia | 0.61 ±0.08 | 21.6 ±7.6 | 0.34 ±0.08 | 1.10 ±0.08 | 430 ±196 | 24.1 ±8.0 | 24.2 ±18.4 |
| Normophosphatemia | 0.97 ±0.13 | 21.7 ±6.6 | 0.72 ±0.09 | 1.14 ±0.05 | 247 ±56 | 33.1 ±12.6 | 27.7 ±17.9 |
| | ** | n.s. | ** | n.s. | * | n.s. | n.s. |

In a previous investigation (4) we found a significant inverse relationship between TmP/GFR and i-PTH in
normophosphatemic transplanted patients (Figure 1). This
relationship was confirmed in the present investigation
(Figure 2). However, in the hypophosphatemic patients no
such relationship could be demonstrated. Despite higher
PTH levels in the hypophosphatemic patients the serum-Ca$^+$
was at the same levels in both groups and in no patient
hypercalcemia was present.

DISCUSSION

     Recent studies (12) have shown that the relation-
ship between TmP/GFR and i-PTH in fact conforms to the
shape of a hyperbola when a wide spectrum of TmP/GFR is
included (Figure 1). A similar correlation was found in
the normophosphatemic transplanted patients, but not in
the hypophosphatemic patients, who showed TmP/GFR values
not correlated with i-PTH (Figure 2). This finding indicates that hypophosphatemic kidney transplanted patients
exhibit a major defect in the PTH-mediated tubular reabsorption of phosphate.
     The finding of identical levels of 25(OH)D$_3$ and 1.25
(OH)$_2$D$_3$ in the two groups of transplanted patients suggests that disturbed vitamin D metabolism after transplantation cannot account for the hypophosphatemia frequently found in such patients.

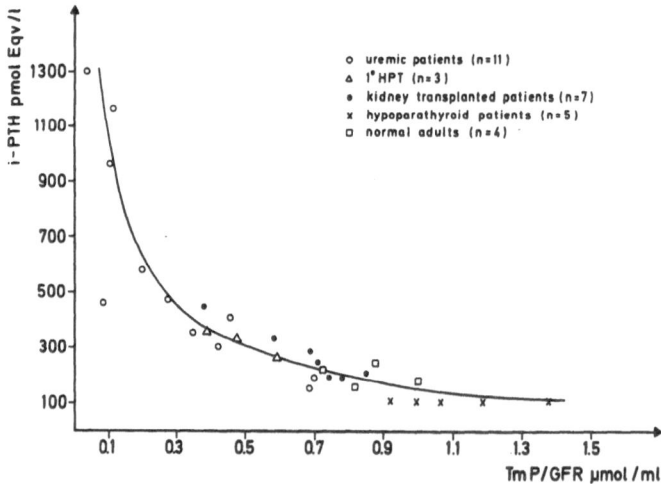

Fig. 1.    Relationship between TmP/GFR and PTH in a wide
           spectrum of patients from a previous investiga-
           tion (12). Note the inverse linear correlation
           in the normophosphatemic transplanted patients.

These results are in accordance with those of Farrington et al. (13). However, since hypophosphatemia stimulates the renal 1-hydroxylase of vitamin D it should be expected that hypophosphatemic patients would exhibit higher levels of 1.25(OH)$_2$D$_3$. As such a difference was not observed in the present study, a relative defect in vitamin D synthesis may exist in the hypophosphatemic transplanted patients. It should therefore be considered whether these patients exhibit a reduced tubular response to vitamin D.

Finally, it should be emphasized that the demonstrated renal phosphate leak may not be the only factor contributing to hypophosphatemia after transplantation since it has recently been shown (13) that also intestinal phosphate absorption frequently remains inappropriately low after transplantation.

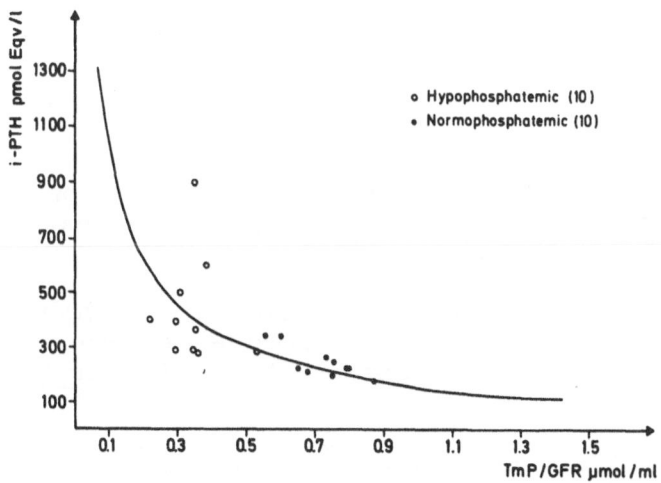

Fig. 2.    Hyperbola from figure 1 and the results of the present investigation in normo- and hypophosphatemic transplanted patients.

REFERENCES

1.  A.Z. Gyory, J.H. Steward, C.R.P. George, D.J. Tiller, and
    K.D.G. Edwards, Renal tubular acidosis, acidosis due to hyper-
    kalaemia, hypercalcaemia, disordered citrate metabolism and
    other tubular dysfunctions following human renal transplantation,
    Quart. J. Med. 38:231 (1969).

2.  J.F. Moorhead, M.R. Wills, K.Y. Ahmed, R.A. Baillod,
    Z. Varghese, and G.L.V. Tatler, Hypophosphataemic osteomalacia
    after cacaveric renal transplantation. Lancet I:694 (1974).

3.  H.E. Nielsen, M.S. Christensen, F. Melsen and S. Tørring,
    Bone disease, hypophosphatemia and hyperparathyroidism after
    renal transplantation, Adv. Exp. Med. Biol. 81:603 (1977).

4.  S. Madsen, K. Ølgaard, and J. Ladefoged, Renal handling of
    phosphate in relation to serum parathyroid hormone levels,
    Acta Med. Scand. 200:7 (1976).

5.  J.B. Puschett, J. Moranz, and W.S. Kurnick, Evidence for a
    direct action of cholecalciferol and 25-hydroxycholecalciferol
    on the renal transport of phosphate, sodium, and calcium.
    J. Clin. Invest. 51:373 (1972).

6.  S. Madsen and K. Ølgaard, Has vitamin D a direct renal effect
    on the tubular reabsorption of phosphate? Adv. Exp. Med. Biol.
    103:111 (1978).

7.  S. Madsen and K. Ølgaard, Evaluation of a new automatic calcium
    ion analyzer. Clin. Chem. 23:690 (1977).

8.  S. Almqvist, B. Hjern, and B. Wästhed, The diagnostic value of
    a radioimmunoassay for parathyroid hormone in human serum.
    Acta Endocrinol. 78:493 (1975).

9.  Bi. Lund, and D.H. Sørensen, Measurement of 25-hydroxyvitamin
    D in serum and its relation to sunshine, age and vitamin D
    intake in the Danish population. Scand. J. Clin. Lab. Invest.
    39:23 (1979).

10. Bj. Lund, Bi. Lund, and O.H. Sorensen, Measurement of circulat-
    ing 1,25-dihydroxyvitamin D in man. Changes in serum concen-
    trations during treatment with 1α-hydroxycholecalciferol.
    Acta. Endocrinol. 91:338 (1979).

11. R.J. Walton, and O.L.M. Bijvoet, Nomogram for derivation of
    renal threshold phosphate concentration. Lancet II:309 (1975).

12. S. Madsen, Calcium and phosphate metabolism in chronic renal failure, with particular reference to the effect of $1\alpha$-hydroxy-vitamin $D_3$. Acta Med. Scand. (1980, in press)

13. K. Farrington, Z. Varghese, S.P. Newman, K.Y. Ahmed, O.N. Fernando, and J.F. Moorhead, Dissociation of absorptions of calcium and phosphate after successful cadaveric renal transplantation. Br. Med. J. 1:712 (1979).

# EFFECT OF ACUTE METABOLIC ACIDOSIS ON PLASMA PHOSPHORUS CONCENTRATION

James R. Oster, Guido O. Perez, Albert Castro and
Carlos A. Vaamonde

Medical and Research Services, Veterans Administration
Medical Center and the Departments of Medicine and
Pathology, University of Miami School of Medicine,
Miami, Florida 33125

ABSTRACT

The effects of acid-base disturbances on plasma phosphorus
concentration remain poorly defined. In a previous study, we infused
anesthetized mongrel dogs with several mineral and non-mineral acids
for one to three hours. HCl and $NH_4Cl$ infusions were not associated
with changes in plasma phosphorus in contrast to the findings with
the organic acids lactic (LA) and beta-hydroxybutyric which increased,
and methylmalonic which decreased phosphorus levels. To evaluate
these observations further and to gain insight into the mechanism(s)
involved we measured plasma phosphorus concentration and renal phosphorus handling in dogs infused with 0.45% NaCl (control), HCl
and LA for six hours. In the control group there was no significant
change in phosphorus levels whereas the increase in phosphorus concentration for LA was significant after hour four. Although with
HCl, phosphorus concentration decreased in the first hour, there
was a tendency for an elevation by five hours. Cumulative six hour
$U_pV$ was significantly lower with HCl than with either LA or NaCl and
the data suggest that the infusion of both acids may have blunted
the augmentation of phosphorus excretion associated with mild volume
expansion. Plasma glucose and insulin measured for three hours
showed no significant differences between the groups. We conclude
that the acid anion provides a major influence of the effect of
mineral acids on plasma phosphorus. The initial differences
in plasma phosphorus concentration between the two acid-infused
groups could not be accounted for by differences in urinary
phosphorus excretion or plasma insulin levels, while the findings

occurring after three hours might have been due, at least in part, to dissimilarities in renal phosphorus handling.


## INTRODUCTION

It has been known for several years that changes in extra-cellular fluid pH may influence serum phosphorus concentration.[1-6] In general, a rise in serum phosphorus concentration may occur during acute metabolic acidosis [2-5] while chronic metabolic acidosis is associated with decreases [4] or no changes [1,5] in serum phosphorus concentration. In addition, there is both experimental [7] and clinical [8,9] evidence suggesting that the blood phosphorus response to acute acidosis depends in part on the nature of the acidifying agent. Recently, we reported that, whereas the one to three hour infusion of HCl and NH4Cl in anesthetized mongrel dogs was not asso-ciated with significant changes in plasma phosphorus concentration, there was a stepwise increment in the blood level during the admin-istration of lactic and beta-hydroxybutyric acids.[7]

The purpose of the present study was to determine if the previously observed varying plasma phosphorus response to organic and mineral acids would obtain during more prolonged acidemia and to attempt to elucidate the pathophysiologic mechanism(s) involved.


## MATERIALS AND METHODS

The studies were performed in thirty-one female mongrel dogs weighing between 14 and 25 kg. The animals received food and water ad libitum until the day of the study. On the morning of the study, the dogs were anesthetized with pentobarbital, 30 mg/kg body weight i.v. (additional small amounts of pentobarbital were administered if necessary). Ventilation was assisted with a Harvard respirator attached to an endotracheal tube in an attempt to keep $Pco_2$ as constant as possible. Cannulas were placed in the right femoral artery for blood sampling and blood pressure monitoring with a Statham transducer connected to a Hewlett-Packard recorder, and in the femoral vein for infusions. Urine was collected using Foley catheters and air washout technique. Glomerular filtration rate (GFR) was estimated by inulin clearance.

After placement of the cannulas, two ml of blood were obtained for arterial blood pH and $Pco_2$ measurements to establish the dog's acid-base status prior to the beginning of the infusions. A 45 minute equilibration period and two 15 minute baseline periods followed. Saline, 0.9%, was infused at a rate of 0.5 ml/min during the equilibration and baseline periods in all animals.

The following groups of dogs received six hour infusions:
a) controls (n=7); b) HCl (analyzed reagent, J.T. Baker Co., 7.5
mEq/kg body weight, n=7); c) lactic acid (LA, Fisher certified reagent,
Fisher Scientific, 15 mEq/kg body weight, n=7). For all groups,
immediately following the second baseline period the infusion was
changed from 0.9% saline to either 0.45% saline (control group) or
the acid solutions. One-third of the total amount of acid was given
in the first hour, one-third in the second and third hours, and one-
third in the last three hours. The acids were diluted in 0.45%
saline. The control and acid infusions were administered at a rate
of five ml/min.

Blood sampling was performed at the end of the equilibration
period and of each baseline period. Since the results of these three
determinations were similar for all the variables measured, these
data were averaged and will be referred to subsequently as the baseline values. Blood was obtained every 30 minutes during the infusions.
Each blood sample was approximately 22 ml and was transferred immediately from polystyrene syringes into heparinized tubes. In all
studies, arterial blood pressure was measured just prior to obtain-
ing the blood samples. Mean arterial pressures were in the range of
120-150 mm Hg and $Po_2$ ranged between 89 and 100 mm Hg throughout the
duration of the experiments.

Determination of blood pH and $Pco_2$ was completed within five
minutes of collection using a Radiometer-Copenhagen acid-base cart
ABC-1. Sodium was measured by flame photometry with a lithium
internal standard (Model 143: Instrumentation Laboratory, Inc.),
phosphorus by an automated method using a modification of the method
of Fiske and Subbarow,[10] and hematocrit using an International Equip-
ment Co. microhematocrit centrifuge. Blood bicarbonate concentration
[HCO3] was calculated from the Henderson-Hasselbalch equation assuming a pK'a of 6.10 and a solubility coefficient of 0.0301. Glucose,[11]
and insulin [12] were measured by standard techniques adapted for automated chemical analysis; inulin was determined by Steele's [13]
modification of the resorcinol method and lactate was measured by
enzymatic analysis.[14]

Statistical evaluation of the data was accomplished by one-way
analysis of variance followed by Fisher's least-significant differences
test when the former indicated that a significant difference ($P<0.05$)
existed, and by other standard techniques.


RESULTS

Blood Acid-Base Status and Plasma Phosphorus (Table 1).

Administration of the acidifying agents resulted in prompt and
substantial declines in arterial blood pH and [HCO3]. Prior to acid

Table 1.   Changes in Acid-Base Status and Plasma Phosphorus Concentration During Acid Infusion

| | | Baseline | Experimental | | | | | |
| | | | 1 hr | 2 hr | 3 hr | 4 hr | 5 hr |
|---|---|---|---|---|---|---|---|
| pH | C | 7.39±.02 | 7.39±.02 | 7.38±.02 | 7.36±.02a | 7.35±.02a | 7.36±.02 |
| | HCl | 7.40±.01 | 7.25±.01bd | 7.23±.02bd | 7.19±.02bd | 7.19±.02bd | 7.15±.03bd |
| | LA | 7.36±.01 | 7.23±.02bd | 7.22±.02bd | 7.22±.02bd | 7.22±.01bd | 7.23±.01bd |
| Pco2 (mm Hg) | C | 34±2 | 32±2a | 33±2 | 34±2 | 36±3 | 33±3 |
| | HCl | 35±2 | 32±2a | 28±2b | 26±2b | 24±2bc | 23±3b |
| | LA | 38±3 | 35±2 | 33±3a | 31±3a | 31±3a | 29±2b |
| HCO3 (mEq/L) | C | 20±1 | 19±1a | 18±1a | 18±1 | 19±1 | 18±1a |
| | HCl | 21±1 | 14±1bd | 12±1bd | 10±1bd | 9±1bd | 8±1bd |
| | LA | 21±2 | 14±1bd | 13±1bd | 12±1bd | 12±1bd | 12±1bd |
| Phosphorus (mg/dl) | C | 4.4±.3 | 4.3±.3 | 4.4±.3 | 4.5±.3 | 4.4±.3 | 4.3±.2 |
| | HCl | 4.7±.4 | 4.1±.3a | 4.2±.3 | 4.5±.3 | 4.9±.4 | 5.3±.4 |
| | LA | 4.9±.1 | 5.0±.3 | 4.9±.3 | 5.3±.2 | 5.7±.2bd | 5.7±.1bd |

Values are means ± SE.   C, control (NaCl)(n=7); LA, lactic acid (n=7); HCl, hydrochloric acid (n=7).
a $p<0.05$; b $p<0.005$ paired data (baseline versus subsequent values).
c $p<0.05$; d $p<0.005$ unpaired data (acid-loading versus C).

infusion there were no significant differences between the plasma
phosphorus concentrations of the three groups.  In the control group,
saline administration was not associated with any change in plasma
phosphorus.  With HCl, the phosphorus concentration initially
declined below the baseline value, and after the first three hours
of infusion returned to baseline, tending to exceed the initial value
at four and five hours.  In contrast, LA administration was not associated with any initial decline in blood phosphorus but rather with
a stepwise increment in the mean concentration which by the fourth
hour was 0.8 ml/dl greater (P<0.005) than the baseline value.  Figure
1 illustrates the relationship between the changes in plasma pH
and phosphorus concentration in each of the three groups.

Renal Phosphorus Handling (Table 2).

The mean baseline inulin clearances of the three groups were
nearly identical.  During the infusions, the inulin clearance
increased significantly in the control and LA groups and remained
unchanged in the dogs given HCl.  Nevertheless, there were no significant differences between the inulin clearances of the three groups
throughout the experiment.

Prior to acid administration, there were no significant differences between the three groups in fractional sodium excretion ($FE_{Na}$)
or in filtered load ($FL_p$), urinary excretion (UpV) or fractional
excretion of phosphorus (FEp).  FLp and UpV increased significantly
in the control and LA groups while the changes in the dogs given
HCl were not statistically significant.  FEp increased significantly
in all three groups.  UpV and FEp tended to be (or in some collection periods were) lower in the acid-infused groups as compared to
the control group.  This was particularly the case with the HCl
group.  Figure 2 illustrates the increments in fractional phosphorus
excretion during acid infusion.  During the first three hours of
infusion the increases in the two acid groups tended to be smaller
than that of the control group but the differences were not statistically significant.  The peak increment in FEp above baseline
occurring during the last three hours of acid administration was
significantly greater in the control animals (28+5%) as compared to
that of the dogs receiving either HCl (11+3%) or LA (11+3%); P<0.025
for both.  Cumulative phosphorus excretion during the six hour
experiment was similar in the control and LA groups and was significantly less in the HCl group (P<0.005, HCl vs LA and vs control;
control 242+42 [SE], HCl 121+88, LA 218+58 mg/6 hour).  During acid
infusion $FE_{Na}$ increased in all three groups but the changes did not
achieve statistical significance in the control group.  The relationship between FEp and $FE_{Na}$ is shown in Figure 3.

Changes in Blood Glucose, Insulin and Lactate Levels (Table 3).

Prior to acid infusion, the plasma glucose concentrations

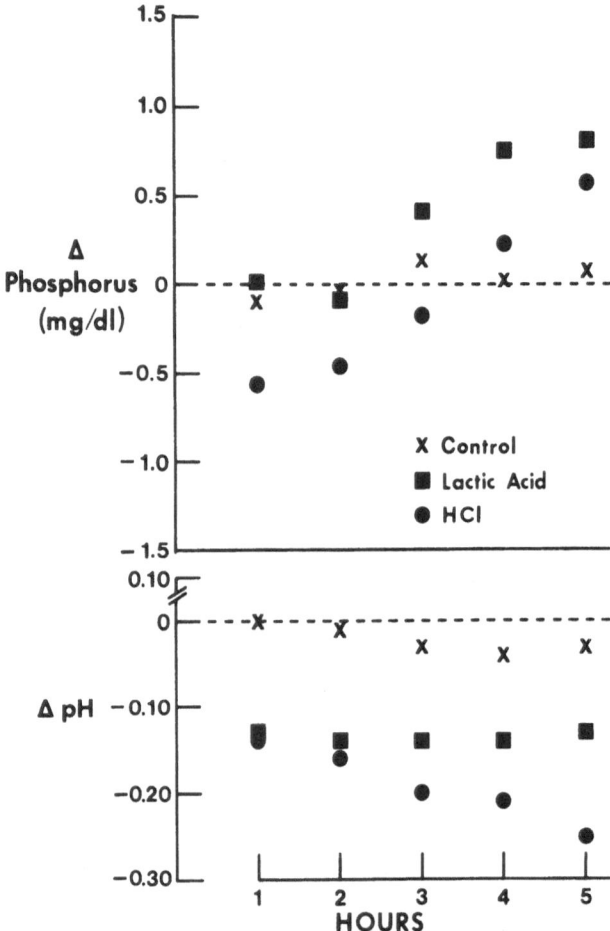

Fig. 1.  Changes (Δ) in plasma pH and phosphorus concentration in control and·acid-infused dogs.  For simplification, standard errors and statistically significant differences are not shown  (see text for details).

Table 2.  Effect of Acid Infusion on Renal Phosphorus Handling

| | | Baseline | Experimental | | | | | |
|---|---|---|---|---|---|---|---|---|
| | | | 1 hr | 2 hr | 3 hr | 4 hr | 5 hr | 6 hr |
| $C_{IN}$ (ml/min) | C | 65+8 | 78+11a | 80+13 | 82+11 | 83+9a | 80+10b | 83+11a |
| | HCl | 66+7 | 67+6 | 71+8 | 73+10 | 70+9 | 63+10 | 60+12 |
| | LA | 64+5 | 61+8 | 66+9 | 71+9 | 79+7a | 78+8a | 76+7a |
| $FL_p$ (μgm/min) | C | 2823+390 | 3359+564 | 3541+727 | 3735+654a | 3807+516a | 3529+529 | 3520+544 |
| | HCl | 2940+391 | 2837+331 | 2897+329 | 3094+373 | 3168+331 | 3094+404 | 2984+448 |
| | LA | 3061+282 | 2849+337 | 3243+409 | 3585+428 | 4301+378b | 4376+434a | 4336+319a |
| $U_pV$ (μgm/min) | C | 175+62 | 197+73 | 245+98 | 606+158a | 811+230a | 1146+169b | 1054+182b |
| | HCl | 314+109 | 231+85 | 215+63 | 278+78 | 385+111 | 520+94c | 654+162 |
| | LA | 392+74 | 384+95 | 413+93 | 503+52 | 724+103 | 887+94a | 978+101b |
| $FE_p$ (%) | C | 6+2 | 6+2 | 6+2 | 15+3a | 26+4b | 33+4b | 31+5b |
| | HCl | 10+3 | 8+3 | 8+3 | 10+3 | 13+4c | 18+4c | 22+5a |
| | LA | 12+1 | 13+2 | 12+2 | 14+1 | 17+2 | 21+3ac | 23+2a |
| $FE_{Na}$ (%) | C | 0.4+0.1 | 0.7+0.2 | 0.9+0.3 | 1.1+0.3 | 1.7+0.6 | 1.8+0.6 | 1.6+0.7 |
| | HCl | 1.1+0.4 | 0.7+0.4 | 1.3+0.6 | 1.8+0.7 | 2.3+0.3 | 2.5+0.6 | 2.9+0.8a |
| | LA | 0.5+0.2 | 0.9+0.4a | 1.0+0.1 | 1.7+0.5a | 2.1+0.5b | 2.5+0.7a | 2.5+0.5b |

Values are means + SE of 7 dogs in each group.  $C_{IN}$ = inulin clearance, $FL_p$ = filtered load of phosphorus, $U_pV$ = urinary phosphorus excretion, $FE_p$ = fractional excretion of phosphorus, $FE_{Na}$ = fractional excretion of sodium.  For explanation of other symbols see Table 1.  There were no statistically significant differences between HCl and LA groups except for the UpV values during the fourth hour (P<0.05).

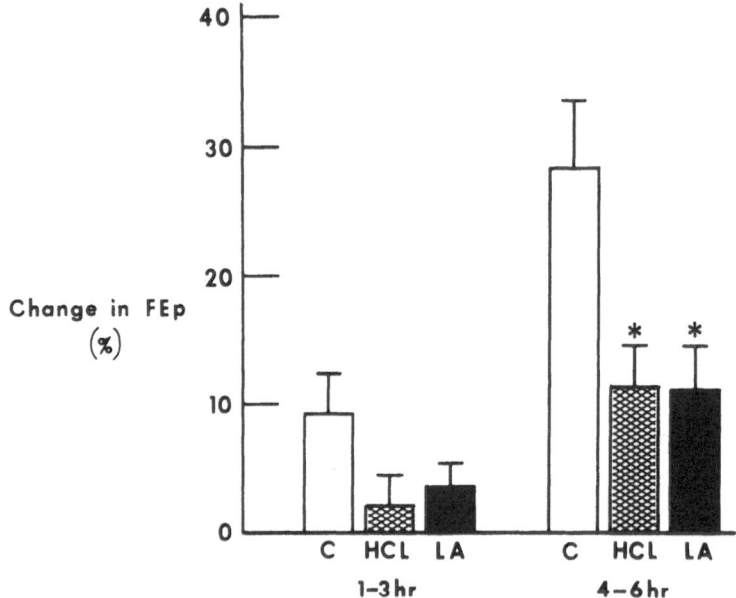

Fig. 2.   Increments in the fractional excretion of phosphorus during acid administration.  Data in left hand panel represent the differences between the peak values in the first
three hours or infusion and the baseline level.  The right
hand panel illustrates the difference between the peak
value for the last three hours of the experimental period
and the baseline level.  C = Control; * P< 0.025 in comparison to control.

Table 3.  Effect of Acid Infusions on Fasting Plasma Glucose,
Insulin and Lactate*

| | n | Baseline | Experimental | | |
|---|---|---|---|---|---|
| | | | 1 hr | 2 hr | 3 hr |
| Glucose (mg/dl) | | | | | |
| C | 6 | 94±4 | 90±4 | 89±7 | 94±7 |
| HCl | 6 | 105±3 | 104±7 | 90±6a | 86±8a |
| LA | 6 | 104±3 | 98±6 | 88±6a | 84±6a |
| Insulin (μU/ml) | | | | | |
| C | 6 | 13±2 | 11±2 | 10±2 | 11±2 |
| HCl | 6 | 17±3 | 15±3 | 13±4 | 13±3 |
| LA | 6 | 21±3c | 20±3 | 18±4 | 16±4 |
| Lactate (mmol/l) | | | | | |
| C | 6 | 1.7±.3 | 1.4±.4a | 1.2±.3 | 1.1±.2b |
| HCl | 6 | 1.9±.4 | 1.9±.6 | 1.5±.4 | 1.3±.3 |
| LA | 6 | 2.0±.2 | 5.3±.3bd | 3.7±.5ad | 3.0±.6c |

Values are means ± SE.  For the insulin and glucose values some of the animals
included in this table are those presented in Table 1 while the remaining are
different dogs.
* Appropriate increases of insulin levels after KCl (n=3) and glucose (n=3)
infusion were exhibited by additional dogs which served as positive controls.
For explanation of symbols see Table 1.

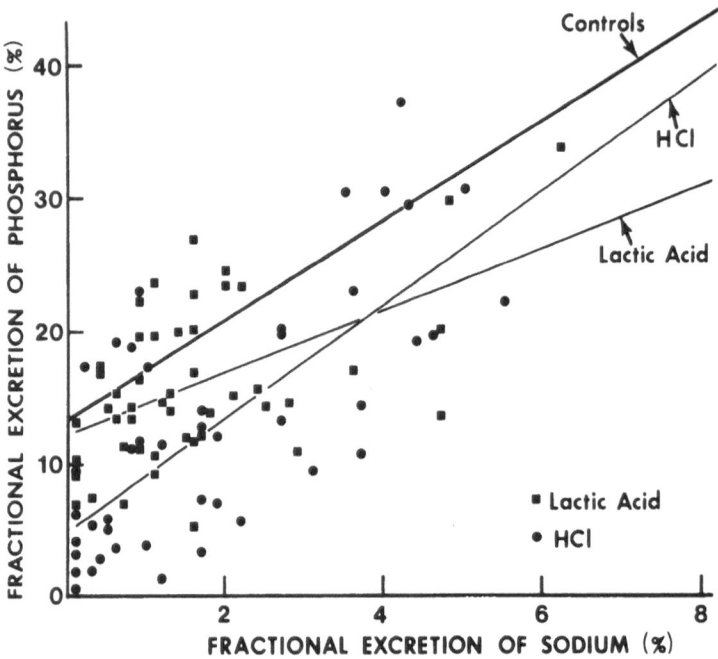

Fig. 3.  Relationship between the fractional excretion of phospho-
         rus (FEp) and fractional excretion of sodium (FE$_{Na}$).  There
         was a significant correlation between FE$_{Na}$ and FEp in all
         groups (C, r=.32, P<.05; HCl, r=.73, P<.01; LA, r=.53,
         P<.01).  There were no significant differences between the
         slope of the regression lines of the control (3.79) versus
         that of either the HCl (4.34) or LA (2.39) group.  The el-
         evation of the regression line of the control animals was
         significantly higher (F 12.2, P<.01) than that of the
         HCl dogs.

of the three groups were similar.  While plasma glucose decreased
significantly below baseline in the two acid-infused groups, the
differences occurring between the three groups during infusion did
not reach statistical significance.  The baseline insulin level of
the LA-infused group was greater ($P<0.05$) than that of the controls.
Although the insulin level tended to decline in the HCl and LA dogs
there were no significant differences between the three groups after
the initiation of acid infusions.

Baseline plasma lactate was similar in all groups.  The level
declined in the control and HCl dogs and increased, as expected, in
the LA dogs, with the increment being the greatest in the first two
hours of lactic acid infusion.  Whereas the excretion rate of lactate
remained stable in the control and HCl dogs, it increased sharply in
the LA group reaching a peak of 40 $\mu$M/min during the first hour (data
not shown).

Effect of $NH_4Cl$ and $CaCl_2$ on Serum Phosphorus in Man.

For comparison with the results obtained in this study, Figure
4 shows the results of the effect of $NH_4Cl$ and $CaCl_2$ ingestion on
serum phosphorus concentration in normal male volunteers.  The data
were evaluated retrospectively from studies performed in 34 volunteers who served as control subjects for other studies conducted in
our laboratory.  A greater degree of acidemia was induced with $NH_4Cl$
than $CaCl_2$.  At two and five hours after acid-loading, serum phosphorus levels were significantly greater than baseline values in the
subjects receiving $CaCl_2$ but not in those given $NH_4Cl$.  In neither
group was there a statistically significant correlation between pH
and phosphorus concentration.


DISCUSSION

Previous studies from this laboratory [7] suggested that the
acute changes in plasma phosphorus concentration induced by metabolic
acidosis depend in part on the nature of the acidifying agent.  The
difference between the effect on plasma phosphorus by three hour
infusion of mineral (HCl) and non-mineral (lactic) acids has been
confirmed in the present studies.  This difference, however, tended
to dissipate by five hours.  Although the varying initial effects
on plasma phosphorus levels could not be explained by dissimilarities
in urinary phosphorus excretion or in plasma insulin concentrations
between the groups, it. is possible that the increase in plasma phosphorus occurring after three hours in the HCl group was related at
least in part to the lower rate of phosphorus excretion in this
group as compared to that of the LA dogs (vide infra).

While acid-base disturbances are known to influence plasma

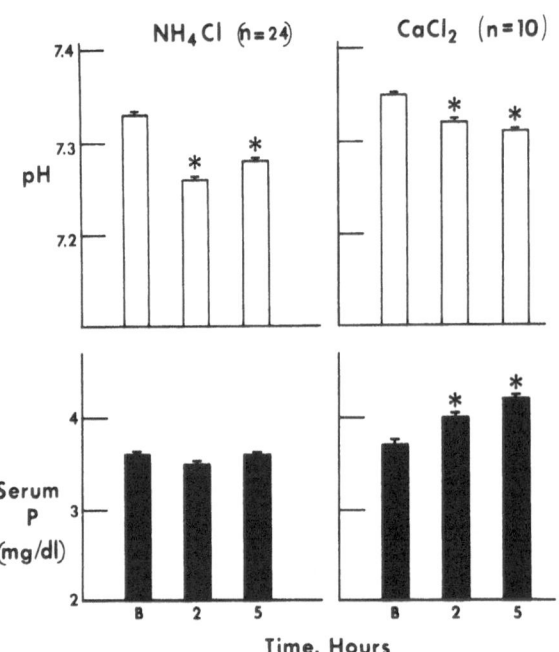

Fig. 4.   Effect of NH4Cl and CaCl2 ingestion on serum phosphorus
          concentration in healthy volunteers previously studied in
          our laboratory.[29-31]  Asterisk denotes statistically sig-
          nificant differences from baseline.

phosphorus levels the available data are limited. Alkalosis, particularly the respiratory variety, is known to produce rather prompt hypophosphatemia probably by stimulation of glycolysis with subsequent translocation of phosphorus out of the extracellular compartment[15-17]. On the other hand, acute acidosis may result in an increase in serum phosphorus concentration which probably results from mobilization of phosphorus from intracellular stores[1-6,18]. Respiratory[1,3,18], as well as metabolic[2,5] acidosis have been reported to be associated with increases in serum phosphorus levels. Despite the above mentioned observations, the effect of acidosis induced by several physiologically-important acidifying agents on blood phosphorus levels has not been systematically evaluated. The results of previous studies, however, suggest that marked hyperphosphatemia may be a concomitant of lactic acidosis[8,9] while other data suggest that $NH_4Cl$-induced metabolic acidosis is[5], or is not[4,15], associated with increases in plasma phosphorus concentration. Of interest, the data of healthy human volunteers presented in Figure 4 demonstrated no significant changes in serum phosphorus concentration following the administratin of $NH_4Cl$. On the other hand, administration of $CaCl_2$, despite the resulting hypercalcemia, was associated with a significant increase in serum phosphorus levels.

In the present study, an increase in UpV occurred in the control as well as the LA group. Thus, the urinary changes cannot be ascribed to acidosis alone and they do not explain the differences in plasma phosphorus levels between control and acid-infused dogs during the first three hours of infusion. Of note, is the finding that the FLp increased in the control and LA group and remained unchanged in the HCl group. The increased FLp in control dogs was due entirely to an increased GFR while that in the LA group was related to increases in both GFR and plasma phosphorus concentration.

Although the FEp increased in all three groups, the increase in the control group was significantly greater than that of the acid-infused groups (Figure 2). This observation suggests that acid administration blunts the phosphaturia associated with mild volume expansion. Furthermore, the finding that the cumulative excretion of phosphorus was signficantly lower in the HCl than in the LA group raises the possibility that a lower rate of phosphorus excretion, concimitant with phosphorus release from cells accounted, at least in part, for the late rise in plasma phosphorus in the former group.

The increment in $FE_{Na}$ in the control dogs suggests that extracellular fluid volume expansion was a factor responsible for the increase in the FEp in all the groups. The relationship between $FE_{Na}$ and FEp is presented in Figure 3. As expected, in each group there was a significant correlation between $FE_{Na}$ and FEp. The equations and correlation coefficients for the regression lines were: C: FEp=3.79 $FE_{Na}$+13.4, r=.32, P<0.05; HCl: FEp=4.34 $FE_{Na}$+4.8, r=73,

$P<0.01$; LA; $FE_p=2.39$ $FE_{Na}+12.2$, $r=.53$, $P<0.01$. The slope of the LA
line was significantly less ($P<0.05$) than that of the HCl group.
Of note, at any given $FE_{Na}$ the $FE_p$ was greater in the control than in
the HCl group. This observation is also consistent with the possibility that HCl administration per se blunted the increase in phosphorus excretion associated with volume expansion.

Other investigators [6,19,20] have noted increments in urinary
phosphorus excretion during acidosis and observed a decrease in
renal tubular reabsorption concomitant with an increase in the filtered load of phosphorus. The basic mechanism(s) by which acid-loading
reduced tubular phosphorus reabsorption was not elucidated. The
changes may have been due to increases in sodium excretion, PTH
secretion or to a direct effect of acidosis on the renal tubules.

Although we have no definitive explanation concerning the pathophysiology of increases in plasma phosphorus during acute acidosis,
it could be explained in part, as discussed above, by movement of
phosphorus out of the intracellular compartment. It is well established that the concentration of organic phosphorus compounds in red
blood cells, especially disphosphoglycerate, is subject to the
influence of various factors affecting the glycolytic system. One
of these factors is the pH of the blood, acidosis favoring the decomposition of diphosphoglycerate in erythrocytes and alkalosis having
the opposite effect.[16,21-23] In addition, hydrogen ions are buffered
in part in bone and perhaps other tissues and metabolic acidosis is
associated with release of phosphorus from bone.[4,5,24]

Hemolysis might be another mechanism whereby phosphorus may be
released from red blood cells raising serum levels. In the present
study, the mean hematocrit levels of the three groups did not differ
significantly from each other prior to acid infusion. During infusion, some hemolysis was noted in both acid-infused groups and there
was a significant decline in hematocrit in the LA but not in either
of the two other groups (baseline: C, $35\pm2$; HCl, $38\pm2$; LA, $39\pm2$
volumes %; hour 5: C, $34\pm2$; HCl, $36\pm3$; L$\overline{A}$, $32\pm2$ volumes %) suggesting
a greater degree of hemolysis in LA dogs. A degree of hemolysis
similar to that found in the present studies was noted by us in in
vitro studies (unpublished observations) using dog red blood cells and
the acidifying agents under investigation. The amount of phosphorus
released during these studies, however, was insufficient to explain
the increases in plasma phosphorus concentration which occurred in
vivo. Furthermore, hemolysis has not been reported in lactic acidosis
in man, a condition which is often associated with hyperphosphatemia.[8,9]

The concentration of inorganic phosphorus of the serum falls
after carbohydrate ingestion or infusion of glucose due to entry of
hexoses into cells and their phosphorylation.[25,26] Pollack et al [25]

demonstrated the marked participation of phosphorus in glucose utilization by the hind limb of the dog. Since our studies were performed on fasted animals and there were no differences in glucose and insulin levels between the acid infused groups it is unlikely that a difference in the rate of entry of glucose into cells was responsible for the observed variations in plasma phosphorus.

The present report is in agreement with the findings of Tranquada et al [8] and O'Connor et al [9] who observed that the serum phosphorus is increased disproportionally in patients with lactic acidosis. The latter authors suggested that hyperphosphatemia in lactic acidosis is due to tissue ischemia since experimental studies suggest that ATP is utilized but not regenerated by ischemic tissues.[27] The findings in the present study do not support this theory since acidosis was produced by lactic acid infusion without hypotension or hypoxia to suggest tissue ischemia. Acidosis, however, appears to be a necessary event since hyperphosphatemia is not present in nonacidemic patients with glycogen storage disease despite marked increases in serum lactate levels.[28]

In summary, the results of the present study confirm and amplify previous observations from this laboratory documenting a temporal difference in the plasma phosphorus response to administration of hydrochloric and lactic acids. The initial differences could not be accounted for by changes in urinary phosphorus excretion or plasma insulin levels, while the findings occurring after three hours might have been due, at least in part, to the more marked blunting of renal phosphorus excretion in the dogs receiving hydrochloric acid.


ACKNOWLEDGMENTS

The technical assistance of Helen Alpert, Kenneth Bailey, Lottie Cason, Raul Rodriguez and Robert Rubin and the secretarial help of Charlene Walbroehl and Louann Rossi are appreciated.

The studies were supported by research funds from the Veterans Administration.


REFERENCES

1.  J.B.S. Haldane, V.B. Wigglesworth, and C.E. Woodrow, The effect of reaction changes on human inorganic metabolism, Proc. Roy. Soc. London Ser. B 96:1-14 (1924).
2.  R.C. Swan and R.F. Pitts, Neutralization of infused acid by nephrectomized dogs. J. Clin. Invest. 34:205-211 (1955).
3.  H.A. Saltzman, A. Herman, and H.O. Sieker, Correlation of clinical and physiologic manifestations of sustained hyperventilation.

N. Engl. J. Med. 268:1431-1436 (1963).

4.  E.J. Lennon and W.F. Piering, A comparison of the effects of glucose ingestion and NH4Cl acidosis on urinary calcium and magnesium excretion in man. J. Clin. Invest. 49:1458-1465 (1970).

5.  F.L. Coe, J.J. Firpo, D.L. Hollandsworth, L. Segil, J.M. Canterbury, and E. Reiss, Effect of acute and chronic metabolic acidosis on serum immunoreactive parathyroid hormone in man. Kidney Int. 8:262-273 (1975).

6.  J.P. Knochel, The pathophysiology and clinical characteristics of severe hypophosphatemia. Arch. Intern. Med. 137:203-220 (1977).

7.  J.R. Oster, G.O. Perez, and C.A. Vaamonde, Relationship between blood pH and potassium and phosphorus during acute metabolic acidosis. Am. J. Physiol. 235:F345-F351 (1978).

8.  R.E. Tranquada, W.J. Grant, and C.R. Peterson, Lactic acidosis. Arch. Intern. Med. 117:192-202 (1966).

9.  L.R. O'Connor, K.L. Klein, and J.E. Bethune, Hyperphosphatemia in lactic acidosis. N. Engl. J. Med. 297:707-709 (1978).

10. C.H. Fiske and Y. Subbarow, The colorimetric determination of phosphorus. J. Biol. Med. 66:375-400 (1925).

11. W.S. Hoffman, Rapid photoelectric method for determination of glucose in blood and urine. J. Biol. Chem. 120:51-55 (1937).

12. A. Castro, J.P. Scott, D.P. Grettie, D. MacFarlane, and R.E. Bailey, Plasma insulin and glucose responses of healthy subjects to varying glucose loads during three hour oral glucose tolerance tests. Diabetes 19:842-851 (1970).

13. T.H. Steele, A modified semi-automated resorcinol method for the determination of inulin. Clin. Chem. 15:1072-1078 (1969).

14. I. Gutmann and A.W. Wahlefeld, L-(+)-lactate determination with lactate dehydrogenase and NAD, in: "Methods of Enzymatic Analysis", 2nd English edition, H.U. Bergmeyer. ed., Academic Press Inc., New York (1974), pp. 1464-1468.

15. G.M. Guest and S. Rapoport, Role of acid-soluble phosphorus compounds in red blood cells. Am. J. Dis. Child. 58:1072-1089 (1939).

16. A.S. Relman, Metabolic consequences of acid-base disorders. Kidney Int. 1:347-359 (1972).

17. M.E. Mostellar and E.P. Tuttle, Effect of alkalosis on plasma concentration and urinary excretion of inorganic phosphate in man. J. Clin. Invest. 43:138-148 (1964).

18. G. Giebisch, L. Berger, and R.F. Pitts, The extrarenal response to acute acid-base disturbances of respiratory origin. J. Clin. Invest. 34:231-245 (1955).

19. R.L. Tannen, The response of normal subjects to the short ammonium chloride test: The modifying influence of renal ammonia production. Clin. Sci. 41:583-595 (1971).

20. J.W. Dubb, M. Goldberg, and Z.S. Agus, Tubular effects of acute metabolic acidosis in the rat. J. Lab. Clin. Med. 90: 318-

323 (1977).

21. A.J. Bellingham, J.C. Detter, and C. Lenfant, Regulatory mechanisms of hemoglobin oxygen affinity in acidosis and alkalosis. J. Clin. Invest. 50:700-705 (1971)

22. S. Rapoport and G.M. Guest, The decomposition of diphosphoglycerate in acidified blood: Its relationship to reactions of the glycolytic cycle. J. Biol. Chem. 129:781-790 (1939).

23. Y. Kanter, J.R. Gerson, and A.N. Bessman, 2,3-Diphosphoglycerate, nucleotide phosphate and organic and inorganic phosphate levels during the early phases of diabetic ketoacidosis. Diabetes 26:429-433 (1977).

24. U.S. Barzel, Parathyroid hormone, blood phosphorus and acid-base metabolism. Lancet I:1329-1331 (1971).

25. N. Pollack, Serum and muscle phosphate changes following glucose injection. Am. J. Physiol. 105:79-80 (1933).

26. R. Levine, S.D. Loube, and H.F. Weisberg, Nature of action of insulin on the level of serum inorganic phosphate. Am. J. Physiol. 159:111-117 (1949).

27. D.A. Hems and J.T. Brosnan, Effects of ischaemia on content of metabolites in rat liver and kidney in vivo. Biochem. J. 120:105-111 (1970).

28. F. Huijing, Hyperphosphatemia and lactic acidosis. N. Engl. J. Med. 298:112 (1978).

29. J.R. Oster, J.L. Hotchkiss, M. Carbon, M. Farmer, and C.A. Vaamonde, A short duration renal acidification test using calcium chloride. Nephron 14:281-292 (1975).

30. J.R. Oster, L.E. Lespier, S.M. Lee, E.L. Pellegrini, and C.A. Vaamonde, Renal acidification in sickle-cell disease. J. Lab. Clin. Med. 88:389-401 (1976).

31. G.O. Perez, J.R. Oster, and C.A. Vaamonde, Incomplete syndrome of renal tubular acidosis induced by lithium carbonate. J. Lab. Clin. Med. 86:386-394 (1975).

# CALCIUM CARBONATE-INDUCED EFFECTS ON SERUM CA X P PRODUCT AND SERUM CREATININE IN RENAL FAILURE: A RETROSPECTIVE STUDY

Mackenzie Walser

Department of Pharmacology and Department of Medicine, Johns Hopkins University School of Medicine, Baltimore, Maryland, U. S. A.

Several lines of evidence, which we have summarized recently elsewhere (1) have lent support to the hypothesis, stated previously by us (2) as well as others, that progression of chronic renal failure may be in part attributable to the vicious circle depicted in Figure 1. The most impressive evidence pertinent to this hypothesis consists of clinical studies in which phosphate intake was restricted early in the course of chronic renal failure in man, in order to prevent renal osteodystrophy (3, 4). An unexpected result of these studies was that progression of renal insufficiency was much slower than in comparable series of patients. In addition, phosphate restriction can prevent the progression to terminal uremia of certain types of experimentally induced renal failure in rats (5, 6).

If this hypothesis is correct, an increase in the serum Ca X P product should hasten the progression of renal insufficiency. Intentional attempts to elevate this product in chronic renal failure would clearly be unethical, but two measures have been used that may lead to an increase as a side effect. These are the use of one form or another of vitamin D and the oral administration of calcium salts.

The literature on the effect of various forms of vitamin D on renal function is somewhat confused, and it will suffice for the present merely to note several reports (7-9) in which accelerated deterioration of renal function has been reported following the use of these agents in pre-dialysis patients. It is reassuring to note that the use of the active form of vitamin D, 1,25-dihydrotachysterol, is approved by the United States Food and Drug Administra-

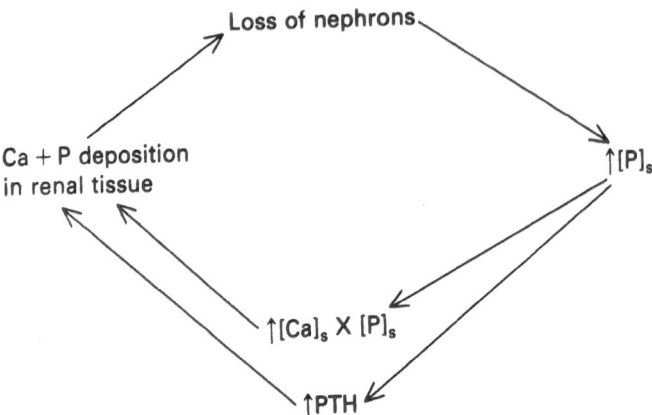

Fig. 1.  Hypothetical vicious circle that may contribute to the
         progression of renal failure.  Following the initial in-
         sult, the population of nephrons is reduced and serum
         phosphate tends to rise, especially postprandially.
         This tends to decrease serum calcium, stimulating para-
         thyroid hormone secretion, but also raises the serum
         Ca X P product.  Both effects tend to cause the deposi-
         tion of calcium (and phosphate) in the kidney, further
         reducing the population of functioning nephrons. Reprint-
         ed by permission from Walser et al, <u>Clin. Nephrol.</u> 11:66,
         1979.

tion only in patients on regular dialysis, and not in patients in
the pre-dialysis phase.

     Calcium supplementation has long been traditional in chronic
renal failure.  Calcium salts are said to reduce phosphate absorption, combat uremic acidosis, and improve hypocalcemia.  There can
be no question that the last-named effect occurs.  Furthermore,
improvement in uremic acidosis has been documented (10, 11).  Paren-
thetically, it should be noted that metabolic acidosis can be ameli-
orated only by increasing the sodiun bicarbonate content of the
extracellular fluid (unless volume contraction is induced).  Calcium
salts can do this only by exchange of calcium for sodium in bone or
other sites outside of the extracellular fluid.  Such a process
would appear to be inherently limited in quantity as well as duration.

     With regard to the effects of calcium salts on phosphate bal-
ance, DeWardener and associates (12, 13) have shown that the diminu-

tion in intestinal phosphate absorption is more than offset by the
reduction which occurs in urinary phosphate excretion, so that
phosphate balance tends to become more positive, whether calcium
citrate (13) or calcium carbonate (12) is employed.  Plasma phosphate in these studies either fell or remained constant.  No consistent change in creatinine clearance was noted.

However, two more recent studies (14, 15) have examined the use
of calcium carbonate in the treatment of uremic acidosis.  In both,
5-7 g of this salt was administered for two to four weeks to
patients with chronic renal failure.  The changes in serum calcium,
phosphorus and creatinine in these patients were noted, but not
commented upon.  On re-examining these data, a positive and
highly significant correlation was noted between the change in
the serum Ca X P product and the change in serum creatinine between
the pre-treatment control values and the values observed after two
to four weeks of calcium carbonate supplementation (Figure 2, Table
1).  In other words, some patients in both series exhibited a rise
in serum creatinine concentration during this brief interval, and
these same patients tended to be those in whom the Ca X P product
rose most.  The similarities between these relationships from two

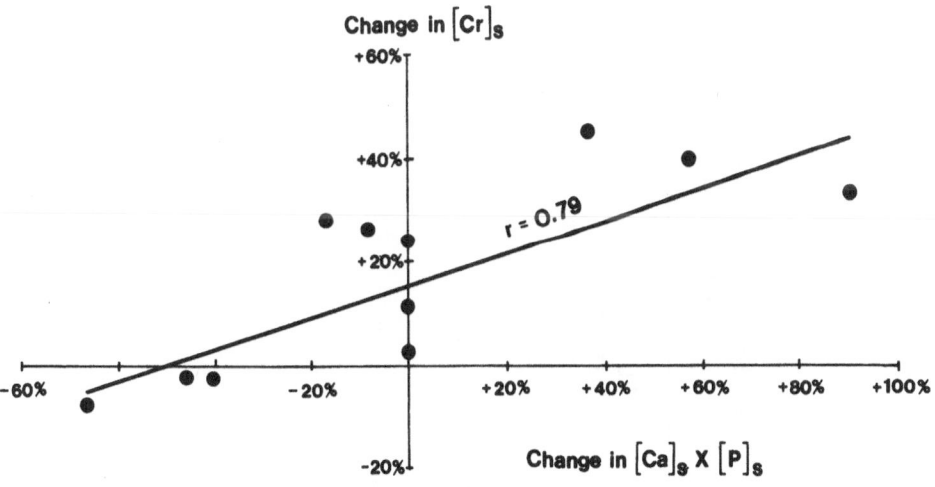

Fig. 2.   Change in serum creatinine as a function of change in
serum Ca X P product in 11 patients treated with calcium
carbonate.  A significant positive correlation is seen
($r = 0.79$, $p < 0.01$).  Calculated from data presented
in ref. (14).

Table 1. Summary of the interdependence of changes in serum creatinine and serum Ca X P product in two studies.

| Reference | No. of patients[a] | Cr mg/dl | Initial serum values | | | Correlation, $y = Cr_1/Cr_2$ on $x = (Ca_2 \times P_2)/(Ca_1 \times P_1)$ | |
| | | | Ca mg/dl | P mg/dl | Ca X P mg²/dl² | r | P |
|---|---|---|---|---|---|---|---|
| Makoff et al (14) | 13 | 8.3 +1.0 | 7.3 +0.3 | 7.9 +1.0 | 55 + 6 | 0.79 | < .01 |
| Berlyne (15) | 12 | 14 + 1 | 8.2 +0.2 | 7.0 +0.5 | 56 + 5 | 0.71 | .01 |

[a] Excluding patients in whom incomplete data for this calculation were presented

independent studies is of particular interest. The studies of DeWardener and associates (12, 13) are not susceptible to this type of retrospective analysis because the serum values before and after calcium supplementation are not reported in detail.

The average rate of decrease in reciprocal creatinine, in dl/mg/month, is a useful quantitative measure of the rate of progression of renal failure (16). In the studies of Makoff et al (14) and Berlyne (15), this value averages -0.036 and -0.015 dl/mg/month during calcium carbonate supplementation. Control observations of these same patients are not available, but in other unselected series of large numbers of patients, this rate averaged -0.0076 (16) and -0.015 dl/mg/month (17). Thus, there is no evidence that calcium carbonate accelerates the deterioration of renal function as a general rule in chronic renal failure. However, such an effect occasionally occurs, and is most prominent in those patients in whom the Ca X P product rises. Examination of these data does not indicate a significant correlation between the increase in serum creatinine and the initial serum Ca X P product or the initial serum calcium or phosphorus concentrations. Thus, there appears to be no way, at present, to predict which patients will exhibit functional deterioration during calcium carbonate therapy. In addition, it cannot be stated with assurance whether the rise in the Ca X P product is the cause or the effect of the rise in serum creatinine.

Despite these reservations, these relationships lend support to the idea that an increase in the serum Ca X P product may accelerate progression, and suggest caution in the use of calcium supplements for this reason.

### Acknowledgments

Supported by Program Project Grant AM 18020 from the National Instititutes of Health.

REFERENCES

1. M. Walser, Does dietary therapy have a role in the pre-dialysis patient? Am. J. Clin. Nutr. In Press (1979).

2. M. Walser, Conservative management of chronic renal failure, Chapter 39 in: "The Kidney", B. Brenner and F. Rector, eds., W. B. Saunders, Philadelphia (1976).

3. W. J. Johnson, R. S. Goldsmith, J. Jowsey, P. P. Frohnert, and C. D. Arnaud, The influence of maintaining normal serum phosphate and calcium on renal osteodystrophy, in: "Vitamin D and Problems Related to Uremic Bone Disease", A. W. Norman, K. Schaefer, H. G. Grigoleit, D. von Herrath, and E. Ritz, eds. Walter de Gruyter, Berlin/New York (1975).

4.  G. Maschio, N. Tessitore, A. D'Angelo, E. Bonucci, A. Lupo, E. Valvo, C. Loschiavo, A. Fabris, P. Morachiello, G. Previato, and E. Fiaschi, Early dietary phosphorus restriction and calcium supplementation in the prevention of renal osteo-dystrophy. <u>Am. J. Clin. Nutr.</u> In Press 1979).

5.  L. S. Ibels, A. C. ALfrey, A. L. Haut, and W. E. Huffer, Preservation of function in experimental renal disease by dietary restriction of phosphate. <u>New Engl. J. Med.</u> 298:122 (1978).

6.  A. C. Alfrey, M. L. Karlinsky, and L. H. Haut. Prevention of functional deterioration in experimental renal disease by dietary phosphorus restriction, <u>in</u>: <u>Proc. IVth International Workshop on Phosphate and Other Minerals</u>, S. Massry, ed. Plenum Publishers, New York (In Press).

7.  S. Winkler, A. S. Brickman, E. G. C. Wong, D. J. Sherrard, R. B. Miller, C. M. Bennett, and J. W. Coburn, Hypercalcemia during treatment with 1,25-hydroxy-vitamin D-3: analysis of 30 cases. <u>Kidney Int.</u> 14:667 (1978).

8.  B. F. C. Nordin, Vitamin D analogues and renal function, Lancet 2:1259 (1978).

9.  C. Christiansen, M. S. Christiansen, B. Hartnal, F. Melsen, I. Transbøl, and P. Rødbro, Vitamin D analogues and renal function. Lancet 1:50 (1979).

10. S. S. Franklin, A. Gordon, C. R. Kleeman, and M. D. Maxwell. The use of a balanced low protein diet in the treatment of chronic renal failure. <u>JAMA</u> 202:141 (1967).

11. M. M. Popovtzer, and J. B. Robinette, Effect of oral calcium carbonate on urinary excretion on Ca, Na, and Mg in advanced renal disease. <u>Proc. Soc. Exp. Biol. Med.</u> 145:222 (1974).

12. E. M. Clarkson, S. J. McDonald, and H. E. DeWardener, The effect of a high intake of calcium carbonate in normal subjects and patients with chronic renal failure. <u>Clin. Sci.</u> 30:425 (1966).

13. S. J. McDonald, E. M. Clarkson, and H. E. DeWardener, The effect of a large intake of calcium citrate in normal subjects and patients with chronic renal failure. <u>Clin. Sci.</u> 26:27 (1964).

14. D. L. Makoff, A. Gordon, S. S. Franklin, A. R. Gerstein, and M. H. Maxwell, Chronic calcium carbonate therapy in uremia, <u>Arch. Intern. Med.</u> 123:15 (1969).

15. G. Berlyne, Calcium carbonate treatment of uremic acidosis, <u>Isr. J. Med. Sci.</u> 7:1235 (1971).

16. W. E. Mitch, G. Buffington, J. Lemann, and M. Walser, A simple method of estimating progression of chronic renal failure, Lancet 2:1326 (1976)

17. W. E. Rutherford, J. Blondin, J. P. Miller, A. S. Greenwalt, and J. D. Vavra, Chronic progressive renal disease: Rate of change of serum creatinine concentration, Kidney Int. 11;62 (1977).

DIVALENT IONS IN BLOOD AND CEREBROSPINAL FLUID:   EFFECT OF
HYPERCALCEMIA, HYPERPHOSPHATEMIA, RENAL FAILURE AND PARATHYROID
HORMONE

David A. Goldstein and Shaul G. Massry

Division of Nephrology and Department of Medicine
University of Southern California School of Medicine
Los Angeles, California 90033

INTRODUCTION

Despite large changes in the electrolyte concentration in blood,
the content of brain electrolyte usually remains quite stable[1,2].
These observations are due to the blood-brain barrier which consists
of the processes involved at the cerebrospinal fluid (CSF)-blood[3],
CSF-brain[4] and blood-brain interfaces[5,6].

The presence of elevated blood levels of parathyroid hormone
(PTH) has been shown to disrupt the blood-brain barrier and increase
the calcium content of the brain[1,2] inducing disturbances in the
electroencephalogram[2].   It is not known at what level of the blood-
brain barrier PTH exerts its effect.

The stability of the electrolyte concentrations in the CSF
should be a critical step in the overall process preventing variations in brain composition.   The concentration of ionized calcium in
the CSF is assumed to be similar to that of blood since under normal
conditions the concentration of calcium in the CSF is similar to
that in the ultrafiltrate of blood[7].   However, information on the
concentration of ionized calcium in CSF is not readily available.
Also, data on the levels of inorganic phosphorus in CSF and its
relationship to its concentration in the blood are rather sparse[8-10].
A rise in the calcium-phosphorus product in blood may be associated
with similar changes in CSF.   Such events may predispose to calcium
deposition in brain.   Also, hyperparathyroidism may be associated
with a rise in CSF calcium.

This investigation was performed in order to evaluate the concentrations of total and ionized calcium and inorganic phosphorus

in CSF and to determine the possible relationships between their
levels in CSF and blood.  These studies were undertaken in normal
conditions and during large alterations in the blood concentrations
of these electrolytes both in the presence and absence of parathyroid
hormone.

METHODS

    The study protocol called for the investigations of both animals
and humans.  Examinations were undertaken in 60 dogs subdivided into
the following groups:  1) 9 normal dogs; 2) 6 animals three days after
thyroparathyroidectomy (TPTX); the success of the removal of the
parathyroid glands was ascertained by a fall in blood calcium of at
least 2 mg/100 ml, 3) 6 dogs after three days of treatment with
parathyroid extract (PTE)  (Eli Lilly & Co., Indianapolis, Indiana)
injection (50 units, twice daily), 4) 16 dogs receiving phosphate
infusion (50 mmoles/hour for 3 hours) for 3 days, 5) 7 dogs in whom
acute uremia was produced by bilateral nephrectomy three days prior
to study, and 6) 12 dogs in whom chronic hypercalcemia (12.0-15.0
mg/100 ml) was produced and maintained for 3 months with oral administration of vitamin D (50,000-100,000 u/day) 2-3 times per week.

    The data from human subjects were obtained from 19 patients with
various neurological disorders other than meningitis.  A lumbar puncture was performed as part of the work-up for the diagnosis of alteration of mental status.  Mild hypophosphatemia was observed in many
of these patients.

    Total and ionized calcium and inorganic phosphorus were measured
in blood and CSF simultaneously.  Total calcium was determined with
a Perkin Elmer Atomic Absorption Spectrophotometer, Model 503;
ionized calcium was measured with Orion calcium electrode SS20 (Orion
Biomedical, Cambridge, Ma.).  Inorganic phosphorus was measured with
a Technicon Autoanalyzer.  In the human studies the concentrations
of diffusible calcium in blood and lactate and citrate in CSF were
also measured.  Diffusible calcium was estimated in ultrafiltrate
of plasma prepared with amicon cones, #CF25 (Amicon Corp., Lexington,
Ma.).  Measurements of protein, lactate and citrate were performed
by previously published methods[11-13].

RESULTS

    The results of our studies appear in Tables I and II and
Figures 1 through 4.  Wide variations in the concentrations of total
calcium in the blood from 5.1 to 14.8 mg/100 ml were accompanied
by minor changes in the CSF concentration of total calcium.  The
relationship between the concentrations of total calcium in blood
and CSF is depicted in Figure 1.  The concentration of calcium in
CSF remained almost stable (4.78±0.05 mg/100 ml) despite a range
of 5.1 to 9.5 mg/100 ml in the level of blood calcium.  When the

blood levels of calcium in CSF were increased from 9.5 to 14.8 mg/ 100 ml, the concentration of calcium in the CSF (5.37±0.06 mg/dl) was modestly but significantly (p <.01) greater than the levels seen in the studies with lower blood concentrations of calcium cited above. Figure 2 shows that the concentration of ionized calcium in CSF also varied only modestly despite a 3.5 fold change in the levels of ionized calcium in blood.

Table 1. Calcium and P levels in blood and CSF

| Group | Blood (mg/100 ml) | | | CSF (mg/100 µl) | | | Ca$_I$:Ca$_T$ (%) |
|---|---|---|---|---|---|---|---|
| | Ca$_T$ | Ca$_I$ | P | Ca$_T$ | Ca$_I$ | P | |
| Animals | | | | | | | |
| Normal (n = 16) | 9.9 ± 0.10 | 4.27 ± 0.10 | 4.5 ± 0.23 | 5.25 ± 0.07 | 2.77 ± 0.08 | 1.4 ± 0.05 | 52.8 ± 1.2 |
| | (9.2–10.7) | (3.64–4.94) | (2.8–6.6) | (4.85–5.90) | (2.36–3.78) | (1.0–1.7) | (48–65) |
| Normal + PTE (n = 6) | 11.6 ± 0.17 | 5.04 ± 0.12 | 4.2 ± 0.26 | 5.24 ± 0.18 | 3.25 ± 0.19 | 1.3 ± 0.05 | 60.0 ± 3.4 |
| | (10.9–11.9) | (4.68–5.36) | (3.4–5.0) | (5.16–5.52) | (2.52–3.84) | (1.1–1.4) | (47–70) |
| TPTX (n = 9) | 6.2 ± 0.31 | 2.56 ± 0.15 | 5.0 ± 0.31 | 4.85 ± 0.08 | 2.67 ± 0.07 | 1.4 ± 0.07 | 55.2 ± 1.9 |
| | (5.1–7.8) | (2.04–3.48) | (3.7–6.5) | (4.41–5.11) | (2.42–2.92) | (1.1–1.7) | (49–65) |
| Uremia (n = 7) | 10.1 ± 0.42 | 4.45 ± 0.20 | 14.5 ± 1.52 | 5.4 ± 0.14 | 3.17 ± 0.05 | 1.5 ± 0.11 | 59.9 ± 1.2 |
| | (8.5–11.5) | (3.74–5.00) | (9.8–21.1) | (4.80–5.80) | (3.00–3.37) | (1.1–1.9) | (54–63) |
| Phosphate infusion (n = 16) | 7.3 ± 0.26 | 3.51 ± 0.09 | 15.1 ± 0.48 | 4.71 ± 0.09 | 2.63 ± 0.06 | 1.2 ± 0.03 | 55.7 ± 0.08 |
| | (5.8–8.8) | (3.10–3.87) | (12.0–18.6) | (4.40–5.30) | (2.60–3.06) | (1.0–1.5) | (49–60) |
| Chronic hypercalcemia (n = 12) | 13.6 ± 0.46 | 6.65 ± 0.16 | 5.8 ± 0.15 | 5.65 ± 0.07 | 3.29 ± 0.11 | 1.3 ± 0.04 | 58.0 ± 1.4 |
| | (11.5–14.8) | (5.7–7.76) | (4.9–6.5) | (5.40–5.80) | (3.24–3.77) | (1.1–1.6) | (49–65) |
| Humans (n = 19) | 9.2 ± 0.35 | 4.10 ± 0.15 | 2.7 ± 0.16 | 4.65 ± 0.26 | 2.76 ± 0.24 | 1.2 ± 0.13 | 63.7 ± 2.2 |
| | (7.1–14.2) | (3.26–5.86) | (1.2–3.9) | (4.26–5.90) | (2.30–4.20) | (1.1–1.9) | (49–77) |

Data are presented as the mean ± 1 SE; the range is in parenthesis. PTE, Parathyroid extract; TPTX, thyroparathyroidectomy. (Goldstein et al., JCE & M 49:60, 1979).

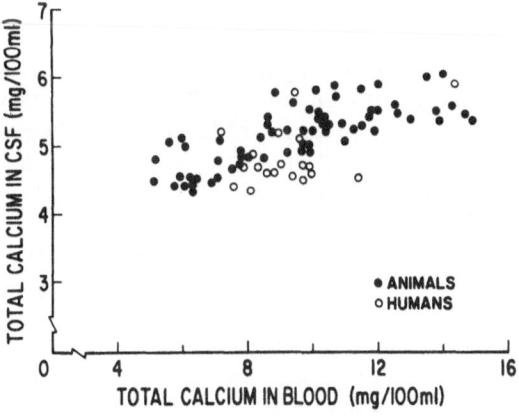

Figure 1. The relationship between the Ca$_T$ in blood and that in CSF. (Goldstein et al., JCE & M 49:59, 1979).

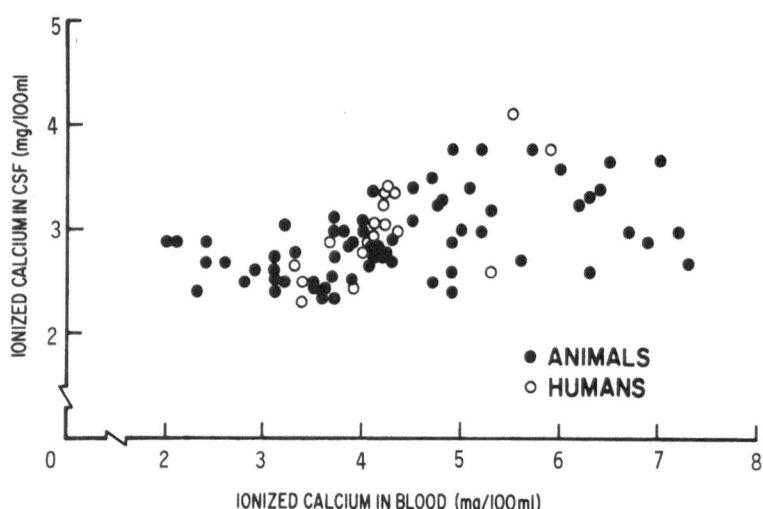

Figure 2.   The relationship between the concentration of $Ca_I$ in
            blood and that in CSF (Goldstein et al., JCE & M 49:59,
            1979).

Figure 3 depicts the mean concentrations of ionized calcium in
CSF which constituted only 50-65% of the total calcium levels.  In
addition, there was a direct and significant correlation between the
concentrations of ionized and total calcium in CSF.  The concentrations of total protein, lactate and citrate in CSF measured in 10
humans were 38.8±9.6 mg/100 ml, 1.87±.33 mmole/l, and .29±.04 mmole/l,
respectively.

The levels of inorganic phosphorus in the CSF ranged between
1.0 and 1.9 mg/100 ml despite marked variations in their concentrations in the blood from 1.2 to 21.1 ml/100 ml.  Figure 4 shows the
relationship between the levels of inorganic phosphorus in CSF and
blood for all of the study protocols.

Table II shows that the product of total calcium and phosphorus
concentrations in blood varied markedly among the different study
groups in dogs from 31.0±1.33 in TPTX animals to 144.0±12.2 in the
uremic dogs.  It is of note that the product of these same substances
in the blood of humans (24.7±1.97) was significantly lower (p<.01)
than in normal dogs (44.1±2.32).  This may be related to the low
levels of inorganic phosphorus present in many of the patients.
Although there was a marked variation in calcium-phosphorus product
in blood, there were no significant differences in this product in

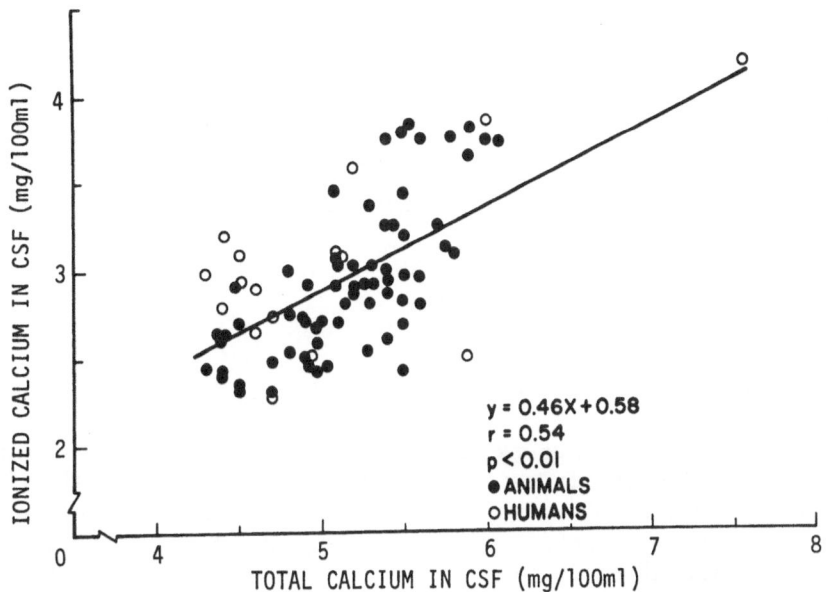

Figure 3.  The relationship between the concentrations of Ca$_T$ and
           Ca$_I$ in CSF (Goldstein et al., JCE & M 49:59, 1979).

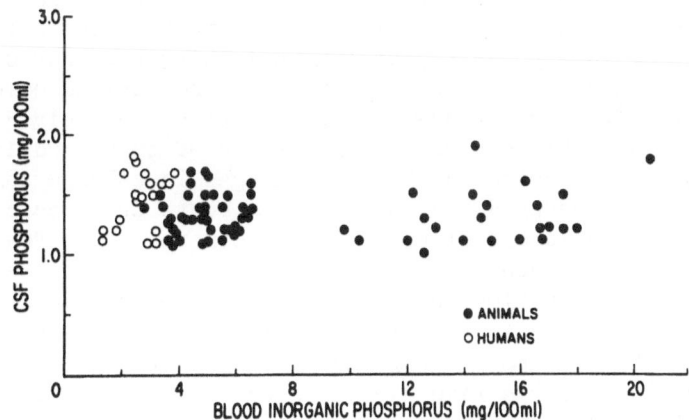

Figure 4.  The relationship between the concentration of inorganic P
           in blood and that in CSF (Goldstein et al., JCE & M 49:60,
           1979).

Table II.  Calcium-P product in blood and CSF

| Animals | Product of $Ca_T$-P | | Product of $Ca_I$-P | |
| | Blood | CSF | Blood | CSF |
| --- | --- | --- | --- | --- |
| Normal | 44.1 ± 2.32 | 7.3 ± 0.30 | 16.8 ± 2.02 | 3.4 ± 2.7 |
| Normal + PTE | 48.5 ± 3.49 | 6.8 ± 0.26 | 19.4 ± 2.78 | 3.7 ± 0.79 |
| TPTX | 31.0 ± 1.33[a] | 6.8 ± 0.34 | 12.7 ± 0.67 | 3.3 ± 0.48 |
| Uremia | 144.0 ± 12.20[a] | 8.1 ± 0.68 | 64.0 ± 6.20[a] | 4.7 ± 0.33[a] |
| Phosphate infusion | 109.0 ± 0.79[a] | 5.7 ± 0.18[a] | 52.5 ± 0.73[a] | 3.2 ± 0.10 |
| Chronic hypercalcemia | 78.1 ± 2.93[a] | 7.3 ± 0.26 | 35.5 ± 3.40[a] | 4.2 ± 0.13[a] |
| Humans | 24.7 ± 1.97[a] | 7.3 ± 0.39 | 10.9 ± 0.79[b] | 4.3 ± 0.19[b] |

Data are presented as the mean ± 1 SE.  PTE, Parathyroid extract;
  TPTX, Thyroparathyroidectomy.
[a]P < 0.01 vs. normal animals.
[b]P < 0.05 vs. normal animals.
(Goldstein et al., JCE & M 49:60, 1979).

the CSF of the various groups under study but was lower in those
animals which received infusions of phosphate.  The calculation of
the calcium-phosphorus product in blood and CSF using the concentrations of ionized calcium showed similar findings in that there
were no significant alterations in this product in the CSF when
there were marked variations in the values of the product in blood.

DISCUSSION

     The results of our study demonstrate that the level of total
calcium in the CSF varies only slightly when the concentration of
calcium in the serum was elevated 2-3 times by means of either the
infusion of calcium, the administration of parathyroid extract, or
chronic treatment with vitamin D.  This is in agreement with other
reports[7,9,10,14,15] on the concentration of total calcium in the CSF.
However, only a few studies in intact or parathyroidectomized
animals[7,14] or in hypoparathyroid humans[10] have been performed.  In
addition, our studies show that both total and ionized calcium levels
in CSF vary only slightly over large variations in their concentrations in blood.  This control of the levels of total and ionized
calcium in CSF was observed when the changes in calcium concentrations in blood were produced in either an acute or chronic fashion
and whether blood levels of parathyroid hormone were normal, increased
or reduced.  These phenomena support the efficiency of the blood-
CSF interface of the blood brain barrier in providing a stable
calcium concentration in the fluid bathing the brain.  Data from
studies in rabbits also support the ability of the blood-CSF interface to maintain stable levels of calcium in the CSF.  These animals
have elevated blood calcium concentrations (12.0-14.5 mg/100 ml) but
the levels of calcium in CSF are not different[16] from those found in
other animals or humans[7,9,15].

An interesting and novel observation of the present study is the demonstration that the concentration of ionized calcium in CSF is 50-65% of the total level; measurements of the levels of ionized calcium in CSF have not heretofore been available and it had been believed that the level of ionized and total calcium in the CSF were equal.  The presence of lactate and citrate in CSF may help provide an explanation for this observation.  These anions have the ability to complex calcium in CSF and produce poorly ionizable compounds. The relevance of this phenomenon is not yet clear, but it is possible that the functional integrity of the brain requires that the concentration of ionized calcium in the fluid bathing it be lower than that of the blood.

A few studies have shown that the concentration of inorganic phosphorus is stable within a narrow range (1.2-2.3 mg/100 ml) in humans other than those suffering from meningitis[8-10].  In the limited data available, there were no wide fluctuations in the concentrations of blood phosphorus, and consequently it was not clear whether the stability of CSF phosphorus could be maintained in the face of rising blood levels of phosphorus.  Our results show that the concentration of phosphorus in the CSF is held within a narrow range despite marked alterations, be they acute or chronic in the level of blood phosphorus.  Thus, our data and those of others[10-12] demonstrate that the blood-CSF interface of the blood brain barrier maintains tight control of the CSF concentration of inorganic phosphorus.  This function does not seem influenced by the presence or absence of PTH.

These observations may have important clinical implications. It appears possible that the CSF maintains a very low calcium-phosphorus product and limits the development of increments in this product during a rise in the concentrations of calcium, phosphorus or both in blood.  Indeed, the results of our study support such a possibility.  The calcium-phosphorus product in CSF remained stable or increased only mildly despite several fold increases in the calcium-phosphorus product of blood.

A rise in the calcium-phosphorus product in extracellular fluid of any organ may lead to calcium deposition[17].  Thus the preservation of a low calcium-phosphorus product in CSF provides a protective mechanism against calcium deposition in brain, which may be deleterious to its functional integrity.

It has been shown that increased calcium deposition in brain occurs in states with elevated blood levels of PTH[1,2].  The results of the present study suggest that this effect of PTH could not be mediated at the blood-CSF or the CSF-brain interfaces since alterations in the concentrations of calcium, inorganic phosphorus, or calcium-phosphorus product in CSF either did not occur or were

slight.  It is more likely that the effect of PTH on brain calcium
is mediated through an effect of the hormone on the blood-brain
interface of the blood-brain barrier.

REFERENCES

1.  A.I. Arieff and S.G. Massry, Calcium metabolism of brain in
        acute renal failure.  Effects of uremia, hemodialysis and
        parathyroid hormone, J. Clin. Invest. 53:387, 1974.
2.  D.A. Goldstein and S.G. Massry, Effect of parathyroid hormone
        administration and its withdrawal on brain calcium and
        electroencephalogram, Min. Elect. Metab. 1:84, 1978.
3.  H. Davson, Physiology of the Cerebrospinal Fluid, Little, Brown
        and Co., Boston, 1967, p. 82.
4.  G.B. Wallace and B.B. Brodie, The distribution of iodine, thio-
        cyanate, bromide and chloride in the central nervous system,
        and spinal fluid.  J. Pharmacol. Exp. Ther. 65:220, 1939.
5.  A. Krough, The active and passive exchanges of inorganic ions
        through the surfaces of living cells and through living mem-
        branes generally, Proc. R. Soc. Lond. (Biol). 133:140, 1946.
6.  C. Crone, The permeability of brain capillaries to non-electro-
        lytes, Acta Physiol. Scand. 64:407, 1965.
7.  A.T. Cameron and V.H.K. Moorhouse, The tetany of parathyroid
        deficiency and the calcium of the blood and cerebrospinal
        fluid, J. Biol. Chem. 63:687, 1925.
8.  H. Cohen, The inorganic phosphorus content of cerebrospinal
        fluid, Q.J. Med. 17:289, 1924.
9.  H.H. Merritt and W. Bauer, The equilibrium between cerebro-
        spinal fluid and blood plasma:  the distribution of calcium
        and phosphorus between cerebrospinal fluid blood serum,
        J. Biol. Chem. 90:215, 1931.
10. H.H. Merritt and W. Bauer, The equilibrium between cerebrospinal
        fluid and blood plasma:  the calcium content of serum, cere-
        brospinal fluid, and aqueous humour at different levels of
        parathyroid activity.  J. Biol. Chem. 90:233, 1931.
11. D.C. Cannon and I. Olitzky, Proteins, In R.J. Henry, (ed.),
        Clinical Chemistry, Principles and Techniques, Harper and
        Row, New York, 1974, p. 423.
12. Z. Gutman and A.W. Wahlefeld, L-Lactate determination with
        LDH and NAD, In H.U. Bergmeyer (ed.), Methods in Enzymatic
        Analysis, Academic Press, New York and London, 1974, p. 1562.
13. S. Dagley, Citrate U.V. spectrophotometric determination, In
        H.U. Bergmeyer, (ed.), Methods in Enzymatic Analysis,
        Academic Press, New York and London, 1974, p. 1562.
14. S. Morguilis, and A.M. Perley, Studies on cerebrospinal fluid
        and serum calcium, with special reference to the parathyroid
        hormone, J. Biol. Chem. 88:169, 1930.
15. W.W. Oppelt, E.S. Owens, and D.P. Rall, Calcium exchange between
        blood and cerebrospinal fluid, Life Sci. 8:599, 1963.

16. L.C.A. Watson and C.R.B. Blackburn, The pressure and calcium concentration of the cerebrospinal fluid of the rabbit, Austria J. Exp. Biol. 34:53, 1956.
17. A.M. Parfitt, Soft tissued calcification in uremia. Arch. Intern. Med. 124:544, 1969.

# EFFECTS OF DISODIUM DICHLOROMETHYLENE DIPHOSPHONATE ($Cl_2MDP$) ON PAGET'S DISEASE OF BONE

P.J. Meunier, M.C. Chapuy, C. Alexandre, C. Bressot,
E. Vignon, U. Trechsel, L. Mathieu, C. Edouard

Laboratoire de Recherches sur l'Histodynamique Osseuse,
Faculté Alexis Carrel, rue G. Paradin, 69008 - LYON and
Clinique de Rhumatologie, Hôpital Ed. Herriot - 69003.
LYON. France

## INTRODUCTION

As first shown by Russell et al[1,2], disodium ethane-1-hydroxy-1, 1 diphosphonate (E.H.D.P.) has a powerful depressive effect on the increased bone turnover which characterizes Paget's disease of bone. When ingested in doses of greater than 5 mg per kg per day, however, it causes a mineralization defect in addition to having a marked antiosteoclastic effect[1-6]. Accordingly, a diphosphonate free of such a side-effect would be preferable for the treatment of not only Paget's disease, but of any other condition of hyperosteoclastosis, whatever the mechanisms of osteoclastic differenciation. To date, two compounds have been suggested in this connection : 3 amino-1-hydroxy-propane-1, 1 diphosphonate (A.H.P.D.P.) investigated by Bijvoet and al.[7], and disodium dichloromethylene diphosphonate ($Cl_2$M.D.P.), a drug similar in structure to E.H.D.P.

In vitro studies using mouse calvaria have demonstrated that $Cl_2$M.D.P. inhibits both parathormone-stimulated and unstimulated bone resorption [8,9]. Furthermore, as well as being the most potent bone resorption inhibitor known, $Cl_2$M.D.P. depresses bone formation less than A.H.P.D.P. and E.H.D.P. do, as demonstrated in both in vitro and in vivo rat studies, and does not inhibit osteoid mineralization[10-15]. The drug was tolerated well in 36 human volunteers who received it orally for 4 weeks at doses ranging from 200 to 3200 mg per day, and acute toxicity studies in animals showed its $LD_{50}$ to be at least 55 times greater than the highest dose administered in this study[16]. This study was undertaken in order to determine the effects that $Cl_2$M.D.P., used here for the first time in human therapeutics, would have on patients exhibiting an active

Paget's disease, this condition being a model of bone hyperremodelling[17].

## MATERIALS AND METHODS

### Patients
        The 19 patients (7 males, 12 females ; ages 46-75 years) were
selected for having clinical symptoms and radiological evidence of
Paget's disease, and elevations of serum alkaline phosphatase (AP)
and/or of urinary hydroxyproline (OHP) to at least 1.5 times the
upper limit of their normal values. Patients previously treated
with E.H.D.P. or having received calcitonin within the preceding
3 months were excluded. An informed consent was obtained from each
patient, and the study was sanctioned by the local ethical committee.

### Treatment
        Supplied in 200 mg capsules, the $Cl_2M.D.P.$ was administered
with water 2 hours after breakfast. The doses were 1600 mg per day
in 10 of the patients (Group I) and 400 mg per day in the remaining
9 (Group II), and treatment lasted for 6 months. Neither the initial mean AP or OHP values differed statistically between the two
groups.

### Methods
        Clinical status was assessed and blood and urine measurements
performed after 1, 2, 3.5, 5 and 6 months of treatment and every
3 months subsequent. To date, 6 patients from group I and 2 from
group II have been followed up for a 9 month post-therapy period.
These figures were 8 and 8 at the 6th post-therapy month, and 10
and 9 (all patients) at the 3rd.

        Blood was obtained for AP (Bodansky Units), calcium (Ca),
phosphorus (P), immunoreactive parathyroid hormone (i P.T.H., measured by an assay sensitive to the C-terminal fragment of P.T.H.
and using a G.P. 6 antibody), calcitonin, 25 OH vitamin D, and
S.G.O. and S.G.P. transaminases measurements ; for blood counts ;
and for a complete Technicon S.M.A. 12 series including creatinine (Cr), glucose, and bilirubin. In addition, $1,25 (OH)_2D3$ was
measured at the Pathophysiologisches Institut of Bern University
in 9 patients during treatment using a competitive binding assay
(normal range : 50 - 170 pmol/l ; mean 101 pmol/l). The upper
limit of the normal serum AP range was 5 Bodansky Units/l, and of
the normal iPTH, 520 pg/ml. (normal values 250 pg/ml $\pm$ 135).

        Urine was collected for 3 consecutive days for OHP, Cr., Ca.,
and P measurements, and mean values were computed. OHP was expressed per gram of urinary Cr. The upper limit of the normal OHP range
was 345 umol/g. Cr./day.

Quantitative bone scans were performed in the pre-treatment period and repeated on the 100th and 180th days. Five hours after the injection of $^{99m}$ Tc-E.H.D.P. count rates were registered and the ratio for pagetic bone over opposite normal bone was computed. The results were expressed for each hyperfixating focus and a thoraco-lumbar reference was taken for unpaired pagetic bones.

A transfixing iliac bone biopsy was performed with an 8 mm trephine prior to therapy and again after 100 days of treatment in pagetic or non-pagetic iliac crests. Prerequisite double labelling was done with demethylchlortetracycline administered (300 mg, b.i.d.) according to a schedule of 2 days on, 12 days off, and then 4 days on. The undecalcified bone biopsies were analyzed quantitatively and the following histomorphometric parameters were evaluated in trabecular bone, all according to previously published methods[17] : trabecular bone volume (T.B.V. in per cent), relative osteoid volume (R.O.V. in per cent), osteoid surfaces (O.S. in per cent), osteoid thickness index (R.O.V./O.S.), number of osteoclasts per mm2 of bone section (N. Ocl.), total resorption surfaces (T.R.S. in per cent), and calcification rate (C.R. in microns per day).

*Statistical methods*
The significance of mean differences between consecutive periods was evaluated using either the Mann-Whitney, signed rank, or contrast Scheffe test.

RESULTS

*Biochemistry*
The changes in OHP and AP are shown in fig. 1 and 2. In the Group I patients (1600 mg/day) there was a striking decline in these two parameters which was significant ($p < 0.01$ for OHP, $p < 0.05$ for AP) by the first month of treatment. The mean pre-treatment OHP and AP levels were reduced by half in about 60 and 70 days respectively. The decline continued significantly and by the 6th month the pre-treatment levels were reduced by about 75 per cent. AP continued to decrease, though only slightly, after the end of treatment (minus 80 per cent after 3 months), and 9 months later there has still been no relapse noted in either parameter. Moreover, when expressed in terms of the per cent of the initial elevation above the upper limits of their normal values (fig. 2), AP and OHP decreased continually throughout the 9 month post-therapy period (minus 95 and 99 per cent respectively). At the end of treatment OHP had normalized in 6 of the 10 Group I patients ($< 345$ $\mu$mol/g. Cr./day), and AP had normalized in one of these ($< 5$ Bodansky Units/l.). Three months after treatment these figures were 7 and 5 respectively.

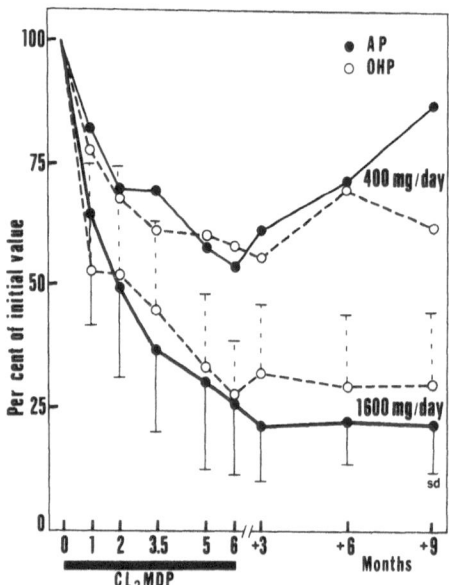

Fig. 1. Reductions in mean percents of pre-treatment serum alkaline phosphatase (AP) and urinary hydroxyproline (OHP) values for 19 pagetic patients treated with $Cl_2$M.D.P. for 6
months in daily doses of 1600 mg (10 patients) and 400 mg
(9 patients). 9 month follow-up.

OHP and AP did not drop significantly (minus 42 per cent and
46 per cent respectively at 6 months) in the Group II patients
(400 mg/day). At the 6th month, OHP had normalized in 3 of the
9 patients, and AP in one of these, but the 3 patients had begun
with only moderately elevated values ( < 760 µmol/g. Cr./day for
OHP and < 10 Bodansky Units/l for AP). Furthermore, within 3 months
after treatment both parameters had already increased markedly.

Evaluated from mean values calculated at each visit, serum
Ca, P., Cr., calcitonin, 25 OH vitamin D, hemoglobin, white blood,
cells, platelets, bilirubin, SGOT, SGPT, glucose, cholesterol and
urinary Cr. did not change in either group. Significant changes
were noted, however, in urinary Ca (insert in fig. 2). In both

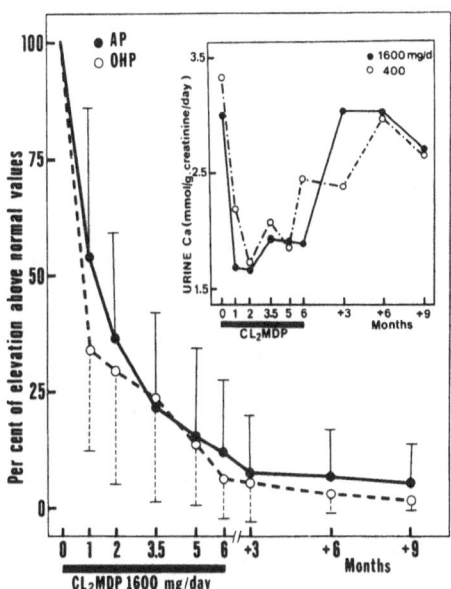

Fig.2. Reductions in percents of elevation above normal values of
serum alkaline phosphatase (AP) and urinary hydroxyproline
(OHP) in 10 pagetic patients treated with 1600 mg per day
of Cl$_2$M.D.P. for 6 months. Insert : reduction of urinary
calcium with both doses (1600 and 400 mg/day).

groups it decreased significantly in the first month (p < 0.01 for
1600 mg dose; p < 0.05 for 400 mg dose) and was reduced from its
initial value by more than 50 per cent by the second, after which
it began to gently reascend.

      Another biochemical response to the Cl$_2$M.D.P. treatment was
a marked increase of iP.T.H. in 6 of the 10 Group I and 7 of the
9 Group II patients (fig. 3), the parathyroid response occurring
at various times after the start of treatment. The earliest and
largest increase was noted in the only patient who developed a
hypocalcemia during treatment, serum calcium dropping from 2.42
to 1.80 mmol/1. OHP also dropped dramatically in this patient,
from 823 μmol/g.Cr./day before treatment to 194 by the first month

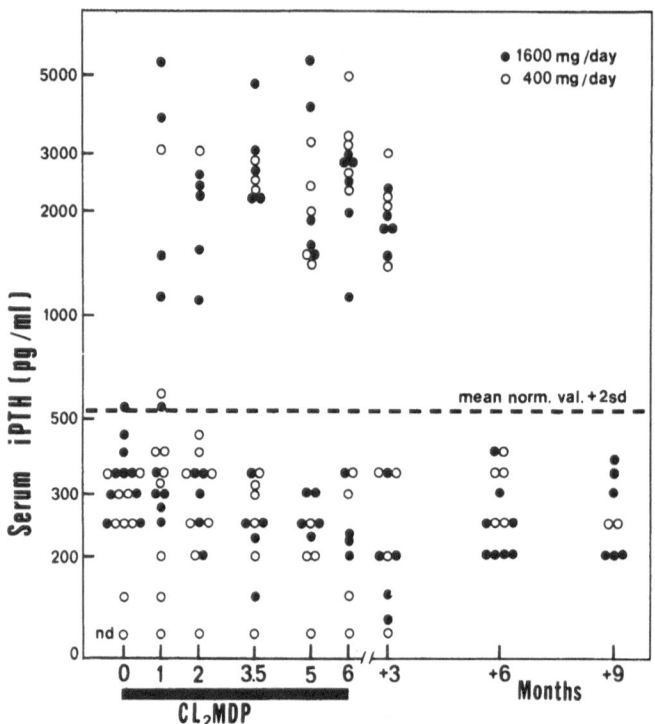

Fig. 3. Changes in serum iPTH during and after treatment with
Cl$_2$M.D.P. for both dose groups.

evincing a rapid inhibition of osteoclastic activity. The hypocalcemia corrected to 2.30 mmol/l. with daily administrations of 1 g.
of elemental calcium and 12.000 I. Units of vitamin D2. iP.T.H.
decreased at the same time and normalized 6 months after treatment,
as was the case with the patients who did not receive any calcium
and/or D. supplementation. The transitory iP.T.H. increase was
much less marked than the mean increase noted in a separate group
of 39 hyperparathyroid patients with parathyroid adenomas (mean :
11,920 pg/ml ± 7,060 ; range 4,800 - 27,000), and was probably responsible for the high 1,25 (OH)2 D3 levels noted in the Group I
patients during treatment. The mean 1,25 (OH)2 D3 value was
251.7 ± 56.7 pmol/l for 6 treated Group I patients (9 assays ;
range 187.3 - 343.9) and 158.2 ± 42.I pmol/l for 3 Group II patients (6 assays ; range 75 - 188). There were no biochemical
signs that Cl$_2$M.D.P. had any liver, renal or hematological toxicity, and serum phosphorus did not increase with the higher, 1600 mg
per day dosage.

*Bone scans*

Table I. Ratio of 99 $Tc^m$ E.H.D.P. uptake in pagetic sites to uptake in opposite normal sites in 19 pagetic patients, before (0) and at the 100th and 180th days of $Cl_2$M.D.P. treatment.

n : number of active sites

* : significantly different from pre-treatment ratio (contrast Scheffe test).

| Daily dose of $Cl_2$M.D.P. | Days | | |
|---|---|---|---|
| | 0 | 100 th | 180 th |
| 1600 mg (Group I) | 6.45 n : 41 | 2.83 * n : 40 | 2.62 * n : 30 |
| 400 mg (Group II) | 4.30 n : 42 | 3.14 n : 41 | 2.41 * n : 23 |

The mean ratio of tracer uptake in pagetic bone to tracer uptake in normal bone, which was calculated using more than 40 active sites from each group, decreased significantly by the 100th day in Group I and at 6 months in Group II.

*Bone histomorphometry*

Post-treatment histological data was gathered on 7 patients from Group I and 9 from Group II, though only the calcification rate was measurable in one of these latter. Of the remaining 15 patients in which all of the parameters were measurable, two from each group were biopsied twice in non-pagetic bone, while the rest (5 and 6 respectively) were biopsied twice in pagetic. After 100 days of 1600 mg/day $Cl_2$M.D.P. treatment, there was a marked reduction both of total resorption surfaces (- 46 per cent of initial mean value) and of the number of osteoclasts per $mm^2$ of bone section (- 59 per cent) in pagetic bone. The antiosteoclastic effect of 400 mg/day seemed to be of equal magnitude (- 40 per cent for T.R.S. and - 74% for N. Ocl.), but the patient sample was not large enough to permit a meaningful statistical analysis. No significant changes were noted in the non-pagetic bone resorption parameters. Trabecular bone volume remained fairly constant, except for in one non-pagetic bone biopsied case in which it increased from its pre-treatment 14.7 % value to 27.2% on the 100th day. Since the osteoid surfaces in this patient were extended and the number of osteoclasts high, it would seem that, like E.H.D.P.[18], $Cl_2$M.D.P. is able to increase bone mass when administered in situations of hyperremodelling. The key question in the histomorphometric analysis was wether $Cl_2$M.D.P. had induced a mineralization defect, as

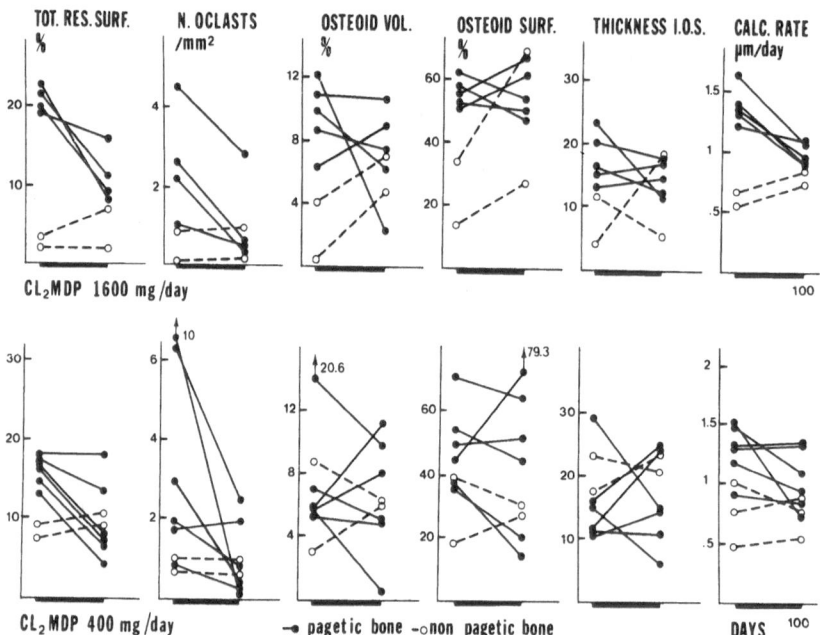

Fig. 4. Bone histology : changes in histomorphometric parameters
        as measured in pagetic and non-pagetic iliac bone biopsies,
        after 100 days of $Cl_2$M.D.P. treatment.

does E.H.D.P. when ingested in doses of greater than 5 mg per kg
per day. With regard to this, there was no increase in any of the
patients in the thickness of pagetic or non-pagetic osteoid seams,
and their calcification rates never fell below normal. The mean
pagetic bone C.R. in Group I was reduced from 1.38 ± .16 µm/day,
the usual pagetic bone value[17], to 0.97 ± 0.10 µm/day. Since this
decrease was not accompanied by an osteoid seam thickness increase,
it represents not a mineralization defect, but a reduction in the
daily "productivity" of pagetic osteoblasts : they stopped synthe-
sizing large amounts of woven bone and began to produce lesser
amounts of lamellar bone. There was no C.R. decrease in non-pagetic
bone.

        Finally, two qualitative histological changes were noted in
pagetic bone after the $Cl_2$M.D.P. treatment : a marked reduction of
both marrow fibrosis and vascularity, and the reappearance, seen
in the bone deposited during treatment, of a normal lamellar texture, as revealed under polarized light.

*Clinical*
        All of the patients receiving the 1600 mg doses exhibited
striking clinical improvements : the intensity of bone pain at
each painful location and the number of painful locations per patients decreased, and in most cases ambulatory capability was increased. These effects were less marked with the 400 mg doses. No

fractures occurred during treatment and no adverse clinical side-
effects, such as gastro-intestinal intolerance or fever,  were noted in either group.

DISCUSSION

    Tested on Paget's disease, a typical situation of bone hyper-
remodelling, Cl$_2$M.D.P. had an obvious antiosteoclastic effect without inhibiting bone mineralization and while being well tolerated
clinically and biochemically. The decreases of AP and OHP were
greater when the daily doses were 1600 mg : the 400 mg treatment
did not have a significant reducing effect on these two parameters.
The decreases were also greater than those noted in a previous study (minus 70 per cent for AP and minus 66 per cent for OHP) in
which equivalent doses of E.H.D.P. (20 mg per kg per day) were administered for six months to 25 pagetic patients[18]. The fall in AP
within  the first two months of treatment occurred about 30 days
after the fall of similar magnitude in OHP, demonstrating that the
osteoclastic effect precedes the reduction in the osteoblastic
population. Moreover, the long-lastingness of the biochemical remission obtained with the 1600 mg per day doses (no relapse having yet
occurred 9 months after treatment) is especially striking.

    By arresting the accentuated bone hyperresorption which cha-
racterizes pagetic remodelling and is responsible for the increased
efflux of calcium from bone, the Cl$_2$M.D.P. induced a marked reduction in the mobilization of calcium from bone. This fact can explain
the drop in urinary calcium, the occasional decrease of serum calcium, and the frequent increases, noted in 13 of 19 patients, of
serum iPTH. This latter normalized by the 6th month after treatment in all cases, while urinary calcium reascended to its pre-
treatment values. The increase of iPTH was very likely the cause
of the high 1,25 (OH)2 D3 levels noted during treatment in 8 of the
9 patients in which this metabolite was measured. It will be interesting to determine if a systematic supplementation of calcium and
vitamin D during Cl$_2$M.D.P. therapy of pagetic patients could prevent this transitory secondary hyperparathyroidism. Increases in
parathyroid secretion have not been observed in pagetic patients
treated with high doses of E.H.D.P., a drug which blocks both bone
calcium efflux and influx by simultaneously inhibiting bone resorption and mineralization[19].

    Cl$_2$M.D.P., even  when ingested in high doses, does not induce
morphological or dynamical osteomalacia, as proven by the absence
of a thickening of osteoid seams or a reduction to subnormal values
of the calcification rate.

    In any case, like A.H.P.D.P.[7,20], Cl$_2$M.D.P. seems promising
for the treatment of all bone diseases characterized by increased
osteoclastic activity, such as multiple myeloma, metastatic bone

disease, hypercalcemias due to these two, disuse osteoporosis, high
remodelling osteoporosis and possibly, localized juxta-articular
bone erosions due to chronic arthritis.

REFERENCES

1. R. Smith, R.G.G. Russell, M.C. Bishop, C.G. Woods, and M. Bishop,
   Paget's disease of bone : experience with a diphosphonate
   (disodium etidronate) in treatment, Quart. J. Med. 42 : 235
   (1973).
2. R.G.G. Russell, R. Smith, C. Preston, R.J. Walton, and C.G. Woods,
   Diphosphonate in Paget's disease, Lancet 894 (1974)
3. R.D. Altman, C.C. Johnston, M.R.A. Khairi, H. Wellman, A.N.
   Serafini, and R.R. Sankey, Influence of disodium etidronate
   on clinical and laboratory manifestations of Paget's disease
   of bone, N. Engl. J. Med. 289 : 1379 (1973)
4. R. Canfield, W. Rosner, J. Skinner, J. Mc Worther, L. Resnick,
   F. Feldman, S. Kammerman, K. Ryan, M. Kunigonis, and W.
   Bohne, Diphosphonate therapy of Paget's disease of Bone,
   J. Clin. Endocrinol. Metab. 44 : 96 (1977)
5. M.R.A. Khairi, P. Meunier, C. Edouard, P. Courpron, J. Bernard,
   G.P. Derosa, C.C. Johnston, Quantitative bone histology in
   Paget's disease of bone : influence of sodium etidronate
   (EHDP) therapy, Calc. Tiss. Res., Suppl. 22 : 355 (1977)
6. P.J. Meunier, C. Alexandre, M.R.A. Khairi, C.C. Johnston, C.
   Edouard, P. Lips, and M.C. Chapuy, Dose dependent effects of
   E.H.D.P. on dynamics of bone remodeling in Paget's disease :
   studies in involved and non involved areas, in "Abstracts
   of 13th Eur. Symp. on Calc. Tissues", Noordwijkerhout, The
   Netherlands, 66 (1977).
7. W.B. Frijlink, O.L.M. Bijvoet, J. Te Velde, and G. Heynen,
   Treatment of Paget's disease with (3-amino-1-hydroxypropy-
   lidene)-1, 1-biphosphonate (A.P.D.), Lancet, 799 (1979).
8. D.B. Morgan, A. Monod, R.G.G. Russell, and H. Fleisch, Influence of $Cl_2M.D.P.$ and calcitonin on bone resorption, lactate
   production and phosphatase and pyrophosphatase content of
   mouse calvaria treated with parathyroid hormone in vitro,
   Calc. Tiss. Res., 13 : 287 (1973)
9. C. Minkin, L. Rabadjija, and P. Goldhaber, Bone remodeling in
   vitro : the effects of two diphosphonates on osteoid synthesis and bone resorption in mouse calvaria, Calc. Tiss. Res.
   14 : 161 (1974).
10. R. Schenk, W.A. Merz, R. Muhlbauer, R.G.G. Russell, and H.
    Fleisch, Effects of EHDP and $Cl_2M.D.P.$ on the calcification
    and resorption of cartilage and bone in the tibial epiphysis
    and metaphysis of rats, Calc. Tiss. Res, 11 : 196 (1973)
11. S.C. Miller and W.S.S. Jee, The comparative effects of $Cl_2MDP$
    and EHDP on growth and modeling of the rat tibia. Calc. Tiss.
    Res. 18 : 215 (1975)

12. J. Gotcher, D. Kimmel, and W.S.S. Jee, A dose response study of Cl₂M.D.P. in a growing rat. IADR Abstract, B.303 : 967 (1976)

13. H. Fleisch, R.G.G. Russell, B. Simpson, and R.C. Muehlbauer, Prevention by a diphosphonate of immobilization "osteoporosis" in rats, Nature 223 : 211 (1969)

14. R.G.G. Russell, and H. Fleisch. Pyrophosphate and diphosphonates in skeletal metabolism. Physiological, clin. and therapeutic aspects, Clin. Orthop. Rel. Res., 108 - 241 (1975)

15. H.H.P.J. Lemkes, P.H. Reitsma, W.B. Frijlink, J. Verlinden, and O.L.M. Bijvoet, Diphosphonates, dissociation between cellular and mineral effects, in "Homeostasis of Phosphate and other Minerals", S.G. Massry, E. Ritz, A. Rapado eds, Plenum, New York, (1977).

16. Unpublished informations in the files of the Procter and Gamble Company, Cincinnati. Ohio. USA.

17. P.J. Meunier, Disturbances in morphology and dynamics of the remodeling process in pagetic bone, in "Human Calcitonin and Paget's disease", I. Mc Intyre ed., Hans Huber, Bern (1977).

18. C. Alexandre, and P.J. Meunier, in "Le traitement de la maladie de Paget par l'E.H.D.P.", ACEML, Lyon (1977).

19. L. David, M.C. Chapuy, and P. Meunier, Parathyroid function and biochemical changes in Paget's disease of bone treated with E.H.D.P., in "Phosphate Metabolism, Kidney and Bone", L. Avioli, P. Bordier, H. Fleisch, S. Massry, E. Slatopolsky ed., Armour Montagu, Paris (1976).

20. F.J.M. Van Breukelen, O.L.M. Bijvoet and A.T. Van Oosterom, Inhibition of osteolytic bone lesions by (3-amino-1-hydroxy-propylene)-1, 1-biphosphonate (A.P.D.). Lancet, 803 (1979).

*ACKNOWLEDGEMENTS*

We thank Pr G. Vignon for his help, Mr. B. van Duzee from the Procter and Gamble Company, Cincinnati, Ohio, USA, for having provided us with Cl₂MDP, Dr. M. Arlot for the statistical analysis, Mr. A. Clark for linguistic suggestions and Mrs. C. Navarro for preparing the typescript.

This work was supported in part by grants from INSERM (CL 76.I.016.4) and the Faculté Alexis Carrel, LYON.

# PHOSPHATE DEPLETION

# FUNCTION OF THE SARCOPLASMIC RETICULUM (SR) IN HYPO-PHOSPHATEMIC MYOPATHY

Wilhelm Kreusser, Eberhard Ritz, Ricardo Boland
Johannes Brachmann

Department Internal Medicine and Max-Planck
Institut für Medizinische Forschung, Heidelberg
Germany

## INTRODUCTION

Changes in the function of skeletal muscle and myocardial performance are well known features of Pi depletion (PD). Asthenia, muscle pain and creatinuria were described in the seminal paper by Lotz et al. (1) in healthy volunteers in whom prolonged Pi deprivation was induced by ingestion of large amounts of Al(OH)$_3$. In patients with chronic alcoholism who exhibit a latent form of metabolic myopathy, Knochel et al. (2) found an increase in plasma CPK and aldolase upon physical exercise; in some cases rhabdomyolysis with acute renal failure ensued. Acute myocardial insufficiency in critically ill patients, reversible upon administration of Pi, was described by O'Connor et al. (3); however, apart from hypophosphatemia a variety of toxic and metabolic derangements may have been present in these patients. Recently, in non-alcoholic patients with pure PD, however, Darsee and Nutter (4) described chronic congestive heart failure which was corrected by administration of Pi.

Corresponding abnormalities of muscular and myocardial function could be reproduced in experimental Pi depletion. In chronically Pi depleted dogs reversible changes in resting transmembrane potential and intracellular electrolyte content were reported by Fuller et al. (5). Furthermore, Fuller et al. (6) observed depressed myocardial contractility, reversible upon administration of Pi, in chronically Pi depleted dogs. These authors proposed the hypothesis that the decrease in cardiac

contractility is associated with an abnormality of $Ca^{2+}$
pumping by the sarcoplasmic reticulum. Such abnormality
could arise either from decreased availability of ATP
or an alteration of the intrinsic membrane transport properties, e.g. by changes in the mebrane lipid composition.
The present experiment was designed to investigate a possible effect of chronic dietary Pi depletion in the rat
on membrane lipid composition, kinetic $Ca^{2+}$ transport
properties, resting transmembrane potential and nucleotide, water and electrolyte composition of skeletal
muscle.

MATERIAL AND METHODS

    Male Sprague Dawley rats (Ivanovas Co., Kisslegg)
with an initial weight of 9o-loo g were housed in single
metabolic ages. After an adaptation phase of 5 days, the
PD rats received a diet containing o.o3% inorganic phosphorous. Control rats (CO) were given a diet containing
o.4% Pi in an amount which maintained body weight at the
same level as in matched PD animals. All rats had free
access to deionised water. After 3 weeks of PD, the following parameters were measured: serum Pi, Ca, Mg; m.
quadriceps Na, K, $H_2O$, Pi, ATP, ADP AMP, creatin    phosphate content as described previously (7). Resting transmembrane potential was measured in the diaphragm as described in Rüdel et al. (8). Sarcoplasmic reticulum (SR)
was prepared from the hind legs according to de Meis and
Hasselbach (9). Initial uptake of Ca $^{2+}$, concentrating ability and storing capacity were determined and calculated
as described by Matthews et al. (lo). In isolated SR,
phospholipid concentration and composition were measured
as described previously (11).

RESULTS

    After 3 weeks of PD, serum Pi was 2.56 + o.48 mg/dl
as compared to 8.o4 $\pm$ o.85 in pair-weighed $\overline{CO}$. At this
stage of PD depletion, the animals were severely asthe-
nic, although muscular force was not quantitated; after
1 further week the rats would begin to die.

    The fall in serum Pi was accompanied by a decrease
in the muscular inorganic phosphorous content. There
were no significant changes with respect to water or electrolyte content of m.quadriceps in PD animals. ATP was
significantly decreased and creatin    phosphate was also
slightly, but not significantly, diminished. These results
are summarized in table 1.

Table 1    The effect of phosphate depletion on
           skeletal muscle water, electrolyte and
           nucleotide content

| | $H_2O$ % wet weight | Na | K | $P_i$ | ATP | CP |
|---|---|---|---|---|---|---|
| | | ——————mmol/g ww—————— | | | umol/mg ww | |
| CO (n=12) | 76.2 $\pm$ o.56 | 21.8 $\pm$ 4.47 | 124 $\pm$ 3.o | 29.9 $\pm$ 2.55 | 5.67 +o.44 | 3.75 +o.49 |
| PD (n=12) | 75.7 $\pm$ o.59 | 21.9 $\pm$ 2.15 | 124 $\pm$ 7.17 | 26.2 $\pm$ 3.28 | 4.9o +o.33 | 3.42 +o.51 |
| p | N.S. | N.S. | N.S. | $<$o.02 | $<$o.ol | N.S. |

All values given as $\bar{x} \pm$ SD; Wilcoxon test for pair differences.

Resting transmembrane potential was measured in the
diaphragm, impaling at least 1o muscle fibers per animal.
The CV for intraindividual measurements was 6.1%.
There was no sig-
nificant difference
between PD and CO
animals (s.figure 1)
This result could be
reproduced in 3 dif-
ferent series of ex-
periments.

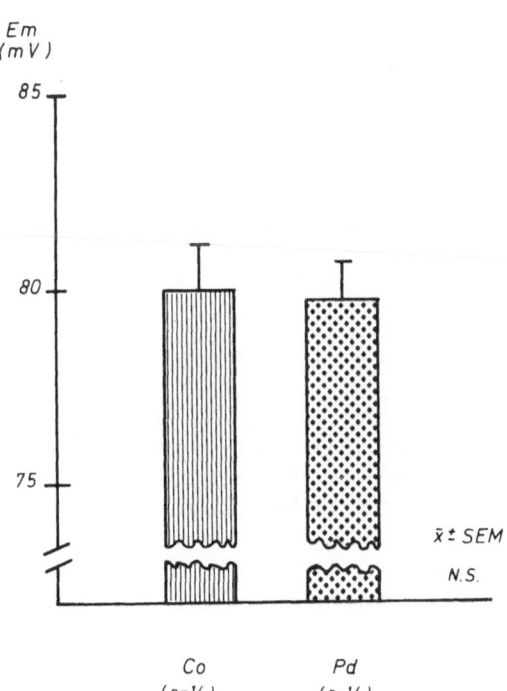

Figure 1
Resting membrane
potential (Em) in
the diaphragm of
phosphate depleted
rats.

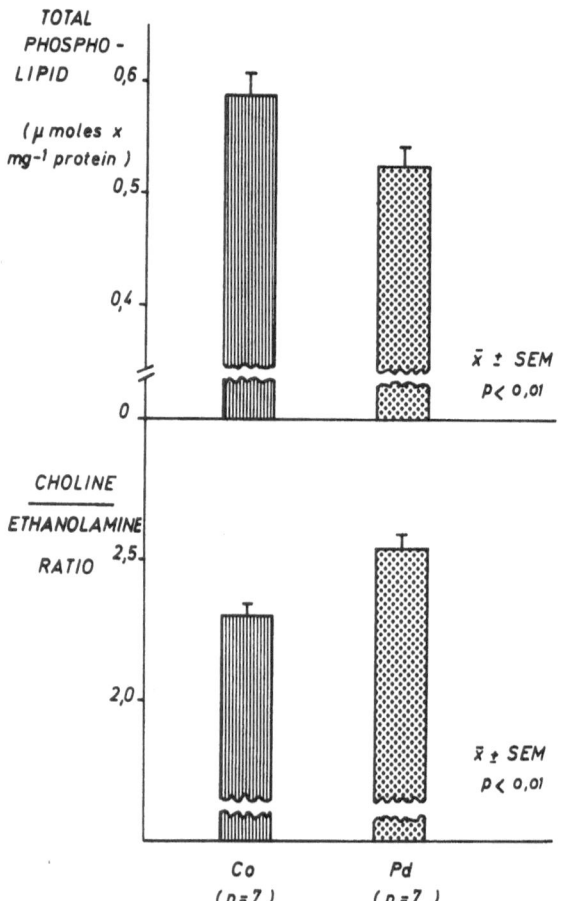

Figure 2

Lipid composition of sarcoplasmic reticulum of phosphate depleted rats.

As shown in figure 2, total phospholipid/protein ratio in isolated SR of PD animals was significantly decreased and the phosphatidyl-choline/phosphatidyl-ethanolamine ratio was significantly elevated.

Concomitantly, as shown in table 2, storing capacity of isolated SR of PD animals, was slightly, but significantly decreased.
In contrast, no significant difference was observed between PD and CO animals with respect to initial rate of uptake of $Ca^{2+}$ and concentrating ability (see table 2).

Table 2    The effect of phosphate depletion on
           sarcoplasmic reticulum

|  | storing capacity $10^{-6}$ mol x mg$^{-1}$ protein | initial rate of uptake $10^{-9}$ mol x mg$^{-1}$ prot x min$^{-1}$ | concentrating ability $10^{-9}$ M |
|---|---|---|---|
| CO (n=12) | 5.41 $\pm$ o.12 | 15o3 $\pm$ 189 | 37.6 $\pm$ 16.o |
| PD (n=12) | 4.7o $\pm$ o.12 | 139o $\pm$ 246 | 45.5 $\pm$ 14.5 |
| p | o.o1 | N.S. | N.S. |

All values given as $\bar{x} \pm$ SD; Wilcoxon test for pair
differences.


DISCUSSION

     The above results provide evidence that severe Pi
depletion in the rat does not cause an intrinsic abnormality of vectorial transport of Ca$^{2+}$ in the sarcoplasmic reticulum isolated from non-exercised muscle, although muscular Pi and nucleotide content are reduced
and although phospholipid content and composition of the
SR are changed.

     In the present study, a severe state of PD in the
experimental animals was evident from inspection of the
rats which were lethargic, weak and unable to fight;Pi
content in m. quadriceps was diminished by 13%, a decrement which is similar in magnitude to that observed in
muscle of PD dogs by Fuller et al. (5). Species differences between dog and rat with respect to the reaction of
muscle to PD are suggested by our failure to observe deviations of muscle electrolyte and water content whereas such changes were clearly demonstrable in PD dogs (5)
Furthermore, in PD rats, repeated efforts to demonstrate
decreased transmembrane resting potential, as described
in PD man (2) and PD dog (5) gave negative results. The
extent to which such species differences may also exist
with respect to the involvement of the SR remains to be
established.

     The present study shows that membrane phospholipid
composition in isolated SR is changed. This corresponds
to findings in human erythrocyte plasma membranes where

Klock et al. (12) also observed an increase in phosphatidyl choline/phosphatidyl ethanolamine ratio. Combined
with the above evidence on muscle Pi and nucleotide content, this finding documents that indeed severe PD existed in the muscles of our experimental animals.

Storing capacity, i.e. the maximum amount of $Ca^{2+}$
taken up under optimal conditions of $Ca^{2+}$ gradient and
ATP supply, was diminished in PD animals. Storing capacity, however, does not necessarily reflect on kinetic
properties of the vesicles and is importantly influenced
by vesicle geometry and completeness of vesicle sealing.
Presence of unsealed empty vesicles or smaller vesicles
would theoretically diminish the maximum amount of $Ca^{2+}$
taken up by a given amount of membrane surface or membrane protein. Phospholipids have indeed been shown to
affect membrane fluidity and sealing properties of SR
(13), but in the light of in vitro reconstitution experiments, it appears unlikely that such minor deviations
of phospholipid content and composition, as observed in
the present study, affect transport characteristics, e.
g. by protein-lipid-interaction.

Kinetic parameters of $Ca^{2+}$ transport in the isolated SR, i.e. initial rate of uptake and concentrating
ability, were both marginally diminished in PD depleted
animals but the difference was not significant. The initial rate of uptake describes the velocity of $Ca^{2+}$ uptake under non-steady state conditions during the first
3o-9o sec of the uptake reaction, which is for all practical purposes equivalent to unidirectional influx because of the tightness of the vesicle membrane. Concentrating ability is assessed by the minimum concentration of
$Ca^{2+}$ outside of the vesicles which can be achieved after
equilibrium is reached. This concentration reflects the
balance between activity of the calcium pump and passive
back leak.

Although the present study fails to demonstrate an
impairment of in vitro $Ca^{2+}$ transport kinetics of SR isolated from non-exercised muscle of severly Pi depleted
rats, several notes of caution are  appropriate. The
above finding does not necessarily exclude that cytosolic $Ca^{2+}$ is changed in muscle of such PD animals, as
postulated by Fuller et al. (6). The uptake reaction as
studied in vitro in the presence of oxalate as anion,
does not necessarily reflect on the rate limiting step
of $Ca^{2+}$ sequestration in vivo which may be represented
by $Ca^{2+}$ binding (14-16) or other processes. Furthermore,
other mechanisms, e.g. mitochondrial $Ca^{2+}$ uptake, may

play a role in setting steady state cytosolic $Ca^{2+}$ (17)
at least under pathological conditions. Finally, conditions may be different in exercised muscle when ATP concentrations presumably fall acutely below the levels used
in the in vitro experiments. This point is particularly
relevant, since superimposition of muscular exercise
upon latent hypophosphatemic myopathy has been shown to
cause severe muscle dysfunction and rhabdomyolysis (18).

SUMMARY

Lipid composition and $Ca^{2+}$ transport properties
were examined in the isolated sarcoplasmic reticulum of
non-exercised muscles of markedly phosphorous depleted
rats. Phosphorous depletion with a fall of plasma Pi from
8.04 + 0.85 to 2.56 + 0.48 mg/dl was accompanied by a decrease in muscle Pi and ATP content and by a significant
decrease in the phospholipid/protein ratio of sarcoplasmic reticulum. The phosphatidyl -choline/phosphatidyl-
ethanolamine ratio in sarcoplasmic membranes was increased. Storing capacity for $Ca^{2+}$ was significantly diminished. In contrast, there was no significant change of
kinetic parameters of $Ca^{2+}$ transport, i.e. of the initial
rate of uptake and concentrating ability. These findings
do not necessarily exclude changes of cytosolic $Ca^{2+}$ concentration in phosphate depletion, but they exclude alterations of intrinsic kinetic  properties of the sarcoplasmic reticulum as a cause of any such potential changes.

Acknowledgement

We thank Professor Hasselbach (Max-Planck Institut
Heidelberg) for permission to use his facilities and for
continued support and stimulation. We also thank Ms.Sis,
Mr. Kretz and Mr. Sommer for excellent technical assistance and Ms. Wolff for secreterial help.

The studies were carried out with the support of
Deutsche Forschungsgemeinschaft (Kr 555/3).

References

1. M. Lotz, E. Zisman, F.C. Bartter, Evidence for a phos-
     phorous depletion syndrome in man, New Engl.J.Med.
     278:4o9 (1968)
2. J.P. Knochel, G.L. Bilbrey, T.J. Fuller, N.W. Carter,
     The muscle cell in chronic alcoholism. The possible

role of phosphate depletion in alcoholic myopathy, Ann.N.Y.Acad.Sci. 252:274 (1975)

3. L.R. O'Connor, W.S. Wheeler, J.E. Bethune, Effect of hypophosphatemia on myocardial performance in man

4. J.R. Darsee, D.O. Nutter, Reversible severe congestive cardiomyopathy in three cases of hypophosphatemia, Ann.Intern.Med. 89:867 (1978)

5. T.J. Fuller, N.W. Carter, C. Barcenas, J.P. Knochel, Reversible changes of the muscle cell in experimental phosphorous deficiency, J.Clin.Invest.57:1o19 (1976)

6. T.J. Fuller, W.W. Nichols, B.J. Brenner, J.C. Peterson, Reversible depression in myocardial performace in dogs with experimental phosphorous deficiency, J.Clin.Invest. 62:1194 (1978)

7. W.J. Kreusser, K. Kurokawa, E. Aznar, S.G. Massry, Phosphate depletion. Effect on renal inorganic phosphorous and adenine nucleotides, urinary phosphate and calcium, and calcium balance, Mineral Electrolyte Metab. 5:3o (1978)

8. R. Rüdel, J. Senges, L. Ehe, A post tetanic decrease of membrane resistance in mamalian skeletal muscle fibers and its antimyotonic effects, Pflügers Arch. 341:121 (1973)

9. D. De Meis, W. Hasselbach, Acetyl phosphate as substrate for $Ca^{2+}$ uptake in skeletal muscle microsomes, J.Biol.Chem. 246: 4759 (1971)

1o. C.Matthews, K.W. Heimberg, E. Ritz, B. Agostini, J. Fritzsche, W. Hasselbach, Effect of 1,25-dihydroxycholecalciferol on impaired calcium transport by the sarcoplasmic reticulum in experimental uremia, Kidney International 11:227 (1977)

11. R. Boland, A. Martinosi, Developmental changes in the composition and function of sarcoplasmic reticulum, J.Biol.Chem. 249:612 (1974)

12. J.C. Klock, S.B. Shohet, Erythrocyte membrane lipid abnormalities in hypophosphatemic hemolysis, abstract, J.Clin.Invest. 52:47 (1973)

13. W. Hasselbach, Sarcoplasmic membrane ATPases, in: "The Enzymes", P.D. Boyer ed., Academic Press, New York-London, p. 431 (1974)

14. W. Hasselbach, Release and uptake of calcium by the sarcoplasmic reticulum, in: "Kolloquium der Gesellschaft für Physiologische Chemie", L. Heilmeyer, ed., Springer, Heidelberg, p. 141 (1977)

15. P.Mermier, W. Hasselbach, The bi-phasic $Ca^{2+}$-uptake by the fragmented sarcoplasmic reticulum, Z.Naturforsch. 3o(c):593 (1975)

16. P. Mermier, W. Hasselbach, The effect of calcium and phosphate on the biphasic calcium uptake by the sarcoplasmic reticulum, Z.Naturforsch. 3o(c):777 (1975)
17. A.L. Lehninger, $Ca^{2+}$-transport by mitochondria and its possible role in the cardiac relaxation cycle Circulation Res. 34 (suppl. II):83 (1974)
18. J.P. Knochel, The pathophysiology and clinical characteristics of severe hypophosphatemia, Archs.Intern.Med. 137:2o3 (1977)

# SELECTIVE PHOSPHORUS DEFICIENCY IN THE HYPERALIMENTED HYPOPHOS-

# PHATEMIC DOG AND PHOSPHORYLATION POTENTIALS IN THE MUSCLE CELL

James P. Knochel, M.D., Ronald Haller, M.D. and Evan
Ferguson, Ph.D.

VA Medical Center, Dallas, Texas and University of Texas
Southwestern Medical School, Dallas,
Texas  75235

## Introduction

Administration of nutrients after underfeeding is associated
with a decline of serum inorganic phosphorus concentration (1).
When nutrients are administered in excess and especially with
inadequate quantities of phosphorus, hypophosphatemia is apt to
become pronounced and is invariably associated with excretion of
only trace quantities of phosphorus in the urine. The decline of
serum phosphorus concentration and its simultaneous disappearance
from the urine suggests that phosphorus is being taken up by
cells. The site of phosphorus uptake with regard to specific
tissues has not been determined. We have examined the effects of
hypophosphatemia induced by hyperalimentation of the underfed
dog. The results show that phosphorus deficiency appears rapidly
in skeletal muscle during hyperalimentation. Significant deficiencies of total phosphorus content were also observed in bone,
parathyroid glands and the liver. Phosphorus content did not
change significantly in other tissues.

## Methods

Eight healthy male fox hounds weighing between 24 and 27 kg.
were placed on a synthetic phosphorus deficient diet in a quantity calculated to provide recommended quantities of carbohydrate, fat and protein, minerals and vitamins in terms of
their body weight. To this diet was added 1.87 grams of elemental phosphorus as sodium phosphate each day. After receiving
this diet for a period of two weeks, blood samples were obtained
and the dogs were thereupon placed on one-half this quantity of
the diet until their weight had declined by 30% of its initial
value. Thereupon the dogs received their full complement of diet

as provided in the control study with additional carbohydrate to
provide a total intake of 140 calories/kg/day.

   Serum phosphorus concentration was measured daily during
hyperalimentation. When it reached 1.0mg/dL or less, the dogs
were studied. Under pentobarbital anesthesia, the dogs were
placed on a Harvard respirator to maintain blood pH within normal
limits. Organs (see Table I) were sampled in order to determine
their total phosphorus content, and contents of sodium,
potassium, chloride, magnesium and calcium. These samples were
processed in accordance with methods previously published from
this laboratory (2-4). In six dogs the posterior edge of the
gracilis muscle was carefully exposed so as to avoid injury to
its nerve or vascular supply. Wallenberg clamps precooled in
liquid nitrogen were employed to obtain frozen sections of the
gracilis muscle for measurement of adenosinetriphosphate, adenosine monophosphate, creatine phosphate and inorganic phosphorus.
Frozen tissues were stored in liquid nitrogen and processed by
the method described by Farrell and Olson (5). In order to avoid
the possibility of misinterpretation by increased content of
collagen in the tissues following weight loss, muscle noncollagen
protein was determined by the method of Lilienthal and his associates (6). By this technique, metabolites in muscle tissue are
expressed in terms of myofibrillar protein. In order to calculate phosphorylation potentials, (7,8) adenine nucleotides and
inorganic phosphorus were expressed in their molar concentrations
estimated by assuming that the intracellular water content was
80% of the total tissue water. The phosphorylation potentials
were expressed as the quotient of the ATP concentration and the
product of ADP and inorganic phosphate concentrations.

TABLE I

TOTAL PHOSPHORUS (mmol/dg FAT FREE DRY WEIGHT)

(DATA ARE MEAN ± SEM)

| | HYPERALIMENTED (n=8) | NORMAL (n=6) | SIGNIFICANCE (p) |
|---|---|---|---|
| SKELETAL MUSCLE | 21.1±0.6 | 28.9±0.3 | <0.001 |
| LIVER | 21.8±3.4 | 29.2±1.3 | <0.001 |
| PARATHYROIDS | 22.8±2.0 | 46.9±3.7 | <0.001 |
| BONE | 98.4±13.1 | 201.8±15.4 | <0.001 |
| CEREBRAL CORTEX | 36.0±1.5 | 36.4±2.0 | NS |
| LEFT VENTRICLE | 28.1±4.1 | 28.8±0.3 | NS |
| ADRENAL | 35.6±1.8 | 38.6±1.3 | NS |
| PANCREAS | 48.3±3.3 | 52.5±1.9 | NS |
| RENAL CORTEX | 32.8±1.0 | 34.1±1.1 | NS |
| RENAL MEDULLA | 31.0±1.1 | 32.2±1.7 | NS |
| THYROID | 15.4±1.2 | 15.5±1.1 | NS |
| SPLEEN | 28.5±0.9 | 32.1±4.1 | NS |

Control values for muscle composition were obtained on six normal fox hounds which had been fed their calculated required diet containing 1.87g of phosphorus for a period of two weeks.

## Results

Each of the dogs consumed and retained the diet. None of the dogs became overtly ill before the final study. Table I illustrates the total phosphorus content of tissues analyzed in these animals. The values for total phosphorus in skeletal muscle, liver, parathyroids and bone were significantly less than those determined on six normal animals. The decline in total muscle phosphorus content was 27%, the decline of liver phosphorus content was 25%. The decline in parathyroid and bone contents of phosphorus were both approximately 50%. Total phosphorus values in all of the other tissues analyzed, viz., cerebral cortex, left ventricle, adrenals, pancreas, renal cortex, renal medulla, thyroid and spleen were numerically less but not statistically different from those values in the normal dogs. Figure 1 shows sequential individual values for inorganic phosphorus concentration immediately before and on each day during hyperalimentation. With the exception of one animal, serum phosphorus had fallen to concentrations less than 1.0mg/dL. The most pronounced depression of serum phosphorus usually occurred by the third or fourth day.

Serum creatine phosphokinase activity was measured on each day of hyperalimentation (Fig. 2). Although the average value for CPK activity rose by the fourth day none exceeded the normal range. Individual values were not significantly different from the control value. Concentrations of serum electrolytes, venous pH and blood $PCO_2$ and $PO_2$ were within normal limits and remained so during the period of hyperalimentation.

Table II lists values for total muscle phosphorus content, serum inorganic phosphorus and muscle contents of adenine nucleotides and creatine phosphate in six control dogs and three after hyperalimentation. Despite phosphorus deficiency in skeletal muscle and pronounced hypophosphatemia, the muscle adenine nucleotides and creatine phosphate did not show a significant change. Table III illustrates comparisons between ATP, ADP and inorganic phosphate concentrations in intracellular water and the calculated phosphorylation potential. Each of these values clearly remained within normal limits despite hypophosphatemia.

Table IV shows that muscle Na content was moderately elevated and K content slightly depressed. Values for chloride, magnesium and calcium content were normal.

## Discussion

Previous studies from this laboratory showed that 28 days of

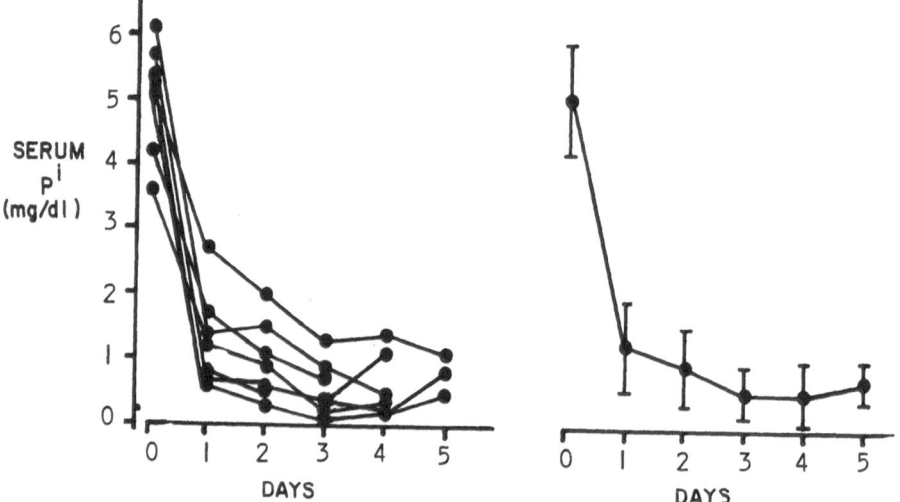

Figure 1.  Individual and average values for serum inorganic phosphate during hyperalimentation of underfed dogs.

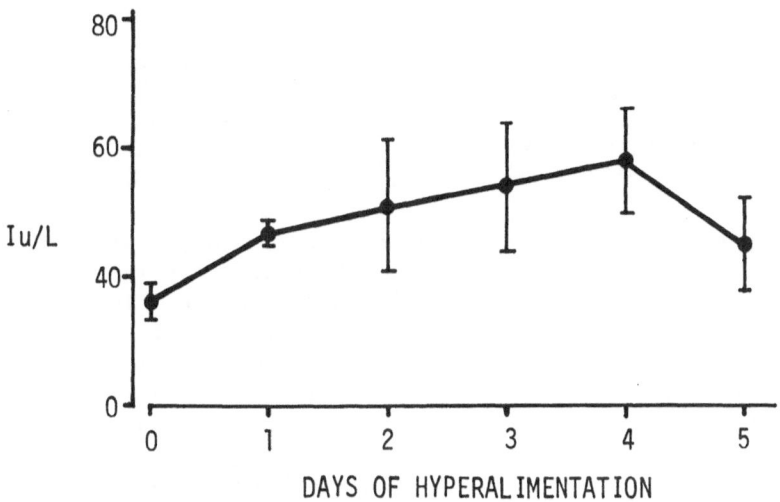

Figure 2.   Serial mean values for CPK activity during hyperalimentation of the underfed dog.   Upper limit of normal is
80 Iu/L.

chronic phosphorus deficiency in the dog induced an electrochemical myopathy characterized by an abnormally low resting muscle

TABLE II
SKELETAL MUSCLE IN UNDERFED, ACUTELY HYPOPHOSPHATEMIC DOGS*

|  |  | CONTROL (n=6) | HYPERALIMENTED (n=3) |
|---|---|---|---|
| Pm | (mmol/Kg FFDW) | 28.1±0.6 | 21.3±0.6 |
| P serum | (mmol/L) | 1.49±0.2 | 0.27±0.13 |
| P muscle | (mmol/Kg NCP) | 64±3.5 | 59±6.0 |
| Adenine Nucleotides (mmol/Kg NCP*) |  |  |  |
| ATP |  | 42.7±1.1 | 37.7±3.7 |
| ADP |  | 4.9±0.6 | 4.6±1.8 |
| Creatine PO |  | 102±26 | 125±20 |

NCP:non-collagen protein
*mean± S.D.

membrane potential of skeletal muscle cells, a depression of
total phosphorus content of muscle of approximately 15%, and elevations of cellular content of sodium and chloride. There was a
slight decline of intracellular potassium concentration. This
abnormality disappeared upon restoration of elemental phosphorus
to the diet. However, if hyperalimentation as conducted in the
studies reported herein were superimposed upon the untreated
electrochemical myopathy in the dog fed a phosphorus-deficient
diet, the animals became extremely ill and florid rhabdomyolysis
occurred within a period of two to five days after initiating
hyperalimentation. In the latter study (9,10) there appeared to
be an inverse relationship between hypophosphatemia and elevation
of CPK activity. In these studies, signs of overt rhabdomyolysis
did not occur.

TABLE III
PHOSPHORYLATION POTENTIAL IN UNDERFED, ACUTELY HYPOPHOSPHATEMIC
DOGS

|  | CONTROL | HYPOPHOSPHATEMIC |
|---|---|---|
| $P^i$serum (mmol/L) | 1.49±0.2 | 0.27±0.13 |
| *ATP | 6.83 | 6.03 |
| *ADP | 0.78 | 0.74 |
| *$p^i$ | 10.24 | 9.44 |
| $\frac{[ATP]}{[ADP] \cdot [P]}$ | 855 M/L$^{-1}$ | 863 M/L$^{-1}$ |

*Concentration term: moles/L intracellular $H_2O \times 10^{-3}$

Administration of a decreased quantity of an otherwise normal diet replete in phosphorus to produce weight loss of the magnitude employed in these studies results in a slight decline of total muscle phosphorus content (Figure 3). However, during

TABLE IV

MUSCLE COMPOSITION IN NORMAL AND HYPERALIMENTED
HYPOPHOSPHATEMIC DOGS (MEAN S.D.)

| | Na | K | Cl | Mg | Ca |
|---|---|---|---|---|---|
| | (mEq/dg FFDW) | | | | mmol/dg FFDW |
| HYPOPHOSPHATEMIC | 18.0 | 37.9 | 7.5 | 7.4 | 1.1 |
| n=8 | ±0.9 | ±0.9 | ±0.3 | ±0.2 | ±0.0 |
| NORMAL | 11.8 | 42.6 | 7.9 | 7.3 | 1.3 |
| n=6 | ±1.9 | ±1.8 | ±1.1 | ±0.5 | ±0.2 |
| P | <0.05 | <0.05 | NS | NS | NS |

hyperalimentation without phosphorus, there occurred a rapid additional decline in total muscle phosphorus content. This pattern suggests that muscle may give up some of its phosphorus to prevent acute depletion in more vital tissues such as the brain and the heart. If it is assumed that the muscle mass in the average dog of 25 Kg was 25% of its weight, and that the fat free dry solid portion of muscle is 25% of its wet weight, an average decline of muscle phosphorus content from 28.9 to 21.1 mmols/dg would imply that about 120 mmols had left skeletal muscle and was taken up by other tissues.

In these studies we attempted to obtain measurements of total tissue phosphorus content and muscle high energy phosphates before significant cellular injury. Thus, by electing to study the animals before the anticipated harmful effects of sustained hypophosphatemia, we could obtain a meaningful assessment of phosphorus distribution. Based upon our observations that sodium content of the tissues rose only slightly and did not become markedly elevated as it does in the face of frank cellular injury and that muscle chloride and serum CPK activity remained within normal limits suggested that the tissues were not seriously injured.

Inorganic phosphorus content of muscle tissue showed only a slight fall despite the coexistence of severe hypophosphatemia. The inorganic phosphorus concentration gradient between the cell contents and extracellular fluid was 6.9 in the control state. After weight loss, hyperalimentation and hypophosphatemia, the gradient rose to 35. This suggests that those vital processes

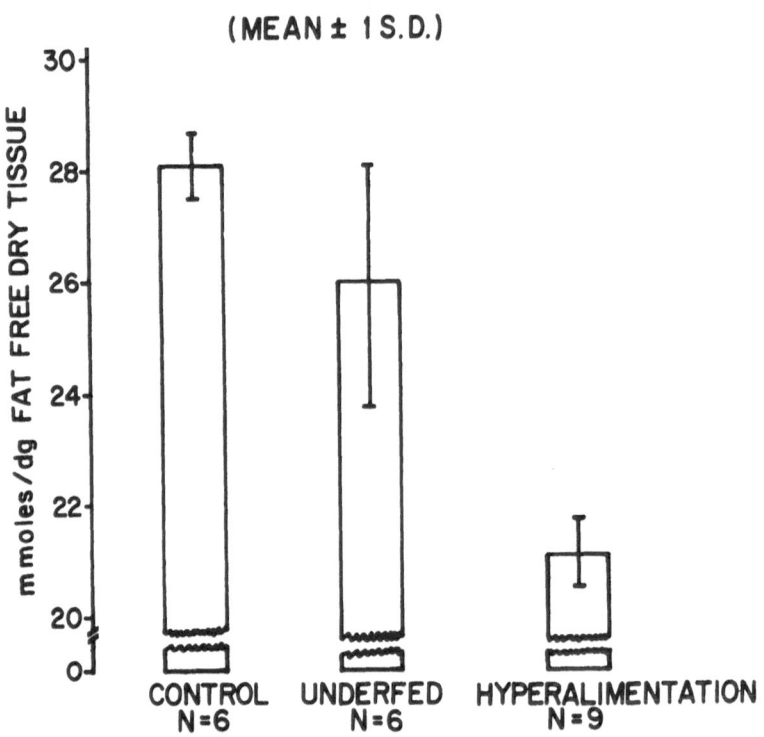

Figure 3. Total muscle phosphorus content in normal, underfed dogs and in dogs hyperalimented without phosphorus. The value in the hyperalimented group was significantly lower than control.

that maintain levels of phosphate ions inside the muscle cell
obviously remained intact despite severe hypophosphatemia and
moderate total phosphorus deficiency of muscle tissue. ATP and
ADP remained normal. Indeed, the phosphorylation potential was
also within normal limits in the hypophosphatemic dogs and was
unchanged from that existing in the control studies. Presumably
this indicates that muscle cells retain their capacity to carry
on phosphorylations despite hypophosphatemia. Nevertheless, it
would seem likely that if hypophosphatemia of such magnitude continued for an indefinite time, energy production within the cell
would have deteriorated and cellular death would have followed
(11).

Although adenine nucleotides, $P^i$ and the phosphorylation
potential of muscle tissue were normal, the cellular content of
Na was elevated. In our previous studies (3,10) similar values
for muscle sodium were observed and were associated with an
abnormally low muscle membrane potential. We interpreted these
findings to mean that ion transport mechanisms might have been
impaired by phosphorus deficiency. However, if ion transport per
se were defective, our current findings that ATP stores are normal suggest that limitation of energy stores is not responsible.
Perhaps other  components of the transport system such as the
plasma membrane or the transport enzyme itself are abnormal.

Hyperalimentation conducted in the manner selected for this
study results in acute massive rhabdomyolysis if an animal is
prepared by feeding a diet similarly restricted in calories but
totally deficient in phosphorus. In further contrast, such animals display overt symptoms of weakness, tremors or even con-
vulsions when hyperalimented without phosphorus. Animals not fed
a phosphorus deficient diet during the phase of weight reduction
do not show these symptoms during hyperalimentation, even though
the hyperalimentation diet is phosphorus deficient. Such differences suggest that a subtle difference must exist in the animal underfed with a phosphorus deficient diet compared to an
animal similarly underfed but provided adequate phosphorus. In
unreported studies by Fuller (12), dogs fed a phosphorus deficient but otherwise nutritious and calorically replete diet for a
period of 28 days develop the classical electrochemical myopathy
as described previously but in addition show a 50% decline in the
concentration of ATP and inorganic phosphorus (as expressed in
terms of whole muscle concentration). The low value for ATP
could imply that such a cell is in jeopardy. Indeed, in the
event of a superimposed insult such as more  pronounced
hypophosphatemia or perhaps anoxia resulting from impaired oxygen
delivery by P-deficient red cells (13), ATP levels would decline
further to critically low values and cellular death would occur.

Hill and his associates (14) studied phosphorus distribution in hyperalimentation induced hypophosphatemia. They studied rats that were fasted for a period of four days and administered a solution intravenously that was devoid of phosphorus. Serum labeled with $^{32}$P was administered on the fourth day of hyperalimentation. These authors found more radioactivity in skeletal muscle and bone than in control animals. These studies, in light of our findings that total bone and muscle phosphorus contents were less than normal, suggest an increased rate of phosphorus turnover in those tissues during hyperalimentation induced hypophosphatemia.

Derr and Zieve (15) examined distribution of phosphate in the underfed rat during total parenteral nutrition. As indicated by the same authors in another study using the same model and treatment,(16) simultaneous values for blood glucose concentration exceeded 1000 mg/dL. Their studies during hypophosphatemia induced by hyperalimentation and hyperglycemia suggested that the bulk of administered radiophosphorus became incorporated into organic compounds in the cell and that most of this occurred in liver, muscle and bone. They did not provide values for adenine nucleotides or phosphorus content.

A large amount of evidence has been published suggesting that depletion of high energy phosphates, particularly ATP, may be the mechanism of cellular destruction in hypophosphatemia (11). The studies reported herein suggest that acute hypophosphatemia, at least in the early stages, is not necessarily associated with a depletion of high energy phosphate compounds in the cell. Of equal importance, muscle tissue apparently serves as a reservoir from which vital quantities of phosphorus can be mobilized to be taken up by more vital tissues such as the brain and heart. Values for total phosphorus in the latter tissues remain normal in phosphorus deficient animals. The precise meaning of lowered phosphorus content of parathyroid glands is obscure. Other studies have shown that phosphorus deficiency is associated with decreased levels of parathyroid hormone in plasma suggesting decreased production (16). It seems possible that decreased phosphorus content of these glands might only reflect decreased hormone production. The deficiency of bone phosphorus is perhaps more easily explained. During phosphorus deprivation, there is mobilization of hydroxyapatite from bone. Preliminary unreported observations from our laboratory show that hyperalimentation is associated with a sharp increase of alkaline phosphatase activity in phosphorus deficient dogs. Whether or not this finding corresponds to increased bone turnover during hyperalimentation induced hypophosphatemia as reported by others is unclear.

References

1. Knochel, J.P.: The pathophysiology and clinical characteristics of severe hypophosphatemia. Arch Int Med
   137:203-220,(1977).
2. Knochel, J.P., Bilbrey , G.L., Fuller, T.J. and Carter, N.W.:
   The muscle cell in chronic alcoholism. The possible role
   of phosphate depletion in alcoholic myopathy. Ann. N.Y. Acad.
   Sci. 252:274-286,(1975).
3. Fuller, T.J., Carter, N.W., Barcenas, C. and Knochel, J.P.:
   Reversible experimental myopathy associated with phosphorus
   depletion. J.Clin.Invest. 57:1019,(1976).
4. Bilbrey, G.L., Carter, N.W., White, M.G. and Knochel, J.P.:
   Potassium deficiency in chronic renal failure. Kidney
   International 4:423-430,(1973).
5. Farrell, P.M. and Olson, R.E.: Creatine phosphate and adenine nucleotides in muscle from animals with muscular
   dystrophy. Amer. J. Physiology 225:1102-1106,(1973).
6. Lilienthal, J.L., Jr., Zierler, K.L., Folk, B.P., Buka, R.
   and Riley, M.J.: A reference base and system for analysis of muscle constituents. J.Biol.Chem. 182:501-
   508,(1950).
7. Krebs, H.A.: Regulation of the concentration of low molecular constituents in compartments. In: Microenvironments
   and Metabolic Compartmentation ed. by P.A.Srere and
   R.W.Estabrook, Academic Press Inc., pp. 3-15,(1978).
8. Veech, R.L.: Regulation of coenzyme potential by near
   equilibrium reactions. In: Microenvironments and
   Metabolic Compartmentation, edited by P.A.Srere and
   R.W.Estabrook, Academic Press Inc., pp.17 64,(1978).
9. Knochel, J.P. Hypophosphatemia and rhabdomyolysis.
   Trans.Assoc. Am.Physicians Vol XCI:156-168,(1978).
10. Knochel, J.P., Barcenas, C., Cotton, J.R., Fuller, T.J.,
    Haller,R. and Carter, N.W.: Hypophosphatemia and
    Rhabdomyolysis. J.Clin.Invest. 62:1240-1246,(1978).
11. Farber, E.: ATP and cell integrity. Fed. Proceedings.
    32:1534-1539,(1973).
12. Fuller, T.J. Personal communication.
13. Jacob, H.S., Yawata, Y., Craddock, P., Hebbel, R.:
    Hypophosphatemia hematologic-neurologic dysfunction due
    to ATP-depletion. Trans. of the Assoc. of American
    Physicians 86:143-153,(1973).
14. Hill, G.L., Guinn, E.J. and Dudrick, S.J.: Phosphorus
    distribution in hyperalimentation induced hypophosphatemia.
    J.Surgical Research 20:527-531,(1976).
15. Derr, R. and Zieve, L.: Intracellular distribution of
    phosphate in the underfed rat developing weakness and
    coma following total parenteral nutrition.
    J.Nutr.106:1398-1403,(1976).

16. Dominguez, J.H., Gray, R.W. and Lemann, J., Jr.:  Dietary
    phosphate deprivation in women and men: Effects on mineral
    acid balances, parathyroid hormone and the metabolism of
    25-OH-Vitamin D:  J. Clin. Endocrinol. Metab. 43:1056,(1976).

This work was supported by the Veterans Administration and
National Institute for Alcohol, and Alcohol Abuse (RO1AA029790).
The authors gratefully  acknowledge the help of Ms. Donna Talmon,
D.L. Morris, J. Long and Martin Calabra.

EFFECTS OF SEVERE PHOSPHATE DEPRIVATION IN GROWING CHICKS AND

POSSIBLE ROLE OF VITAMIN D

D. Harold Copp, Scott A. Lang and Stephanie W.Y. Ma

Department of Physiology
University of British Columbia
Vancouver, B. C., Canada

## INTRODUCTION

When growing rats are restricted to a diet very low in phosphate, they develop hypophosphatemia, hypercalcemia, hypercalciuria and almost complete suppression of phosphate excretion in the urine and there is progressive loss of calcium and phosphate from the skeleton[1,2,3]. There would appear to be potent homeostatic mechanisms to ensure a supply of phosphate for the growing soft tissues. Since hypophosphatemia stimulates the synthesis of the active metabolite of vitamin $D_3$, 1,25 dihydroxycholecalciferol,[4] the question arises as to whether vitamin D is essential for the homeostatic changes associated with severe phosphate deprivation. The following studies were carried out on young chicks, which are particularly sensitive to the effects of vitamin D.

## PROCEDURES

In Experiment I, the skeleton of day old cockerels was labelled by two daily injections i.p. of 4 µCi [45]Ca per chick. They were then fed a synthetic diet containing 0.7% P and 400 U vitamin $D_2$/kg for 6 days. The composition of the diet is given in Table I. To make it palatable to the young chicks, it was moistened, baked light, and ground to give a coarse consistency similar to that of chick starter mash. On this diet, the chicks grew as well as those fed on regular chicken feed. After 6 days, half were changed to the same diet without phosphate supplement and containing less than 0.04% Pi. Blood and excreta samples were collected at 1, 3, 6, 12, 24, 72 and 120 hours after initiating the low phosphate diets, and were analyzed for Ca, P and [45]Ca. The left femur was also removed and the fat-free dry weight, ash weight and Ca and P were determined.

## Table I

### Synthetic Diets

A)  Low Phosphorus Diet (1 Kilogram)

| | | | |
|---|---|---|---|
| Peanut Oil | 50 g. | $CuSO_4 \cdot 5H_2O$ | 16 mg. |
| Iodized Salt | 6 g. | Sodium Selenite | 0.2 mg. |
| Choline Chloride | 1.5 g | Thiamine·HCl | 1.8 mg. |
| Egg Albumin | 300 g | Riboflavin | 3.6 mg. |
| Starch | 561 g. | Calcium Pantothenate | 10 mg. |
| Alphacel | 42 g. | Niacin | 25 mg. |
| $CaCO_3$ | 27 g. | Pyridoxine HCl | 3 mg. |
| KCl | 6.47 g. | Folic Acid | 0.55 mg. |
| KI | 0.05 g. | Biotin | 0.6 mg. |
| $MgSO_4 \cdot 7H_2O$ | 5 g. | Vitamin B-12 | 0.01 mg. |
| NaBr | 0.02 g. | Vitamin K-1 | 0.55 mg. |
| $Na_2MO_4$ | 0.01 g. | Vitamin A | 5000 units |
| Ethoxyquin | 125 mg. | Vitamin $D_2$ | 400 units |
| $MnSO_4 \cdot 5H_2O$ | 170 mg. | Vitamin E | 10 units |
| Ferric Citrate·$5H_2O$ | 500 mg. | | |

B)  Normal Phosphorus Diet (0.7%)

1)  Add 37.33 grams of $Na_2HPO_4$
2)  Reduce Alphacel to 4.67 grams

C)  Vitamin D Deficient Diets

1)  Omit vitamin D from the vitamin mix
2)  Add or omit phosphate as desired

In Experiment II, the newborn chicks were labelled with [45]Ca as above, and after feeding a normal diet for 2 days, they were fed the normal phosphate diet with (+D) or without (-D) vitamin D supplement for 14 days.  Half the chicks in each group were then changed to a low phosphate diet (.04% P) with or without D supplement.  After 6 days on these regimens, they were sacrificed and blood was taken by heart puncture for determination of plasma Ca and P, and [45]Ca was determined on the previous 24 hour collection of excreta.  The left femur was analyzed as above.

RESULTS

A.  Experiment I.  Changes in plasma phosphate following initiation of the low phosphate diet (-P) are shown in Figure 1, and compared with values for chicks receiving the control diet (+P).  It will be noted that a significant drop occurred at the first hour, indicating the rapidity of the response to phosphate deprivation. Similar changes in plasma calcium are shown in Figure 2. There was a small but significant rise in plasma calcium in the -P chicks at the first hour. The rate of excretion of $^{45}$Ca, expressed as C.P.M./ hour, is shown in Figure 3. In the phosphate deprived group, this increased 75% in the first 3 hour collection and over 6-fold by 6 hours. Since this presumably reflects bone resorption, it indicates a very rapid response to the phosphate depletion.

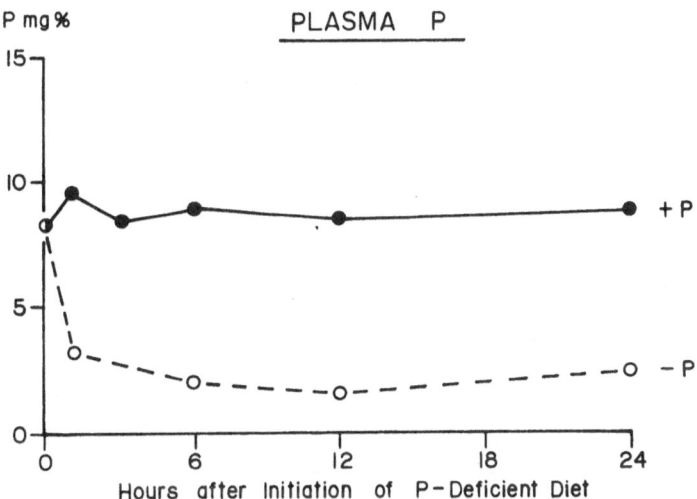

Figure 1.  Changes in plasma phosphate following initiation of the low phosphate diet.

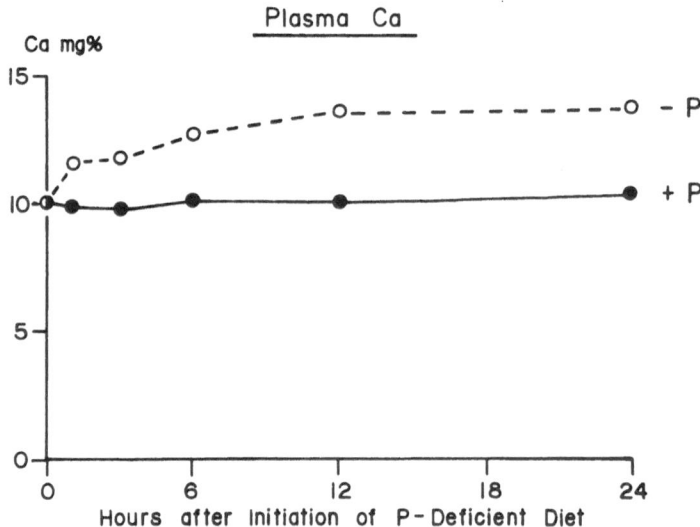

Figure 2.    Changes in plasma calcium following initiation of the
             low phosphate diet.

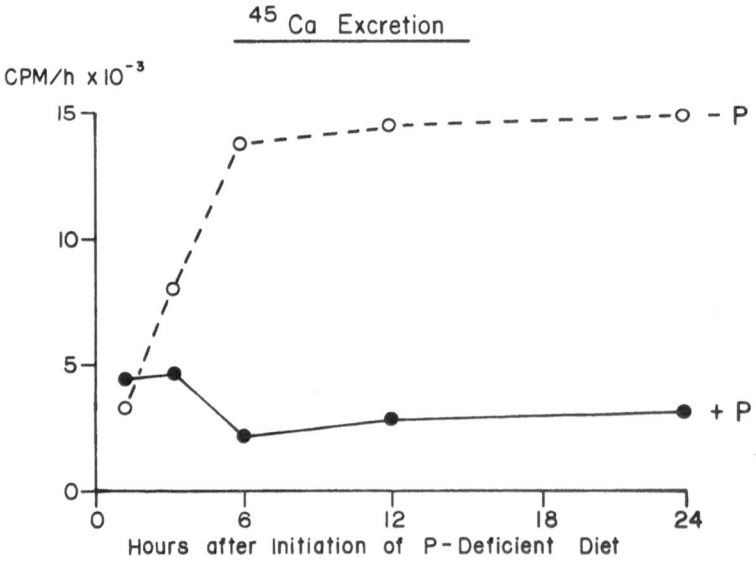

Figure 3.    Rate of $^{45}$Ca excretion (CPM/hr) following initiation of
             the low phosphate diet.

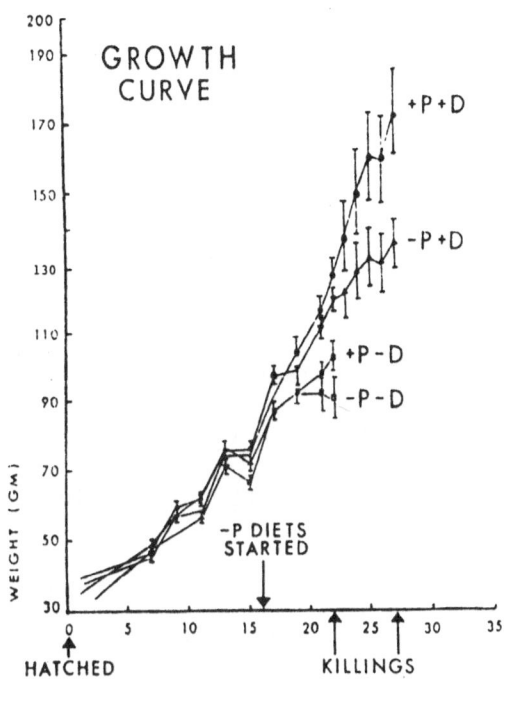

Figure 4.  Growth curves for chicks fed +P+D; +P-D; -P+D and
           -P-D Diets.


B.  Experiment II.  The growth curves for the chicks on the D deficient and D supplemented diets are shown in Figure 3.  It will be
noted that growth was retarded on the D deficient diet and on the
low phosphate diet.  This would reduce the demand for phosphate.
The changes in plasma P and Ca after 6 days on the experimental
diets are shown in Table II.

### Table II

| Diet | Plasma P mg.% | | Plasma Ca mg.% | |
|------|-----|-----|-----|-----|
|      | +D  | -D  | +D  | -D  |
| +P   | 7.08±0.20 | 7.72±0.29 | 11.5±0.2 | 11.1±0.1 |
| -P   | 1.61±0.11 | 1.45±0.23 | 17.0±0.4 | 11.0±0.3 |

The fall in plasma phosphate was independent of vitamin D, but hypercalcemia occurred only when vitamin D was present. This may be the result of high conversion to the active metabolite 1,25 dihydroxy-$D_2$ and high absorption of calcium from the gut.

Changes in excretion of [45]Ca are shown in Table III. There was a large increase in [45]Ca excretion in the -P group, particularly in the presence of vitamin D.

Table III

Rate of [45]Ca excretion (% dose/chick/hr x 100)

| Diet | 24 hr prior to -P Diet | | Final 24 hr collection (6 days on diet) | |
|------|------|------|------|------|
|      | +D   | -D   | +D   | -D   |
| +P   | 1.93 | 1.73 | 1.17 | 1.63 |
| -P   | 1.71 | 2.27 | 11.4 | 4.60 |

The differences in the mineral and [45]Ca contents of the left femur after 6 days on the experimental diets are shown in Table IV, expressed in terms of fat-free dry weight (FFDW)

Table IV

| Diet | Phosphate (%P/FFDW) | | Calcium (%Ca/FFDW) | |
|------|------|------|------|------|
|      | +D   | -D   | +D   | -D   |
| +P   | 8.47±0.12 | 8.08±0.13 | 17.5±0.4 | 17.6±0.4 |
| -P   | 6.01±0.14 | 5.90±0.10 | 13.6±0.4 | 12.7±0.3 |

| Diet | % Ash weight/FFDW | | [45]Ca (% dose/femur) | |
|------|------|------|------|------|
|      | +D   | -D   | +D   | -D   |
| +P   | 46.9±4.0 | 45.4±4.0 | 3.83±0.12 | 3.72±0.19 |
| -P   | 36.5±8.0 | 35.0±5.0 | 2.74±0.08 | 3.42±0.13 |

There was a significant reduction in bone mineral content, P and Ca in the chicks fed the low phosphate diet, and an enhanced loss of [45]Ca which was most pronounced in the birds receiving vitamin D.

DISCUSSION

As is the case in young rats, feeding growing chicks a diet very low in phosphate results in retarded growth, hypophosphatemia, hypercalcemia and increased mineral loss from bone as indicated by an increase in excretion of [45]Ca from the prelabelled skeleton. On the vitamin D free diet, phosphate deprivation caused a more marked retardation of growth and although the fall in plasma phosphate was similar, there was no significant hypercalcemia. Release of bone mineral was also reduced. Since hypophosphatemia is associated with enhanced conversion of vitamin D to the active metabolite 1,25 dihydroxy-$D_2$, this may account for the greater mobilization of phosphate from bone to permit growth of new tissues. This would also account for the hypercalcemia which was observed in the D supplemented chicks.

CONCLUSIONS

Even in the absence of vitamin D supplements, chicks fed a diet low in phosphorus (0.04%) rapidly develop hypophosphatemia and enhanced bone resorption. Thus the basic homeostatic mechanism to provide P for growing tissues does not require vitamin D, but is enhanced in its presence.

REFERENCES

1.    Day, H.G., and McCollum, E.V., 1939, Mineral metabolism, growth and symptomatology of rats on a diet extremely deficient in phosphorus, J.Biol.Chem., 130:269.

2.    Baylink, D.J., Wergedal, J., and Stauffer, M., 1971, Formation, mineralization and resorption of bone in hypophosphatemic rats, J.Clin.Invest., 50:2519.

3.    Copp, H., 1971, Effets d'un regime pauvre en phosphore sur l'homeostasie du calcium et de l'ion phosphate chez le rat jeune, in: "Phosphate et Metabolisme Phosphocalcique", D.J. Hioco, ed., Sandoz Publications, Paris.

4.    Tanaka, Y. and DeLuca, H.F., 1973, The control of 25-hydroxy-vitamin $D_3$ metabolism by inorganic phosphate, Arch.Biochem., 154:566.

ACKNOWLEDGEMENTS

The work presented in this paper was supported by a grant from the Medical Research Council of Canada. The authors would also like to acknowledge the assistance of Mrs. Mary Forsyth and Mr. Kurt Henze in preparation of the manuscript.

# ABNORMALITIES OF GLYCOGEN METABOLISM IN CARDIOMYOPATHY

# OF PHOSPHOROUS DEPLETION

Walter H.Hörl, Wilhelm Kreusser, August Heidland, and Eberhard Ritz

Depts. Internal Medicine Univ. Würzburg and Heidelberg/Germany

## INTRODUCTION

Changes in myocardial performance are an important and clinically relevant consequence of phosphorous depletion (PD) both in man (1,2) and in experimental animals (3).O'Connor et al.(1) found in acutely phosphorous depleted alcoholic patients that stroke volume was low and reverted to normal upon administration of phosphate despite no change or even reduction of preload.Furthermore, Darsee and Nutter (2) described reversible congestive heart failure in chronically phosphorous depleted patients.These findings would indicate that PD interferes with the inotropic state of the myocardium.However, for obvious reasons, a number of parameters which might influence myocardial performance cannot be controlled in such severely ill patients.Fuller et al.(3) were able to reproduce experimentally reversible depression of myocardial performance in dogs with experimental PD.When inorganic serum phosphorous was lowered from 5,1 to 0,9 mg/dl with an associated 20% fall in muscular phosphorous concentration, stroke volume, peak blood flow and dP/dt were abnormally low and returned to normal upon administration of phosphate.

These observations clearly indicate abnormal myocardial function in PD.Cellular phosphorous and calcium concentration play important direct and indirect roles in the control of glycogen synthesis and breakdown. Therefore, in the present study, we examined whether glycogen content and the activities of key enzymes in-

343

volved in glycogen synthesis or glycogenolysis are altered in rats with experimental PD.

MATERIAL AND METHODS

Male Sprague Dawley rats(Ivanovas Co.Kisslegg)
with an initial weight of 90-100 g were housed in single metabolic cages.After an adaptation phase of 5 days,
the phosphorous depleted(PD)rats received a diet which
contained 0,03% inorganic phosphorous.Control rats(CO)
were given a diet containing 0,4% $P_i$ in an amount which
maintained body weight at the same level as in matched
PD animals. All rats had free access to deionised water.
The animals were killed under Nembutal[R] anesthesia.The
heart was quickly (3sec) removed and quick-frozen on
dry ice.A crude extract was prepared as described by
Hörl et al(4). Glycogen was determined with a modified
procedure after Montgomery (5).Protein was assayed with
the Lowry method (6).Phosphorylase activity was determined according to Hedrick and Fischer (7) and glycogen synthetase according to Thomas et al (8). cAMP dependent and independent protein kinase were measured
according to Reimann et al (9).

RESULTS

The above feeding protocol lowered serum $P_i$ from
$7.23 \pm 0.7$ mg/dl (CO) to $2.9 \pm 0.7$ mg/dl (PD).This was
accompanied by a 23% decrease of myocardial $P_i$ content (CO: $1309 \pm 257$ nmol $P_i$/mg protein; PD: $977 \pm 174$;
$p < 0.05$).

There was no change of glycogen content in non-
exercised skeletal muscle (CO:$1.82 \pm 1.12$ ug glycogen/mg
protein;PD:$1.46 \pm 0.99$;N.S.).In contrast, a significant
decrease in myocardial glycogen content was observed in
PD animals (CO  $28.6 \pm 8.1$ ug glycogen/mg protein;
PD $14.9 \pm 7.0$; $p < 0.01$) (figure 1)

The activity of glycogen synthetase (I-form) was
significantly decreased in PD animals (CO: $4.68 \pm 0.90$
nmol/min/mg protein; PD: $2.25 \pm 1.42$; $p < 0.01$). The same
was true for total glycogen synthetase activity (I+D-
forms) (figure 2)

In contrast, glycogen phosphorylase activity was
increased in PD animals (a-form - CO: $0.49 \pm 0.14$ umol/
min/mg protein; PD: $1.69 \pm 0.33$, $p < 0.01$; b-form - CO:
$1.18 \pm 0.30$ umol/min/mg protein; PD: $4.00 \pm 1.17$; $p < 0.01$)
(figure 3).

In contrast, no such difference between PD and CO animals with respect to glycogen synthetase and phosphorylase was observed in skeletal muscle (glycogen synthetase-I-form: CO: $6.94 \pm 1.97$ nmol/min/mg protein; PD: $5.94 \pm 2.35$; N.S.).

D+I-form; CO: $8.98 \pm 1.90$ nmol/min/mg protein; PD: $8.21 \pm 2.11$; N.S.; phosphorylase a CO: $2.71 \pm 0.51$ µmol/min/mg protein; PD: $2.44 \pm 0.54$; N.S. phosphorylase b CO: $5.72 \pm 0.88$ µmol/min/mg protein; PD: $5.91 \pm 1.02$; N.S.).

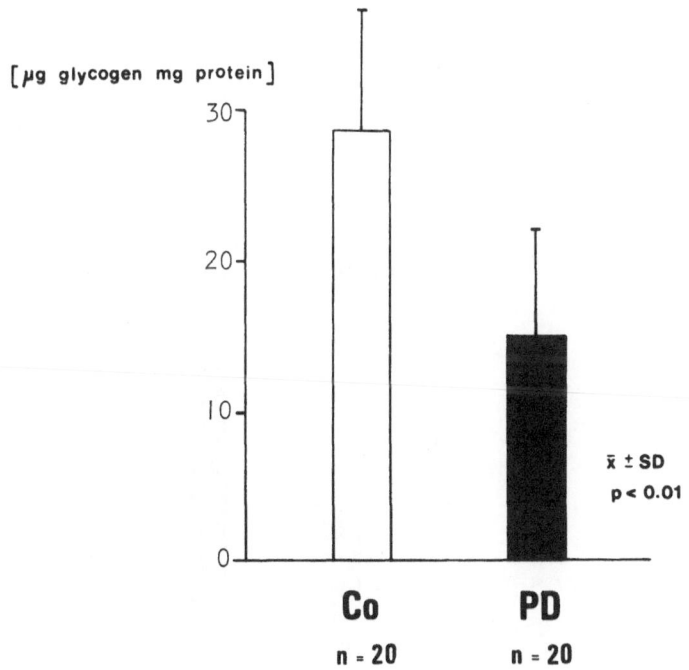

figure 1

Glycogen content of heart muscle in $P_i$ depleted rats

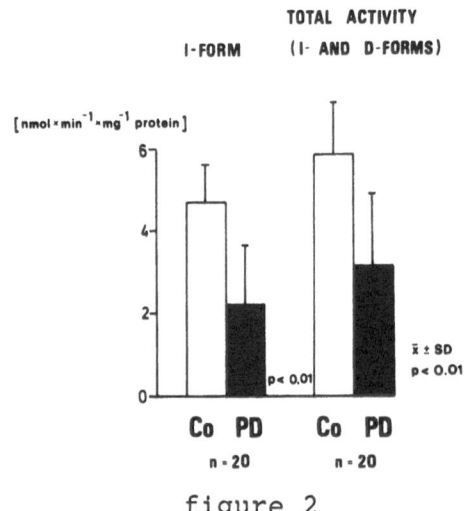

figure 2

Glycogen synthetase activity in heart muscle in PD rats

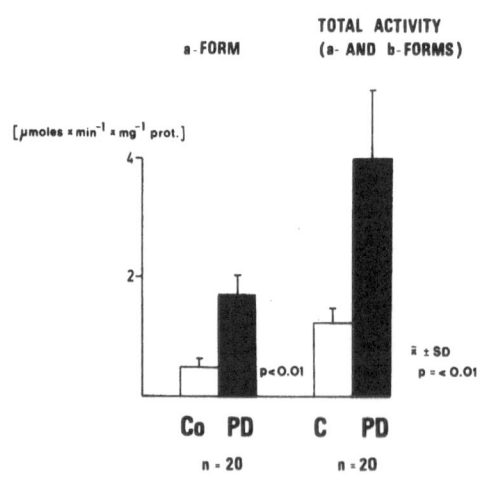

figure 3

Glycogen phosphorylase activity of heart muscle in PD rats

DISCUSSION

For the purpose of this discussion, the pathways of glycogen synthesis and glycogen breakdown are depicted in figure 4.

Phosphorylase, the enzyme which cleaves glycogen by phosphorolysis, is present in 2 forms, an active phosphorylated form (phosphorylase a) and an inactive form (phosphorylase b). Activation can occur either through ionic control via Ca or through hormonal signals via cAMP. Hormonal signals are mediated through a sequence comprising cAMP, protein kinase (= phosphorylase kinase kinase) and phosphorylase kinase, which are arranged in the fashion of a cascade.

Glycogen synthesis is brought about by the activity of glycogen synthetase. This enzyme is relatively inactive in its phosphorylated form and is activated upon dephosphorylation which is catalysed by specific phosphatases. Phosphorylation of synthetase is mediated by cAMP dependent protein kinase. For review see Larner (10).

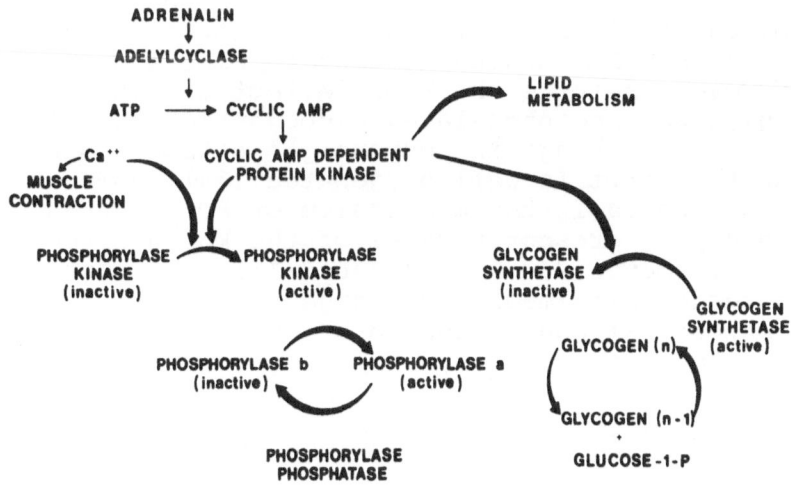

figure 4

The above study shows that in the rat PD leads to
a similar decrease of $P_i$ content in non-exercised skeletal muscle and in heart muscle. In contrast, glycogen
content remains unchanged in skeletal muscle and is
decreased in heart muscle. This observation shows that
the change in glycogen content is not a direct consequence of the depletion of cellular $P_i$ stores.

The decrease in myocardial glycogen content was
paralleled by increased activity of glycogenolysis and
decreased activity of glycogen synthesis. As outlined
in the above schema (figure 4),   phosphorylase may be
activated either by ionic or by hormonal signals. One
could argue that PD leads to changes in cytosolic $Ca^{2+}$.
$Ca^{2+}$ is known to activate glycogen breakdown. An increase in cytosolic $Ca^{2+}$ in PD would be anticipiated on
the basis of the model of intracellular Ca control as
proposed by Rasmussen (11). If myocardial $P_i$ stores are
used to raise lowered cytosolic $P_i$ levels, cytosolic
$Ca^{2+}$ must rise, at least transiently, secondary to the
concomitant mobilisation of mitochondrial Ca.

Alternatively, one has to consider the possibility
of altered insulin metabolism. PD is known to affect
the action of insulin (12) so that a state of insulin
resistance ensues. Changes of insulin (or possibly glucagon) action are one possible cause of altered myo-
cardialglycogen metabolism.

Finally, in view of the known negative inotropic
effect of PD (3), one could entertain the possibility
that low cardiac output activates the sympathetic nerve
system. Catecholamines are known to increase glycogenolysis via the cAMP dependent protein kinase mechanism
(13).However, despite the known effect of catecholamines on glycogen phosphorylase, glycogen content of the
heart does not change in response to catecholamines as
long as the heart is well oxygenated (14). However,
tissue hypoxemia in the myocardium of PD depleted
animals may be present because of the known effect of
PD on erythrocyte 2,3-DPG content (15). The possibility
of a catecholamine mediated change in myocardial glycogen metabolism can be tested by analysing the effect
of beta-blockade.

SUMMARY

In severely phosphorous depleted rats, no change
of glycogen content or activities of enzymes catalysing

glycogen synthesis or breakdown was observed. In contrast in heart muscle, a decrease of myocardial glycogen content was observed which was accompanied by increased activity of phosphorylase and decreased activity of synthetase. It is assumed that these changes result from increased catecholamine action secondary to an activation of the sympathetic nerve system resulting from impaired contractile state of the myocardium. The changes observed are analogous to those found in heart failure.

REFERENCES

1. O'Connor, L. R., Wheeler, W. S., and Bethune, J. E., 1977, Effect of hypophosphatemia on myocardial performance in man, N. Engl. J. Med., 297:901.
2. Darsee, J. R., and Nutter, D. O., 1978, Reversible severe congestive cardiomyopathy in three cases of hypophosphatemia, Ann. Intern. Med.,89:867.
3. Fuller, T. J., Nichols, W. W., Brenner, B. J., and Peterson, J. C., 1978, Reversible depression in myocardial performance in dogs with experimental phosphorus deficiency, J. Clin. Invest., 62:1194.
4. Hörl, W. H., Sperling, J., and Heidland, A., 1978, Enhanced glycogen turnover in skeletal muscle of uremic rats - cause of uncontrolled actomyosin ATPase? Am. J. Clin. Nutr., 31:1861.
5. Montgomery, R., 1957, Determination of glycogen, Arch. Biochem. Biophys., 67:378.
6. Lowry, O. H., Rosebrough, N. J., Farr, A. L., and Randall, R. J., 1951, Protein measurements with the folin phenol reagent, J. Biol. Chem., 193:265.
7. Hedrick, J. L., and Fischer, E. H., 1965, On the role of pyridoxal 5'-phosphate in phosphorylase.I.Absence of classical vitamin $B_6$-dependent enzymatic activities in muscle glycogen phosphorylase, Biochemistry, 4:1337.
8. Thomas, J. A., Schlender, K. K., and Larner, J., 1968, A rapid filter paper assay for UDP glucose-glycogen glucosyltransferase, including an improved biosynthesis of UDP-$^{14}$C-glucose, Anal. Biochem. 25: 486.
9. Reimann, E. M., Walsh, D. H., and Krebs, E. G., 1971, Purification and properties of rabbit skeletal muscle adenosine 3',5' monophosphate-dependent protein kinases, J. Biol. Chem., 246:1986.
10. Larner, J., 1976, I. Regulation of intermediary metabolism. Mechanisms of regulation of glycogen synthesis and degradation, Supp. 1, Circ. Res., 38:I-2.

11. Rasmussen, H., and Bordier, P., 1974, The physiolo-
    gical and cellular basis of metabolic bone disease,
    The Williams & Wilkins Company, Baltimore.
12. Harter, H. R., Santiago, J. U., Rutherford, W. E.,
    Slatopolsky, E., and Klahr, S., 1976, The relative
    roles of calcium, phosphorous and parathyroid hor-
    mone in glucose and tolbutamide mediated insulin re-
    lease, J. Clin. Invest., 58:359.
13. Yeaman, S. J., and Cohen, P., 1975, The hormonal con-
    trol of activity of skeletal muscle phosphorylase
    kinase. Phosphorylation of the enzyme at two sites
    in vivo in response to adrenalin, Eur. J. Biochem.,
    51:93
14. Mommaerts, W. F. H. M., 1974, Current problems in
    myocardial metabolism, Supplements to Circ. Res. 34
    and 35 (suppl.III) III-2.
15. Travis, S. F., Sugerman, H. J., Tuberg, R. L., Du-
    drick, S. J., Delivoria-Papadopoulos, M., Miller, L.
    D., and Oski, F. A., 1971, Alterations of red-cell
    glycolytic intermediates and oxygen transport as a
    consequence of hypophosphatemia in patients recei-
    ving intravenous hyperalimentation, N. Engl. J. Med.,
    285:763.

ALTERED VITAMIN D, CYCLIC NUCLEOTIDE AND TRACE MINERAL METABOLISM

IN THE X-LINKED HYPOPHOSPHATEMIC MOUSE

Ralph A. Meyer, Jr.[1], Richard W. Gray[2], Gary M. Kiebzak[1] and Paul M. Mish[1]

[1]Department of Basic Science, Marquette University School of Dentistry, 604 North 16th St., Milwaukee, WI 53233

[2]Departments of Medicine and Biochemistry, Medical College of Wisconsin, 8701 Watertown Plank Rd., Milwaukee, WI 53226

## INTRODUCTION

Human X-linked hypophosphatemia is a genetic disease in which the mutant gene is dominant and sex-linked[1]. It is the most common form of vitamin D-resistant rickets[1]. The study of this disease has been aided by the discovery of the Hyp gene in mice[2]. This gene is also X-linked and dominant. Hyp mice have reduced tubular reabsorption of phosphate[2,3] which leads to hypophosphatemia and osteomalacic bone disease[4]. Their intestinal phosphate transport is resistant to 1,25-(OH)$_2$-vitamin D therapy [5].

The Hyp mouse should prove useful not only in exploring this poorly understood human disease but also in gaining insights into the regulation of phosphate metabolism. This mutant has the first known alteration in endogenous phosphate metabolism and may provide insights into the functioning of as yet unknown phosphate-regulating systems.

Three experiments were undertaken to detect additional abnormalities in the Hyp mice. The status of vitamin D metabolites was explored, and possible alterations in the control system for 1,25-(OH)$_2$-vitamin D formation were studied. Cyclic AMP and cyclic GMP were measured to test their possible involvement in the reduced renal tubular reabsorption of phosphate. Since there are alterations in phosphate, calcium[2] and magnesium[4] metabolism, the more abundant trace minerals were measured to test for additional alterations.

Table 1.  Plasma Vitamin D Metabolites in Normal and Hyp Mice

| Metabolite[1] | n[2] | Normal | Hyp | P |
|---|---|---|---|---|
| 25-OH-D (nM) | 6 | 59 ± 4 | 37 ± 4 | < 0.01 |
| 1,25-(OH)$_2$-D (pM) | 8 | 70 ± 4 | 66 ± 4 | NS |

[1]Units are nanomoles (nM) or picomoles (pM) per liter.  Each value is $\bar{X}$ + SE.
[2]n is the number of samples.  Each sample is the pooled plasma from the exsanguination of 10-15 mice at 13 weeks of age.

VITAMIN D

Vitamin D metabolites were measured in the plasma of Hyp and normal mice to test whether X-linked hypophosphatemia of mice is a pseudovitamin D-deficiency disease with low plasma 1,25-(OH)$_2$-vitamin D.  Mice were exsanguinated and the plasma from 10-15 mice was pooled to give each 4.0 ml sample.  25-OH-vitamin D was measured by a modification of the competitive binding assay of Haddad, and 1,25-(OH)$_2$-vitamin D was measured by a modification of the Eisman method [6].  Both male (+/Y or Hyp/Y) and female (+/+ or Hyp/+) mice were used.  Since no sex difference was apparent the data were pooled

As shown in Table 1 there was no significant difference in plasma 1,25-(OH)$_2$-vitamin D between normal and Hyp mice[7].  This ruled out pseudovitamin D deficiency.  However, the normal levels in Hyp mice were surprising since hypophosphatemia is usually associated with elevated plasma 1,25-(OH)$_2$-vitamin D[8].  Plasma 25-OH-vitamin D, while lower in Hyp mice, seems adequate to support the synthesis of normal levels of 1,25-(OH)$_2$-vitamin D.  This differs from the human disease in which no difference in 25-OH-vitamin D is reported [9].

The failure of 1,25-(OH)$_2$-vitamin D to be elevated in Hyp mice suggested that there was a defective control system over vitamin D metabolism which was not responsive to changes in plasma phosphate.  Dietary-induced hypophosphatemia usually causes elevated plasma 1,25-(OH)$_2$-vitamin D[8].  To test this, mice were exposed to a low P diet (ICN Pharmaceutical Inc., #902206) for 3 or 6 days or to the same diet to which enough phosphate was added to give 0.6% P in the

Table 2.  Effect of Low P Diet for 3 or 6 Days on Plasma Vitamin
          D Metabolites in Hyp Mice

| Metabolite[1] | n[2] | Normal Mice | | Hyp Mice |
|---|---|---|---|---|
| | | Normal P diet | Low P diet | Low P diet |
| 25-OH-D  (nM) | 8 | $47.8 \pm 2.7$ | $48.9 \pm 2.0$ | $34.0 \pm 1.4$[3] |
| 1,25-(OH)$_2$-D  (pM) | 6 | $108 \pm 9$ | $182 \pm 9$[4] | 5 of 6 not detectable |

[1] Units are nanomoles (nM) or picomoles (pM) per liter.
[2] n is the number of samples collected as in Table 1.
[3] Significantly less than normal mice on low P diet (p < 0.001).
[4] Significantly greater than normal mice on normal P diet
    (p < 0.01).

diet (40g Na$_2$HPO$_4 \cdot$7H$_2$0 and 6.2g KH$_2$PO$_4$ per kg).  The diet was fed
ad libitum with deionized water.

     Low P diet caused a significant increase in plasma 1,25-(OH)$_2$-
vitamin D in normal mice (Table 2).  However Hyp mice on the low P
diet showed non-detectable levels of 1,25-(OH)$_2$-vitamin D[10].  This
demonstrates a difference between Hyp and normal mice.  Hyp mice do
not respond to low P stimulus with elevated plasma 1,25-(OH)$_2$-
vitamin D.  We conclude that the regulatory system for the renal
25-hydroxyvitamin D-1α-hydroxylase is defective.

     While this would explain the failure of Hyp mice to increase
1,25-(OH)$_2$-vitamin D, it would not explain the observed decrease.
The synthesis of 1,25-(OH)$_2$-vitamin D is thought to be principally
regulated by phosphate and parathyroid hormone[8].  If Hyp mice are
not recognizing P as a stimulus, this leaves only parathyroid hormone to control its synthesis.  Since low P diet raised plasma
calcium, this may have caused a decrease in circulating parathyroid
hormone[11].  We hypothesize that a drop in plasma parathyroid hormone
may have decreased the level of plasma 1,25-(OH)$_2$-vitamin D in Hyp
mice on low P diet.

     As a result of the low P diet, plasma inorganic phosphate fell,
and calcium and magnesium rose in both genotypes (Table 3).  Urinary
magnesium rose and urinary phosphate fell to quite low values.

Table 3.   Effect of Low P Diet for One Day on Plasma and Urine
           Minerals in <u>Hyp</u> Mice

|  | Normal Mice | | <u>Hyp</u> Mice | |
|---|---|---|---|---|
|  | Normal P diet | Low P diet | Normal P diet | Low P diet |
| $n^1$ | 16 | 16 | 11 | 9 |
| | Plasma (mmoles/liter) | | | |
| Ca | 2.21 + 0.03 | $2.42 + 0.04^2$ | 2.12 + 0.04 | $2.39 + 0.06^2$ |
| Mg | 0.81 + 0.03 | $1.00 + 0.04^2$ | 0.78 + 0.02 | $0.97 + 0.03^2$ |
| P | 2.22 + 0.11 | $0.83 + 0.08^2$ | 1.09 + 0.05 | $0.34 + 0.10^2$ |
| | Urine (mmoles/liter) | | | |
| Mg | 5.9 + 0.9 | $18.6 + 1.2^2$ | 12.6 + 2.1 | $24.8 + 1.6^2$ |
| P | 55.0 + 5.5 | $3.7 + 0.6^2$ | 81.3 + 15.1 | $3.8 + 1.4^2$ |
| Creatinine | 2.6 + 0.4 | 2.7 + 0.2 | 2.8 + 0.4 | 3.3 + 0.3 |

[1]n is the number of individual male mice.
[2]Differs significantly from mice of the same genotype on a normal P
 diet (p < 0.01).

Urinary creatinine was unchanged (Table 3).  Similar data (not shown)
were found after 6 days on the experimental diet.  These changes in
Mg metabolism reflect the changes reported earlier for <u>Hyp</u> mice[4].
This suggested that the hypophosphatemia rather than an independent
expression of the mutant gene causes the altered Mg metabolism in
<u>Hyp</u> mice.   25-OH-vitamin D was unaffected by low P diet (Table 2).
There was no change in normal mice and <u>Hyp</u> mice had a decrease which
was similar to the change seen on stock diets (Table 1).


CYCLIC NUCLEOTIDES

     Parathyroid hormone-induced phosphaturia is thought to be
mediated by elevated renal production of cyclic AMP[12].  Administration of exogenous cyclic AMP will cause phosphaturia [13].  Altered
cyclic GMP is also reported to accompany high doses of parathyroid
hormone[14].

     It is possible that the phosphaturia of <u>Hyp</u> mice might be

Table 4.  Cyclic Nucleotides in the Plasma and Urine of Normal
and Hyp Male Mice[1]

|  | Normal | Hyp | P |
|---|---|---|---|
| | cyclic AMP | | |
| plasma (nM) | 66.5 + 8.7 (12) | 51.0 + 4.7 (10) | NS |
| urine (µM) | 20.3 + 1.1 (23) | 30.8 + 2.0 (21) | < 0.01 |
| FE[2] | 3.8 + 0.5 (12) | 6.2 + 0.6 (10) | < 0.01 |
| | cyclic GMP | | |
| plasma (nM) | 7.6 + 1.4 (10) | 3.8 + 1.0 (8) | < 0.05 |
| urine (µM) | 4.9 + 0.4 (21) | 8.9 + 0.6 (18) | < 0.01 |
| FE | 9.1 + 1.5 (10) | 29.6 + 7.5 (8) | < 0.01 |

[1]Units are nanomoles (nM) or micromoles (µM) per liter.  Each value
is $\bar{X}$ + SE with the number of mice in parentheses.
[2]FE is fractional excretion:  the urine/plasma ratio of the cyclic
nucleotide divided by the urine/plasma ratio of creatinine.

mediated by altered production of cyclic nucleotides.  Tenenhouse
et al.[3] reported elevated urinary cyclic AMP in Hyp mice.  However,
in the absence of plasma cyclic AMP data it was not shown whether
the increased cyclic AMP came from renal cells or from renal clearance of elevated plasma cyclic AMP.  Also, cyclic GMP was not
measured.

Conscious 12 week old male mice, normal and Hyp, were held,
and the spontaneously voided urine was collected.  Plasma samples
were collected from the orbital sinus under ether anesthesia.
Fractional excretion (FE) was calculated by the urine/plasma (U/P)
ratio of cyclic nucleotide divided by U/P for creatinine.  Cyclic
nucleotides were measured by radioimmunoassay[15] with reagents purchased from New England Nuclear (Boston, MA).

As shown in Table 4, urinary cyclic nucleotides are elevated
for both cyclic AMP and cyclic GMP[16].  Fractional excretion was also
elevated for both nucleotides.  The data were normalized to fractional excretion values by dividing by U/P creatinine.  This eliminated any changes caused by Hyp mice producing a more or less dilute
urine than normal mice.  Also, fractional excretion gives insight
into the origin of elevated urinary cyclic nucleotides.

Table 5.  Trace Minerals in Normal and Hyp Male Mice[1]

| Mouse | n | Cu | Fe | Mn | Zn |
|-------|---|-----|-----|-----|-----|
| | | | Liver[2] | | |
| Normal | 12 | 5.8 + 0.2 | 66 + 3 | 1.11 + 0.8 | 29.4 + 0.6 |
| Hyp | 13 | 5.4 + 0.1 | 78 + 4 | 1.16 + 0.9 | 29.7 + 0.4 |
| P | | NS | 0.01 | NS | NS |
| | | | Muscle[2] | | |
| Normal | 12 | 0.94 + 0.04 | 11.7 + 0.6 | 0.124 + 0.004 | 10.9 + 0.3 |
| Hyp | 13 | 1.08 + 0.08 | 12.1 + 0.4 | 0.125 + 0.006 | 12.1 + 0.3 |
| P | | NS | NS | NS | < 0.01 |
| | | | Femur[3] | | |
| Normal | 11 | - | 563 + 30 | - | 353 + 9 |
| Hyp | 11 | - | 715 + 4 | - | 505 + 7 |
| P | | - | < 0.01 | - | < 0.001 |
| | | | Feces[4] | | |
| Normal | 9 | 65 + 2 | 1841 + 117 | 587 + 93 | 438 + 46 |
| Hyp | 9 | 69 + 2 | 2037 + 39 | 917 + 27 | 366 + 20 |
| P | | NS | NS | < 0.02 | NS |

[1]Each value is $\bar{X}$ + SE.  Samples were ashed[21] and analyzed by
atomic absorption spectroscopy in an air-acetylene flame.
[2]µg per g wet weight.
[3]µg per g ash.  Cu and Mn were too low to be measured.
[4]µg per g dry weight.

If a substance is merely secreted from the renal blood into
the tubules, the maximum possible fractional excretion is the FE
for p-aminohippuric acid (PAH).  FE for PAH is the inverse of the
filtration fraction, which is 0.2 for a variety of mammals[17].  Thus,
the maximum FE for substances cleared from the blood is about 5.
Values markedly above 5 indicate that the substance could not have
totally originated from the renal blood flow but must have been
synthesized by the renal cells.  In Hyp mice the high values for
fractional excretion of both cyclic AMP and cyclic GMP indicated
that the nucleotides originated in renal tissue. This seems to be
a significant difference between the mouse disease and the human

disease in which cyclic nucleotide production is reported to be not
significantly altered[18].

Brunette et al. [19] have reported a hypersensitivity to calcitonin in cyclic AMP production by Hyp kidney tubules in vitro. The
significance of these changes to the reduced renal tubular reabsorption of phosphate is currently being explored.


TRACE MINERALS

O'Doherty[5] reported the resistance of phosphate transport in
the gut of Hyp mice to the administration of $1,25-(OH)_2$-vitamin D.
This would suggest low intestinal absorption of phosphate which
might contribute to the animal's phosphate deficiency. This implies
that fecal phosphate should be high. To test this fecal pellets
were collected from normal and Hyp male mice and were analyzed for
mineral content. There was no significant difference in the fecal
content of normal vs. Hyp mice for calcium ($1.50 + 0.05$ vs. $1.58 +$
$0.05$ mmol/g dry wt., n = 9, NS) or phosphate ($1.07 + 0.03$ vs. $1.11$
$+ 0.05$ mmol/g dry wt., n = 9, NS). However fecal Mn was found to
be high (Table 5). This led to an examination of other abundant
trace minerals in liver, muscle and femur. Significant accumula-
tions of minerals were found in certain tissues: Fe in liver and
femur and Zn in muscle and femur (Table 5).

These data can be interpreted to suggest that the diet remains
in the gut long enough to permit adequate absorption of Ca, P, Cu,
Fe and Zn. The Hyp mice may consume more food per g body weight
than normal mice. Since dietary Mn is reported to be poorly absorbed in normal animals[20] and since the soft tissues are not Mn
deficient (Table 5), this could lead to the raised fecal Mn data.
Higher food intake would also explain the increased organ content
of Fe and Zn. Further work with carefully controlled balance
studies are needed to test this interpretation.


SUMMARY

Hyp mice have a defective control system for the synthesis of
$1,25-(OH)_2$-vitamin D that does not respond to a low phosphate
stimulus. While the plasma levels of 25-OH-vitamin D are reduced
somewhat, this seems to be not a serious defect since plasma $1,25-$
$(OH)_2$-vitamin D levels are normal. Hyp kidneys synthesize and excrete elevated levels of cyclic AMP and cyclic GMP. The elevated
tissue levels of trace minerals suggests increased food intake with
normal intestinal absorption of the minerals. In addition there is
the reduced renal tubular reabsorption of phosphate[2] caused by a
change in the brush border transport of phosphate[3]. This leads to

hypophosphatemia[2], osteomalacic bone disease[4] and altered Mg metabolism[4]. There is intestinal resistance to $1,25-(OH)_2$-vitamin D
stimulation[5].

Many of these defects seem unrelated to the reduced renal
tubular reabsorption of phosphate. Yet all are derived from one
mutation in the Hyp gene. The underlying explanation must account
for all abnormalities by a single mutation in a single gene product.
The near normal phosphate levels in soft tissues and the multiple
defects argue against a genetic change in the phosphate pump as an
ultimate explanation. Still to be explored are possible changes in
a phosphate recognition site on a cell membrane or a change in an
as yet unknown phosphate regulating system.

ACKNOWLEDGEMENTS

This work was supported in part by research grants from the
Kroc Foundation and the N.I.H. (AM-22014, RR-00058) and by an N.I.H.
Biomedical Research Development Grant (RR-09016). We wish to thank
Ms. Dawn Braatz for her technical assistance.

REFERENCES

1. C.E. Dent, J.M. Round and T.C.B. Stamp, Treatment of sex-linked
   hypophosphatemic rickets, in: "Clinical Aspects of Metabolic
   Bone Disease", B. Frame, A.M. Parfitt and H. Duncan, eds.,
   Excerpta Medica, Amsterdam, p. 427 (1973).
2. E.M. Eicher, J.L. Southard, C.R. Scriver, and F.H. Glorieux,
   Hypophosphatemia: mouse model for human familial hypophosphatemic (vitamin D-resistant) rickets, Proc. Natl. Acad. Sci.
   USA 73: 4667 (1976).
3. H.S. Tenenhouse, C.R. Scriver, R.R. McInnes, and F.H. Glorieux,
   Renal handling of phosphate in vivo and in vitro by the X-
   linked hypophosphatemic male mouse: Evidence for a defect in
   the brush border membrane, Kidney Int. 14: 236 (1978).
4. R.A. Meyer, Jr., J. Jowsey, and M.H. Meyer, Osteomalacia and
   altered magnesium metabolism in the X-linked hypophosphatemic
   mouse, Calcif. Tissue Int. 27: 19 (1979).
5. P.J.A. O'Doherty, H.F. DeLuca, and E.M. Eicher, Lack of effect of
   vitamin D and its metabolites on intestinal phosphate transport in familial hypophosphatemia of mice, Endocrinology 101:
   1325 (1977).
6. A.E. Caldas, R.W. Gray, J. Lemann, Jr., The simultaneous
   measurement of vitamin D metabolites in plasma: studies in
   healthy adults and in patients with calcium nephrolithiasis,
   J. Lab. Clin. Med. 91: 840 (1978).
7. R.A. Meyer, Jr., R.W. Gray and M.H. Meyer, Paradoxical normal

levels of vitamin D metabolites in the plasma of the X-linked hypophosphatemic mouse, in: "Program and Abstracts", 60th Annual Meeting. The Endocrine Society, p. 486 (1978).

8.  H.F. DeLuca and H.K. Schnoes, Metabolism and mechanism of action of vitamin D, Annu. Rev. Biochem. 45: 631 (1976).

9.  J.G. Haddad, Jr., K.J. Chyu, T.J. Hahn and T.C.B. Stamp, Serum concentrations of 25-hydroxyvitamin D in sex-linked hypophosphatemic vitamin D-resistant rickets, J. Lab. Clin. Med. 81: 22 (1973).

10. R.A. Meyer, Jr., R.W. Gray, and M.H. Meyer, Abnormal vitamin D metabolism in the X-linked hypophosphatemic mouse, Submitted for publication.

11. J.I. Rader, D.J. Baylink, M.R. Hughes, E.F. Safilian, M.R. Haussler, Calcium and phosphorus deficiency in rats: effects on PTH and 1,25-dihydroxyvitamin $D_3$, Am. J. Physiol. 236: E118 (1979).

12. L.R. Chase and G.D. Aurbach, Parathyroid function and the renal excretion of 3',5'-adenylic acid, Proc. Natl. Acad. Sci. USA 58: 518 (1967).

13. H. Rasmussen, M. Pechet and D. Fast, Effect of dibutyryl cyclic adenosine 3',5'-monophosphate, theophylline, and other nucleotides upon calcium and phosphate metabolism, J. Clin. Invest. 47: 1843 (1968).

14. N.L. Kaminsky, A.E. Broadus, J.G. Hardman, D.J. Jones, Jr., J.H. Ball, E.W. Sutherland and G.W. Liddle, Effects of parathyroid hormone on plasma and urinary adenosine 3',5'-monophosphate in man, J. Clin. Invest. 49: 2387 (1970).

15. A.L. Steiner, C.W. Parker, and D.M. Kipnis, Radio-immunoassay for cyclic nucleotides. I. Preparation of antibodies and iodinated cyclic nucleotides, J. Biol. Chem. 247: 1106 (1972).

16. G.M. Kiebzak and R.A. Meyer, Jr., Increased urinary excretion of cyclic nucleotides in the X-linked hypophosphatemic mouse, manuscript in preparation.

17. P.L. Altman and D.S. Dittmer, eds., "Biology Data Book" Volume III, 2nd edition, Federation of American Societies for Experimental Biology, Bethesda, p. 1992 (1974).

18. F.H. Glorieux and C.R. Scriver, Loss of a parathyroid hormone-sensitive component of phosphate transport in X-linked hypophosphatemia, Science 175: 997 (1972).

19. M.G. Brunette, D. Chabardes, M. Imbert-Teboul, A. Clique, M. Montegut, and F. Morel, Hormone-sensitive adenylate cyclase along the nephron of genetically hypophosphatemic mice. Kidney Int. 15: 357 (1979).

20. E.J. Underwood, "Trace Elements in Human and Animal Nutrition", Academic Press, New York, p. 170 (1977).

21. M. Meyer and R.A. Meyer, Jr., Unsuitability of porcelain crucibles for dry ashing of biological tissues for calcium analysis, Clin. Chem. 22: 1396 (1976).

CATION EFFECTS ON PHOSPHATE HOMEOSTASIS

IN HYPOPHOSPHATEMIC SUBJECTS

Steven R. Goldring and Stephen M. Krane

Harvard Medical School, Massachusetts General Hospital
New England Deaconess Hospital
Boston, Massachusetts 02114

INTRODUCTION

X-linked hypophosphatemia and sporadic hypophosphatemic osteo-malacia are disorders characterized by inappropriately high renal clearance of phosphate ($P_i$). Although the results of some studies have suggested an additional defect in intestinal $P_i$ absorption[1,2], excessive urinary $P_i$ excretion is generally considered to be the major determinant of the hypophosphatemia. Treatment with oral $P_i$ salts alone or in combination with vitamin D has resulted in increased serum $P_i$ levels and improvement in bone disease[3]. Oral $P_i$ supplements have most often been administered in the form of the neutral sodium (Na) salts or as a combination of neutral Na and potassium (K) salts. Frick[4] has demonstrated that expansion of extracellular fluid volume by the infusion of isotonic saline re-sults in increased $P_i$ excretion in the rat. Similar effects of saline infusion on $P_i$ excretion have been observed in dogs[5,6] and normal human subjects[7]. Recently Tenenhouse et al[8] in studies of the X-linked hypophosphatemic mouse, have suggested the presence of a selective $P_i$ transport defect in the Na dependent transport system of the kidney brush border membrane. In order to evaluate the effects of high Na intake in individuals receiving oral $P_i$ supple-ments, we have compared the effects of neutral Na and K salts of $P_i$ on levels of serum $P_i$, renal $P_i$ clearance, immunoreactive para-thyroid hormone (PTH) and urinary cAMP clearance in three adults with hypophosphatemic osteomalacia. In all three subjects, serum $P_i$ levels were higher while receiving the neutral K salt of $P_i$ than while receiving equivalent quantities of the neutral Na salt. In one subject with X-linked hypophosphatemia, a high Na diet reversed the beneficial effects of the K salt on serum $P_i$ levels. These studies suggest that $P_i$ excretion is markedly affected by

Na intake in individuals with hypophosphatemic osteomalacia.

METHODS

    Three subjects were studied on the metabolic ward at the
Massachusetts General Hospital:  Subject RC, a male, age 27, with
classical X-linked vitamin D resistant rickets; subject AD, a
female, age 50, with short stature, childhood rickets with typical
skeletal deformities, but no hypophosphatemia in other members of
a large kindred; and subject GS, a male, age 25, of normal stature
without developmental skeletal deformities with spontaneous onset
of hypophosphatemia and osteomalacia at age 22 and no hypophosphatemia in other family members.

    Subjects were placed on a low gelatin diet approximating pre-
admission diets.  Daily intakes of Na, K, calcium (Ca) and $P_i$ were
maintained within a range of approximately 10%.  Study periods consisted of four or five consecutive 24 h periods of oral supplement
with either Na, K or mixed Na - K neutral salts of $P_i$.  Subject RC
was also studied on the neutral K salt of $P_i$ while receiving a high
Na diet.  During each of the treatment periods 24 h urine samples
were collected for measurement of Ca, $P_i$, creatinine, Na and K.
Daily fasting serum levels of Ca, $P_i$, Na, K, chloride, bicarbonate
and plasma levels of PTH were also determined.  At the end of each
treatment period a single oral dose of the $P_i$ salt employed during
the preceding treatment period was administered and $P_i$ "tolerance"
assessed.  The subjects received 500 ml of water 2 h before the test
and then 200 ml every 2 h until completion of the study.  A single
2 h urine sample was obtained before administration of the $P_i$ supplement and then three consecutive 2 h urine samples collected for Ca,
$P_i$, Na, K, creatinine and cAMP.  Blood samples were obtained every
1 h during the study for Ca, $P_i$, PTH, creatinine, cAMP, Na and K.
All subjects were receiving dihydrotachysterol prior to hospital
admission and were maintained on the same dose throughout the study.

RESULTS

    In Table 1 is illustrated representative determinations of 24 h
urinary $P_i$, Na and K in subject GS.  During study Period I he
received the neutral Na salt of $P_i$ orally in divided doses throughout the day.  Calculated 24 h dietary Ca and $P_i$ intakes averaged 1800
and 2100 mg respectively, during Period I and throughout the remainder of the study.  Dietary Na averaged 200 mEq/24 h and K averaged
125 mEq/24 h.  During Period II he was switched to the neutral K
salt of $P_i$, at a reduced $P_i$ level in order to allow gastrointestinal
accomodation.  Urinary excretion of $P_i$ was comparable despite lower
$P_i$ intake.  During Period II, 24 h urinary Na remained high presumably reflecting the high Na intake during the preceding period.
During Period III,  24 h urinary Na fell and urine K increased
reflecting the change from the Na to the K salt of $P_i$.  Fasting

Table 1.   Effect of Oral Supplementation with the Neutral
           Phosphate Salts of Na or K on Urinary Na, K and
           $P_i$ Excretion[a]

| Period | Supplement | | | Urine | | |
|--------|------|------|------|------|------|------|
|        | $P_i$ mg/24h | Na mEq/24h | K | $P_i$ mg/24h | Na mEq/24h | K |
| I   | 3750 | 257 | -   | 2793 | 296 | 73  |
| II  | 2250 | -   | 128 | 3110 | 241 | 185 |
| III | 3750 | -   | 257 | 3222 | 116 | 296 |

[a]Subject GS was receiving 0.4 mg dihydrotachysterol
daily.

serum $P_i$ levels averaged 2.3 mg/dl while on the Na salt (Period I)
and increased to 3.0 during Period III.  Serum Ca values averaged
9.0 and 8.8 mg/dl during Periods I and III, respectively.

Since isolated fasting serum $P_i$ and Ca values may not
accurately reflect serum levels during a 24 h period, $P_i$ "tolerance"
was assessed following a single oral $P_i$ load over a six hour period.
In Table 2 are compared the $P_i$ "tolerance" during Periods I (on
neutral Na salt of $P_i$, 3750 mg $P_i$/24 h) and Period III (on the
neutral K salt of $P_i$, 3750 mg $P_i$/24 hr).  After a single oral dose
of the Na salt (1250 mg $P_i$), serum $P_i$ increased to 3.1 mg/dl and
rapidly decreased to 1.7 mg/dl 5 h after the $P_i$ load.  In contrast,
during Period III an equivalent oral load of the K salt of $P_i$ (1250
mg $P_i$) resulted in an increase in serum $P_i$ level to 4.7 mg/dl.  Five
h after the oral load of $P_i$, serum $P_i$ level was 2.7 mg/dl compared
to 1.7 mg/dl during the comparable period while receiving the Na
salt.  PTH levels, although slightly higher during Period III, than
during Period I were comparable (ave. 6.7 µlEq/ml and 8.5 µlEq/ml,
respectively).  Although serum $P_i$ levels were lower during the $P_i$
"tolerance" test in Period I, the $P_i$ creatinine clearance ratios
were considerably higher during each of the 2 h periods when compared to comparable intervals during Period III.

In Table 3 is illustrated the $P_i$ "tolerance" test in subject AD.
During Period I (not shown) she received a combination of the neutral Na and K salts of $P_i$.  Results of study Periods II and III
while receiving the K and Na salts (1750 mg $P_i$/24 h) are shown.
Renal clearance ratios of $P_i$/creatinine were high during Period III
after receiving the Na salt, despite lower serum $P_i$ levels.  PTH
levels during all study periods were elevated above normal range
(>10 µlEq/ml).  The higher $P_i$/creatinine ratios while receiving the
Na salt of Pi could not be accounted for by changes in PTH levels.

Table 2.   Effect of an Oral Phosphate Load (Neutral Na or K Salts)
           on Urinary Phosphate Clearance and Levels of Serum $P_i$
           and Plasma PTH[a]

| | Period I | | | Period III | | |
|---|---|---|---|---|---|---|
| Collection time | $\dfrac{Cl_{P_i}}{Cl_{C_r}}$ | Serum $P_i$ mg/dl | PTH μlEq/ml | $\dfrac{Cl_{P_i}}{Cl_{C_r}}$ | Serum $P_i$ mg/dl | PTH μlEq/ml |
| 0400–0600 | 0.64 | 2.3 | 7.0 | 0.18 | 3.0 | 6.5 |
| 0600–0800 | 1.04 | 3.1 | 8.0 | 0.41 | 4.7 | 7.0 |
| 0800–1000 | 0.89 | 2.4 | 6.5 | 0.37 | 3.5 | 11.0 |
| 1000–1200 | 0.78 | 1.7 | 5.5 | 0.48 | 2.7 | 9.5 |

[a]Subject GS was consuming either Na($P_i$) (Period I) or K($P_i$)
   (Period III) equivalent to 3750 mg $P_i$ daily in three divided
   doses at the time of each study.  A load of oral $P_i$ (1250 mg)
   was administered either as Na($P_i$) or K($P_i$) at 0600 h.

In Table 4 is illustrated the results of $P_i$ "tolerance" tests
in subject RC.  During each of the study periods he received 3750
mg $P_i$/24 h as either Na or K salts of $P_i$.  During the Period II he
received supplements of neutral Na($P_i$) equivalent to 214 mEq Na/24 h.
During Period III he received the neutral K salt of $P_i$ but his diet
was supplemented with 214 mEq/Na to approximate the Na intake during
Period II.  Serum levels of $P_i$ after oral $P_i$ supplements averaged
3.3 mg/dl during Period I.  The apparent beneficial effect of the
neutral K salt of $P_i$ was abbrogated by supplemental dietary Na.
Serum Ca levels during the three periods averaged 8.8, 8.3 and
8.8 mg/dl, respectively.  PTH levels were considerably higher during
Period I while receiving the neutral K salt of $P_i$.

DISCUSSION

In all three subjects, serum $P_i$ levels were higher while receiving the neutral K salt of $P_i$ than while receiving an equivalent
quantity of the neutral Na salt of $P_i$.  In subjects GS and AD $P_i$/
creatinine clearance ratios were higher while on the neutral Na
salt compared to values during treatment with equivalent amounts of
the neutral K salt.  The relative increases in clearance of $P_i$ are
especially striking when one considers that the serum $P_i$ levels were
lower during the Na treatment period.  These findings suggest that
individuals with hypophosphatemic osteomalacia do respond to volume
expansion which accompanies Na loading with an increase in renal $P_i$

Table 3.  Effect of an Oral Phosphate Load (Neutral K or Na Salts)
          on Urinary Phosphate Clearance and Levels of Serum $P_i$
          and Plasma PTH[a]

|  | | PERIOD II | | | PERIOD III | |
|---|---|---|---|---|---|---|
| Collection time | $\dfrac{CL_{Pi}}{Cl_{Cr}}$ | Serum $P_i$ mg/dl | PTH μleq/ml | $\dfrac{CL_{Pi}}{Cl_{Cr}}$ | Serum $P_i$ mg/dl | PTH μlEq/ml |
| 0400-0600 | - | 2.0 | 12.5 | 0.52 | 1.8 | 14.0 |
| 0600-0800 | 0.58 | 2.8 | 12.0 | 0.93 | 2.4 | 17.0 |
| 0800-1000 | 0.43 | 3.1 | 16.5 | 1.11 | 2.7 | 16.0 |
| 1000-1200 | 0.48 | 2.7 | 13.0 | 1.08 | 1.7 | 14.5 |

[a]Subject AD was consuming either K (Period II) or Na (Period III)
phosphate equivalent to 1750 mg $P_i$ in divided doses daily at the
time of each study.  A load of oral $P_i$ (500 mg) was administered
either as $K(P_i)$ (Period II) or $Na(P_i)$ (Period III) at 0600 h.

clearance.  Although ionized serum Ca levels were not measured, the
absence of significant changes in PTH in these two subjects suggest
that the increased $P_i$ clearance was not secondary to stimulation of
PTH secretion as has been suggested,[9,10] but rather a direct effect
of high Na intake and extracellular volume expansion.  It is also
possible that the increased $P_i$ clearance while receiving $Na(P_i)$
reflects a specific effect of Na on $P_i$ transport as suggested in
studies of the hypophosphatemic mouse[8].  Condon[1] has employed
similar tests of $P_i$ tolerance and has demonstrated impaired intestinal $P_i$ absorption in individuals with vitamin D resistant rickets.
We can not exclude a possible difference in intestinal absorption
of the two salts of $P_i$.  However, the high clearance ratios of $P_i$/
creatinine in subjects GS and AD, while receiving the Na salt of
$P_i$ suggest that the major cause of hypophosphatemia was related to
increased renal $P_i$ excretion.

In subject RC. serum $P_i$ levels were significantly higher while
receiving the K salt than during treatment with equivalent amounts
of $P_i$ in the form of the neutral Na salt.  Dietary Na supplement
while receiving the K salt resulted in a lowering of serum $P_i$ to
values comparable to those achieved while on the neutral Na salt.
Unlike subjects GS and AD, the clearance ratios of $P_i$/creatinine
were comparable during all of the treatment periods.  Higher $P_i$/
creatinine clearance might have been expected in the face of the
higher serum $P_i$ levels during treatment with $K(P_i)$.  Unlike subjects

Table 4.  Effect of an Oral Phosphate Load (Neutral K or Na Salts) on Urinary Phosphate Clearance and the Levels of Serum $P_i$ and Plasma PTH[a]

| Collection time | Period I | | | Period II | | | Period III | | |
|---|---|---|---|---|---|---|---|---|---|
| | $\dfrac{Cl_{P_i}}{Cl_{C_r}}$ | Serum $P_i$ mg/dl | PTH μlEq/ml | $\dfrac{Cl_{P_i}}{Cl_{C_r}}$ | Serum $P_i$ mg/dl | PTH μlEq/ml | $\dfrac{Cl_{P_i}}{Cl_{C_r}}$ | Serum $P_i$ mg/dl | PTH μlEq/ml |
| 0600–0800 | — | 3.2 | 27 | 0.77 | 2.4 | 22 | 0.82 | 2.8 | 17 |
| 0800–1000 | 0.91 | 3.5 | 49 | 0.74 | 2.7 | 29 | 0.83 | 2.8 | 24 |
| 1000–1200 | 0.74 | 3.1 | 28 | 0.60 | 2.3 | 25 | 0.57 | 2.7 | 22 |
| 1200–1400 | 0.63 | 3.2 | 30 | 0.59 | 2.5 | 25 | 0.60 | 2.8 | 27 |

[a] Subject RC was receiving either K (Periods I and III) or Na (Period II) phosphate equivalent to 3750 mg $P_i$ daily at the time of each study.  In addition, NaCl was added to K($P_i$) supplements during Period III.  A load of oral $P_i$ (750 mg) was administered either as Na($P_i$)(Period II) or K($P_i$) (Periods I and III) at 0800 h.

GS and AD subject RC demonstrated markedly elevated PTH levels while receiving the K salt. Although levels of PTH were also evaluated during the two other treatment periods, the absolute values were lower. Riggs et al[11] have suggested that PTH plays a permissive role in $P_i$ transport in individuals with vitamin D-resistant rickets. Short et al[12] have suggested that individuals with this disorder have an exaggerated phosphaturic response to this hormone. It is possible that in subject RC the high circulating levels of PTH while receiving the K salt of $P_i$ were responsible for the high $P_i$ excretion. Although the mechanism of the PTH stimulation is uncertain, it may be related to the high serum $P_i$ levels which indirectly stimulated PTH secretion via an effect on serum Ca levels. An effect of the various salts on intestinal $P_i$ transport can also not be excluded.

Recently, Cowgill et al[13] have presented evidence obtained from studies employing mice with genetic hypophosphatemic rickets suggesting that a defect in $P_i$ transport exists in both proximal convoluted tubules and more distal sites. Studies in several species have demonstrated distal sites of PTH transport[14]. Our studies help define factors controlling $P_i$ homeostasis in individuals receiving neutral salts of $P_i$, and the results have obvious therapeutic implications for individuals with hypophosphatemic osteomalacia.

ACKNOWLEDGEMENTS

This work was supported by USPHS grants AM-03564, AM-0450 and RR-010616. PTH immunoassays were performed in the laboratories of the Endocrine Unit, Massachusetts General Hospital under the supervision of J.T. Potts, Jr.

BIBLIOGRAPHY

1.  J.R. Condon, J.R. Nassim, and A. Rutter, Pathogenesis of rickets and osteomalacia in familial hypophosphatemia, Arch. Dis. Child. 46:269 (1971).

2.  E.M. Short, H.J. Binder, and L.E. Rosenberg, Familial hypophosphatemic rickets: Defective transport of inorganic phosphate by intestinal mucosa, Science 179:700 (1973).

3.  C. Nagant de Deuxchaisnes and S.M. Krane, The treatment of adult phosphate diabetes and Fanconi syndrome with neutral sodium phosphate, Am. J. Med. 43:508 (1967).

4.  A. Frick, Mechanism of inorganic phosphate diuresis secondary to saline infusions in the rat, Pflugers Arch. 313:106 (1969).

5.  W.N. Suki, M. Martinez-Maldonado, D. Rouse, and A. Terry,
    Effect of expansion of extracellular fluid volume on renal
    phosphate handling, J. Clin. Invest. 48:1888 (1969).

6.  S.G. Massry, J.W. Coburn, and C.R. Kleeman, The influence of
    extracellular volume expansion on renal phosphate reabsorption
    in the dog, J. Clin. Invest. 48:1237 (1969).

7.  T.H. Steele, Increased urinary phosphate excretion following
    volume expansion in normal man, Metabolism 19:129 (1970).

8.  H.S. Tenenhouse, C.R. Scriver, R.R. McInnes, and F.H.
    Glorieux, Renal handling of phosphate in vivo and in vitro by
    the X-linked hypophosphatemic male mouse:  Evidence for a
    defect in the brush border membrane, Kidney International
    14:236 (1978).

9.  A. Frick, Parathyroid hormone as a mediator of inorganic phos-
    phate diuresis during saline infusion in the rat, Pflugers
    Arch. 325:1 (1971).

10. E.G. Schneider, R.S. Goldsmith, C.D. Arnaud, and F.G. Knox,
    Role of parathyroid hormone in the phosphaturia of extracellular
    fluid volume expansion, Kidney International 7:317 (1975).

11. B.L. Riggs, R.G. Sprague, J.J. Jowsey, and F.T. Maher, Adult-
    onset vitamin D-resistant hypophosphatemic osteomalacia.
    Effect of total parathyroidectomy, New Engl. J. Med. 281:762
    (1969).

12. E. Short, R.C. Morris, Jr., A. Sebastian, and M. Spencer,
    Exaggerated phosphaturic response to circulating parathyroid
    hormone in patients with familial X-linked hypophosphatemic
    rickets, J. Clin. Invest. 58:152 (1976).

13. L.D. Cowgill, S. Goldfarb, K. Lau, E. Slatopolsky, and Z.S. Agus,
    Evidence for an intrinsic renal tubular defect in mice with
    genetic hypophosphatemic rickets, J. Clin. Invest. 63:1203
    (1979).

14. F.G. Knox, H. Osswald, G.R. Marchand, W.S. Spielman, J.A. Haas,
    T. Berndt, and S.P. Youngberg, Phosphate Transport along the
    nephron, Am. J. Physiol. 233:F261 (1971).

# INTESTINAL ABSORPTION

# OF CALCIUM AND PHOSPHATE

# TRANSMUCOSAL $^{45}$Ca-FLUX AND Ca-ATPase SPECIFIC ACTIVITY IN BASOLATERAL PLASMA MEMBRANES OF THE SMALL INTESTINAL MUCOSA IN RESPONSE TO DIURETICS

I.C. Radde, J. Sheepers, D. Davis, H.G. McKercher

Research Institute, The Hospital for Sick Children and Department of Paediatrics, University of Toronto, Toronto, Canada

## INTRODUCTION

A relationship between the effects of certain diuretics, such as ethacrynic acid (EA) and furosemide (F), on renal $(Na^+ + K^+)$-ATPase specific activity and renal $Na^+$-transport in vivo and in vitro has been established (1, 2). Both these diuretics inhibit the specific activity of the renal NaK-ATPase as well as the rates of renal tubular reabsorption of Na (3).

Our interest in diuretics affecting Ca-transport phenomena was aroused in the early seventies when we found that EA also inhibited Ca-ATPase specific activity in plasma membrane preparations of placental tissue (4). Since EA and benzothiadiazine diuretics affect renal Ca-excretion in opposite directions (5, 6), we carried out the experiments reported here in which we attempted to correlate small intestinal Ca-flux with Ca-ATPase specific activity under the influence of two types of diuretics, EA and F as examples of high-ceiling diuretics, and hydrochlorothiazide (HCT), a benzothiadiazine diuretic. We wanted to investigate the following hypotheses:
(a) that the intestinal mucosa serves as a useful model to test correlations between in vitro Ca-ATPase specific activity and bidirectional Ca-flux following the administration of diuretics;
(b) that the two types of diuretics, EA and F vs. HCT, affect Ca-ATPase activity and $^{45}$Ca-fluxes in specific and coupled ways;
(c) that the effects of the two classes of diuretics on urinary Ca-excretion can be explained on the basis of their action on Ca-ATPase specific activity; and
(d) that there are age-related changes of the intestinal response to various diuretics.

These hypotheses were tested in the young piglet. We chose this animal species because:
(a) piglets respond to diuretics in a manner qualitatively similar to man;
(b) their calcium homeostasis is also very similar to that described for man, particularly as it pertains to intestinal Ca-absorption, plasma calcium, phosphorus and vitamin D levels, and
(c) their renal function and response to various stress tests are comparable to those seen in man.

In addition, we have some basal information from previous studies in young piglets in which we have determined the effect of diuretics on renal Ca-ATPase specific activity and on in vivo urinary excretion of cations and anions.

MATERIAL AND METHODS

The experimental protocol was as follows: The piglets serving as donors of intestinal mucosa and basolateral plasma membrane fraction were 3 to 35 days old. They were suckled by the sow until the morning of the experiment when they were anaesthetized with Na-pentobarbital (50 mg/kg). The desired measured segment of the small bowel was removed in standardized fashion, the mucosa stripped from underlying tissue and placed in Ussing chambers for measurement of $^{45}$Ca-fluxes. Adjacent pieces, their conductance matched within 30% of each other, were used for measurement of mucosal to submucosal ($J_{MS}$) and submucosal to mucosal $^{45}$Ca-fluxes ($J_{SM}$); the net flux ($J_{net}$) being the difference between the two. After measurement of basal flux rates the diuretic was added to the mucosal side in 0.22 mM concentration, and serial flux measurements continued. The principles of the set-up and the calculations were those according to Schultz & Zalusky (7) and to Walling and Kimberg (8).

For Ca-ATPase specific activity measurements, the basal plasma membranes were prepared from homogenates of mucosal cells and cell sheets by differential and sucrose gradient centrifugation using a modification of the methods of Forstner et al. (9) and Quigley and Gotterer (10). For measurement of Ca-ATPase specific activity, we added to the incubation solution (1.0 ml, containing 70 mM NaCl, 20 mM Tris-HCl, pH 7.8, and either 5 or 0 mM CaCl$_2$), the plasma membrane suspension (0.1 ml, containing 10-20 µg protein, in 5 mM ethylene-glycol-bis(β aminoethyl ether)N,N'-tetraacetic acid (EGTA), pH 7.8) and diuretic (in 0.1 ml EGTA, 0 to 2 mM, adjusted to pH 7.8). After addition of 0.1 ml 5 mM Na$_2$ATP, pH 7.8, the samples were incubated at 37°C for 1 hr and the reaction terminated by plunging the tubes into an ice-water bath and adding 1.0 ml of a 10% (w/w) trichloracetic acid solution. As an index of ATP hydrolysis, the inorganic phosphate released in each sample was measured by the method of Gomori (11). The protein concentration was determined by the procedure of Lowry et al. (12).

RESULTS

$^{45}$Ca-flux

Segments and Age.  The basal $J_{MS}$ $^{45}$Ca-flux rates were slightly higher in the duodenum than in the jejunum during the first two
weeks of life but the difference was not significant.  No differences between segments and age groups were observed in $J_{SM}$ and $J_{net}$-
fluxes.  In the jejunum a higher $J_{MS}$ and $J_{net}$ was noted during the
first week of life (p<0.05) compared to weeks 2 and 3 (Fig. 1).

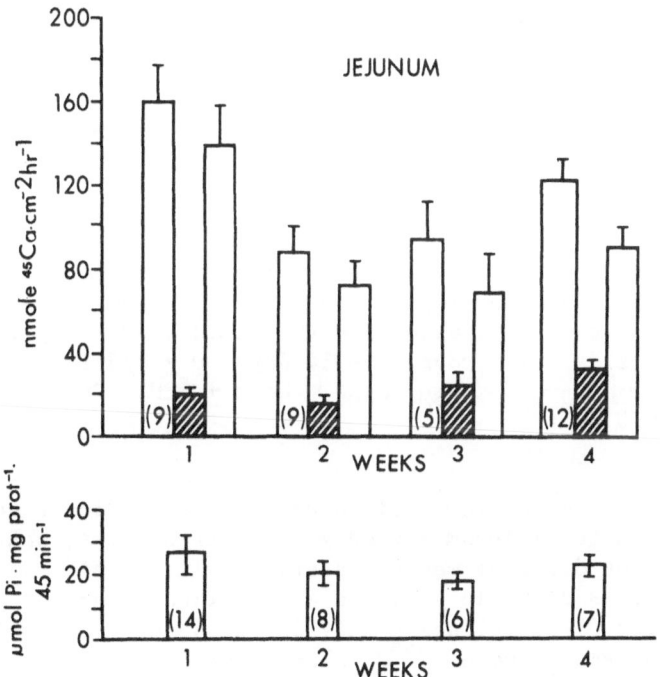

Fig. 1.   Upper panel:  $^{45}$Ca-flux (nmole · cm$^{-2}$ · hr$^{-1}$) in jejunum
during the first four weeks of life.⌐□ ▨ □¬= $J_{MS}$,
$J_{SM}$, $J_{net}$ · Mean ± SEM.   Lower panel:  Ca-ATPase specific
activity (µmole Pi released · mg protein$^{-1}$ · 45 min$^{-1}$) in
basolateral plasma membrane fraction of jejunum.  Mean ±
SEM.  Number in parentheses = n.

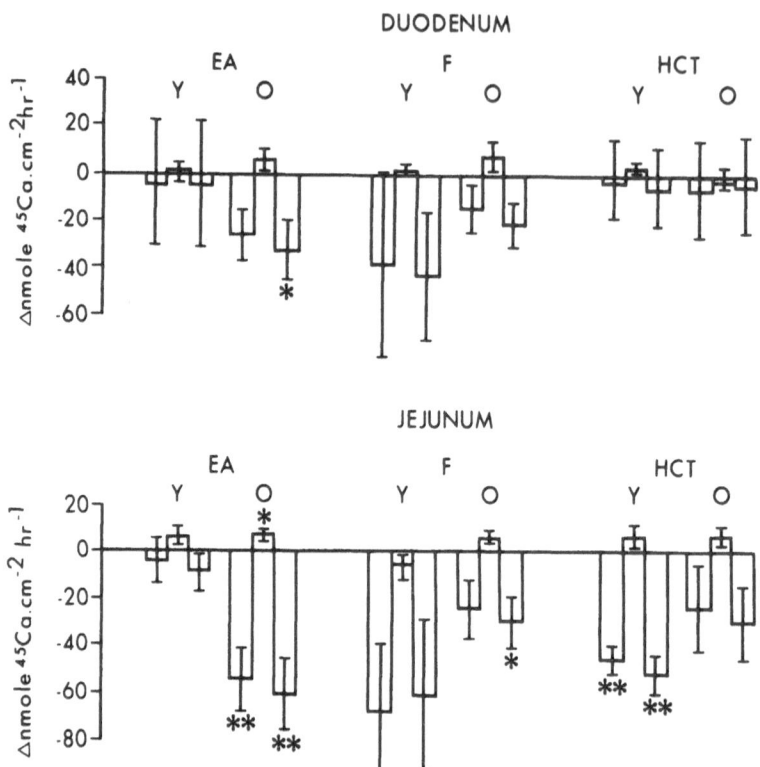

Fig. 2.  Changes in $^{45}$Ca-fluxes following the addition of diuretics in duodenum (upper panel) and jejunum (lower panel).
EA = ethacrynic acid, F = furosemide, HCT = hydrochlorothiazide.  Y = young 1 - 14 days; O = old 15 - 35 days.
$J_{MS}$, $J_{SM}$, $J_{net}$ · Mean ± SEM.  *p<0.05;
**p<0.005.

     Diuretics.  Ethacrynic acid produced a significant decrease
in $J_{MS}$ only in the jejunum and only in older animals, whereas the
decrease in the duodenum was not statistically significant (Fig.2).
Conversely, this diuretic produced a significant increase in $J_{SM}$,
i.e. secretory flux, but again only in the jejunum and only in
the older animals.  The net $^{45}$Ca-fluxes were significantly
depressed only in the older animals but this occurred in both
duodenum and jejunum.

     Furosemide produced a greater inhibition of $J_{MS}$ and $J_{net}$
$^{45}$Ca-fluxes in the jejunum compared to duodenum; secretory ($J_{SM}$)
fluxes were not affected by this diuretic. Net $^{45}$Ca-fluxes were
significantly inhibited in older animals in the jejunum only.

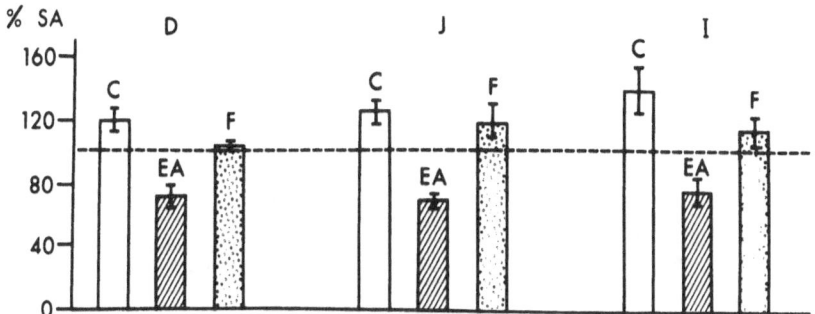

Fig. 3.  Ca-ATPase specific activity as % of basal specific activ-
         ity in basolateral plasma membrane preparations.  Mean +
         SEM.  D = duodenum, J = jejunum, I = ileum.  C = chloro-
         thiazide; EA = ethacrynic acid; F = furosemide.


Hydrochlorothiazide did not affect duodenal $^{45}$Ca-fluxes, but
inhibited $J_{MS}$ and $J_{net}$ in the jejunum of younger animals significantly.

Ca-ATPase specific activity.

    Segments and Age.  The basal specific activity of Ca-ATPase
showed no change with age in the duodenum, but decreased in the
jejunum between birth and 4 weeks of age (Fig. 1) in parallel with
changes in $^{45}$Ca-flux.

    Diuretics.  Figure 3 shows the change in Ca-ATPase specific
activity following addition of diuretics to the in vitro system.
It decreased significantly following the addition of EA, and was
enhanced following chlorothiazide (2 mM).

    Furosemide produced either no change or slight enhancement.
There were no significant differences seen between intestinal
segments in response to the diuretics tested.


DISCUSSION

    Figure 4 shows the transport rates of Ca and Na across the
renal tubular cell and the urinary excretion rates of these two
ions following the in vivo administration of diuretics to young
piglets.  Analogous to these findings and assuming that one of our
working hypothesis is correct and there exists a direct correlation between the transport rate of Ca and the specific Ca-ATPase
activity, one would expect the following changes with EA and HCT.
Ethacrynic acid, inhibiting the Ca-ATPase specific activity of

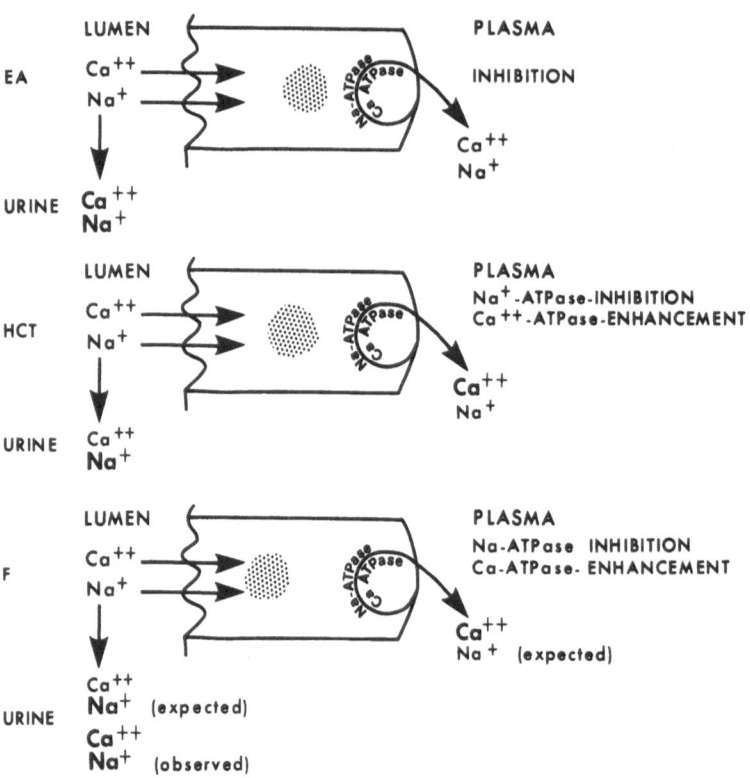

Fig. 4.  Effects of diuretics on Ca$^{++}$ and Na$^{+}$ transport from lumen
          to plasma in the kidney and on urinary excretion rates
          of Ca$^{++}$ and Na$^{+}$.  EA = ethacrynic acid; HCT = hydrochloro-
          thiazide, F = furosemide.

basolateral plasma membranes could interfere with absorptive $^{45}$Ca-
fluxes in the small intestine.  This was indeed the case.  HCT,
on the other hand, which has been shown to enhance the specific
Ca-ATPase activity in basolateral plasma membranes, should lead to
an increase in absorptive Ca-fluxes in the small intestine.  However, we did not find this but observed an inhibition of absorptive Ca-fluxes.  A similar discrepancy between Ca-ATPase specific
activity of basolateral plasma membranes and Ca-fluxes (absorptive
or net fluxes) was also found on testing F in these two in vitro
systems.  This diuretic enhanced Ca-ATPase activity but inhibited
Ca-flux in the jejunum although not to the same degree as did EA.

Thus, although the EA effect on jejunal and renal Ca-fluxes
and Ca-ATPase specific activity were correlated and could thus be
causally related, such a relationship did not hold with respect
to HCT and F.

Benzothiadiazine diuretics are said not only to diminish the rate of reabsorption of Ca in the distal renal tubule (13), but also to decrease small intestinal absorption of the ion (14). Thus, our finding of inhibition of absorptive Ca-fluxes following the application of HCT would be in agreement with earlier in vivo findings in man. However, the mechanism by which HCT inhibits intestinal absorption of Ca is unlikely to involve the Ca-ATPase located predominantly in the basolateral plasma membranes of the intestinal mucosal cell.

As to the second working hypothesis that diuretics act on different segments of the small intestine similar to their differential effect in various segments of the nephron, we found almost no effect on the duodenum, but differing responsiveness to diuretics in the jejunum. We did not report here our experience with the ileum since absorptive Ca-fluxes were seen only during the first few days of life in the piglet (15) and the effects of diuretics on $^{45}$Ca-flux rates were minimal after day 7 in this species.

Finally, we observed that tissues from young piglets were generally less responsive to the in vitro addition of the high-ceiling diuretics than those originating from older animals close to or after weaning. This finding could be related to postnatal development of absorptive functions in the intestine. Ca-absorption from the gut is especially high in very young animals (16) but seems to be dependent mainly on the Ca content in the intestinal lumen. Responsiveness of Ca-absorption to modulating factors, such as hormones and diuretics, probably increases with postnatal age.

SUMMARY AND CONCLUSIONS

The intestinal mucosa may serve as a useful model to examine the effects of modulators of renal Ca and Na transport. Changes in Ca-transport rates following the application of diuretics to the in vitro system corresponded qualitatively to those seen in renal systems.

Only EA produced similar changes in Ca-ATPase specific activity, intestinal Ca-fluxes and renal Ca-excretion to suggest that it may produce its inhibitory effect on renal Ca-reabsorption through an inhibition of Ca-ATPase activity. The other two diuretics tested (F, HCT) gave discrepant results between in vitro Ca-transport, in vivo Ca-absorption and Ca-ATPase activity.

REFERENCES

1.  A. E. Györy, U. Brendel, and R. Kinne, Effect of cardiac glyco-
    sides and sodium ethacrynate on transepithelial sodium
    transport in in vivo micropuncture experiments and on iso-
    lated plasma membrane Na-K-ATPase in vitro of the rat.
    Pfluegers Arch. 335:287 (1972).
2.  R. H. Kessler, D.Landwehr, A. Quintanilla, S. A. Weseley,
    W. Kaufmann, H. Arcila, and B. K. Urbaitis, Effects of
    certain inhibitors on renal sodium reabsorption and ATPase
    specific activity, Nephron, 5:474 (1968).
3.  S. P. Banerjee, V. K. Khanna, and A. K. Sen, Inhibition of
    sodium-and potassium-dependent adenosine triphosphatase by
    ethacrynic acid.  Two modes of action, Molec. Pharmacol.
    6:680 (1970).
4.  Y. Shami, and I. C. Radde, Calcium-stimulated ATPase of guinea
    pig placenta, Biochim. Biophys. Acta, 249:345 (1971).
5.  C. G. Duarte, Effects of ethacrynic acid and furosemide on
    urinary calcium, phosphorus and magnesium, Metabolism,
    17: 867 (1968).
6.  B. R. Edwards, P. G. Baer, R. A. L. Sutton, and J. H. Dirks,
    Micropuncture study of diuretic effects on sodium and
    calcium reabsorption in the dog nephron, J. Clin. Invest.
    52:2418 (1973).
7.  S. G. Schultz, and R.Zalusky, Ion transport in isolated rabbit
    ileum.  I.  Short circuit current and $Na^+$-fluxes, J. Genl.
    Physiol.  47:567 (1964).
8.  M. W. Walling, and D. V. Kimberg, Active secretion of calcium
    by adult rat ileum and jejunum in vitro, Am. J. Physiol.
    225:415 (1973).
9.  G. G. Forstner, S. M. Sabesin, and K. J. Isselbacher, Rat
    intestinal microvillus membranes.  Purification and bio-
    chemical characterization, Biochem. J. 106:381 (1968).
10. J. P. Quigley, and G. S. Gotterer, Properties of a high spe-
    cific activity $(Na^+ + K^+)$-stimulated ATPase from rat intes-
    tinal mucosa, Biochim. Biophys. Acta, 173:469 (1969).
11. G. Gomori, A modification of the colorimetric phosphorus deter-
    mination for use with the photoelectric colorimeter,
    J. Lab. Clin. Med., 27:955 (1942).
12. O. H. Lowry, N. J. Rosebrough, A. L. Farr, and R. J. Randall,
    Protein measurement with the Folin reagent, J. Biol. Chem.
    193:265 (1951).
13. L. S. Costanzo, and L M. Weiner, On the hypocalciuric action
    of chlorothiazide, J. Clin. Invest., 54:628 (1974).
14. U. Ehrig, J. E. Harrison, and D. R. Wilson, Effect of long-
    term thiazide therapy on intestinal calcium absorption in
    patients with recurrent renal calculi, Metabolism, 23: 139
    (1974).

15. I. C. Radde, D. Davis, J., Sheepers, and H. G. McKercher, Bidirectional transmucosal $^{45}$Ca and $^{32}$P-fluxes across the small intestine of the young piglet. Relationship to intestinal Ca$^{2+}$-Mg$^{2+}$-ATPase activity and postnatal age, In: <u>Pediatric Diseases Related to Calcium</u>, Eds., H.F. DeLuca, L. Finberg, C.S. Anast., Elsevier North-Holland, Excerpta Medica, New York City, (1979). (In press).
16. H. H. Harrison, Factors influencing calcium absorption, <u>Fed. Proc.</u>, 18:1085 (1959).

## ACKNOWLEDGEMENTS

This work was supported in part by the Medical Research Council of Canada (MA 1797). The hydrochlorothiazide used in the investigation was a generous gift of Dr. W. D. Dorian, Merck Frosst Laboratories, Pointe Claire, Dorval, Quebec, Canada.

INTESTINAL PHOSPHATE TRANSPORT

Renate Fuchs and Meinrad Peterlik

Department of General and Experimental
Pathology, University of Vienna,
A-1090 Vienna, Austria

INTRODUCTION

Previous studies on inorganic phosphate ($P_i$) absorption by chick intestine have established some characteristics of transepithelial $P_i$ transport and its regulation by vitamin $D_3$ (1-4). Uptake of $P_i$ from the lumen is accomplished by a "phosphate pump" located on the mucosal surface of the intestinal epithelium. The well known stimulation of intestinal $P_i$ absorption is due to action of the sterol on this active transport system, its maximal velocity ($V_{max}$) being raised about threefold above levels observed in vitamin D-deficient animals.

The action of vitamin $D_3$, or of its metabolite 1,25-dihydroxyvitamin $D_3$, on the $P_i$ absorptive system can be blocked by inhibition of protein synthesis at both the transcriptional and translational level (1,4) indicating that intact protein synthesis is required for full expression of the sterol's effect on phosphate transport. It is attractive to speculate that the increase in the number of carrier sites - as revealed by the increase in $V_{max}$ - may be the result of vitamin D-induced synthesis of proteins constituting the phosphate-carrier complex.

Stimulation of $P_i$ transport is apparently one of the earliest results of vitamin D repletion in vitamin D-deficient chicks (5,6), preceeding other well known

responses to the sterol, e. g. induction of the vitamin D-dependent calcium-binding protein, or stimulation
of alkaline phosphatase activity.

The adaptive increase in $P_i$ transfer across the
gut wall due to dietary restriction of phosphate or
calcium has been linked to the modulation of transport
efficiency by 1,25-dihydroxyvitamin $D_3$ under physiological conditions (1,6).

The purpose of the present study was to characterize possible routes of basal (vitamin D-independent)
and vitamin D-induced phosphate transfer in chick jejunum, their dependence on extracellular sodium, and
their sensitivity towards substances known to interfere
with phosphate transport in other tissues.


MATERIALS AND METHODS

One day old White Leghorn cockerels were raised on
a vitamin D-free diet for 4 weeks.

Everted gut sacs (4 cm long) were prepared from the
jejunum of either vitamin D-deficient (-D) or vitamin D-
replete (+D) chicks. The latter received 1000 I.U. vitamin $D_3$ in 0.2 ml propylene glycol by intramuscular injection 48 h before the experiment.

Preparation of everted gut sacs, buffer composition,
and analytical procedures have been described in detail
elsewhere (1,2). Standard incubation medium was Krebs-
Henseleit buffer (KHB). Radiotracers (0.2 μCi/ml P-32
or 0.5 μCi/ml Ca-45) were added to the mucosal solution.

Unidirectional $P_i$ fluxes were determined from
total P-32 transfer/mean specific activity. Calcium
fluxes were calculated accordingly.

M, S, and C in Fig. 1 and 2 denote mucosal, cellular and serosal compartment, respectively. Fluxes between these compartments were termed according to previously used designations (2).

Statistical comparisons were based on Student's
t-test.

RESULTS AND DISCUSSION

## Active $P_i$ Translocation Across the Mucosal Surface

Tab. 1 documents the effect of vitamin D repletion on active $P_i$ entry which is about threefold higher in the +D than in the -D group. A further indication that $P_i$ uptake is mediated by an active transport mechanism is that flux rates are heavily reduced by addition of the uncoupler carbonyl cyanide m-chlorophenylhydrazone (mClCCP) to the mucosal bathing solution (Tab. 1).

Phosphate transport in chick jejunum (3) and rat duodenum (7) depends on the presence of sodium in the bathing solution. Isosmolar substitution of sodium by choline reduces $P_i$ uptake to a level comparable to that observed under metabolic inhibition (Tab. 1). This suggests that $P_i$ active transport across the mucosal surface entirely depends on extracellular sodium.

The indol alkaloid harmaline and the local anesthetic dibucaine have been shown to interfere with $Na^+$-linked transport mechanisms in intestine and liver (8,9).

Table 1: Vitamin D-independent (-D) and vitamin D-induced (+D) $P_i$ entry across mucosal boundary

| Incubation buffer | Addition to mucosal buffer | Flux rate (nmol/min/g tissue) | |
|---|---|---|---|
| | | -D | +D |
| KHB | none | $82 \pm 34$ | $223 \pm 35^{[a]}$ |
| KHB | mClCCP 50 µM | $22 \pm 5$ | $55 \pm 7^{[b]}$ |
| $Na^+$-free | none | $52 \pm 7$ | $31 \pm 12^{[b]}$ |
| KHB | harmaline 4.0 mM | $48 \pm 15$ | $114 \pm 20^{[a,b]}$ |
| KHB | dibucaine 1.6 mM | $14 \pm 22$ | $87 \pm 10^{[a,b]}$ |

Data are means $\pm$ S.E. from 9–18 gut sacs per group; a, statistically significant difference between +D and -D group, $P < 0.05$; b, significantly different from uninhibited control, $P < 0.05$

As expected, both drugs reduced $P_i$ influx to diffusional levels.

## Influence of $Na^+$ on Kinetics of $P_i$ Transport

The concentration dependence of $P_i$ entry was measured at various $Na^+$ concentrations in the incubation medium ( 143, 96, 48, 24, and 0 mM). In the -D group, saturable $P_i$ uptake was observed at levels above 24 mM $Na^+$; in the +D group, saturation of $P_i$ influx was abolished only at 0 mM $Na^+$. $P_i$ uptake at these low $Na^+$ concentrations is therefore considered to be simply diffusional.

Kinetic constants of $P_i$ influx at normal and low $Na^+$ were calculated from linearized plots after subtraction of the diffusional term (Tab. 2). The +D and -D $P_i$ transfer systems are modulated by extracellular sodium in a different manner: Basal, i. e. vitamin D-independent $P_i$ transport is stimulated by $Na^+$ through a change in the binding affinity as evidenced by alteration of $K_m$. On the other hand, the predominant effect of $Na^+$ on vitamin D-induced $P_i$ transport is a dramatic increase in the maximal velocity.

Table 2: Kinetic constants of active $P_i$ entry across
the mucosal surface at normal and low $Na^+$

|  | $V_{max}$ (nmol/min/g tissue) | | $K_m$ (mM) | |
|---|---|---|---|---|
|  | normal $Na^+$ | low $Na^+$ | normal $Na^+$ | low $Na^+$ |
| -D | 125 | 105 | 0.15 | 1.13 |
| +D | 314 | 182 | 0.18 | 0.53 |

## Effect of Glucose and cAMP on Mucosal $P_i$ Influx

Inhibition by glucose of phosphate reabsorption in the proximal tubule of the kidney has been linked to competition for the energy available from the sodium gradient (10). This may occur also in the intestine, since 10 mM glucose significantly depresses $P_i$ influx in the +D group (Tab. 3).

Tubular reabsorption of phosphate is inversely related to cellular levels of cAMP (11). As shown in Tab. 3, neither 0.1 mM dibutyryl cAMP nor 10 mM theo-

Table 3: Effect of glucose, dibutyryl cAMP, and theophylline on $P_i$ influx in everted chick jejunum

| Addition to mucosal buffer | $P_i$ influx (nmol/min/g tissue) | |
|---|---|---|
| | -D | +D |
| none | 109 ± 25 | 258 ± 34 |
| glucose 10 mM | 70 ± 4 | 130 ± 16[*] |
| db-cAMP 0.1 mM | 160 ± 32 | 296 ± 25 |
| db-cAMP 1.0 mM | 95 ± 27 | 129 ± 23 |
| theophylline 10 mM | 123 ± 25 | 289 ± 39[*] |

Data are means ± S.E. from 12 everted gut sacs per
group. Asterisk indicates statistically significant
difference from control group (at least at $P < 0.05$).

phylline had any significant effect on intestinal $P_i$
transport. A substantial reduction of +D phosphate influx was observed only at an unphysiologically high
dibutyryl cAMP concentration of 1.0 mM.


Transepithelial Phosphate and Calcium Transport

Transmural $P_i$ transport can be separated into two
distinct phases (Fig. 1): A non-delayed mucosal-to-
serosal $P_i$ movement (M-S$_1$) is followed after a lag time
of about 15 min by a rapid increase in serosal phosphate
acquired from the contralateral side (M-S$_2$ flux).

The transepithelial M-S$_1$ flux represents only a
small fraction of total transmural $P_i$ transport, is
not subject to vitamin D-action and is also not dependent on extracellular Na$^+$ (Fig. 1, Tab. 4). Further,
the M-S$_1$ flux displays linear dependence on initial $P_i$
concentration (not shown) and is unaffected by metabolic
inhibition through mClCCP (Tab. 4). These characteristics of a passive, low permeability pathway indicate
a paracellular shunt rather than a transcellular route.

A substantial mucosal-to-serosal transfer of $P_i$
(M-S$_2$ flux) is observed only after vitamin D repletion
and in the presence of Na$^+$, suggesting transcellular

transport via the vitamin D-dependent sodium-linked phosphate pump (Fig. 1).

As opposed to $P_i$ transport, transepithelial calcium transport in everted chick jejunum is clearly monophasic (Fig. 1), has a significant vitamin D increment at every time point, and is not dependent on the presence of extracellular $Na^+$ (Tab. 5). These results provide further evidence for the separation of calcium and $P_i$ pathways in chick jejunum.

Table 4: Non-delayed mucosal-to-serosal $P_i$ flux (M-S$_1$)

| Incubation buffer | Addition to buffer | Flux rate (nmol/min/g tissue) | |
|---|---|---|---|
| | | -D | +D |
| KHB | none | 8.8 ± 1.2 | 8.5 ± 1.9 |
| $Na^+$-free | none | 8.7 ± 0.8 | 8.0 ± 0.8 |
| KHB | mClCCP 50 µM | 9.2 ± 2.3 | 13.6 ± 2.6 |

Data are means ± S.E. from 9-18 segments per group.

Table 5: Accumulative transfer of luminal $P_i$ and calcium into the serosal compartment

| Inhibition by | $P_i$ (nmol/g tissue) | | Ca | |
|---|---|---|---|---|
| | -D | +D | -D | +D |
| - | 153 ± 6 | 334 ± 40[a] | 61 ± 8 | 122 ± 12[a] |
| $Na^+$-free | 174 ± 16 | 160 ± 60[b] | 64 ± 8 | 150 ± 10[a] |
| Cyto. B 50 µM | 144 ± 20 | 123 ± 11[b] | 54 ± 8 | 78 ± 8[a,b] |

Data are expressed as mean ± S.E. of 12-14 determinations. a, significantly different from -D group at least at P<0.05. b, significantly different from respective control group at least at P < 0.05

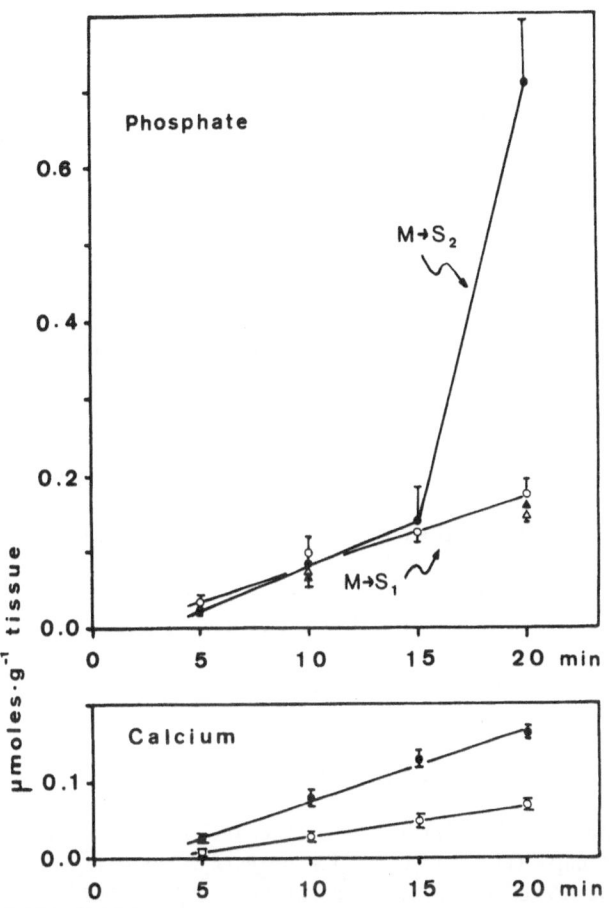

Figure 1: Accumulation of luminal $P_i$ (upper panel)
and calcium (lower panel) in the serosal
compartment of everted chick jejunum
•, +D, 143 mM $Na^+$ in incubation solution;
o, −D, 143 mM $Na^+$;
▲, +D, $Na^+$-free incubation buffer
△, −D, $Na^+$-free;
Each data point is the mean ± S.E. from
9−18 determinations.

Transcellular Movement of Phosphate and Calcium

As shown before, vitamin D-induced mucosal-to-
serosal $P_i$ transfer is via a transcellular route. This
pathway can be completely blocked by addition of 50 μM
cytochalasin B to the mucosal bathing solution (Tab. 5).
The inhibitor which is known to disrupt microfilaments
at this dose level (12) does not affect $P_i$ influx (data
not shown). Whether blocking of subsequent intracellular
migration of $P_i$ is due to disintegration of the entero-
cytic microfilamentous system or by cytochalasin B
action on $P_i$ release across the serosal surface, is not
known at present.

While vitamin D-induced $P_i$ transfer is abolished by
cytochalasin B, calcium transfer in the +D group is reduced only by 30 percent (Tab. 5).


CONCLUSIONS

The data presented in this study allow to establish
a tentative model of intestinal phosphate transport
(Fig. 2). The immediate appearance of a small fraction
of luminal phosphate on the serosal side suggests the
possibility of a direct exchange between the two compartments which may take place across the intercellular
junctions (M-$S_1$ flux). In vitamin D-deficient animals,
mucosal-to-serosal $P_i$ transport occurs mainly via this
diffusional, low permeability pathway.

Uptake of $P_i$ from the lumen through the mucosal
phosphate pump (M-$C$ flux) is insufficient to match the
simultaneous backflux of cellular $P_i$, resulting in net
secretion into the lumen in –D animals (2). After repletion with vitamin $D_3$, the activity of the phosphate
pump is effectively increased to channel $P_i$ into a
cytochalasin B-sensitive intracellular pathway for final
release into the serosal compartment (M-$S_2$ flux).

Vitamin D regulates the activity of the mucosal
phosphate pump, its actual efficiency being controlled
by luminal $Na^+$. $P_i$ entry can be blocked by either inhibitors of sodium-linked transport processes or by
competition for the energy provided by the $Na^+$-gradient.
Unlike the renal system, intestinal phosphate transport
is apparently not regulated by cellular cAMP.

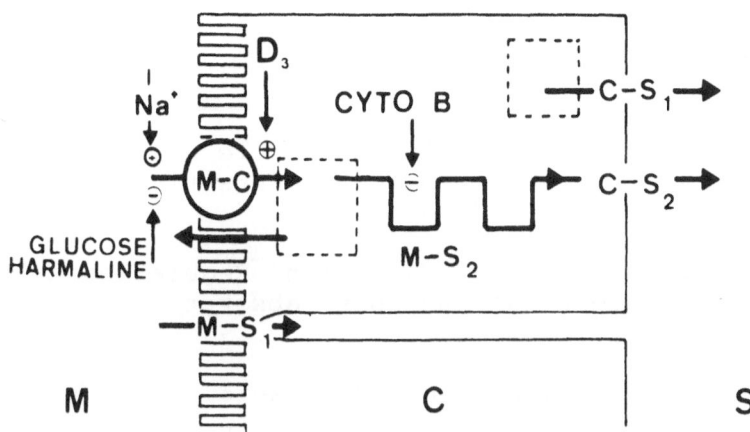

Figure 2: Tentative model of intestinal $P_i$ transport. Stimulatory or inhibitory action is indicated by positive or negative sign, respectively.

ACKNOWLEDGEMENTS

These investigations were supported by Grant No. 3031 of the Fonds zur Förderung der wissenschaftlichen Forschung in Österreich. The capable technical assistance of Peter Wyskovsky is thankfully acknowledged.

REFERENCES

1. M. Peterlik and R. H. Wasserman, Effect of vitamin $D_3$ and 1,25-dihydroxyvitamin $D_3$ on intestinal transport[3] of phosphate, in: "Phosphate Metabolism", S. G. Massry and E. Ritz, eds., Plenum Press, New York (1977)

2. M. Peterlik and R. H. Wasserman, Effect of vitamin D on transepithelial phosphate transport in chick intestine, Am. J. Physiol. 234:E379 (1978)

3. M. Peterlik, Vitamin D-dependent phosphate transport
   by chick intestine: inhibition by low sodium and
   N-ethyl maleimide, in: "Homeostasis of Phosphate and
   Other Minerals", S. G. Massry, E. Ritz and A. Rapado,
   eds., Plenum Press, New York (1978)

4. M. Peterlik, Phosphate transport by embryonic chick
   duodenum: stimulation by vitamin $D_3$, Biochim. Biophys. Acta 514:164 (1978)

5. S. J. Birge and R. Miller, The role of phosphate in
   the action of vitamin D on the intestine, J. Clin.
   Invest. 60:980 (1977)

6. M. Peterlik and R. H. Wasserman, Regulation by vitamin D of intestinal phosphate absorption, Horm.
   Metab. Res., in press

7. M. W. Walling, Intestinal inorganic phosphate transport, in: "Homeostasis of Phosphate and Other Minerals", S. G. Massry, E. Ritz and A. Rapado, eds.,
   Plenum Press, New York (1978)

8. F. V. Sepúlveda and J. W. L. Robinson, Harmaline, a
   potent inhibitor of sodium-dependent transport,
   Biochim. Biophys. Acta 373:527 (1974)

9. M. Peterlik, Experimentelle Cholestase durch Nuper-
   cain und Harmalin: Wirkungen auf die Gallesekretion
   und auf den aktiven Transport von Gallensäuren,
   Ethacrynsäure und g-Strophanthin in der isolierten
   Leber, Wien. klin. Wschr. 89:414 (1977)

10. V. W. Dennis and P. C. Brazy, Phosphate and glucose
    transport in the proximal convoluted tubule: mutual
    dependence on sodium, in: "Homeostasis of Phosphate
    and Other Minerals", S. G. Massry, E. Ritz and
    A. Rapado, eds., Plenum Press, New York (1978)

11. L. R. Chase and G. D. Aurbach, Parathyroid function
    and the renal excretion of 3',5'-adenylic acid,
    Proc. Natl. Acad. Sci. USA 58:518 (1967)

12. S. Lin, D. C. Lin and M. D. Flanagan, Specificity
    of the effects of cytochalasin B on transport and
    motile processes, Proc. Natl. Acad. Sci. USA 75:329
    (1978)

GUT ABSORPTION OF CALCIUM:   INTERACTIONS BETWEEN PHOSPHATE AND

VITAMIN D

N. Brautbar, M.W. Walling and J.W. Coburn

Department of Medicine, Division of Nephrology,
Wadsworth V.A. Hospital, and the Department of Medicine,
University of California, Los Angeles School of Medicine,
Los Angeles, California, 90024

INTRODUCTION

The role of dietary phosphorus (P) in the gut absorption of
calcium (Ca) has been investigated in vitamin D-replete animals and
vitamin D-deficient animals receiving exogenous vitamin D[1,2].
However, these studies did not differentiate the role of dietary P,
independent of the role of vitamin D.

Birge and Miller[3], utilizing in vitro studies, have suggested
that intracellular P is an important mediator of intestinal Ca
transport.

We have recently reported a decreased intestinal absorption of
Ca in rats fed a P-deficient diet[4].  Ribovitch et al[2] have shown
that rats fed a low-P diet have a higher intestinal Ca transport
than rats fed a normal-P diet, when both groups are given either
vitamin $D_3$, $25(OH)D_3$, or $1,25(OH)_2D_3$.  These authors suggested that
low dietary P has an effect on the intestinal Ca transport in addition to its stimulation of $1,25(OH)_2D_3$.  Thus, it seems that these
in vitro and in vivo data conflict with regard to the role of P in
the mediation of intestinal calcium transport.

We designed this study to evaluate the role of dietary P in
intestinal Ca transport and to study the interaction of dietary P
with vitamin D sterols.

METHODS

Weanling male Holtzman rats (Holtzman Co., Madison, WI) were

fed an artificially prepared, vitamin D-deficient diet[5] containing
0.3% P and 0.5% Ca for six weeks.  When hypocalcemia was prominent--
serum calcium 1.70±0.05 mM (mean±SE)--and the animals weighed
between 140 and 160 grams, they were randomly separated into diet
groups and housed in individual metabolic cages.  Three-day pooled
fecal samples were collected and blood samples were obtained from
the tail vein on alternate days.  The animals were divided into
two groups:  those receiving a low-phosphorus (0.03%) diet (LP) and
those receiving a normal-phosphorus (0.3%) diet (NP).  After the
animals had received the vitamin D-deficient diet (LP or NP) for
three days, each group was subdivided into three subgroups of 8-10
animals.  These animals then received a vitamin D sterol or equivalent amount of vehicle as indicated in Table 1.  The quantity of
vitamin $D_3$ given was that considered to be a normal replacement
dose[6], while the quantity of $1,25(OH)_2D_3$ given was that needed for
maintenance of growth and normal serum calcium levels[7].  The vitamin D sterol or vehicle was injected intraperitoneally at 9:00 A.M.
on days 3,5,7, and 8.  Vitamin $D_3$ was obtained from N.V. Phillips-
Dupher (Weesp, The Netherlands); $1,25(OH)_2D_3$ was provided by
Dr. M. Uskokovic (Hoffman-LaRoche, Nutley, New Jersey).

    Serum Ca was analyzed by EGTA titration utilizing the Automatic
Calcium Analyzer (Calcette[R], Precision Scientific Instruments,
Chicago) and fecal Ca by spectrometry (Perkin-Elmer Model 303,
Perkin-Elmer Corp., South Pasadena, Ca).  Serum P was measured by

### TABLE 1.  TREATMENT GROUPS AND ABBREVIATIONS

| TREATMENT | DOSE | DIETARY PHOSPHORUS | |
|---|---|---|---|
| | | 0.03% (LP) | 0.3% (NP) |
| | | DESIGNATION | |
| Vehicle (IP)* | 0.20 ml every other day | LP+D | NP+D |
| Vitamin $D_3$* | 1.25 µg/0.20 ml** every other day | LP+D | NP+D |
| $1,25(OH)_2D_3$ | 54 ng every other day | LP+D | NP+D |

 *Vehicle=ethanol:propanediol, 1:1

**Equivalent to 50 IU

the malachite green micromethod[8] and fecal P by the standard Technicon Autoanalyzer method[5]. The fecal pools were dried overnight, ashed at 400°C for 8 hours, dissolved in 6 ml of 70% hydrochloric acid and analyzed for Ca and P.

The rats were pair-fed and dietary P and Ca were related to the daily food intake. Intestinal absorption of Ca is expressed as percentage utilization and is calculated by the formula:

dietary CA/day-fecal Ca/day $\div$ fecal Ca X 100.

The statistical analysis included one-way analysis of variance, Dunnett's test for multiple group comparison[9], and multiple correlations performed in a manner previously described[10].

RESULTS

Intestinal Utilization of Calcium

Ca utilization in the LP-D and LP+D rats is shown in Figure 1. Although D-deficient, with adequate dietary P the NP rats had low but positive intestinal Ca utilization in the range of 15-20%. However, with LP diets significant Ca malabsorption developed (Figure 1) ($p < 0.01$).

The intestinal response of the LP rats to vitamin $D_3$ or to $1,25(OH)_2D_3$ administration is shown in Figure 1. The overt malabsorption of Ca induced with dietary P restriction was corrected with administration of either $D_3$ or $1,25(OH)_2D_3$. With $D_3$ administration, a 60% intestinal utilization was reached by days 7-9. With $1,25(OH)_2D_3$, the response was rapid, reaching a level of 59% and suggesting a positive response of the gut to the action of $D_3$ or $1,25(OH)_2D_3$ even in the absence of luminal P.

The intestinal utilization of Ca in response to $D_3$ or $1,25(OH)_2D_3$ in NP rats is shown in Figure 1. The adminstration of either of these compounds caused an immediate and significant increase as early as the second fecal pool collection (days 4-6).

Relation Between Serum P and Intestinal Utilization of Calcium

From Table 2 it can be seen that the increase in intestinal utilization of calcium in the LP rats occurred in the face of significant hypophosphatemia whether the rats were treated with $1,25(OH)_2D_3$ or vitamin $D_3$.

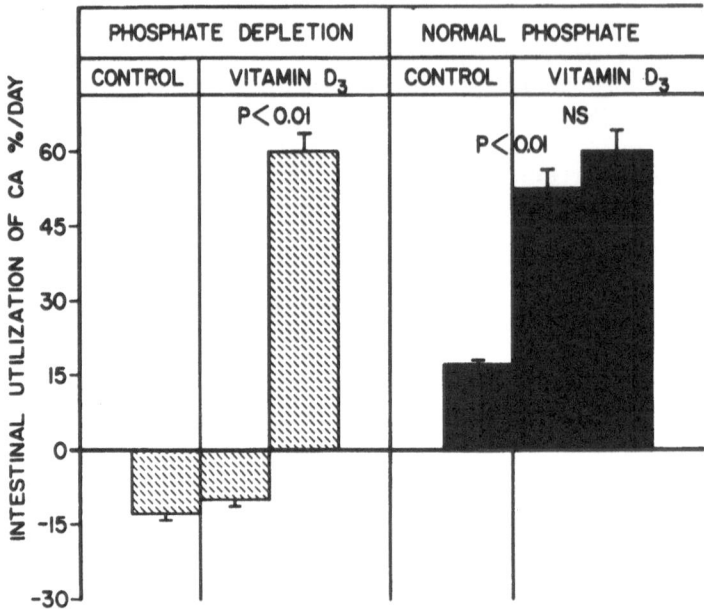

Figure 1.   Intestinal utilization of calcium (Ca) in D deficient rats
during phosphate depletion (-P diet).   Control (Day 1-3) and administration of vitamin $D_3$ and $1,25(OH)_2D_3$.   Each group represents 8-10
rats.   Results expressed as MEAN±SEM.

<u>Relationship between Dietary Intake of Calcium and Intestinal Utili-</u>
<u>zation of Calcium:</u>

     The dietary intake of Ca expressed as mg/day was 54.3±36.2 (SEM)
in the -D+P rats, as compared to 62.7±7.5 (SEM; p> 0.05) in the
-D-P rats.   These results suggest no relation between the dietary
intake of calcium and intestinal utilization of calcium.

DISCUSSION

     A significant malabsorption of Ca develops if P is not present
in the gut, in the D-deficient rat.   This malabsorption of Ca is not
a function of dietary Ca, since the amount of Ca consumed per day
was the same, and is not attributable to growth differences since no
significant differences were noted in the growth rates between the
groups.   Since both LP and NP groups were D-deficient, it seems
that a mechanism independent of vitamin D is operable.

     The only differences between these LP and NP rats are dietary P
and serum P concentrations.   Intestinal calcium transport has been
shown to be an energy dependent process that moves Ca against

TABLE 2.   CHANGES IN SERUM PHOSPHORUS

| Diet | | Control | Vitamin D Administration | | |
| --- | --- | --- | --- | --- | --- |
| | | | Day 2 | Day 6 | Day 9 |
| LP | Vehicle | | | 0.3 ±0.1 | 0.4 ±0.2 |
| LP | $D_3$ | 2.0 ±0.1 | 0.21 ±0.03 | 1.7 ±0.11 | 1.0 ±0.11 |
| LP | 1,25 | | | 1.5 ±0.21 | 1.21 ±0.12 |
| NP | Vehicle | | | 1.91 ±0.14 | 2.25 ±0.12 |
| NP | $D_3$ | 2.0 ±0.1 | 2.15 ±0.18 | 3.81 ±0.21 | 2.71 ±0.18 |
| NP | | | | 3.31 ±0.16 | 0.16 ±0.18 |

concentration gradients[11,12]. It is possible that P may influence the energy stores of the intestinal cells. Phosphate depletion has been associated with a significant decrease in intracellular inorganic P and ATP in muscle and in kidney, as well as in red blood cells[13,14]. We did not measure intestinal brush border ATP or inorganic P concentration, but it is possible that intracellular energy stores were depleted and thus Ca transport was affected. That this defect is specific for Ca and is not a nonspecific malfunction of the intestinal mucosa is suggested from short-circuit current studies in these rats[15]. These observations suggest that while the intestinal mucosa is intact as far as short-circuit current, there may be a specific defect for Ca transport.

It seems logical to assume that P affects a specific mechanism for Ca transport in the absence of intraluminal P. This postulate is in agreement both with early observations (9,16), suggesting that intraluminal P is crucial for intestinal absorption of Ca, and with the recent observation that intracellular P concentration influences transcellular Ca transport[1].

With administration of vitamin $D_3$ or $1,25(OH)_2D_3$ to LP rats this malabsorption is improved, and significantly positive intestinal absorption of Ca develops.

We conclude that intestinal absorption of calcium in the vitamin D-deficient rat is phosphate dependent and probably represents a mechanism specific for calcium transport mediated by intracellular P concentrations. A generalized mucosal defect cannot be excluded, since fecal analysis for sodium, amino acids and glucose are not available.

REFERENCES

1.  M.L. Ribovich and H.F. DeLuca, Effects of dietary calcium and phosphate on intestinal calcium absorption and vitamin D metabolism. Arch. Biochem. Biophys. 188:145 (1978).
2.  M.L. Ribovich and H.F. DeLuca, The influence of dietary calcium and phosphorus on intestinal calcium transport in rats given vitamin D metabolites. Arch. Biochem. Biophys. 170:529 (1975).
3.  S.J. Birge and R. Miller, The role of phosphate in the action of vitamin D on the intestine. J. Clin. Invest. 60:980 (1977).
4.  D.N.B. Lee, N. Brautbar, M.W. Walling, J.W. Coburn and C.R. Kleeman, Evidence against intestinal calcium hyperabsorption in phosphorus depleted rats. Am. J. Physiol. (in press).
5.  J.W. Coburn and S.G. Massry, Changes in serum and urinary calcium during phosphate depletion: Studies on mechanisms. J. Clin. Invest. 49:1073 (1970).
6.  H. Steenbock and C. Herting, Vitamin D and growth. J. Nutr. 57: 449 (1955).
7.  U. Trohler, J.P. Bonjour and H. Fleisch, Inorganic phosphate homeostasis. Renal adaptation to the dietary intake in intact and thyroparathyroidectomized rats. J. Clin. Invest. 57:264, (1976).
8.  W. Hohenwallner and E. Wimmer, The malachite green micromethod for the determination of inorganic phosphate. Clinica Chim. Acta 45:169 (1973).
9.  C.W. Dunnett, A multiple comparison procedure for comparing several treatments with a control. Am. Statis. Assoc. J. 50: 1096 (1955).
10. M.W. Walling and D.V. Kimberg, Active secretion of calcium by adult rat ileum and jejunum in vitro. Am. J. Physiol. 225: 415 (1968).
11. S.J. Birge, H.R. Gilbert and L.V. Avioli, Intestinal calcium transport: The role of sodium. Science 176:168 (1972).
12. M.W. Walling and S.S. Rothman, Phosphate independent, carrier-mediated active transport of calcium by rat intestine. Am. J. Physiol. 217:1144 (1969).
13. W.J. Kreusser, K. Kurokawa, E. Aznar and S.G. Massry, Phosphate depletion: Effect on inorganic phosphorus and adenine nucleotides, urinary phosphate and calcium, and calcium balance. Miner. Elect. Metab. 1:30 (1978).

14.  M.W. Lichtman, D.R. Miller, J. Cohen, and C. Waterhouse, Red-
       wall red cell glycolysis, 2,3-diphosphoglycerate and adenosine
       triphosphate concentration, and increased hemoglobin oxygen
       affinity caused by hypophosphatemia.  Ann. Intern. Med. 74:
       562 (1971).
15.  M.W. Walling, N. Brautbar, and J.W. Coburn, Jejunal phosphate
       active transport:  Effects of phosphorus depletion of vitamin
       D.  Fed. Proc. 36:1097 (1977).
16.  K.M. Henry and S.K. Kon, The effect of age and the supply of
       phosphorus on the assimilation of calcium by the rat.
       Biochemical J. 41:169 (1947).

# CHARACTERIZATION OF PHOSPHATE UPTAKE IN ISOLATED CHICK INTESTINAL CELLS

Richard Avioli, Ruth A. Miller, and Stanley J. Birge

The Jewish Hospital of St. Louis, Washington University
School of Medicine, St. Louis, Missouri  63110

The action of vitamin D on phosphate homeostasis and, specifically, intestinal phosphate transport has assumed an increasingly prominent role in the overall physiologic action of vitamin D.  More rapid advances in this area are limited by the available experimental models for the study of intestinal phosphate transport.  In vitro tissue preparations are required to eliminate the systemic metabolism of vitamin D to both active and inactive derivatives.  In the past, such in vitro preparations have involved intact tissue (1-3).  The interpretation of those studies utilizing these preparations is complicated by the large extracellular space and paracellular transport.  Secondly, the physiologic site of vitamin D action, the basal-lateral membrane, is not accessible to the vitamin in these in vitro incubations.  For these reasons a preparation of isolated intestinal cells was evaluated as an experimental model for the study of phosphate transport and the influence of vitamin D on the cellular accumulation of phosphate.

## Methods and Materials

Preparation of cells was essentially by the method of Harrison and Webster (4) utilizing the isolation buffer of Kimmich (5). White leg-horn chicks were maintained on a rachitogenic diet supplemented with 0.4% phosphate.  Everted sacs of the proximal intestine were incubated in a physiologic salt solution with 1 mM glucose, buffered with 30 mM HEPES at pH 7.4, containing 0.01% bovine hyaluronidase and gased with 95% $O_2$ for 15 min. at $34^\circ C$.  The intestine epithelial cells were dislodged from the intestine by sliding the everted intestinal sac over a vibrating stirring rod.  The rod was oscillated at an amplitude of 4 mm for 3 min. at $4^\circ C$ in the above incubation buffer without hyaluronidase but containing 4.5%

ficol.  The resulting cell suspension was collected by centrifugation at 400 x g for 8 min.  The cells were resuspended in incubation
buffer to give 400,000 cells/ml.  A 0.5 ml aliquot of the cell suspension was delivered onto a Whatman #541 filter supported by a
2.5 cm Millipore filter apparatus over a gentle vacuum.  This filter
was selected because it did not retain broken cell fragments and
nuclei.

Incubation of cells was carried out in 60 x 15 mm Falcon #3011
organ culture dishes under an atmosphere of 95% $O_2$ and 5% $CO_2$ at
34°C.  Prior to the determination of $^{32}P$ uptake the filter and cells
were incubated for 10 min. in a 0.01% hyaluronidase buffer.  The
filters were then transferred to buffer containing $^{32}P$-phosphate
for the appropriate time interval and at various phosphate concentrations.  Linear rates of phosphate uptake were approximated for
the first 6 to 7 min. depending upon the phosphate concentration.
Accordingly, 6 min. incubations were used for these studies.  The
uptake was terminated by blotting the filters, briefly emersing
them in 10 mM phosphate in saline at pH 6.8 at 4°C then washing the
filters on the Millipore filter support with 80 ml of the above
phosphate buffer.

Results and Discussion

The viability of the cells established by trypan blue exclusion
and measuring the initial rate of $^{32}P$ uptake by the incubated cells.
At 34°C this rate of uptake was constant up to 120 min. of incubation.  The characteristics of the uptake process at .02 and 2.0 mM
phosphate was determined with respect to the dependence of phosphate
accumulation on $Na^+$, and $Ca^{++}$ (Table 1).  Phosphate uptake at both

Table 1.  Characteristics of Isolated Intestinal
Cell Uptake of Phosphate

$^{32}P$-uptake (cpm/mg protein)
% control $\pm$ % S.E.M.[*]

| Conditions | .02 mM $P_i$ | 2.0 mM $P_i$ |
|---|---|---|
| Control | 100 | 100 |
| $-Na^+$ | 26 $\pm$ 8 | 46 $\pm$ 7 |
| $+ Na^+$ + ouabain (1.0 mM) | 46 $\pm$ 8 | 61 $\pm$ 8 |
| $- Ca^{++}$ | 93 $\pm$ 5 | 31 $\pm$ 6 |

Cells were isolated from vitamin D deficient chicks treated
48 hrs. prior to sacrifice with oral vitamin $D_3$   (1000
units).  Pre-incubations for 30 min. were performed in the
complete incubation buffer.  Sodium was replaced by

equimolar concentrations of choline chloride and $Ca^+$
eliminated in the $^{32}P$-uptake incubations only as indicated.
*% S.E.M. is the average of the % S.E.M. of the 4-6 experi-
ments used to derive the $^{32}P$-uptake response to each of
the conditions indicated.

the high and low phosphate concentrations requires $Na^+$ and $K^+$ for
optimum activity.  Although the removal of $Ca^{++}$ from the medium
reduced the uptake of $^{32}P$ at the low phosphate concentration, this
inhibition of $^{32}P$ uptake was several-fold greater at the high phosphate concentration.

The influence of pH on the uptake process was also examined at
different phosphate concentrations by varying the pH of the $^{32}P$
uptake buffer.  Unexpectedly, the influence of pH on $^{32}P$-uptake was
found to be a function of the phosphate concentration (Fig. 1).

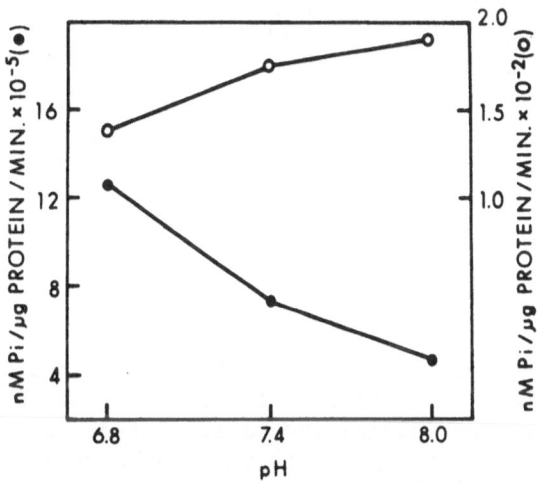

Fig. 1.   The influence of pH on $^{32}P$-uptake by isolated intestinal
          cells.   The cell preparation was preincubated for 30 min.
          in 0.5 mM phosphate and 10 min. in the hyaluronidase
          buffer before transfer to the $^{32}P$-uptake buffer at vary-
          ing pH and phosphate concentrations.

At 0.02 mM phosphate, optimum uptake was observed at pH 6.8 consistent with the observations of others.  However, at phosphate
concentrations of 2.0 mM optimum uptake was at pH 8.0, thus

similar to the renal phosphate transport mechanism (6).   The diver-
gent dependence on Ca$^{++}$ and pH suggests that more than one transport
process may be involved in the accumulation of phosphate by the
isolated intestinal cells.   A double reciprocal plot of the rate of
phosphate uptake as a function of phosphate concentration also
suggested the presence of two saturable processes with a Km .08 mM
and 1.67 mM, respectively.   The addition of 40 ng/ml of 25-hydroxy-
cholecalciferol to the incubation buffer results in the stimulation
of $^{32}$P uptake both in the presence and absence of 1.4 mM Ca$^{++}$.
Although in the presence of Ca$^{++}$, this stimulation was more
pronounced (Fig. 2).

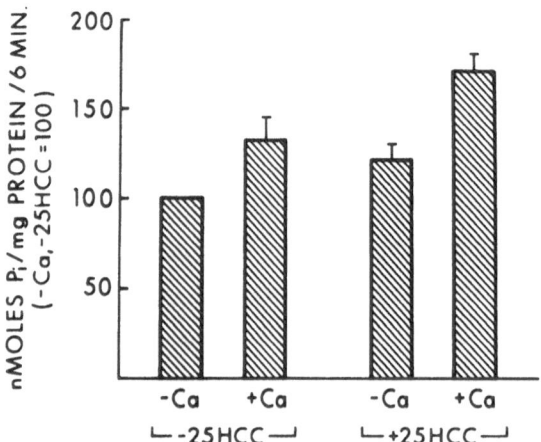

Fig. 2.   The influence of 25-hydroxycholecalciferol on $^{32}$P-uptake
          by isolated intestinal cells from vitamin D deficient
          chicks.   The initial incubation buffer contained the
          vitamin (40 ng/ml) or its vehicle, partially purified
          human vitamin D binding protein (70 μg/ml).   The cells
          were incubated for 60 min. before transfer to hyaluroni-
          dase buffer and the $^{32}$P-uptake conditions.

     These observations suggest that in the isolated intestinal
cell there are at least two mechanisms for the uptake of phosphate,
a low affinity, calcium dependent transport process which is facilitated by alkaline pH and a high affinity, calcium independent transport process which is enhanced by acidic pH.   These studies do not
address the question as to the localization of the two transport
processes with respect to the basal-lateral or brush-border

membranes.  Transport of phosphate across brush-border vesicles
has essentially all the features which characterize the high
affinity transport process in the isolated cell (7).  Localization
of the low affinity process is more difficult.  Several investigators have demonstrated a dependence of phosphate uptake on $Ca^{++}$ in
intact intestinal tissue which should limit, if not exclude, transport across the basal-lateral membranes (8-10).  However, other
investigators have reported no requirement for $Ca^+$ in similar
experimental models (11-13).  At this point, there is insufficient
data to permit the localization of this low affinity transport
process.  These studies clearly indicate, however, that in
characterizing intestinal phosphate transport, it is necessary to
monitor the uptake process over a range of phosphate concentrations.
Some of the discrepancies in the literature may therefore be the
result of experimental designs which would not permit the appreciation of more than one phosphate transport mechanism.

## Summary

A preparation of isolated intestinal cells has been developed
which permits the incubation of these cells in culture for 90 min.
with preservation of viability and responsiveness to vitamin D
analogues added in vitro.  Characterization of phosphate transport
suggested the presence of two transport processes which differed
in their affinity for phosphate, calcium stimulation, and pH
dependence.  Both processes were facilitated by sodium transport.
This cell preparation promises to be a valuable experimental model
for the elucidation of the action of vitamin D on phosphate
transport.

## References

1.   S. J. Birge and R. A. Miller, The role of phosphate in the
      action of vitamin D in the intestine, J. Clin. Invest. 60:
      980 (1977).
2.   R. L. Morrissey, D. T. Zolock, D. D. Bikle, R. N. Empson, and
      T. J. Bucci, Intestinal response to 1α, 25-dihydroxychole-
      calciferol I. RNA polyurase, alkaline phosphatase, calcium
      and phosphorus uptake in vitro, and in vivo calcium transport
      and accumulation, Biochim. Biophys. Acta 538:23  (1978).
3.   M. Peterlik, Phosphate transport by embryonic chick duodenum,
      Biochim. Biophys. Acta 514:164 (1978).
4.   D. D. Harrison and H. L. Webster, The preparation of isolated
      intestinal crypt cells, Exp. Cell Res. 55:257 (1969).
5.   A. Kimmich, Preparation and properties of mucosal epithelial
      cells isolated from small intestine of the chicken, Biochem.
      9:3659 (1970).
6.   N. Hoffmann, M. Thees, and R. Kinne, Phosphate transport by
      isolated renal brush border vesicles, Pflugers Arch. 362:
      147 (1976).

7.  W. Berner, R. Kinne, and H. Murer, Phosphate transport into
    brush border membrane vesicles isolated from rat small
    intestine, Biochem. J. 160:467 (1976).
8.  H. E. Harrison and H. C. Harrison, Intestinal transport of
    phosphate-action of vitamin D, calcium and potassium, Am. J.
    Physiol. 201:1007 (1961).
9.  T. C. Chen, L. Castillo, M. Korycka-Dahl, and H. F. Deluca,
    Role of vitamin D metabolites in phosphate transport of rat
    intestine, J. Nutr. 104:1056 (1974).
10. E. Neville and E. S. Holdworth, Phosphorus metabolism during
    transport of calcium, Biochim. Biophys. Acta 163:362 (1968).
11. R. H. Wasserman and R. N. Taylor, Intestinal absorption of
    phosphate in the chick: effect of vitamin D3 and other
    parameters, J. Nutr. 103:586 (1973).
12. M. W. Walling, Intestinal calcium and phosphate transport:
    differential responses to vitamin D3 metabolites, Am. J.
    Physiol. 233:E488 (1977).
13. S. Kowarski and D. Shachter, Effects of vitamin D on phosphate
    transport and incorporation into mucosal constituents of rat
    intestinal mucosa, J. Biol. Chem. 244:211 (1969).

ROLE OF PHOSPHATE IN THE RESISTANCE TO INTESTINAL EFFECTS OF

PARATHYROID HORMONE IN RATS WITH CHRONIC RENAL FAILURE

T. Drüeke, B. Lacour, and J. Chanard

INSERM U 90, Hôpital Necker, Paris
and CHU Reims
France

INTRODUCTION

PTH decreases phosphate reabsorption in the proximal renal
tubule and also at more distal tubular sites (1). In contrast
to this in vivo effect, PTH has been reported to increase
cellular uptake of $^{32}PO4$ in vitro in a number of tissues
including intestine (2) and kidney (3,4), possibly by stimulating an active, energy-dependent "phosphate-pump" (5). This
apparent discrepancy between observations made in vivo and in
vitro is not well understood at present. In the intestine, PTH
stimulates phosphate absorption indirectly via an increased
formation of 1,25 (OH)2 vitamin D3 (6). A direct effect of PTH
on intestinal transport remains controversial. We have previously reported an acute, inhibitory effect of PTH on intestinal
absorption of sodium, calcium, and water in normal (7) as well
as acutely thyroparathyroidectomized (8) rats.

The purpose of the present study was to investigate in rats
a) whether PTH could also acutely inhibit intestinal phosphate
absorption, b) whether the acute inhibitory effect of PTH on
intestinal electrolyte transport was also observed in chronically uremic rats, and c) whether the phosphorus concentration of

405

the intestinal perfusion played a role in the magnitude of
intestinal electrolyte transport.


MATERIAL AND METHODS

   Chronic renal failure was created in male Wistar AF rats by
cortical electrocoagulation (10) three to four weeks before
study. An identical number of rats were sham operated. Their
diet contained protein 24%, cellulose 6.5%, lipids 4.5%,
vitamin D 200 I.U.%, salt mix 7-9%, and water 12%. The salt
mix contained 0.7% potassium, 0.4% sodium, 1.5% calcium, 0.2%
magnesium, and 0.95% phosphorus. The uremic animals were
allowed free access to food and water. The sham operated
animals had also free access to water but were pair-fed with
the uremic rats. The experimental procedure of jejunal perfusion in situ was performed as described previously (7). The
composition of the jejunal perfusion solution was NaCl 137,
Na HCO3 11.9, KCl 3.4, CaCl2 1.4, MgCl2 0.1, and glucose 5.0 mM,
respectively. The concentration of NaH2 PO4 was either 0.4 mM
("low P" solution) or 3.0 mM ("high P" solution). Initial osmolality of the solution was 296 mOsm/kg and 301 mOsm/kg, respectively ; pH was maintained constant (7.0) by previous bub-
bling of the solution with CO2 (5%) and air (95%). Group I and
II rats received a "low P" jejunal perfusion, group III and IV
rats a "high P" jejunal perfusion. Group I and III animals
were sham-operated control rats while group II and IV rats were
uremic. Half of each group's rats received an intravenous infusion of parathyroid hormone (PTH)(designed by letter a) while
the other half received the PTH vehicle only (designed by
letter b). Each period of PTH or vehicle infusion (corresponding to 4 x 15 min "experimental" jejunal collection periods)
was preceded by a control period of infusion of isotonic ·
Ringer's solution at a rate of 20 µl/min (3x15 min "control"
jejunal collection periods). The i.v. infusion of PTH (0.8 I.U.

1-84 bovine PTH/100 g body weight.hr) was done using an ice-
cold vehicle solution at an infusion rate of 0.32 ml/hr, after
an i.v. priming dose of 0.16 ml (0.4 I.U. 1-84 bovine PTH/100 g
body weight). Following the priming dose, an equilibration
period of 15 min was allowed before experimental collection
periods. The preparation of PTH and vehicle solutions was done
as previously described (7). The degree of uremia was comparable
in group II a and II b rats : their mean ($\pm$ SEM) plasma creatinine concentrations were 1.85$\pm$ 0.16 and 1.6 $\pm$ 0.17 mg/dl, respectively (P = N.S.). Similarly, plasma creatinine concentrations in group IV a and IV b rats were 2.12 $\pm$ 0.31 and 2.2 $\pm$
0.28 mg/dl, respectively (P = N.S.). Mean body weight at time
of study was comprised between 200 and 310 g for uremic rats
and between 240 and 360 g for sham rats.

The analysis of samples was done as follows : sodium concentration by flame photometry, calcium in triplicate by atomic
absorption spectrophotometry (model 403, Perkin-Elmer), phosphate by an automated colorimetric method (9). The pH was determined using a Tacussel pH meter (type TS 4N). Phenolsulfo-
nephtalein (PSP) concentration in jejunal fluid (a marker of
volume changes) was measured in triplicate in alkaline solution
at a wave length of 555 nm using an automated procedure. Calculations were performed as previously described (7). Statistical
analysis of the changes was done using paired Student's t test
comparing intra-series values, and unpaired Student's t test
for inter-series values. The results have been expressed as
means $\pm$ SEM.

RESULTS

The effects of bPTH or its vehicle on jejunal electrolyte
absorption during the two types of phosphate concentration of
the jejunal perfusion solution are shown in Fig.1-3.

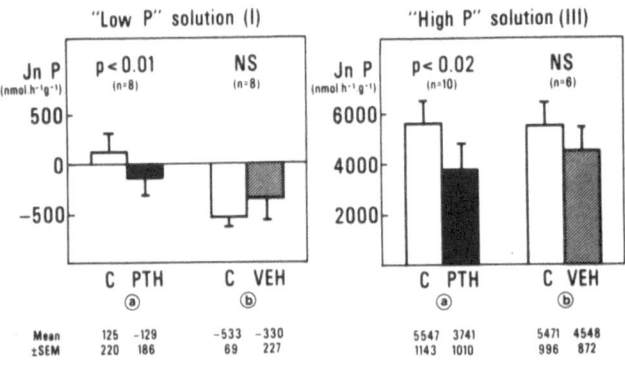

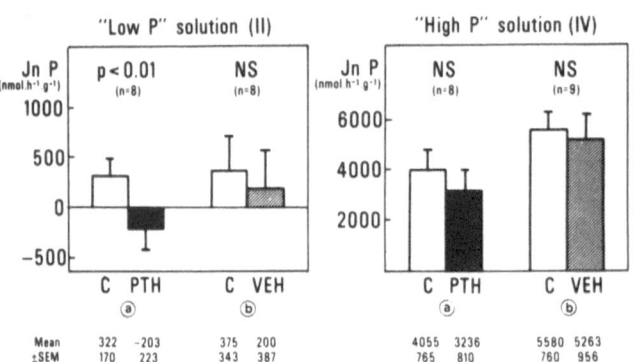

Fig. 1 : Mean (± SEM) net jejunal transport of phosphorus
during 3 control periods (C) and during 4 experimental
periods following either parathyroid hormone infusion
(PTH) or only PTH vehicle (VEH).(+)indicates net absorption from the lumen, (-) indicates net secretion into
the lumen.

"Low P" solution. When using a jejunal perfusion solution
containing 0.4 mM phosphorus ("low P" solution) a significant,
acute decrease in mean net jejunal phosphorus as well as sodium
and calcium absorption was observed after intravenous infusion
of bPTH when compared to the respective mean absorption rates
observed during the preceding control periods. Such decreases
were noted in normal (group I a) as well as in uremic (group
II a) animals. No such effects were found in normal or uremic
animals that received the bPTH vehicle only (groups I b and
II  b, respectively).

"High P" solution. When using a jejunal perfusion solution containing 3.0 mM phosphorus ("high P" solution) the magnitude of
mean net jejunal absorption of phosphorus during control periods
was tenfold higher in normal groups III a and b and in uremic
groups IV a and b rats than in those receiving the "low P" perfusion solution. No substantial difference was observed in the
amount of mean net phosphorus absorption during control periods
between normal (groups III a and b) and uremic (groups IV a and
b) rats. A significant acute decrease in mean net jejunal
absorption of phosphorus and sodium (but not of calcium) was
also observed after i.v. administration of bPTH in normal animals (group III a) when compared to control periods. However,
no such decrease was noted in uremic animals that were infused
identical amounts of bPTH (group IV a). In vehicle infused rats
(groups IIIb and IVb, respectively), the mean absorption rates
of phosphate, sodium and calcium did not change significantly
during experimental periods when compared to their preceding
control periods.

Plasma biochemistry. Mean plasma phosphorus concentration at the
end of experiments was 2.11 $\pm$ 0.15 and 2.1 $\pm$ 0.16 mM in group I a
and I b rats, and 2.21 $\pm$ 0.02 and 2.17 $\pm$ 0.06 mM in group III a
and III b rats respectively. Thus, no difference was observed in

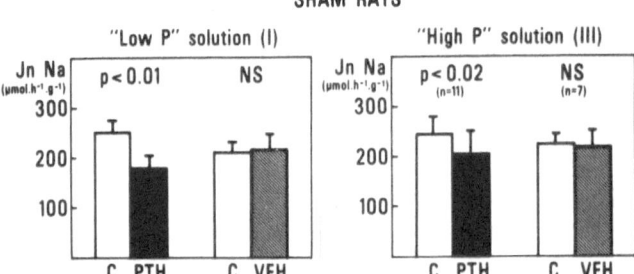

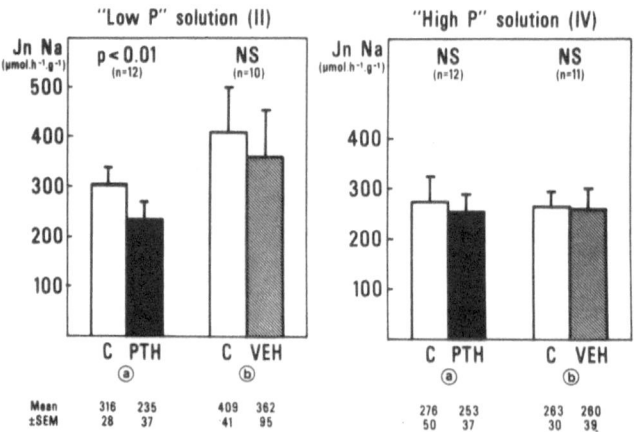

Fig. 2: Mean (± SEM) net jejunal transport of sodium.
Legend as in Fig. 1.

normal rats whether treated by bPTH or not. In uremic rats, differences were noted between rats receiving a jejunal perfusion of
"low P" solution and those receiving "high P" solution : group
II rats ("low P") had a mean plasma phosphorus concentration at
the end of experiments of 3.03 ± 0.20 mM (group II a) and
2.97 ± 0.14 mM (group II b) while group IV rats ("high P") had
3.46 ± 0.24 mM (group IV a) and 3.46 ± 0.13 mM (group IV b)(the
difference reached level of statistical significance only for
group II b vs group IV b rats, p<0.025). Mean plasma phosphorus
concentrations at the end of experiments were significantly
higher in uremic rats than in non-uremic animals independent of
whether bPTH or vehicle was infused. Similarly, mean plasma
calcium concentration at the end of experiments was higher in
uremic animals receiving "low P" perfusion solution (2.45 ± 0.04
mM, group II a ; and 2.56 ± 0.06 mM, group II b) than in uremic
animals receiving "high P" perfusion solution (2.31 ± 0.02 mM,
group IV a ; and 2.32 ± 0.07 mM, group IV b). However , the
difference did not reach level of statistical significance.
In sham operated animals, plasma calcium levels at the end of
experiments were comparable for all four groups : 2.38 ± 0.07 mM
(group I a), 2.32 ± 0.09 mM (group I b), 2.32 ± 0.04 mM (group
III a), and 2.30 ± 0.08 mM (group III b). No significant differences in plasma total protein concentration at the end of experiments were observed between uremic and normal animal groups.


DISCUSSION

 The present data indicate that bPTH can acutely decrease jejunal
absorption of phosphorus as well as that of sodium in normal rats
that undergo a jejunal perfusion using a solution with either
0.4 or 3.0 mM phosphorus. However, in uremic rats bPTH exerted
its inhibitory effect on sodium and phosphorus absorption only
when the jejunal perfusion solution contained 0.4 mM phosphorus
("low P" solution). The inhibitory effect was not observed when
perfusing the 3.0 mM phosphorus ("high P" solution). The cause of

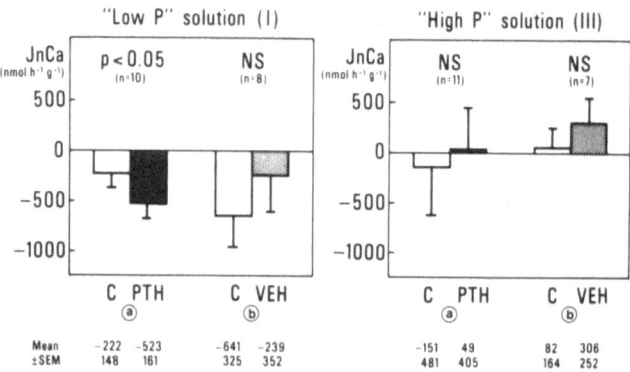

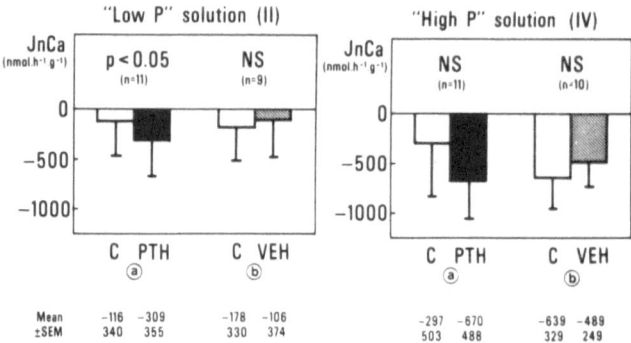

Fig. 3 : Mean (± SEM) net jejunal transport of calcium.
Legend as in Fig. 1.

the blunted  PTH effect in uremic animals perfused with the
"high P" jejunal solution is not clear. Resistance to the calcemic and phosphaturic action of PTH in uremia has been reported
previously : decreased production of 1,25(OH)2 D3, circulating
uremic toxins, and the existence of autoantibodies directed
against cellular PTH receptors have all been incriminated (11-14).
Resistance to the phosphaturic and calcemic action of PTH has
also been reported for other disturbances of phosphorus metabolism such as chronic phosphate depletion (15). However, in one
recent study (16) no resistance to the phosphaturic action of
PTH has been found in uremic dogs fed a normal phosphorus diet
while interestingly the dogs fed a reduced phosphorus diet had
even an exaggerated phosphaturia. Possibly, the difference in
the phosphaturic action of PTH between this study and previous
studies reporting a resistance to PTH action is due to different
PTH doses administered.

In the present experiments a high (but not a low) phosphate concentration of the jejunal perfusion solution prevented exogenous
PTH to induce its acute inhibitory effect on jejunal phosphate
and sodium absorption in uremic animals. In addition to uremia
the phosphate ion must have played a role in the resistance to
PTH. Even in the non-uremic animals, the per cent decrease in
jejunal electrolyte absorption after PTH injection  was less
pronounced in those groups receiving the "high P" than in those
receiving the "low P" perfusion solution. Possible mechanisms
include changes in plasma phosphate and calcium concentration
and/or intracellular phosphate distribution inducing directly or
indirectly changes in phosphate and sodium transport. Indeed,
at the end of experiments plasma calcium tended to be lower, and
plasma phosphate to be higher, in the uremic animals receiving
the "high P" perfusion solution when compared to the uremic animals receiving the "low P" solution. Therefore, circulating endogenous PTH would be expected to be higher in the former than in

the latter. Moreover, similarly to the greater increase in plasma
PTH observed in uremic when compared to normal dogs after an a-
cute oral phosphorus load (17), the increase in circulating endogenous PTH might have been more pronounced in our uremic rats
receiving the "high P" perfusion solution when compared to the
non-uremic animals receiving the same perfusion solution. Such
an increase in endogenous PTH could have contributed to the observed resistance to the action of exogenous PTH. It is possible
that the influence of PTH on jejunal phosphate absorption was
secondary to that on sodium absorption. In our study, changes of
phosphate transport paralleled that of sodium transport. Studies
on brush-border membrane vesicles isolated from rat small intestine (18) and intestinal perfusion studies in man (19) have supported the concept of a sodium dependence of phosphate transport.
The question whether differences in intracellular ion distribution after the two jejunal perfusion procedures may have played
a role in the resistance to PTH action cannot be solved on the
basis of the present experiments.

In conclusion : A resistance to exogenous parathyroid hormone
action was observed in uremic rats in the presence of a phospho-
rus-rich, but not of a phosphorus-poor, jejunal perfusion solution. Whether the phosphate ion plays a more general role in the
resistance to parathyroid hormone on its target cells in uremia
remains to be elucidated.

REFERENCES

1. F.G. Knox, R.F. Greger, F.C. Lang, and G.R. Marchand : Renal
   handling of phosphate : Update, in Phosphate Metabolism, (Advances in Experimental Medicine and Biology, volume 81), edited
   by S.G. Massry and E. Ritz, Plenum Press, New York and London,
   1976, p. 3

2. A.B. Borle, H.T. Kentman, and W.F. Neuman : Role of parathyroid hormone in phosphate transport across rat duodenum. Am.
   J. Physiol. 204 : 705 (1963)

3. J. Egawa and W.F. Neuman : Effect of parathyroid extract on the metabolism of radioactive phosphate in the kidney. Endocrinology 74 :90 (1964)

4. E.M. Rosenberg, S.W. Lee, J. Lee, and L.V. Avioli : Effect of parathyroid hormone, cyclic AMP, dibutyryl cyclic AMP and theophylline on phosphate transport in isolated renal tubular preparations. Proc. Endocrinol. Soc. 1975, p. 322

5. C.P. Geary and F.B. Cousin : Effect of parathyroid extract and glycerol on $^{32}$P uptake in rat renal tissue. Austral. J. Biol. Sci. 49 : 463 (1971)

6. M. Garabedian, Y. Tanaka, M.F. Holick and H.F. De Luca : Responses of intestinal calcium transport and bone calcium mobilization to 1,25-dihydroxyvitamin D3 in thyroparathyroidectomized rats. Endocrinology 94 :1022, (1974)

7. T. Drüeke, J. Chanard, B. Lacour, E. Pujade-Lauraine, and J.L. Funck-Brentano : Effects of hyperoncotic albumin and parathyroid hormone infusion on jejunal electrolyte and water absorption in the rat. Pflügers Arch. 373 : 249 (1978)

8. T. Drüeke, J. Chanard, B. Lacour and J.L. Funck-Brentano : Effects of parathyroid hormone and thyrocalcitonin on jejunal transport of sodium, calcium, and water in rats, in Procedings of the 27 th International Congress of Physiological Sciences, Paris, 1977, volume 13, p. 196

9. C.C. Mabry, I.E. Roeckel , R.E. Gevedon, J.A. Koepke : Automated submicrochemistries. In : Recent advances in pediatric clinical pathology, Grune and Stratton Corp. eds, New York, London, 1968, p. 63.

10.J. Boudet, N.K. Man, P. Pils, A. Sausse and J.L. Funck-Brentano : Experimental chronic renal failure in the rat by electrocoagulation of the renal cortex. Kidney Internat. 14 : 82 (1978)

11.S.G. Massry, J.W. Coburn, D.B.N. Lee, J. Jowsey, C.R. Kleeman: Skeletal resistance to parathyroid hormone in renal failure: Studies in 105 human subjects. Ann. Int. Med 78 : 357 (1973)

12. S.G. Massry, R. Stein, J. Garty, A.I. Arieff, J.W. Coburn, A.W. Norman and R.M. Friedler : Skeletal resistance to the calcemic action of parathyroid hormone in uremia : Role of 1,25(OH)2 D3. Kidney Internat. 9 : 467, (1976)

13. P.J. Somerville and M. Kaye : Resistance to parathyroid hormone in renal failure : Role of vitamin D metabolites. Kidney Internat. 14 : 245 (1978)

14. H. Jüppner, Bialasiewicz A.A. and R.D. Hesch : Autoantibodies to parathyroid hormone receptor. Lancet 2 : 1222 (1978)

15. H.J. Gloor, J.P. Bonjour, J. Caverzasio and H. Fleisch : Resistance to the phosphaturic and calcemic actions of parathyroid hormone during phosphate depletion. J. Clin. Invest. 63 : 371 (1979)

16. M.A. Kaplan, J.M. Canterbury, G. Gavellas, D. Jaffe , J.J. Bourgoignie, E. Reiss, and N.S. Bricker : The calcemic and phosphaturic effects of parathyroid hormone in the normal and uremic dog. Metabolism 27 : 1785 (1978)

17. M.A. Kaplan, J.M. Canterbury, G. Gavellas, D. Jaffe, Bourgoignie J.J., E. Reiss and N.S. Bricker : Interrelations between phosphorus, calcium, parathyroid hormone, and renal phosphate excretion in response to an oral phosphorus load in normal and uremic dogs. Kidney Internat. 14 : 297 (1978).

18. W. Berner, R. Kinne, and H. Murer : Phosphate transport into brush-border membrane vesicles isolated from rat small intestine. Biochem. J. 160 : 467 (1976)

19. J. Walton and T.K. Gray : Absorption of inorganic phosphate in the human small intestine. Clin. Sci. 56 : 407 (1979)

ACKNOWLEDGMENT

The authors wish to thank Mrs D. Coraboeuf and E. Pierandrei for the technical assistance and Mrs D. Mavroyannis for excellent secretarial help.

# METABOLIC STUDIES OF THE CYTOSOLIC CALCIUM-BINDING PROTEIN OF THE RAT

Felix Bronner, T.-H. Ueng and Michael Buckley

Department of Oral Biology, The University of Connecticut
Health Center, Farmington, CT 06032 (USA)

Biosynthesis of the calcium-binding protein (CaBP) found in
mucosal scrapings or isolated cells of rat intestinal mucosa (1)
requires 1,25-dihydroxyvitamin $D_3$ (1,25-$(OH)_2$-$D_3$), the dihydroxylated metabolite of vitamin D (2). Studies of this process have
suggested (3,4) that it is akin to steroid hormone induced protein
synthesis, involving a sequence of two cytosolic and one nuclear
receptor for 1,25-$(OH)_2$-$D_3$, with CaBP synthesis the ultimate
result. Cell-free translation of the chick CaBP, a larger molecule,
and of the pig CaBP (MW $\approx$ 10,000, like that of the rat [5]) has
been effected (6,7). In addition to an absolute requirement for
1,25-$(OH)_2$-$D_3$, CaBP biosynthesis is also regulated by calcium,
inasmuch as animals on high calcium intakes have low levels of
CaBP, while low calcium intakes are associated with much higher
CaBP levels (5,8,9). Moreover, in vitro studies with isolated
intestinal cells have suggested (10) that raising the calcium
concentration of the medium depresses the amount of CaBP that can
be synthesized. In addition, the calcium status of the whole
animal affects the amount of circulating 1,25-$(OH)_2$-$D_3$, with
larger amounts circulating and reaching the intestinal target
cells in animals on low calcium intakes (11).

The mechanism by which calcium status affects 1,25-$(OH)_2$-$D_3$
production in the kidney is not understood; it may involve a
direct effect of calcium (12), as well as parathyroid hormone (13).
Thus regulation of CaBP biosynthesis is a function of the amount
of circulating 1,25-$(OH)_2$-$D_3$ and of the calcium status, each of
which independently appears to affect CaBP biosynthesis. In addition, a feedback loop appears to exist between calcium intake and
1,25-$(OH)_2$-$D_3$ production. The studies to follow were done in an

417

F. BRONNER ET AL.

attempt to by-pass in vivo the feedback loop between calcium intake
and $1,25-(OH)_2-D_3$ production so as to be able to assess independently
the effects of $1,25-(OH)_2-D_3$ and calcium status.  As will be shown,
response to exogenous $1,25-(OH)_2-D_3$ is a function of the calcium
status of the animal, while rate of biosynthesis of CaBP is a
function of the animal's vitamin D status.


MATERIALS AND METHODS

     Male Sprague-Dawley rats, purchased from ARS, Madison, WI
were either placed on vitamin D-deficient diets at weaning (35-50g)
or on D-replete semisynthetic regimens when they weighed 120-140g.
The diets, described previously (5,14,15), contained either 0.06% Ca,
0.2% P (I) or 1.5% Ca, 1.5% P (III) and 2200 i.u. vitamin $D_2$/kg.
The vitamin D-deficient diet, 1.5% Ca, 1.5% P, contained no added
vitamin D (III-D).  The diets were purchased from Teklad Mills,
Madison, WI under the following codes:  I:  TD78245; III:  TD78349;
III-D:  TD78250.  Vitamin D deficiency was established from plasma
calcium measurements done by atomic absorptiometry (14) and from
duodenal CaBP levels, determined by means of an equilibrated column
procedure (1).  CaBP content is expressed as nmol $Ca_b$/gm mucosa,
with 1 nmol Ca $\rightleftharpoons$ 0.5 nmol CaBP.


RESULTS

     Fig. 1 shows the results of an experiment in which two groups
of vitamin D-replete animals were treated with increasing doses of
$1,25-(OH)_2-D_3$.  The untreated animals on diet III had a base level
of 43.3 ± 2.1 (SE) nmol $Ca_b$/gm mucosa.  Progressive doses of
$1,25-(OH)_2-D_3$ led to a concentration-dependent increase in CaBP.
The response appears to have reached a plateau with a dose of 0.5µg,
as CaBP levels of animals treated with 0.75µg did not increase beyond
those of animals treated with 0.5µg.

     In the case of the animals fed the low-calcium diet I, the
situation was different.  Their base level of CaBP was more than
double that of the animals fed diet III, i.e., 112 ± 3.7 nmol $Ca_b$/gm
mucosa, but treatment with $1,25-(OH)_2-D_3$ failed to increase CaBP
levels which, as can be seen from Fig. 1, averaged 105.6 ± 3.1 nmol
$Ca_b$/gm mucosa in the five groups of two treated animals each, a
value that does not differ statistically from the control level of
the animals fed diet I.  It therefore appears that when animals fed
a high calcium diet are treated with $1,25-(OH)_2-D_3$, their CaBP level
can be increased to near the level found in animals fed a low calcium
diet, but that treatment of the latter is ineffective in raising
the CaBP concentration further.  The response to exogenous $1,25-$
$(OH)_2-D_3$ thus appears to depend on prior calcium intake.

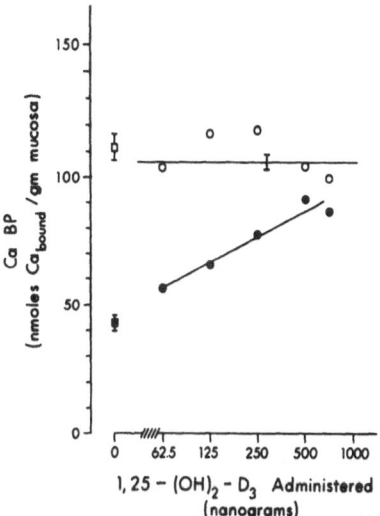

Fig. 1. CaBP response of vitamin D-replete animals on a low calcium diet (open symbols) or a high calcium diet (closed symbols) to the intraperitoneal injection of varying doses of 1,25-(OH)$_2$-D$_3$. The animals were sacrificed 3 hr after treatment. The square symbols represent CaBP levels in controls, two groups of two animals each, shown as the means with standard error bars. The circles represent values on pooled samples derived from two animals each. The line through the closed circles was derived by a least squares procedure; the line through the open circles is the mean, shown with its standard error bar. It does not differ significantly from the mean value of the low-calcium controls.

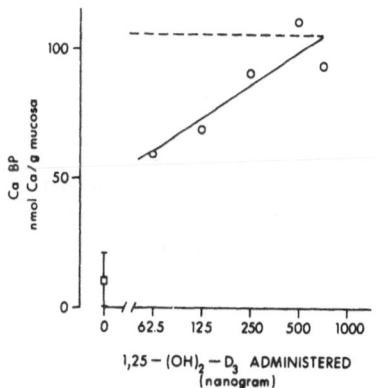

Fig. 2. CaBP response of vitamin D-deficient animals, placed from weaning on a high calcium diet without added vitamin D (III-D). The square symbol (with its standard error bar) refers to the mean CaBP level of two groups of untreated animals, killed at the beginning and end of the experiment. The open circles refer to CaBP values of groups of two animals each, treated as shown. The solid line was derived by a least squares procedure. The dashed line refers to the mean CaBP levels of the vitamin D-replete animals on a low calcium diet.

To determine whether vitamin D status affects the quantitative response to exogenous $1,25-(OH)_2-D_3$, animals that had been depleted of vitamin D while fed a high calcium diet (III-D) were treated with the same increasing doses of the metabolite. Fig. 2 shows that the CaBP base level of the untreated, D-deficient animals was $10.3 \pm 5.9$ nmol $Ca_b$/gm mucosa, a value typical of vitamin D-deficiency (5,11,14). The figure also indicates that the lowest dose administered, 0.0625µg, raised CaBP levels to that found in similarly treated D-replete animals (59.7 nmol $Ca_b$/gm mucosa in the -D group vs 56.4 nmol/gm mucosa in the +D group). Again the response to 0.750µg $1,25-(OH)_2-D_3$ was no greater than the response to 0.50µg of the metabolite. The dashed line in Fig. 2 represents the average CaBP level of the +D animals fed a low calcium diet (Fig. 1). As can be seen, the CaBP levels of the -D animals treated with $1,25-(OH)_2-D_3$ did not exceed the high CaBP levels found in the replete rats fed the low calcium diets. The amount of CaBP found in the latter group thus appears to constitute a maximum.

More than 8 hr elapsed between injection of $1,25-(OH)_2-D_3$ into vitamin D-deficient animals and the first detectable increase of CaBP (Fig. 3). Maximum CaBP activity was found between 16 and 24 hr after dosing, in conformance with the report by others (17). In contrast, injection of $1,25-(OH)_2-D_3$ into D-replete animals fed on the same intake of calcium led to near-doubling of CaBP in about two hours. As shown in Fig. 4, the first measurement, 2 hr after dosing, was 83 nmol $Ca_b$/gm mucosa; the mean CaBP value for 7 measurements (2,4,8,12,16 and 24 hr after dosing) was $89.1 \pm 1.3$ nmol $Ca_b$/gm mucosa. Thereafter the CaBP level began dropping and had returned to the preinjection level by 48 hr after dosing.

Fig. 5 represents the results of an experiment in which the early time points after $1,25-(OH)_2-D_3$ treatment were studied in similar D-replete animals. The figure indicates that by 30 min after dosing CaBP levels had increased by 50 per cent and had reached the new plateau level 1 hr after dosing. The figure also shows that absolute CaBP levels had about doubled following treatment with 0.5µg $1,25-(OH)_2-D_3$, as had been observed in the first time-course experiment (Fig. 4) or in the dose experiment (Fig. 1).

DISCUSSION

The experiments described here show there exists an upper limit to the amount of CaBP that the D-replete rat can synthesize, even when treated with large doses of $1,25-(OH)_2-D_3$. This limit appears to correspond to the amount of CaBP found in D-replete animals fed a low-calcium diet, since treatment of the latter did not lead to an increase in their duodenal CaBP (Fig. 1). This observation recalls earlier studies (1) which showed that D-replete neonatal rats have no detectable CaBP and that when these animals

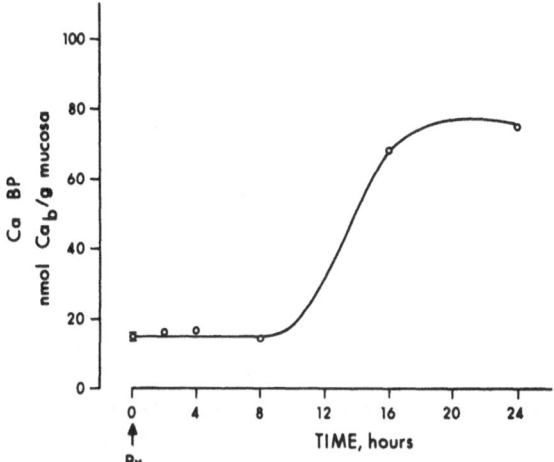

Fig. 3.  Time course of CaBP response in vitamin D-deficient animals.
At weaning the animals were placed on diet III-D.   Approximately
6 wk later, when hypocalcemic (5.5 ± 0.1 mg/dl), they received by
i.p. injection 0.5μg 1,25-(OH)₂-D₃ and were killed in groups of two
at the times shown.  The square symbol refers to the mean of two
groups of untreated animals.

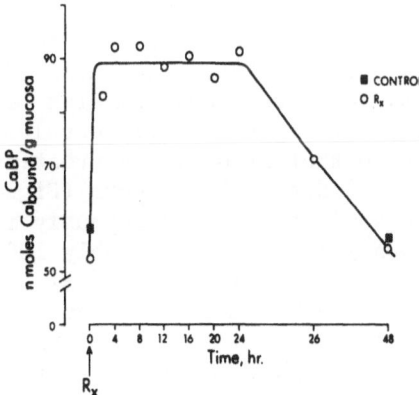

Fig. 4.  Time course of CaBP response in vitamin D-replete animals.
The rats were fed a high calcium diet (III).   14 days later they
received by i.p. injection 0.5μg 1,25-(OH)₂-D₃ (Rx) and were killed
in groups of two at the times shown.  The solid squares refer to
untreated controls killed at the beginning and end of the experiment.

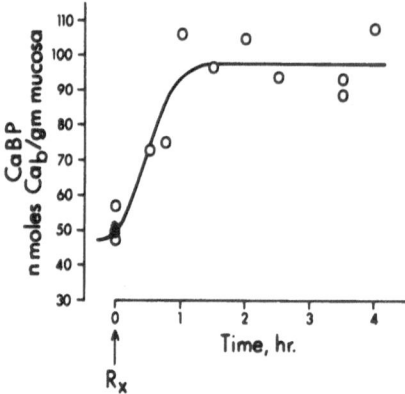

Fig. 5. *Detailed time course of the CaBP response of vitamin D-replete animals. Rats, fed diet III, received by i.p. injection 0.5μg 1,25-(OH)₂-D₃ (Rx) and were killed in groups of two at the times indicated. The solid circle represents the CaBP content of two animals killed 3 days before the experiment.*

were treated with $1,25-(OH)_2-D_3$, no CaBP was formed. Older animals, however, show an age-dependent rise in their duodenal CaBP and responded to $1,25-(OH)_2-D_3$ treatment. It was therefore suggested that CaBP levels are developmentally programmed and that the maximum amount of CaBP that can be induced is independent of the amount of administered $1,25-(OH)_2-D_3$. The experiments reported here confirm these observations.

In addition, these experiments, like previous studies (5,16), show that the amount of steady-state CaBP varies inversely with intake. When an animal fed a high calcium diet is shifted to a low calcium diet, its CaBP level approximately doubles in 24 hr (5) an increase comparable to that produced by treating the animals on a high calcium diet with 0.5μg $1,25-(OH)_2-D_3$ (Fig. 1). The amount of $1,25-(OH)_2-D_3$, if distributed instantaneously in the plasma, would correspond to about 100ng/ml, a value probably 100 times greater than that of a rat on a low calcium intake (18). Therefore the exogenous amount of $1,25-(OH)_2-D_3$ needed to overcome the calcium intake-related regulation seems quite large. However, a fuller understanding of the relationship between $1,25-(OH)_2-D_3$ and CaBP requires quantitative knowledge of how much and what proportion of circulating $1,25-(OH)_2-D_3$ becomes bound to the tissue.

Of major interest is the finding that net CaBP biosynthesis was much slower in D-deficient than in D-replete animals. Much more work is needed before the underlying mechanisms can be understood. A reasonable explanation is that a step or molecule needed for CaBP biosynthesis is present in the D-replete, but absent in the D-deficient intestinal cell. If this step were a CaBP-specific messenger that needs to be synthesized before CaBP can be translated, then $1,25-(OH)_2-D_3$ may have post-translational as well as transcriptional effects. Such a possibility is consistent with the reports that $1,25-(OH)_2-D_3$ can stimulate calcium transport before CaBP synthesis occurs (19,20).

## ACKNOWLEDGMENTS

This work was supported by NSF grants PCB76-00709 and PCM78-23366, NIH grant 4R01 AM 14251, and the University of Connecticut Research Foundation. Part of this material has been submitted by Michael Buckley in partial fulfillment of the requirements for a Master of Science degree in Biomaterials. We thank Dr. M. Uskokovic of Hoffman-LaRoche, Nutley, NJ for generous gifts of $1,25-(OH)_2-D_3$.

## REFERENCES

1. T.-H. Ueng, E. E. Golub and F. Bronner. The effect of age and 1,25-dihydroxyvitamin D treatment on the intestinal calcium-binding protein of suckling rats. Arch. Biochem. & Biophys. In Press (1979).
2. H. F. DeLuca and H. K. Schnoes. Metabolism and mechanism of action of vitamin D. Ann. Rev. Biochem. 45: 631 (1976).
3. M. Haussler. Vitamin D: Mode of action and biomedical applications. Nutr. Rev. 32: 257 (1974).
4. M. Haussler and T. A. McCain. Basic and clinical concepts related to vitamin D metabolism and action. N.E.J. Med. 297: 1041 (1977).
5. T. Freund and F. Bronner. Regulation of intestinal calcium-binding protein by calcium intake in the rat. Am. J. Physiol. 228: 861 (1975).
6. J. S. Emtage, D.E.M. Lawson and E. Kodicek. Vitamin D-induced synthesis of an RNA for calcium-binding protein. Nature 246: 100 (1973).
7. S. Tomlinson, H. Mellersh and R. Ross. In vitro synthesis of vitamin D-dependent porcine intestinal calcium-binding protein by translation of messenger RNA in a cell-free system. Calcified Tiss. Intl. Suppl. 27: A4 (1979).
8. R. L. Morrissey and R. H. Wasserman. Calcium absorption and calcium-binding protein in chicks on differing calcium and phosphorus intakes. Am. J. Physiol. 220: 1509 (1971).

9.  S. Edelstein, A. Harell, A. Bar and S. Hurwitz. The functional metabolism of vitamin D in chicks fed low-calcium and low-phosphorus diets. Biochem. Biophys. Acta 385: 438 (1975).

10. E. E. Golub, M. Reid, C. Bossak, L. Wolpert, L. Gagliardi and F. Bronner. Calcium-dependent induction of calcium-binding protein in vitro, in: "Calcium-Binding Proteins and Calcium Function," R. H. Wasserman, R. A. Corradino, E. Carafoli, R. H. Kretsinger, D. H. MacLennan and F. D. Siegel, eds. North Holland, New York (1977) p. 364.

11. S. Edelstein, D. Noff, L. Sinai, A. Harell, J. B. Puschett, E. E. Golub and F. Bronner. Vitamin D metabolism and expression in rats fed on low-calcium and low-phosphorus diets. Biochem. J. 170: 227 (1978).

12. K. W. Colston, P. J. Butterworth, I.M.A. Evans and J. MacIntyre. The regulation of vitamin D metabolism, in: "Phosphate Metabolism," S. G. Massry and E. Ritz, eds. Plenum, New York (1977) p. 251.

13. M. Garabedian, Y. Tanaka, M. F. Holick and H. F. DeLuca. Response of intestinal calcium transport and bone calcium mobilization to 1,25-dihydroxyvitamin $D_3$ in thyroparathyroidectomized rats. Endocrinology 94: 1022 (1974).

14. F. Bronner and T. Freund. Intestinal CaBP: A new quantitative index of vitamin D deficiency in the rat. Am. J. Physiol. 229: 689 (1975).

15. T. Freund and F. Bronner. Stimulation in vitro by 1,25-dihydroxyvitamin $D_3$ of intestinal cell calcium uptake and calcium-binding proteins. Science 190: 1300 (1975).

16. T.-H. Ueng and F. Bronner. Cellular and luminal forms of rat intestinal calcium-binding protein as studied by counter ion electrophoresis. Arch. Biochem. Biophys. In Press (1979).

17. H. J. Armbrecht, T. V. Zenser and B. B. Davis. Effect of 1,25-dihydroxyvitamin $D_3$ on intestinal calcium transport and calcium-binding protein in young and adult rats. Fed. Proc. 38: 385 (1979).

18. M. Haussler, M. Hughes, D. Baylink, E. T. Littledike, D. Cork and M. Pitt. Influence of phosphate depletion of the biosynthesis and circulating level of 1α,25-dihydroxyvitamin $D_3$, in: "Phosphate Metabolism," S. G. Massry and E. Ritz, eds. Plenum, New York (1977) p. 233.

19. R. Spencer, M. Chapman, P. W. Wilson and D. Eric M. Lawson. The relationship between vitamin D-stimulated calcium transport and intestinal calcium-binding protein in the chicken. Biochem. J. 170: 93 (1978).

20. D. D. Bikle, D. J. Zolock, R. L. Morrissey and R. H. Herman. Independence of 1,25-dihydroxyvitamin $D_3$-mediated calcium transport from de novo RNA and protein synthesis. J. Biol. Chem. 253: 484 (1978).

# NEPHROLITHIASIS AND PHOSPHATE

IS THERE A DISORDER OF PHOSPHATE METABOLISM IN IDIOPATHIC HYPER-

CALCIURIA?

Jacob Lemann, Jr., Richard W. Gray, Donald R. Wilz,
and Nancy D. Adams

Departments of Medicine and Biochemistry and the Clin-
ical Research Center, Medical College of Wisconsin and
Milwaukee County Medical Complex, 8700 West Wisconsin
Avenue, Milwaukee, Wisconsin 53226 U.S.A.

Albright, Henneman and their associates (Albright et al.,
1953; Henneman et al., 1958; Melick and Henneman, 1958) introduced
the term idiopathic hypercalciuria to describe a group of patients
who had formed calcium containing kidney stones and who exhibited
hypercalciuria without hypercalcemia, increased intestinal calcium
absorption, normal skeletal radiographs and hypophosphatemia. Most
of the patients were men. These investigators emphasized that this
group of patients did not give a history of vitamin D use or exhibit
evidence of sarcoidosis, hyperthyroidism, Cushing's syndrome, malig-
nant tumor, rapid bone loss or renal tubular acidosis. The repetitive demonstration that serum calcium concentrations were normal
excluded the diagnosis of primary hyperparathyroidism. Subsequent
studies of patients with calcium nephrolithiasis have also demonstrated that these patients frequently exhibit lower serum phosphate
levels than do healthy adults. Data from several studies are summarized in Table I (Henneman et al., 1958; Coe et al., 1973; Gray
et al., 1977; Shen et al., 1977; Bordier et al., 1977). In each
of these studies, the serum phosphorus levels among the patients
with idiopathic hypercalciuria were significantly below those of
healthy control subjects, the mean differences in the several
series ranging from 0.15 to 0.32 mmol/L. Although other investigators, notably Pak and associates (1974), have failed to even
observe such mild hypophosphatemia among patients with idiopathic
hypercalciuria, the data in Table I appear to unequivocally document that this is a very common finding among this group of patients
with calcium nephrolithiasis. Perhaps the difficulty in detecting
mild hypophosphatemia in stone formers is a consequence of the
broad range for serum phosphorus concentrations in normal subjects.
Fasting serum phosphorus concentrations in a large number of healthy

TABLE I

Serum P Levels in Healthy Adults and in Patients with Idiopathic
Hypercalciuria

| | Normal Subjects | | Idiopathic Hypercalciurics | | p |
|---|---|---|---|---|---|
| | N | Serum P mmol/L | N | Serum P mmol/L | |
| Henneman et al., 1958 | – | 1.10 (range 0.90–1.26) | 35 | 0.90 (range 0.77–1.06) | – |
| Coe et al., 1973 | 77 | 1.24 ± 0.17* | 48 (normal PTH) | 1.08 ± 0.18 | <0.01 |
| | | | 72 (high PTH) | 1.05 ± 0.22 | <0.01 |
| Shen et al., 1977 | 17 | 1.19 ± 0.10 | 15 | 0.94 ± 0.19 | <0.001 |
| Gray et al., 1977 | 45 | 1.25 ± 0.19 | 26 | 1.10 ± 0.18 | <0.001 |
| Bordier et al., 1977 | – | 1.13 ± 0.13 | 22 (high PTH) | 0.81 ± 0.10 | – |
| | | | 25 (normal PTH) | 0.81 ± 0.10 | – |

*Mean ± standard deviation

adults and calcium stone formers that we have studied are depicted
in Fig. 1 and emphasize the overlap in the ranges for the two
groups.  In addition, although we have regularly measured serum
phosphate concentrations fasting in the morning hopefully thereby
obviating any variation due to the tendency for serum phosphorus
levels to fall during the morning hours (Carruthers et al., 1964),
it is also important to note  that the serum phosphorus concentrations in normal subjects can be reduced after meals (Annino and
Relman, 1959) or during short periods of hyperventilation (Okel
and Hurst, 1961).

Since the serum phosphorus concentration is determined by the
rates of input of phosphorus from the intestine and from bone relative to the rates of losses of phosphorus in the urine, we have
undertaken an evaluation of components of the phosphate balance in
13 calcium stone formers with hypercalciuria as compared to 16

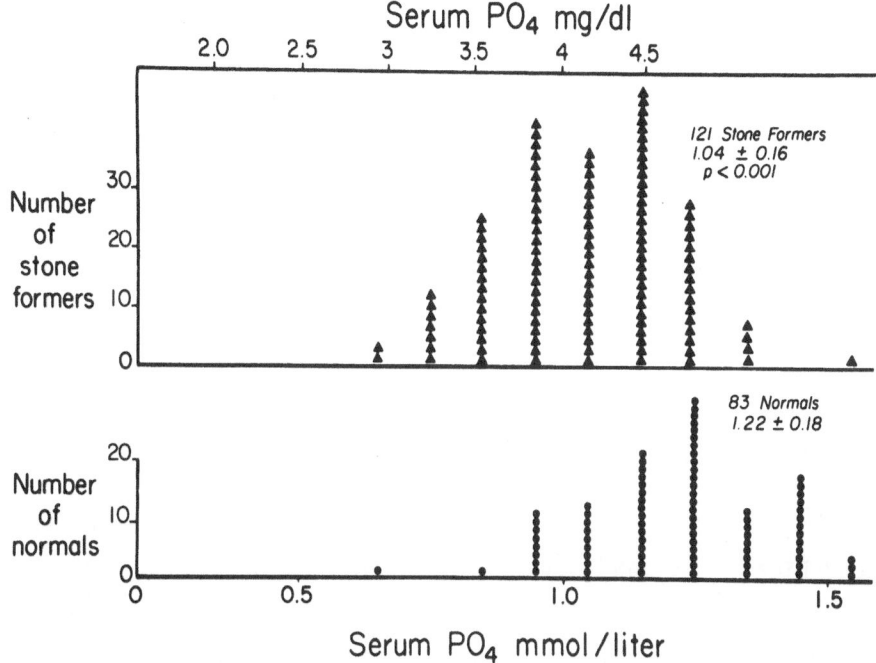

Fig. 1.   Distribution of fasting morning serum PO$_4$ concentrations
among healthy adults (●) and among Ca-stone formers (▲)

healthy adults.   These data are summarized in Table II.   As can be
seen, there were no differences in dietary phosphate intake or
fecal phosphate excretion and hence, net intestinal phosphate absorption between the groups.   This confirms prior observations by
Nordin and associates (1976) who found that intestinal phosphate
absorption as measured by $^{32}$P was normal among patients with calcium nephrolithiasis.   In our studies (Table II), urinary phosphate
excretion and phosphorus balance were not different in stone formers
as compared to normal subjects.   Thus, since the stone formers exhibited lower mean serum phosphorus concentrations than did the
normal subjects but similar glomerular filtration rates, these data
indicate that the stone formers as a group must have a defect in
renal tubular phosphate reabsorption that sets their serum phosphate concentration at a lower than normal level.

Since parathyroid hormone is well known to inhibit renal
tubular phosphate reabsorption, the lower serum phosphorus concentrations in idiopathic hypercalciurics could, first of all, be the
consequence of secondary hyperparathyroidism (primary hyperparathyroidism is excluded because of persistent absence of hypercalcemia among these patients).   Evidence in support of such a
defect was first presented by Coe and associates (1973 and Table
I) who observed high PTH levels among almost two-thirds of a group

TABLE II

Phosphate Balances in Ca Stone Formers and in Healthy Adults

|  | Healthy Adults 16 | Ca Stone Formers 13 | p |
|---|---|---|---|
| N |  |  |  |
| Diet PO$_4$ mmol/day | 54.0 $\pm$ 14.4 SD | 51.7 $\pm$ 5.2 | NS |
| Fecal PO$_4$ mmol/day | 18.2 $\pm$ 5.7 | 15.4 $\pm$ 3.8 | NS |
| Net Intestinal PO$_4$ Absorption mmol/day | 35.8 $\pm$ 11.9 | 36.3 $\pm$ 6.0 | NS |
| Percent Diet PO$_4$ Absorbed | 66 $\pm$ 9 | 70 $\pm$ 8 | NS |
| Urine PO$_4$ mmol/day | 32.9 $\pm$ 8.9 | 33.1 $\pm$ 5.3 | NS |
| PO$_4$ Balance mmol/day | + 3.2 $\pm$ 5.7 | + 3.1 $\pm$ 4.4 | NS |
| Serum PO$_4$ mmol/liter | 1.44 $\pm$ 0.17 | 1.28 $\pm$ 0.13 | <0.025 |
| Urine Ca mmol/day | 4.4 $\pm$ 1.7 | 7.7 $\pm$ 3.1 | <0.005 |

of patients with calcium nephrolithiasis and hypercalciuria. In these patients, evidence was presented that the hyperparathyroidism was secondary to a defect in renal tubular calcium reabsorption since the elevated serum PTH levels returned to normal when urinary calcium excretion was suppressed by the administration of thiazide diuretics. Bordier et al. (1977) have also presented evidence for such a defect in the pathogenesis of the hypophosphatemia among some patients with idiopathic hypercalciuria (Table I; their Type 2 patients). In addition to observing elevated PTH levels among this group of patients, those investigators also observed that this group of idiopathic hypercalciurics exhibited a reduction in Tm$_{PO_4}$/GFR, an increase in urinary hydroxyproline excretion together with bone biopsies showing coupled increases in osteoclastic resorption surfaces and osteoblastic surfaces, consistent with the hyperparathyroid state. Thus, hypophosphatemia as a consequence of secondary hyperparathyroidism in turn due to a renal calcium leak appears to be a reasonably well documented defect among a subset of the patients with hypercalciuria and nephrolithiasis traditionally described as having idiopathic hypercalciuria.

By contrast, it is also apparent that another subset of the patients with hypercalciuria and calcium nephrolithiasis exhibit hypophosphatemia but without evidence of hyperparathyroidism. Coe and associates (1973 and Table I) observed that patients with idiopathic hypercalciuria but normal PTH levels were nevertheless on the average hypophosphatemic. Those observations have been subsequently confirmed by Shen and associates (1977 and Table I) who observed hypophosphatemia and a low $Tmp_{O4}$/GFR despite low serum PTH concentrations in their patients and by Bordier et al. (1977 and Table I; their Type 3 patients) who exhibited hypophosphatemia a low $Tmp_{O4}$/GFR and a low serum PTH concentration. The latter investigators extended the observations in this group of patients by observing that they also exhibited increased urinary excretion of hydroxyproline as well as bone biopsies showing increased osteoclastic resorption surfaces as is observed during experimental dietary phosphate deprivation (Baylink et al., 1971).

In a larger group of recurrent calcium stone formers (N = 121), we have also observed that serum phosphate averaged only 1.04 ± 0.16 SD mmol/L compared to 1.22 ± 0.18 mmol/L in 83 healthy adults; p <0.001. Since creatinine clearances (stone formers 166 ± 30 L/day and normal subjects 155 ± 33 L/day; NS) and urinary phosphate excretion (stone formers 32 ± 9 mmol/day and normal subjects 31 ± 10 mmol/day; NS) were not different, the fractional urinary excretion of filtered phosphate was obviously higher in the stone formers (stone formers 22 ± 4 percent, normal subjects 16 ± 5 percent; p <0.001). In this large group of patients, serum PTH levels averaged 6.5 ± 2.2 SD µlEq/ml as compared to 5.8 ± 1.8 SD µlEq/ml in the normal subjects (p <0.05) suggesting that our stone formers included both subjects with a renal calcium leak and secondary hyperparathyroidism as well as subjects with a separate defect in renal tubular phosphate reabsorption, independent of parathyroid hormone.

In a further effort to characterize the magnitude of defective renal tubular phosphate reabsorption in calcium stone formers, we have evaluated the response of 9 male stone formers to 3 days of dietary $PO_4$ deprivation in comparison to similar studies in 13 healthy men. The results of these studies are summarized in Table III. The stone formers as a group exhibited distinct hypercalciuria in comparison to the normal subjects. Although control serum phosphorus levels among the stone formers were not significantly different in comparison to the normals in these small groups, after 3 days of phosphate deprivation, serum phosphorus fell significantly

TABLE III

Response of Healthy Men and Male Ca-Stone Formers to Dietary P
Deprivation

|  | Normal Men | Male Stone Formers | $p^+$ |
|---|---|---|---|
| N | 13 | 9 | |
| **Control Conditions** | | | |
| Serum P mmol/L | 1.30 ± 0.06* | 1.28 ± 0.06 | NS |
| Serum Ca mmol/L | 2.42 ± 0.02 | 2.38 ± 0.05 | NS |
| Serum iPTH μlEq/ml | 5.5 ± 0.4 | 5.7 ± 0.8 | NS |
| Urine P mmol/day | 32.0 ± 1.9 | 27.9 ± 2.3 | NS |
| Urine Ca mmol/day | 3.8 ± 0.6 | 8.2 ± 0.7 | <0.001 |
| E/F PO$_4$ | 16 ± 1 | 16 ± 1 | NS |
| **Third Day of Low P Diet** | | | |
| Serum P mmol/L | 1.35 ± 0.06 | 1.10 ± 0.07 | <0.001 |
| p$^X$ | NS | <0.01 | |
| Serum Ca mmol/L | 2.40 ± 0.01 | 2.36 ± 0.04 | NS |
| p | NS | NS | |
| Serum iPTH mmol/L | 4.8 ± 0.6 | 5.4 ± 0.8 | NS |
| p | NS | NS | |
| Urine P mmol/day | 1.7 ± 0.5 | 4.5 ± 1.0 | <0.02 |
| p | <0.001 | <0.001 | |
| Urine Ca mmol/day | 7.5 ± 1.1 | 12.6 ± 1.0 | <0.005 |
| p | <0.001 | <0.001 | |
| E/F PO$_4$ | 1.0 ± 0.3 | 3.0 ± 0.6 | <0.001 |
| p | <0.001 | <0.001 | |

[+]p comparison of normals and stone formers

*Mean ± SEM

[X]p comparison of low P and control data

among stone formers but did not change in the normal subjects. Moreover, maximum urinary phosphate conservation appeared to be impaired among the stone formers since 24-hour urinary phosphate excretion on the 3rd day of the low phosphorus diet remained significantly higher in that group in comparison to normal subjects. Thus, fractional renal excretion of phosphate on the 3rd day of the low phosphorus diet was also higher among the stone formers. Since we could not discern any difference in PTH levels between the two groups, this defect would appear to be independent of parathyroid hormone.

TABLE IV

Composition of Saliva, Blood and Urine in Normal Subjects and Ca-Stone Formers

|  | Normals 27 | Stone Formers 26 | p |
|---|---|---|---|
| N |  |  |  |
| Salivary Flow Rate ml/min | 1.3 ± 0.1 | 1.5 ± 0.2 | NS |
| Salivary [Ca] mmol/liter | 1.16 ± 0.04 | 1.38 ± 0.07 | <0.01 |
| Serum [Ca] mmol/liter | 2.41 ± 0.01 | 2.40 ± 0.02 | NS |
| Saliva/Serum [Ca] | 0.48 ± 0.02 | 0.59 ± 0.02 | <0.001 |
| Salivary [PO$_4$] mmol/liter | 3.56 ± 0.15 | 4.25 ± 0.25 | <0.02 |
| Serum [PO$_4$] mmol/liter | 1.17 ± 0.04 | 1.02 ± 0.02 | <0.01 |
| Saliva/Serum [PO$_4$] | 3.1 ± 0.2 | 4.8 ± 0.2 | <0.002 |
| Salivary [K] mmol/liter | 18.5 ± 0.4 | 19.0 ± 0.7 | NS |
| Serum [K] mmol/liter | 4.2 ± 0.1 | 4.2 ± 0.1 | NS |
| Salivary [Na] mmol/liter | 15.0 ± 2.1 | 16.8 ± 2.1 | NS |
| Serum [Na] mmol/liter | 140 ± 1 | 140 ± 1 | NS |
| Salivary [Mg] mmol/liter | 0.17 ± 0.01 | 0.18 ± 0.02 | NS |
| Serum [Mg] mmol/liter | 0.87 ± 0.01 | 0.89 ± 0.02 | NS |
| Urine Ca mmol/day | 4.3 ± 0.2 | 7.6 ± 0.7 | <0.001 |
| Serum PTH µlEq/ml | 5.7 ± 0.2 | 6.7 ± 0.5 | NS |

In an effort to determine whether a defect in phosphate transport in calcium stone formers is limited solely to the kidney or
whether such an abnormality might be present in other tissues, we
have compared the composition of saliva in calcium stone formers
and in healthy adults.  Mixed saliva was collected after overnight
fasting from 26 untreated stone formers and 27 normal subjects.
Each subject rinsed their mouth with deionized water and then
chewed a square of paraffin.  Saliva produced during the first
minute of chewing was discarded.  The saliva was then collected
during two subsequent and consecutive 3 minute periods and the
results of the two collections averaged for each subject.    Blood
was drawn immediately after the saliva was collected.  The results
are summarized in Table IV.    Serum phosphate concentrations were
lower among the stone formers despite which salivary phosphate
concentrations were higher so that the salivary to serum phosphate
concentrations ratios were also higher in stone formers than among
the normal subjects.  Salivary calcium concentration was also
higher among the stone formers so that despite normal serum calcium
concentrations their salivary to serum calcium concentrations were
also elevated.  There were no differences between the groups with

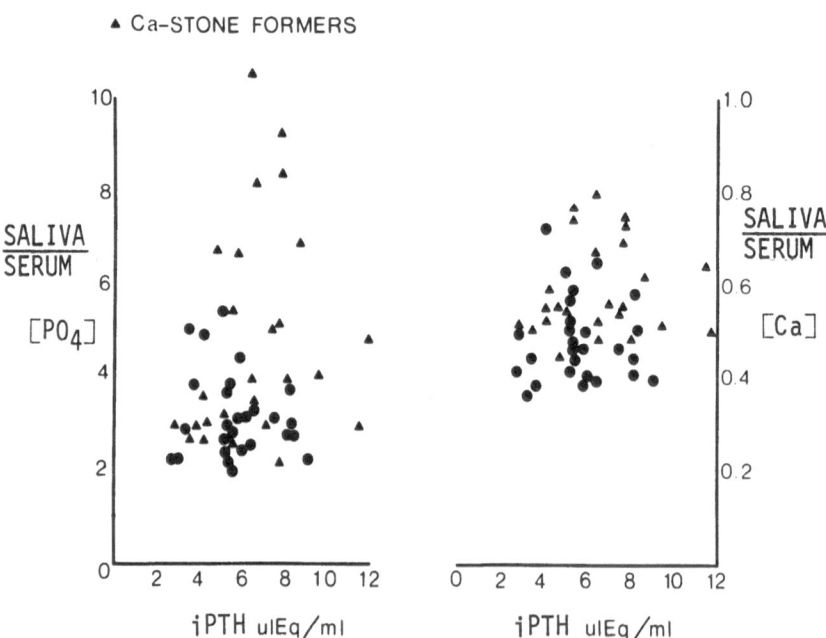

Fig. 2.    Salivary/serum concentration ratios for PO4 and for Ca
in relation to simultaneously measured serum PTH concentrations in healthy adults (●) and Ca-stone formers (▲).

respect to salivary or serum sodium, potassium or magnesium. Despite the hypercalciuria demonstrated by the stone formers, we
could not detect a significant difference in serum PTH levels in
this group as compared to the normal subjects. Although Weinberger
and associates (1974) have previously demonstrated that subjects
with primary hyperparathyroidism have elevated salivary calcium
and phosphate concentrations and that patients with idiopathic
hypercalciuria likewise have a tendency toward elevation of salivary calcium and phosphorus concentrations, we have not been able
to demonstrate a relationship between the salivary to serum concentration ratios for phosphate and calcium and the simultaneously
measured serum PTH levels. These data are depicted in Fig. 2. It
thus appears that in addition to a renal leak for phosphate, stone
formers as a group have a salivary leak for phosphate that is independent of parathyroid hormone. Moreover, there is also frequently a salivary calcium leak.

In our view, therefore, the data summarized here provides
firm evidence for the existence of a defect in phosphate metabolism in patients with idiopathic hypercalciuria. In some patients,
secondary hyperparathyroidism as a consequence of a renal calcium
leak as described by Coe (1973), Pak (1974), and Bordier (1977)
and associates results in diminished renal tubular phosphate reabsorption and hypophosphatemia. In other hypercalciuric stone
formers, it appears that hypophosphatemia is a consequence of a
primary renal phosphate leak since serum PTH levels are normal
or in some cases low (Bordier et al., 1977; Shen et al., 1977).

Both of these pathogenetic sequences play important roles in
the initiation and maintenance of so-called idiopathic hypercalciuria. Among the patients who exhibit a renal calcium leak and
secondary hyperparathyroidism (Coe et al., 1973; Pak et al., 1974;
Bordier et al., 1977), the resulting elevation of serum PTH concentrations either directly, or because of the accompanying hypophosphatemia, stimulates renal synthesis of $1,25-(OH)_2$-vitamin D
that in turn augments intestinal calcium absorption thereby sus-
taining the hypercalciuria that is the initial result of the renal
calcium leak (Kaplan et al., 1977). Such a formulation is consistent with the observation that serum $1,25-(OH)_2$-D levels are often
elevated in patients with primary hyperparathyroidism (Haussler
et al., 1976; Gray et al., 1977). Among the subset of patients
with idiopathic hypercalciuria who exhibit hypophosphatemia but
normal serum PTH concentrations, the defect in phosphate metabolism directly leads to augmentation of renal $1,25-(OH)_2$-D synthesis and elevation of plasma levels of the hormone (Gray et al.,
1977; Shen et al., 1977; Caldas et al., 1978). Such a pathogenetic
sequence is consistent with the observation that dietary phosphate
deprivation in parathyroidectomized rats raises the plasma concentrations of $1,25-(OH)_2$-D (Hughes et al., 1975) and the observation

that, as serum phosphate levels fall during short term dietary phosphate deprivation in healthy women, plasma $1,25-(OH)_2-D$ levels also rise despite a fall in serum PTH concentrations (Gray et al., 1977). Once again, the elevations in plasma $1,25-(OH)_2-D$ levels are responsible for an increase in intestinal calcium absorption and hypercalciuria. Whether or not the increased plasma concentrations of $1,25-(OH)_2-D$ are responsible for the acceleration of osteoclastic bone resorption in such patients (Bordier et al., 1977) or whether the bone disease is a direct consequence of the primary defect in phosphate metabolism remains to be determined.

In summary, hypophosphatemia either as a consequence of secondary hyperparathyroidism or as a consequence of a primary defect in phosphate metabolism appears to be a well established abnormality among subsets of patients with idiopathic hypercalciuria and nephrolithiasis. The detailed biochemical events that lead to hypophosphatemia in those patients who exhibit a primary abnormality of phosphate metabolism remain to be clarified.

## ACKNOWLEDGEMENTS

Supported in part by USPHS RR-00058, AM-15089, HL-05949 and AM-22014.

## REFERENCES

Albright, F., Henneman, P., Benedict, P. H., and Forbes, A.P., 1953, Idiopathic hypercalciuria, Proc. Royal Soc. Med., 46: 1077.

Annino, J. S., and Relman, A. S., 1959, The effect of eating on some of the clinically important chemical constituents of the blood, Am. J. Clin. Path., 31:155.

Baylink, D., Wergedal, J., and Stauffer, M., 1971, Formation, mineralization and resorption of bone in hypophosphatemic rats, J. Clin. Invest., 50:2519.

Bordier, P., Ryckewart, A., Gueris, J., and Rasmussen, H., 1977, On the pathogenesis of so-called idiopathic hypercalciuria, Am. J. Med., 63:398.

Caldas, A. E., Gray, R. W., and Lemann, J., Jr., 1978, The simultaneous measurement of vitamin D metabolites in plasma: Studies in healthy adults and in patients with calcium nephrolithiasis, J. Lab. Clin. Med., 91:840.

Carruthers, B. M., Copp, D. H., and McIntosh, H. W., 1964, Diurnal variations in urinary excretion of calcium and phosphate and its relation to blood levels, J. Lab. Clin. Med., 63:959.

Coe, F. L., Canterbury, J. M., Firpo, J. J., and Reiss, E., 1973, Evidence for secondary hyperparathyroidism in idiopathic hypercalciuria, J. Clin. Invest., 52:134.

Gray, R. W., Wilz, D. R., Caldas, A. E., and Lemann, J., Jr., 1977, The importance of phosphate in regulating plasma 1,25-$(OH)_2$-vitamin D levels in humans: Studies in healthy subjects, in calcium-stone formers and in patients with primary hyperparathyroidism, J. Clin. Endocrinol. Metab., 45:299.

Haussler, M. R., Baylink, D. J., Hughes, M. R., Brumbaugh, P. F., Wergedal, J. E., Shen, F. H., Nielsen, R. L., Counts, S. J., Bursac, K. M., and McCain, T. A , 1976, The assay of 1α-25-dihydroxyvitamin $D_3$: Physiologic and pathologic modulation of circulating hormone levels, Clin. Endocrinol., 5:151S.

Henneman, P. H., Benedict, P. H., Forbes, A. P., and Dudley, H. R., 1958, Idiopathic hypercalciuria, N. Engl. J. Med., 259:802.

Hughes, M. R., Haussler, M. R., Wergedal, J., and Baylink, D. J., 1975, Regulation of serum 1α,25-dihydroxyvitamin $D_3$ by calcium and phosphate in the rat, Science, 190:578.

Kaplan, R. A., Haussler, M. R., Deftos, L. J., Bone, H., and Pak, C. Y. C., 1977, The role of 1α,25-dihydroxyvitamin D in the mediation of intestinal hyperabsorption of calcium in primary hyperparathyroidism and absorptive hypercalciuria, J. Clin. Invest., 59:756.

Melick, R. A., and Henneman, P. H., 1958, Clinical and laboratory studies of 207 consecutive patients in a kidney-stone clinic, N. Engl. J. Med., 259:307.

Nordin, B. E. C., 1976, "Calcium, Phosphate and Magnesium Metabolism," Churchill Livingstone, Edinburgh.

Okel, B. B., and Hurst, J. W., 1961, Prolonged hyperventilation in man, Arch. Int. Med., 108:157.

Pak, C. Y. C., Ohata, M., Lawrence, E. C., and Snyder, W., 1974, The hypercalciurias: Causes, parathyroid functions, and diagnostic criteria, J. Clin. Invest., 54:387.

Shen, F. H., Baylink, D. J., Nielsen, R. L., Sherrard, D. J., Ivey, J. L., and Haussler, M. R., 1977, Increased serum 1,25-dihydroxyvitamin D in idiopathic hypercalciuria, J. Lab. Clin. Med., 90:955.

Weinberger, A., Sperling, O., and DeVries, A., 1974, Calcium and inorganic phosphate in saliva of patients with primary hyperparathyroidism, Clin. Chim. Acta, 50:5.

# HYPERURICOSURIC CALCIUM OXALATE NEPHROLITHIASIS

Fredric L. Coe, M.D.

Director, Renal Division, Michael Reese Hospital;
Professor of Medicine and Physiology, University of
Chicago, Chicago, Illinois

Patients with calcium oxalate urolithiasis excrete in their
urine a larger amount of uric acid than normal subjects. For example, the proportion of 24-hr urine collections from patients with
calcium stones that contain more than 800 mg of uric acid is much
higher than that seen in normal people; and the entire distribution
of values among patients is shifted upwards (Table 1).

Table 1
Frequency of Various Uric Acid
Excretion Rates Among
Calcium Oxalate Stone Formers (P)
and Normal Subjects (N)

| Urine Urate (mg/24 hr) | Men | | Women | |
|---|---|---|---|---|
| | N (128) | P (1046) | N (77) | P (302) |
| <200 | 0 | 0 | 0 | 0 |
| 200-400 | 2 | 1 | 36 | 25 |
| 400-600 | 38 | 17 | 54 | 53 |
| 600-800 | 48 | 50 | 9 | 8 |
| 800-900 | 6 | 14 | 0 | 6 |
| 900-1000 | 4 | 11 | – | 5 |
| >1000 | 2 | 7 | – | 3 |

* Numbers are the percentage of 24-hour urine samples containing
the amounts of urate indicated. Total number of urine samples
in each group is shown in parentheses.

There is now an impressive body of evidence that hyperuricosuria
induces calcium stones in a significant proportion of patients and
that its treatment can prevent stone recurrence (1,2,3,4). We have
considered hyperuricosuria to be present when 24-hr uric acid excretion exceeds 800 mg in men or 750 mg in women. Thus defined, hyperuricosuria occurred alone, or in combination with idiopathic hypercalciuria, in 26 percent of 460 patients with calcium oxalate stone
disease. Hypercalciuria and hyperuricosuria coexisted at a frequency
compatible with chance alone (Table 2).

Table 2
Metabolic and Clinical Disorders in
460 Consecutive Calcium Stone Formers

|  | Number of Patients | Per cent |
|---|---|---|
| Idiopathic Hypercalciuria | 95 | 20.7 |
| Marginal Hypercalciuria† | 53 | 11.5 |
| Hyperuricosuria | 67 | 14.6 |
| Hypercalciuria and Hyperuricosuria* | 54 | 11.7 |
| Hyperuricemia Alone | 26 | 5.7 |
| Primary Hyperparathyroidism | 24 | 5.2 |
| Renal Tubular Acidosis‡ | 17 | 3.7 |
| Inflammatory Bowel Disease** | 21 | 4.6 |
| Medullary Sponge Kidney | 7 | 1.5 |
| Sarcoidosis | 3 | .7 |
| No Disorder Found | 93 | 20.2 |
| Total | 460 | |

† , Urine calcium  140 mg/gm creatinine
 *, Marginal hypercalciuria not included
‡ , Distal, hereditary form
**, Regional enteritis, ulcerative colitis, granulomatous ileocolitis

Hyperuricosuria was due largely to excessive dietary purine
intake (Fig. 1).

Urinary uric acid excretion (y axis) normally varies with dietary
purine intake (x axis) as depicted by the shaded confidence band.
Seven of 10 patients appeared to be hyperuricosuric solely because of
a high purine intake. The other 3, who excreted more uric acid than
would be expected given their diet, and who also excreted excessive
amounts of uric acid after 7 days of a purine-free diet, had a mixture of purine excess and endogenous uric acid overproduction. The
foods that provided the excess purine were mainly meat, fish, and
poultry (Fig. 2).

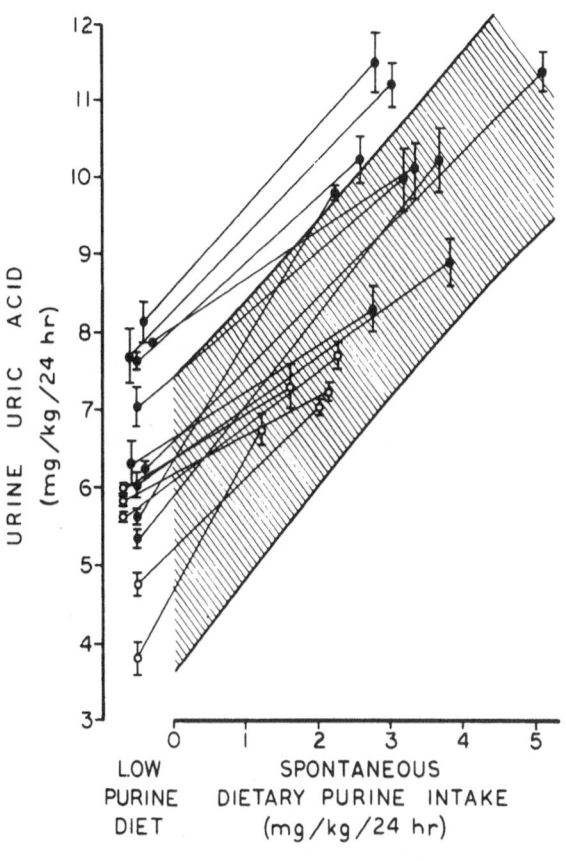

Figure 1

Compared to 5 age- and sex-matched controls, 10 hyperuricosuric
calcium stone formers consumed approximately 300 calories of additional meat and other purine-rich foods, mainly at the expense of
breads, grains, and starches (5).  This pattern appears to be an
exaggeration of a general change in the American diet; since 1910,
daily per capita intake of breads, grains, and starches has decreased from 22 to 11 oz, whereas per capita, daily, consumption of
meat, fish, and poultry rose from 7 to 11 oz.

Hyperuricosuria increases urinary supersaturation, mainly with
respect to undissociated uric acid (Table 3).

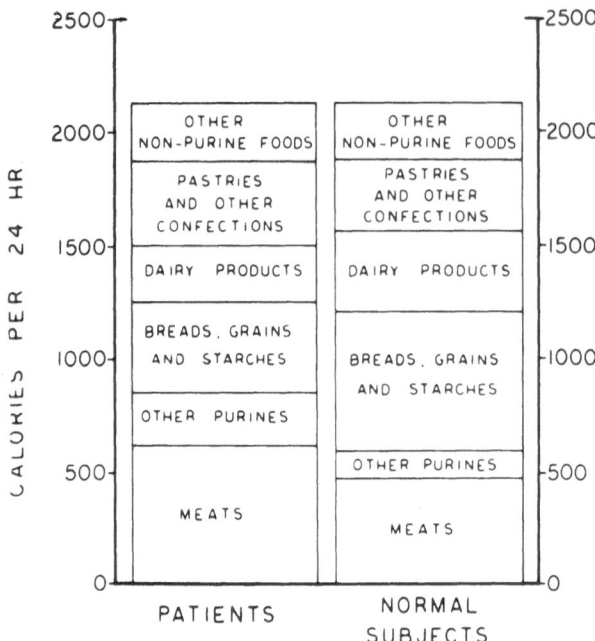

Figure 2

Table 3
Summary of Urine Uric Acid
Saturation Measurements

| 24-HR URINE VALUES | METABOLIC GROUP | | | | |
|---|---|---|---|---|---|
| | NORMAL (20) | IH (24) | HU (12) | BOTH (14) | NEITHER (17) |
| Samples | 24 | 69 | 36 | 42 | 51 |
| T(mg/L) | 503±32 | 421±23 | 575±28 | 616±27** | 462±32 |
| V(ml) | 1268±65 | 1717±133 | 1501±79* | 1397±70 | 1387±90 |
| pH | 6.22 | 5.92 | 5.62** | 5.74** | 5.67*** |
| U(mg/L)‡ | 57±8 | 84±11 | 155±21*** | 150±16**** | 128±18** |
| CPR | 2.8±.3† | 2.2±.2 | 2.7±.2 | 3.1±.2 | 2.2±.2 |
| Na(mEq/L) | 131±8 | 118±7 | 130±7 | 149±7 | 132±7 |

All values except for the numbers of samples and the numbers of people in each metabolic group (in parentheses) are means ±1 SEM. Abbreviations: IH, Idiopathic Hypercalciuria; HU, Hyperuricosuria; CPR, Concentration Product Ratio; [Na], sodium concentration (mEq/L); T, Total Uric Acid Concentration; V, Urine Volume; U, Undissociated Uric Acid Concentration.
*, Differs from control, p<.05; **, p<.02; ***, p<.01; ****, p<.001.
†, Based on the study of 16 normal subjects with CPR measurements.

‡, The mean equilibrium value, determined in 25 urine samples of pH below 5.6, after 48 hours of incubation with crystals of uric acid, was 90±5 (SEM) mg/L.

The average value of urine pH among 19 normal subjects was 6.21; undissociated urinary uric acid, calculated from the dissociation constant of uric acid, urine pH, and total uric acid concentration, averaged 77 mg/L. Saturation of the urine with respect to sodium hydrogen urate was estimated using the concentration product method of Pak. In this measurement, a value of 1 indicates a urine at the solubility product; values above 1 indicate supersaturation. Among normal subjects, the mean value for the CPR was 2.8.

In patients with idiopathic hypercalciuria, urine pH, undissociated uric acid concentration, and CPR with respect to sodium hydrogen urate were indistinguishable from normal. Patients with hyperuricosuria, studied on their own diets, elaborated a more acid urine than normal subjects; the CPR for sodium hydrogen urate was not elevated, mainly because the lower pH reduced the concentration of urate available for crystallization; but the concentration of undissociated uric acid was very elevated. Patients with a combination of hyperuricosuria and hypercalciuria displayed an equivalent pattern. The solubility of undissociated uric acid, measured by seeding urine from these patients with uric acid crystals, was 98±4 mg/L, and uric acid supersaturation (y axis) increased smoothly with the undissociated uric acid concentration (x axis) (Fig. 3); therefore, the values observed in hyperuricosuric patients reflect significant supersaturation. In a previous study, Pak (7) and his colleagues have shown that if urine pH is fixed at 6.2, hyperuricosuria increases supersaturation mainly with respect to sodium hydrogen urate. In a parallel series of experiments, in which we fixed the urine pH at 6.2, we were readily able to reproduce his results. The reason for the lower urine pH values in our patients with hyperuricosuria may well have been their high meat diets, which impose a considerable load of metabolic acids for elimination by the kidney.

Two mechanisms have been proposed to link hyperuricosuria to calcium oxalate nephrolithiasis. The lattice dimensions of uric acid or sodium hydrogen urate crystals and crystals of calcium oxalate correspond well enough that seed crystals of one could act as heterogeneous nuclei for the other (Table 4).

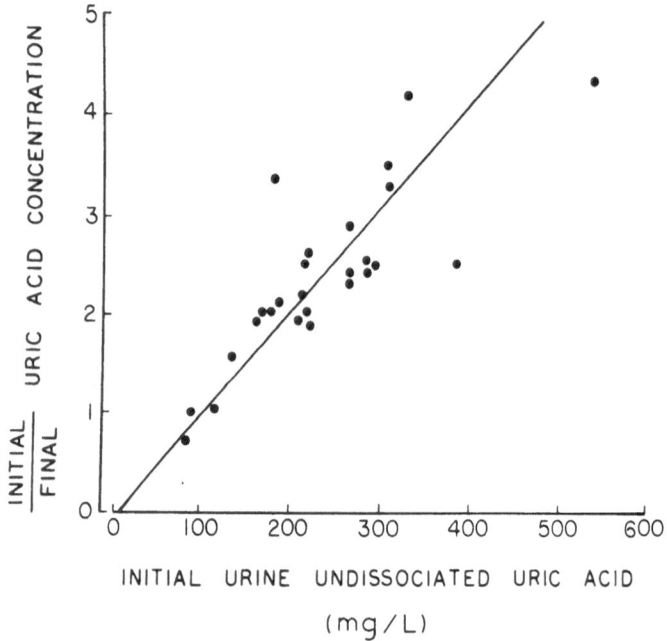

Figure 3

Table 4
Geometrical Correspondences Between
Naturally Occurring Faces of Uric Acid
and Calcium Oxalate Crystals

|  | Face | Dimensions (Å) |
|---|---|---|
| Uric acid | 100 | 6.21 X 7.40 |
| Uric acid·2H$_2$O | 100 | 6.35 X 7.40 |
| CaOx·H$_2$O* | 001 | 6.28 X 14.57 |
| CaOx·2H$_2$O† | 101 | 12.30 X 7.34 |
| NaH urate·H$_2$O | 100 | 3.567 X 8.693 |
|  | 010 | 9.097 X 3.567 |

*, Whewellite, calcium oxalate monohydrate
†, Weddellite, calcium oxalate dihydrate

In general, efficient heterogeneous nucleation can occur when unit
cell dimensions match within 1-3% or are integral multiples of each
other (8,9). This is the case for uric acid and calcium oxalate mono
and dihydrate. The match for the sodium hydrogen urate crystal is
not as good. Addition of seed crystals of anhydrous uric acid to a
metastable solution of calcium oxalate leads, after a lag period, to
loss of calcium oxalate from the liquid phase (open circles) (Fig.
4).

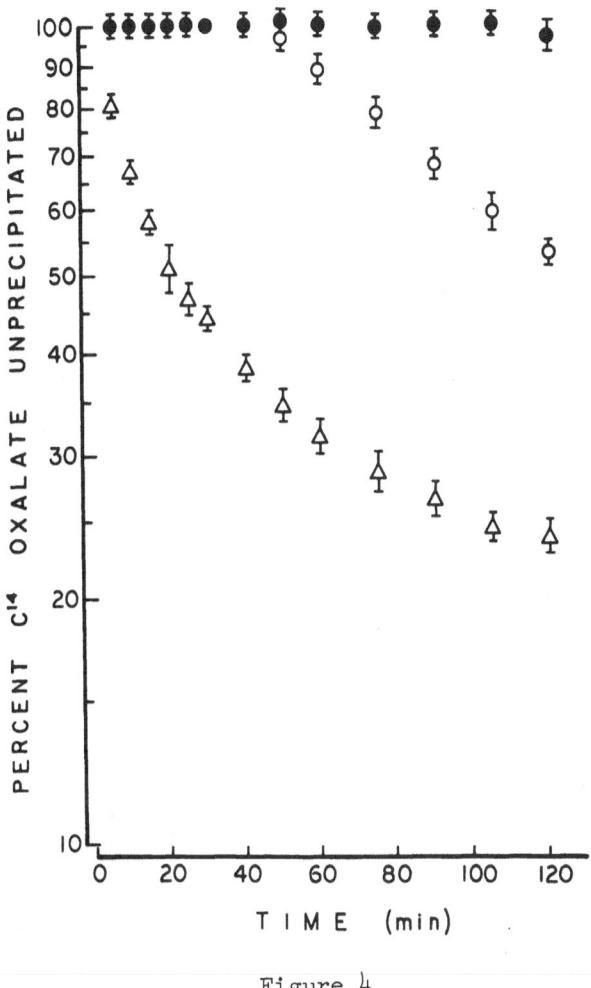

Figure 4

Crystals of calcium oxalate monohydrate (triangles) were more effective and worked without a lag period. Crystals of sodium hydrogen
urate produced equivalent heterogeneous nucleation (Fig. 5).
Effects of 2 concentrations of urate crystals are shown as circles
and squares, effects of corresponding concentration of calcium
oxalate crystals by triangles.

It is very unlikely that heterogeneous nucleation by uric acid
or sodium hydrogen urate produces calcium renal stones in the flowing
urine. If anything, this would lead to gravel and bladder stones
because the total transit time through the renal tubules and upper

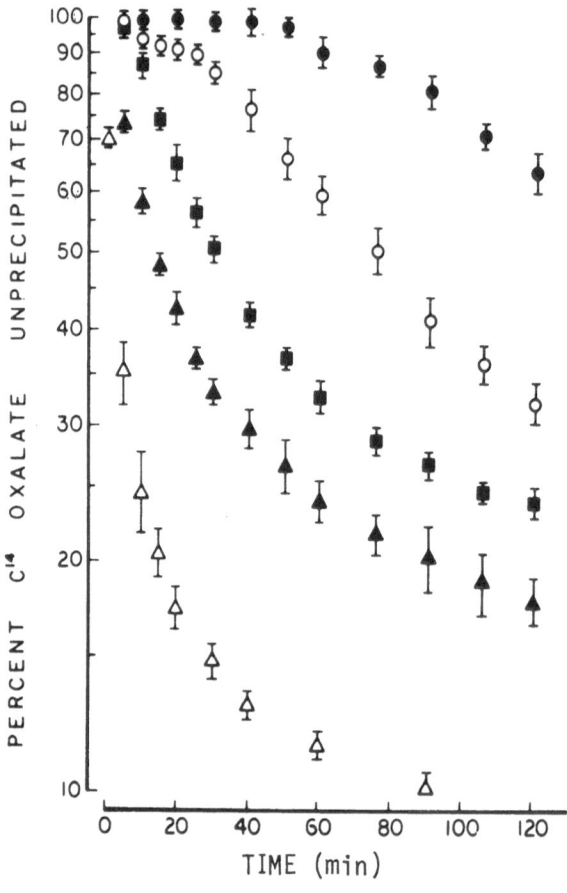

Figure 5

urinary tract is only about 5 minutes, whereas the residence time of urine in the bladder is many hours. A more likely hypothesis is that crystals of uric acid tend to plug occasional terminal collecting ducts. The open end of such a plug, bathed perpetually by the film of urine that covers the papillary tip, could serve as an anchored nidus upon which crystals of calcium oxalate could deposit at leisure, gradually developing a calcium oxalate plaque on the surface of the papillum, which could then grow into an organized stone.

An alternative hypothesis, proposed by Robertson (10), is that hyperuricosuria promotes the formation of a uric acid or urate gel phase in urine that adsorbs naturally occurring macromolecular crystal growth inhibitors, thereby removing from the urine an important

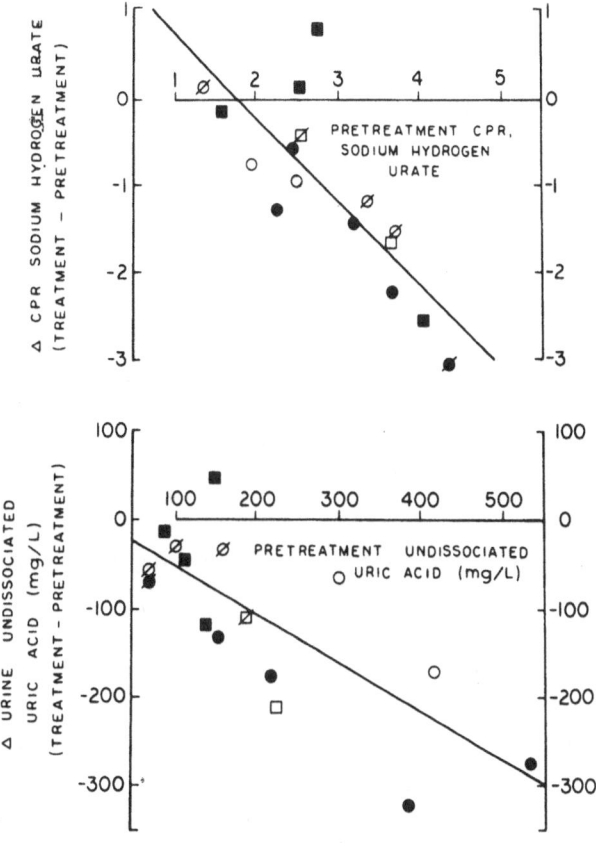

Figure 6

normal protection against crystallization. In support of this hypothesis, Robertson has shown that hyperuricosuria lowers the ability
of urine to inhibit calcium oxalate crystal growth (10). In other
experiments, Pak and colleagues have not found a reduction of crystal
growth inhibition by hyperuricosuria, but have found, instead, a
reduction of the calcium oxalate ion product at which spontaneous
crystallization of calcium oxalate occurred (11). This reduction
could have been due to heterogeneous nucleation of calcium oxalate by
a solid phase of sodium hydrogen urate or uric acid, or to depletion
of inhibitors of crystallization that normally raise the formation
product in urine far above that seen in salt solutions. A complete
evaluation of the challenging hypothesis of Robertson has not yet
been concluded.

Either hypothesis predicts that reducing urinary supersaturation

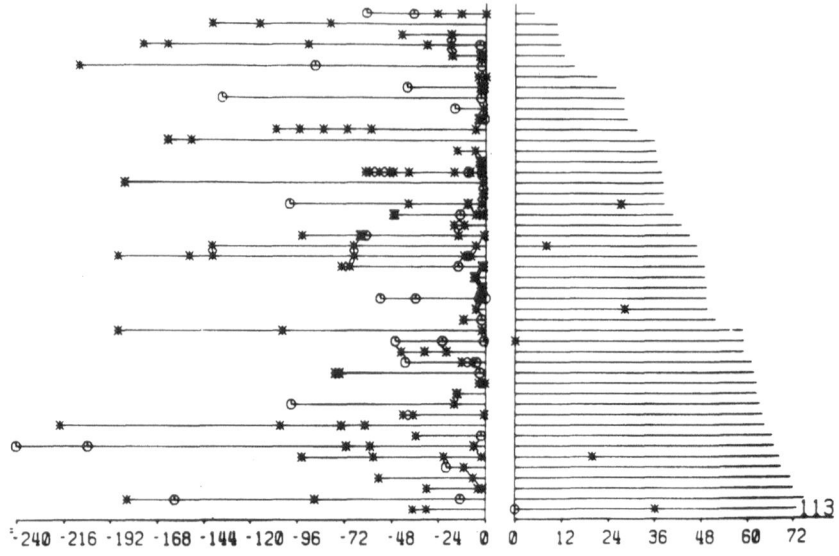

MONTHS BEFORE TREATMENT          MONTHS AFTER TREATMENT

Figure 7

with respect to both solid phases of uric acid would prevent recurrent calcium stones, and 2 studies have provided evidence for such
a protective action. We have found that allopurinol, which reduces
uric acid production, lowers urinary supersaturation with respect to
both solid phases (Fig. 6).

The reduction in the CPR (y axis, upper panel) was proportional to
the initial, or pretreatment, CPR (x axis). A similar pattern was
observed for undissociated uric acid, shown in the lower panel. The
regression line is less perfect because allopurinol does not raise
the pH of the urine, and low urine pH elevates the undissociated
urinary uric acid concentration even in the absence of hyperuricosuria.

     The effect of long-term allopurinol treatment on stone formation
is shown in Fig. 7. During the pretreatment interval of 298 patient
years, these patients formed 51 recurrent stones/100 patients/year.
During the follow-up interval of 186 patient years, they should have
formed 95 new stones; in contrast, they formed 8. Smith and his
colleagues (4) have published a similar study, which employed a
placebo control group and a double-blind design (Table 5).

Table 5
Effects of Allopurinol on New Stone
Production by Recurrent Calcium Oxalate
Stone Formers with Serum Urate Levels
Above 6 mg/100 ml*

| Year of Follow-up | Allopurinol-Treated Patients-New Stones | | | Placebo-Treated Patients-New Stones | | | $X^{2\dagger}$ | $p^{\ddagger}$ |
|---|---|---|---|---|---|---|---|---|
| | Yes | No | All | Yes | No | All | | |
| 0.5 | 21 | 28 | 49 | 30 | 13 | 43 | 6.57 | <.01 |
| 1 | 11 | 27 | 38 | 24 | 3 | 27 | 20.70 | <.001 |
| 2 | 10 | 20 | 30 | 19 | 1 | 20 | 16.84 | <.001 |
| 3 | 6 | 17 | 23 | 12 | 1 | 13 | 14.54 | <.001 |
| 4 | 4 | 15 | 19 | 11 | 1 | 12 | 14.73 | <.001 |
| 5 | 2 | 10 | 12 | 4 | 1 | 5 | 5.97 | <.02 |

*, Adapted from Smith (4). Numbers are patients who have or have not formed new stones at each follow-up interval.

†, Includes patients remaining in the study; some were lost due to failure of treatment compliance, personal decisions to leave the study or drug intolerance. Patients entered the study at different times and therefore had varying lengths of total follow-up.

‡, Calculated $X^2$ for placebo vs. allopurinol treated patients; p values are for 1 degree of freedom.

They selected recurrent calcium oxalate stone formers whose serum urate levels exceeded 6 mg/100 ml, and in whom hypercalciuria, hyperparathyroidism, hyperoxaluria, or other known cause could be excluded. Patients were not uniformly hyperuricosuric. During the first 6 months of follow-up, 28 of 49 allopurinol-treated patients were stone-free compared to 13 of 43 placebo-treated patients. At one year, 27 of 28 treated patients were stone-free compared to only 3 of 27 placebo controls. Thereafter, more than 2/3 of the allopurinol-treated patients remained stone-free, compared to only 1 of the placebo-treated patients. Our study and that of Smith both show a dramatic effect of allopurinol to prevent recurrence of calcium oxalate stones.

Overall, there appears to exist a well-defined syndrome that we have termed hyperuricosuric calcium oxalate urolithiasis. It is characterized by the coexistence of hyperuricosuria and recurrent calcium oxalate renal stones and the absence of any other established causes of stones. Such patients tend to develop excessive urinary supersaturation with respect to undissociated uric acid, because of uric acid overexcretion and a tendency towards a low urine pH, the latter due to an acid-ash diet; they presumably form a solid phase of uric acid or its salt in the renal tubules and urine. Because of either heterogeneous nucleation or adsorption and subsequent depletion of protective macromolecular crystal growth inhibitors from the urine, a calcium oxalate crystal phase eventually forms and produces stones. Treatment with allopurinol tends to prevent the formation of new stones and is therefore a rational therapy for this condition.

Obviously, the ideal treatment would be diet, which could eliminate both the hyperuricosuria and the abnormally acid urine pH. Unfortunately, dietary treatment is difficult to achieve, because hyperuricosuria appears to be a reflection of a widespread dietary pattern that has manifested itself during the 20th century and has come to be viewed as desirable. If subsequent studies continue to confirm a strong link between dietary purine overconsumption, hyperuricosuria, and calcium oxalate urolithiasis, public education and a restoration of an earlier dietary pattern, based more upon grains and less upon meat, may offer the hope of a significant, widespread, reduction in upper tract calcium oxalate urolithiasis.

## References

1.  Coe, F.L.: Hyperuricosuric calcium oxalate nephrolithiasis. Kid. Intern. 13:418-426, 1978.
2.  Coe, F.L.: Nephrolithiasis, Pathogenesis and Treatment. Year Book, Chicago, 1978, p. 95-114.
3.  Coe, F.L.: Treated and untreated recurrent calcium nephrolithiasis in patients with idiopathic hypercalciuria, hyperuricosuria, or no metabolic disorder. Ann. Intern. Med. 87:404-410, 1977.
4.  Smith, M.J.V.: Placebo vs. allopurinol for renal calculi. J. Urol., 1977, in press.
5.  Coe, F.L., Moran, E., and Kavalich, A.G.: The contribution of dietary purine over-consumption to hyperuricosuria in calcium oxalate stone formers. J. Chron. Dis. 29:793-800, 1976.
6.  Brewster, L. and Jacobson, M.F.: The Changing American Diet. Center for Science in the Public Interest, Washington, D.C., 1978, p. 77.
7.  Pak, C.Y.C., Waters, O., Arnold, L., Holt, K., Cox, C., and Barilla, D.: Mechanism for calcium urolithiasis among patients with hyperuricosuria. J. Clin. Invest. 52:134-142, 1977.
8.  Lonsdale, K.: Human stones. Science 159:1159-1207, 1968.
9.  Lonsdale, K.: Epitaxy as a growth factor in urinary calculi and gallstones. Nature 217:56-58, 1968.
10. Robertson, W.G., Knowles, F., Peacock, M.: Urinary acid mucopolysaccharide inhibitors of calcium oxalate crystallization, in Urolithiasis Research, edited by Fleisch, H., Robertson, W.G., Smith, L.H., Vahlensieck, W., London, Plenum Press, 1976, pp. 331-334.
11. Pak, C.Y.C., Barilla, D.E., Holt, K., Brinkley, L., Tolentino, R., and Zerwekh, J.E.: Effect of oral purine load and allopurinol on the crystallization of calcium salts in urine of patients with hyperuricosuric calcium urolithiasis. Am. J. Med. 65:593-599, 1978.

A CRITICAL EVALUATION OF TREATMENT OF CALCIUM STONES

Charles Y.C. Pak

The University of Texas Health Science Center at Dallas
5323 Harry Hines Blvd.
Dallas, Texas 75235

Although various treatment programs have been introduced for
the medical management of calcium urolithiasis, their therapeutic
efficacy has been difficult to appraise critically, because of failure to define clearly indications for treatment, limited double-
blind clinical trials and over-reliance on retrospective stone history. However, recent progress concerning pathogenesis of stone
formation has provided an improved understanding of mechanism of
drug action, and of indications for treatment. Moreover, some
objective data have been gathered supporting clinical efficacy of
certain treatment regimens, despite continued problems in initiation
of controlled (double-blind) clinical studies.

### DEFINITION OF INDICATIONS FOR EACH TREATMENT PROGRAM

It is reasonable to speculate that the optimum treatment regimen should satisfy the following criteria:[1] (a) the treatment
"reverses" the underlying physiological and physicochemical derangements, which characterize the given cause of stone disease, (b) it
is effective in inhibiting new stone formation, and (c) it is
associated with minimum or tolerable side effects. Because of the
recognition that calcium urolithiasis is a heterogeneous entity with
different etiologies, the optimum treatment program should ideally
be defined for each cause. Recent advances in urolithiasis research
provides a sufficient background for the adoption of such a rational
approach to treatment. This chapter reviews our current format for
optimum therapy, admittedly preliminary and subject to further
refinement pending new data.

The first criterion for optimum therapy represents the definition of indications for each treatment program, and entails (a) an
appreciation of different causes of calcium urolithiasis, (b) an
understanding of mechanism of drug action, and (c) selection of
particular treatment directed specifically at ameliorating the cause.

## Causes of Calcium Urolithiasis:  Physiological Derangements.

Calcium urolithiasis may be categorized on the basis of major
physiological abnormalities, -hypercalciuria, hyperuricosuria and
hyperoxaluria (Table 1).[2]  Hypercalciuria is the most common

Table 1.  Causes of Calcium Urolithiasis

I.    Hypercalciuria
      1.    Resorptive (primary hyperparathyroidism)
      2.    Absorptive
            a.    Vitamin D-independent
            b.    Vitamin D-dependent
      3.    Renal
II.   Hyperuricosuria
      1.    Hyperuricosuric calcium oxalate nephrolithiasis
      2.    Hyperuricosuria with hypercalciuria
III.  Hyperoxaluria
      1.    Primary
      2.    Enteric
IV.   No "metabolic" abnormality
      1.    Inhibitor deficiency (and/or promoter excess)
      2.    Acquired
            a.    Infection
            b.    Structural abnormality
            c.    Low fluid volume

abnormality.  In a recent series of Coe,[3] it was encountered in 49%
of patients with calcium urolithiasis.  In 151 consecutive patients
evaluated by us in an ambulatory setting[4] over a 2-year period,
hypercalciuria was disclosed in 76%.  Hypercalciuria is comprised of
three principal subtypes,[5] -primary hyperparathyroidism (resorptive
hypercalciuria), absorptive hypercalciuria and renal hypercalciuria.
The cause for the increased calcium absorption in the majority of
patients with absorptive hypercalciuria is the apparent vitamin D-
independent intestinal hyperabsorption, involving calcium and not
magnesium, and localized to jejunum but not ileum.[6]  In some
patients, a primary renal phosphate "leak" may augment intestinal
calcium absorption via stimulation of the renal synthesis of 1,25-
dihydroxyvitamin D.[7]  Sarcoidosis may represent another vitamin D-
dependent variant of the absorptive hypercalciuria.

The cause for the impaired renal tubular reabsorption of calcium in renal hypercalciuria is not known. Moreover, the possibility that this condition may be accompanied by other abnormalities in renal tubular function has not been excluded. Secondary hyperparathyroidism is invariably present,[8] and intestinal calcium absorption may be sometimes increased, consequent to the parathyroid hormone-dependent stimulation of the synthesis of 1,25-dihydroxyvitamin D. Medullary sponge disease, though speculated to be a cause for the renal calcium leak,[9] is infrequently encountered[3] in either renal or absorptive hypercalciuria. Medullary sponge disease was encountered in less than 5% of our patients with calcium urolithiasis. The principal metabolic abnormality associated with this condition was absorptive hypercalciuria and not renal hypercalciuria. Distal renal tubular acidosis, though an uncommon cause of calcium urolithiasis, may be considered as a form of renal hypercalciuria, at least before the development of significant renal functional impairment.

Hyperuricosuria may be the only recognizable physiological abnormality in some patients with calcium nephrolithiasis.[10] Such an abnormality (hyperuricosuric calcium oxalate nephrolithiasis) comprised 15% of calcium stone-formers in Coe's series,[3] and 9% in our series. The hyperuricosuria is usually the result of dietary overindulgence with purine-rich foods, and sometimes is the sequelae of a primary overproduction of uric acid. The urinary pH is typically greater than the $pK_a$ for the first proton of uric acid (5.47), though reported to be lower than in non-stone forming subjects. Clinical gout is rare. Hyperuricosuria may coexist with all three forms of hypercalciuria.

Although primary hyperoxaluria is a rare cause of calcium urolithiasis, enteric hyperoxaluria,[11,12] associated with an inflammatory disease of the small bowel or with an intestinal bypass surgery, may account for 1-5% calcium urolithiasis.[3] An increased intestinal absorption of oxalate is present and accounts for the hyperoxaluria. Two influences probably combine to cause the intestinal hyperabsorption of oxalate.[13] The intestinal transport of oxalate may be primarily increased from the action of bile salts on the permeability of intestinal mucosa to oxalate. The total amount of oxalate absorbed may also be increased because of an enlarged luminal pool of oxalate available for absorption. The intestinal fat malabsorption characteristic of ileal disease may exaggerate the soap formation with divalent cations, limit the amount of "free" divalent cations to complex oxalate, and thereby raise the available oxalate pool. The intestinal absorption and renal excretion of calcium are often decreased in enteric hyperoxaluria. Urine output may be substantially reduced consequent to an excessive fluid loss from the intestinal tract. Citrate excretion may be impaired.

In remaining patients, constituting 20% in Coe's series  and
9% in ours, no underlying "physiological" or "metabolic" abnormality
could be found.  This category may include the heretofore unproven
hypothetical cause, characterized by an impaired renal excretion of
inhibitors of crystallization, and/or an exaggerated excretion of
promoters.[14]  Such an abnormality may coexist with some of the recognized causes of calcium urolithiasis.  For example, a reduced renal
excretion of pyrophosphate has been reported in male subjects with
idiopathic hypercalciuria (consisting primarily of absorptive and
renal hypercalciurias) and in patients with primary hyperparathyroidism.

Causes of Calcium Urolithiasis:  Physicochemical Derangements

It is recognized that important determinants for stone formation from the physicochemical standpoint include:  urinary supersaturation with respect to stone-forming salts, reduced limit of
metastability, and facilitated nidus growth via crystal growth,
heterogeneous nucleation and crystal aggregation.  Available data,
albeit preliminary, indicate that this requirement is largely met
in most causes of calcium urolithiasis discussed previously.

In all three forms of hypercalciuria, the urinary environment
is characteristically supersaturated with respect to calcium oxalate
and brushite, owing principally to the high urinary concentration
of calcium.[14,15]  Moreover, the formation product ratio (limit of
metastability) of both calcium salts is often decreased.[14]  These
effects combine to enhance the propensity for the spontaneous
nucleation (or heterogeneous nucleation by naturally occurring
nuclei) of calcium salts.  Besides reduced metastable limit, the
crystal growth and aggregation may sometimes be exaggerated,[14] a
finding indicating the operation of a low inhibitor activity and/or
a high promoter activity.  The above physicochemical profile is not
unique to any one form of hypercalciuria, although the reduced
limit of metastability is more commonly encountered in primary
hyperparathyroidism.

The essential finding in hyperuricosuric calcium oxalate
nephrolithiasis is the urinary supersaturation of monosodium urate,
which results from a high urinary content of uric acid and a favorable pH range (>5.5) in which this urate phase is stable.[16,17]
Though not yet proven conclusively, it has been suggested that
either a colloidal or crystalline monosodium urate forms from such a
supersaturated environment, and initiates formation of calcium
stones (a) by a direct induction of heterogeneous nucleation of calcium oxalate,[18,19] or (b) indirectly by adsorption of certain muco-
polysaccharides (thereby attenuating the inhibitory action of muco-
polysaccharides on crystal aggregation[20] or on spontaneous nuclea-

tion[21]of calcium oxalate).

In calcium oxalate nephrolithiasis associated with enteric hyperoxaluria, there is an increased saturation of urine with respect to calcium oxalate[13] because of high oxalate concentration, even though urinary calcium is low. Urinary inhibitor or promoter activity has not been systematically measured.

There is limited available data concerning physical chemistry of stone formation in patients without discernible physiological abnormality. A preliminary study indicates that the urinary limit of metastability of calcium salts is often reduced,[14] a finding suggesting that certain patients may suffer from a deficiency of inhibitors and/or an excess of promoters.

## Mechanism of Action of Therapeutic Modalities.

For many treatment programs recommended for calcium urolithiasis, sufficient information is now available to characterize their physiological and physicochemical actions.[1] From these effects, specific indications may be defined for each treatment regimen; i.e., a particular program may be selected for each cause, based on its ability to most optimally correct the physiological and physicochemical derangements which characterize that disorder. Table 2 summarizes available data concerning the mode of action of parathyroidectomy, various forms of phosphates, thiazide, allopurinol, and divalent cations. Though admittedly preliminary and controversial, their optimal indications are also provided.

The sole indication for parathyroidectomy is primary hyperparathyroidism.[1] Following a successful parathyroid surgery, a normal urinary calcium is restored, commensurate with a decline in serum calcium and in intestinal calcium absorption. Physicochemical changes include a decreased saturation of urine with respect to calcium oxalate and brushite, and an increased limit of metastability of calcium oxalate. The latter finding suggests that normal inhibitor and/or promoter activity may be restored upon parathyroidectomy.

The use of sodium cellulose phosphate, a non-absorbable ion-exchange resin with a high affinity for calcium, should be restricted to absorptive hypercalciuria.[1] This drug represents the only established available regimen which restores normal urinary calcium by directly inhibiting intestinal calcium absorption. However, it is not the ultimate therapy for the absorptive hypercalciuria, since it does not alter the basic abnormality in calcium transport. The amount of absorbed calcium is reduced, simply by a restriction in the available calcium pool. This particular mode of action of sodium cellulose phosphate probably accounts for the

Table 2.  Mode of Action of Therapeutic Modalities

| | PTX | SCP | $PO_4$ | DiP | TZ | Allop | Mg |
|---|---|---|---|---|---|---|---|
| Urin Ca | ↓↓ | ↓↓↓ | ↓ | - | ↓↓ | - | ↑ |
| Urin P | - | ↑ | ↑↑↑ | - | ↑/- | - | ↓ |
| Urin Ox | -/↓ | ↑ | ↑/- | ↑/- | ↑/↓ | - | ↓ |
| Urin Citr | ? | - | ↑ | - | ↓ | - | ? |
| Urin $P_2O_7$ | ? | - | ↑↑ | - | ↑ | ↑/- | ? |
| Brushite APR | ↓ | ↓↓ | ↑ | - | ↓ | - | ↑ |
| FPR | ↑ | - | ↑ | ↑ | ↑ | ↑/- | - |
| CG | ↓ | - | ↓/- | ↓ | - | - | - |
| CaOx APR | ↓ | ↓/- | ↓ | - | ↓ | - | - |
| FPR | ↑ | - | ↑ | ↑ | ↑ | ↑ | - |
| CG | ↓ | - | ↑/- | ↓ | - | ↓ | - |
| Aggr | ? | ? | ↓ | ↓ | ? | ? | ? |
| Indications | PHPT | AH | AH-P ID | ?ID | RH ID,?AH | HU | ? |

Abbreviations:  ↓, decrease;   -, no change;  ↑, increase; PTX,
parathyroidectomy; SCP, sodium cellulose phosphate; $PO_4$, orthophosphate; DiP, diphosphonate; TZ, thiazide; Allop, allopurinol; Ox, oxalate; Citr, citrate; $P_2O_7$, pyrophosphate; APR,
activity product ratio or state of saturation; FPR, formation
product ratio or limit of metastability; CG, crystal growth;
Aggr, aggregation; PHPT, primary hyperparathyroidism; AH,
absorptive hypercalciuria; AH-P, hypophosphatemic absorptive
hypercalciuria; ID, inhibitor deficiency, RH, renal hypercalciuria; HU, hyperuricosuric calcium oxalate nephrolithiasis.

slight-moderate increase in oxalate excretion encountered during
treatment, particularly during a calcium restricted diet.[22]  The
reduced luminal content of "free" calcium, resulting form binding
of calcium to the resin, lowers calcium-oxalate complexation, and
augments the luminal pool of oxalate available for absorption.
Physiocochemically, the treatment reduces the urinary saturation of
brushite dramatically,[23] and to a lesser extent lowers that of
calcium oxalate.[22]  The treatment probably does not affect the
inhibitor or promoter activity, since no changes are found in the
limit of metastability or in the renal excretion of known inhibitors
such as pyrophosphate or citrate.

Soluble orthophosphate given orally reduces the renal excretion
of calcium, probably by interfering with the renal tubular reabsorption of phosphate.  It does not affect the intestinal absorption
of calcium in the vitamin D-independent variant of absorptive
hypercalciuria.[24]  In hypophosphatemic absorptive hypercalciuria
with an increased production of 1,25-dihydroxyvitamin D, phosphate

therapy may theoretically restore normal intestinal calcium absorption by inhibiting the synthesis of the vitamin D metabolite. This scheme, if proven, should provide a physiological rationale for the selection of orthophosphate in the management of this form of absorptive hypercalciuria. Besides its effect on calcium absorption and excretion, orthophosphate causes a marked enhancement of urinary phosphate excretion, a finding attesting to the solubility and absorbability of phosphate. Moreover, the treatment increases the renal excretion of certain inhibitors, including pyrophosphate and citrate.[25] Its physicochemical effects are represented by a reduced saturation of calcium oxalate, and a stimulated inhibitor activity as reflected by a rise in the limit of metastability of calcium oxalate.[26] While there is an increased saturation of brushite, a concurrent rise in the limit of metastability usually compensates for this potentially negative effect. The ability of orthophosphate to augment inhibitor activity and to stimulate urinary excretion of certain inhibitors provides a justification for the use of this treatment in patients without discernible physiological derangements in whom an inhibitor deficiency (or a promoter excess) is suspected. [25]

The urinary inhibitor activity may also be stimulated by an exogenous inhibitor, such as diphosphonate. Following an oral administration of disodium ethane-1-hydroxy-1,1-diphosphonate, a sufficient amount of the compound may appear in urine to inhibit nucleation and growth of calcium oxalate and brushite.[27] While the potential usefulness of diphosphonate in patients with a presumed inhibitor deficiency is attractive, a long-term treatment with this drug is precluded by attendant serious hazards, particularly an induction of osteomalacia.

A well-established action of thiazide is the augmentation of renal tubular reabsorption of calcium.[28] It is particularly indicated in renal hypercalciuria, since it has been shown to correct the renal leak of calcium and secondary hyperparathyroidism and restore normal circulating concentration of 1,25-dihydroxyvitamin D and intestinal calcium absorption.[29] In absorptive hypercalciuria, however, the intestinal hyperabsorption of calcium is maintained during thiazide therapy, despite an equivalent fall in urinary calcium.[29] Thus, thiazide may not be ideally suited physiologically for the management of absorptive hypercalciuria, until the fate of "retained" calcium is clarified. Physicochemically, thiazide reduces the urinary saturation of calcium oxalate and brushite and increases the limit of metastability of these salts.[30] The latter effect is probably the result of the stimulation of urinary excretion of certain inhibitors, including pyrophosphate and zinc. This inhibitor property of thiazide forms the basis for its use in normocalciuric patients with presumed inhibitor deficiency.

   Allopurinol is the physiologically meaningful drug of choice
in hyperuricosuric calcium oxalate nephrolithiasis[3] resulting from
uric acid overproduction, because of its ability to reduce uric
acid synthesis and lower urinary uric acid.  Its use in hyperuricosuria associated with dietary purine overindulgence is also
reasonable, since dietary purine restriction is impractical.  Physicochemical changes ensuing from restoration of normal urinary uric
acid include a reduction in urinary saturation of monosodium urate
and a commensurate increase in the urinary limit of metastability of
calcium oxalate.[17]  Thus, the spontaneous nucleation of calcium
oxalate is retarded by treatment, probably via inhibition of monosodium urate-induced stimulation of calcium oxalate crystallization.

   The available data do   not justify the use of oral magnesium
oxide in calcium urolithiasis.  There is no evidence for magnesium
deficiency in the vast majority of patients with calcium urolithiasis.  While this treatment slightly reduces urinary oxalate, it
augments calcium excretion.  Thus, urinary saturation of calcium
salts is not reduced by this therapy.[32]  Furthermore, the urinary
inhibitors activity is not significantly altered, a finding attesting to the low inhibitor action of magnesium.  In enteric hyperoxaluria, oral magnesium or calcium therapy may reduce oxalate excretion, probably by promoting divalent cation- oxalate complexation.
However, the concurrent rise in urinary calcium compensates for the
decline in urinary oxalate, and maintains urinary supersaturation
of calcium oxalate.[13]

## REVIEW OF CLINICAL TRIALS

   Numerous reports have appeared concerning the effect of long-
term treatment with various drugs on renal stone formation.  The
appraisal of the results of these clinical trials should be made
in the following context:  (a) patients selected for treatment were
often heterogeneous suffering from different causes, and sometimes
included those in whom the particular treatment chosen was not
optimally indicated on physiological or physicochemical grounds,
(b) few double-blind clinical trials are available, because of
inherent problems in conducting them, and (c) there may be a positive placebo effect on the clinical course of nephrolithiasis.

   The rationale for the selection of a certain treatment program
according to its ability to reverse physiological and physicochemical abnormalities as outlined previously, is the assumption that the
particular physiological and physicochemical aberrations identified
with the given disorder are etiologically important in the formation
of renal stones, and that the correction of these disturbances
would prevent stone formation.  Moreover, it is assumed that such
a selected treatment program would be more effective and safe,
than a "random" treatment.  Despite a lack of conclusive experimen-

tal verification, these hypotheses appear reasonable and logical. However, it is acknowledged that certain randomly-chosen treatments may be clinically useful because they may ultimately prove to be physiologically "sound". Moreover, some treatments may be efficacious because of their positive physicochemical effects, even though they may not alter physiological aberrations.

There are only two reports of double-blind clinical trials, with an imposition of a placebo control group, for the assessment of the treatment of calcium urolithiasis, one involving orthophosphate[33] and another with allopurinol.[34] This limited information stems partly from the constraints of human experimentation which often does not permit a denial of treatment which is essential for the inclusion of a placebo group, and partly from the difficulty in the preparation of placebo medications which cannot be readily identified by the patient. For this reason, most of clinical trials have compared prospective data during treatment with retrospective data before treatment. Unfortunately, factors other than the particular therapy itself may be introduced during treatment; these factors include changes in dietary habits, fluid intake and physician's care.

The importance of these non-specific effects on the course of calcium urolithiasis has been amply illustrated by the two double-blind clinical trials. In the study of Ettinger,[33] stone passage rate decreased from 0.78 - 0.33/patient year during placebo treatment, and 70% of patients remained in remission (no new stone formation) after 3 years of placebo treatment. In patients with hyperuricemia (>6 mg/dl) and calcium oxalate nephrolithiasis,[34] Smith found that 48% of patients in the placebo group formed fewer stones. Moreover, Coe followed 34 patients without detectable metabolic abnormality while they were not receiving any specific treatment.[10] New stone formation declined to 63% of the predicted rate; 65% of patients did not form new stones over a mean follow-up of 3.2 years.

In assessing the results of clinical trials which lack placebo control, the response to therapy should be substantially better than the placebo response for the treatment to be considered effective. We shall review data from some of the representative clinical trials. These studies will be discussed in order of decreasing conformity to the optimum indications outlined previously.

Sodium cellulose phosphate and allopurinol have been employed for the treatment of absorptive hypercalciuria and hyperuricosuric calcium oxalate nephrolithiasis respectively, the conditions for which these drugs are optimally indicated from both physiological and physicochemical grounds. Pak et al.[23] reported that sodium cellulose phosphate produced a decline in stone passage rate from 3.84 - 0.27/patient year, and remission in 81% of patients

over a mean treatment period of 2.6 years.  Similar findings were
found by Pietrek  and Kokot[35] and by Blacklock and MacLeod[36] in
patients with idiopathic hypercalciuria, most of whom probably had
absorptive hypercalciuria.  Although these studies lack placebo
control group, they nevertheless indicate a probable effectiveness
of this drug regimen since the response obtained is substantially
better than that reported for placebo treatment.  Moreover, no
significant side-effects have been reported.

     In the study of Coe et al. involving patients with hyperurico-
suric calcium oxalate nephrolithiasis, allopurinol treatment (over
3.9 years/patient)  reduced the stone passage rate from 0.67 - 0.04/
patient year, and maintained 85% of patients in remission.[3]  Smith
evaluated patients with hyperuricemia (>6 mg/dl), some of whom may
not have had hyperuricosuric calcium oxalate nephrolithiasis.[34] A
smaller portion of patients (61%) were in remission during allopurinol treatment, than was shown by Coe et al., a finding which
emphasizes the importance of a rigid patient selection.  However,
allopurinol therapy was probably effective, since the placebo
control group showed a remission rate of only 8%.

     Thiazide was used by Yendt et al.[28],[31] for the treatment of a
mixed group of patients with calcium urolithiasis, most of whom
had idiopathic hypercalciuria.  In those without pre-existing stones,
stone passage rate decreased from 0.24 - 0.03/patient  year and 94%
of patients were in remission during a mean treatment period of
2.2 years.[28]  Similar results were obtained by Coe[3] with thiazide in
patients with idiopathic hypercalciuria.  The rate of stone passage
decreased from 0.32 -0.02/patient year, and 95% of patients did not
form new stones (over a mean treatment period of 2.9 years).  In a
recent study, Yendt and Cohanim[31] reported that none of normocalciuric patients receiving thiazide formed new stones, a finding
which emphasizes the importance of the promotion of endogenous
inhibitor activity for thiazide action.

     These results support the probable indication and efficacy of
thiazide in renal hypercalciuria and normocalciuric nephrolithiasis
with inhibitor deficiency.  However, a similar evidence is not yet
available for absorptive hypercalciuria and hyperuricosuric calcium
oxalate nephrolithiasis.  It has been reported that the intestinal
hyperabsorption of calcium is maintained during thiazide therapy
(up to 3 years) in absorptive hypercalciuria, despite a reduction in
urinary calcium.[29]  Although there are no reports of metastic calcification or increased bone density ensuing from thiazide therapy,
the fate of "retained" calcium remains unresolved.  Yendt and
Cohanim[31] suggested that the intestinal calcium absorption may be
ultimately restored to normal by a continued thiazide therapy.
However, their study was based on two patients, in whom the
diagnosis of absorptive hypercalciuria was not firmly established.

It is acknowledged that thiazide may prove to be an appropriate indication for absorptive hypercalciuria on physiological grounds, if the observation of Yendt and Cohanim is confirmed.  In hyperuricosuric calcium oxalate nephrolithiasis, the treatment with thiazide alone may have a limited utility, since it may augment uric acid excretion.[37]   Moreover, Yendt and Cohanim[31] found that an important feature of treatment failure to thiazide was a high urinary excretion of uric acid.

The use of orthophosphates has not been restricted to those with hypophosphatemia or with inhibitor deficiency.  Berstein and Newton[38] found a remission rate of 78% in patients with idiopathic hypercalciuria receiving orthophosphate (1.9 years/patient).  In a mixed group of hypercalciuric and normocalciuric patients, Thomas[39] reported that orthophosphate therapy caused a cessation of stone formation in 86% of patients.  Smith et al.[40]  showed a similar favorable finding.  However, in a double-blind controlled study conducted by Ettinger[33]   involving patients with hypercalciuria as well as with normocalciuria, orthophosphate (given over 3.1 years/patient) altered stone passage rate from 0.67 - 0.54/patient year and produced remission in 52% of patients.  These responses were not substantially different from those of the placebo control group of 0.78 - 0.33/patient year and 70% respectively.  A similar treatment failure was reported by Ettinger and Kolb[41] in a non-double-blind study.  The apparent ineffectiveness in the last two reports may have partly resulted from the use of marginally effective dose of orthophosphate, and the employment of an acid rather than neutral or alkaline form of phosphate.  Some workers have reported significant side-effects of therapy, including extraskeletal calcification, renal functional deterioration, and parathyroid stimulation.  However, others have not been able to confirm these observations.  Thus, the clinical trials of orthophosphate in a diverse group of patients have yielded conflicting data.

Melnick et al. treated a mixed group of patients identified as "idiopathic recurrent calcium oxalate stone formers" with magnesium oxide.[42]  Magnesium oxide treatment produced a 78% reduction in stone passage; however, the control group who received no treatment showed a reduction of 49% (from data obtained retrospectively).  A complete remission was obtained in 63% of patients receiving magnesium oxide, a rate which is not substantially different from that obtained in untreated patients.

## CONCLUSION

It is apparent from the previous discussion of clinical trials that those treatment programs which meet the physiological and physicochemical criteria for optimum indications are seemingly more effective in the prevention of stone formation and/or are

associated with fewer side-effects than those regimens in which
conditions chosen for treatment are less rigidly selected.  This
finding, albeit based on preliminary data, provides a justification
for the selective approach to treatment, whereby a particular regimen is specifically chosen for the amelioration of the underlying
physiological and physicochemical abnormalities characteristic of
the given disorder.

It is anticipated that a further confirmation of this "rational"
approach to treatment would be obtained even in the present con-
strainsts of human experimentation, if the subjective response
(rate of stone passage or remission) were shown to be correlated
with the objective response (physiological or physicochemical
measures), and if a modified study design for treatment efficacy,
based on stone "relapse" rate after drug withdrawal, were found to
be applicable.

ACKNOWLEDGEMENT

This work was supported by grants from the USPHS R01-AM16061,
M01-RR00633 and P50-AM20543.

REFERENCES

1.  C.Y.C. Pak, "Calcium Urolithiasis:  Pathogenesis, Diagnosis,
    and Management,"  Plenum Publishing Company, New York (1978).
2.  C.Y.C. Pak, Idiopathic renal lithiasis:  New developments in
    evaluation and treatment, in:"Urolithiasis Research," H.
    Fleisch, W.G. Robertson, L.H. Smith, and W. Vahlensieck, eds.,
    Plenum Press, New York, (1976).
3.  F.L. Coe, Treated and untreated recurrent calcium nephrolith-
    iasis in patients with idiopathic hypercalciuria, idiopathic
    hyperuricosuria, or no metabolic disorder, Ann. Int. Med. 87:
    404 (1977).
4.  C.Y.C. Pak, C. Fetner, J. Townsend, L. Brinkley, C. Northcutt,
    D.E. Barilla, M. Kadesky, and P. Peters, Evaluation of calcium
    urolithiasis in ambulatory patients.  Comparison of results
    with those of inpatient evaluation, Am. J. Med. 64:979 (1978).
5.  C.Y.C. Pak, M. Ohata, E.C. Lawrence, and W. Snyder, The hyper-
    calciurias:  Causes, parathyroid functions and diagnostic
    criteria, J. Clin. Invest. 54:387 (1974).
6.  P.G. Brannan, S. Morawski, C.Y.C. Pak, and J.S. Fordtran,
    Selective jejunal hyperabsorption of calcium in absorptive
    hypercalciuria, Am. J. Med. 66:425 (1979).
7.  R.W. Gray, D.R. Wilz, A.E. Caldas, and J. Lemann, Jr., The
    importance of phosphate in regulating plasma $1,25\text{-}(OH)_2$-vitamin
    D levels in humans:  Studies in health subjects, in calcium
    stone formers and in patients with primary hyperparathyroidism,
    J. Clin. Endocrinol. Metab. 45:299 (1977).

8.  F.L. Coe, J.M. Canterbury, J.J. Firpo, and E. Reiss, Evidence for secondary hyperparathyroidism in idiopathic hypercalciuria, J. Clin. Invest. 52:134 (1973).

9.  P.W. Dlabal, R.M. Jordan, and S.G. Dorfman, Medullary sponge kidney and renal-leak hypercalciuria: A link to the development of parathyroid adenoma? JAMA 241:1490 (1979).

10. F.L. Coe, Hyperuricosuric calcium oxalate nephrolithiasis, Kidney Int. 13:418 (1978).

11. L.H. Smith, H. Fromm, and A.F. Hofmann, Acquired hyperoxaluria, nephrolithiasis and intestinal disease: Description of a syndrome. N. Eng. J. Med. 286:1371 (1972).

12. D.L. Earnest, H.E. Williams, and W.H. Admirand, A physicochemical basis for treatment of enteric hyperoxaluria, Trans. Assoc. Am. Physicians 88:224 (1975).

13. D.E. Barilla, C. Notz, D. Kennedy, and C.Y.C. Pak, Renal oxalate excretion following oral oxalate loads in patients with ileal disease and with renal and absorptive hypercalciurias: Effect of calcium and magnesium. Am. J. Med. 64:579 (1978).

14. C.Y.C. Pak and K. Holt, Nucleation and growth of brushite and calcium oxalate in urine of stone-formers, Metabolism 25:665 (1976).

15. W.G. Robertson, M. Peacock, and B.E.C. Nordin, Activity products in stone-forming and non-stone-forming urine, Clin. Sci. 34:579 (1968).

16. C.Y.C. Pak, O. Waters, L. Arnold, K. Holt, C. Cox, and D. Barilla, Mechanism for calcium urolithiasis among patients with hyperuricosuria: Supersaturation of urine with respect to monosodium urate, J. Clin. Invest. 59:426 (1977).

17. C.Y.C. Pak, D.E. Barilla, K. Holt, L. Brinkley, R. Tolentino, and J.E. Zerwekh, Effect of oral purine load and allopurinol on the crystallization of calcium salts in urine of patients with hyperuricosuric calcium urolithiasis, Am. J. Med. 65:593 (1978).

18. F.L. Coe, R.L. Lawton, R.B. Goldstein, and V. Tembe, Sodium urate accelerates precipitation of calcium oxalate in vitro, Proc. Soc. Exp. Biol. Med. 149:926 (1975).

19. C.Y.C. Pak and L.H. Arnold, Heterogeneous nucleation of calcium oxalate by seeds of monosodium urate, Proc. Soc. Exp. Biol. Med. 149:930 (1975).

20. W.G. Robertson, F. Knowles, and M. Peacock, Urinary acid mucopolysaccharide inhibitors of calcium oxalate crystallization, in:"Urolithiasis Research," H. Fleisch, W.G. Robertson, L.H. Smith, and W. Vahlensieck, eds. Plenum Press, New York (1976).

21. C.Y.C. Pak, K. Holt, and J.E. Zerwekh, Attenuation by monosodium urate of the inhibitory effect of mucopolysaccharide on calcium oxalate nucleation, Invest. Urol. In press.

22. Y. Hayashi, R.A. Kaplan, and C.Y.C. Pak, Effect of sodium cellulose phosphate therapy on crystallization of calcium oxalate in urine, Metabolism 24:1273 (1975).

23. C.Y.C. Pak, C.S. Delea, and F.C. Bartter, Successful treatment of recurrent nephrolithiasis (calcium stones) with cellulose phosphate, N. Eng. J. Med. 290:175 (1974).

24. D.E. Barilla, J.E. Zerwekh, and C.Y.C. Pak, A critical evaluation of the role of phosphate in the pathogenesis of absorptive hypercalciuria, Min. & Elec. Metab. In press.

25. W.C. Thomas, Use of phosphates in patients with calcareous renal calculi, Kidney Int. 13:390 (1978).

26. C.Y.C. Pak, K. Holt, J. Zerwekh, and D.E. Barilla, Effects of orthophosphate therapy on the crystallization of calcium salts in urine, Min Elec. Metab. 1:147 (1978).

27. M. Ohata and C.Y.C. Pak, The effect of diphosphonate on calcium phosphate crystallization in urine in vitro, Kidney Int. 4:401 (1973).

28. E.R. Yendt, G.F. Guay, and D.A. Garcia, The use of thiazides in the prevention of renal calculi, C.M.A. J. 102:614 (1970).

29. D.E. Barilla, R. Tolentino, R.A. Kaplan, and C.Y.C. Pak, Selective effect of thiazide on the intestinal absorption of calcium in absorptive and renal hypercalciurias, Metabolism 27:125 (1978).

30. A. Woelfel, R.A. Kaplan, and C.Y.C. Pak, Effect of hydrochlorothiazide therapy on the crystallization of calcium oxalate in urine, Metabolism 26:201 (1977).

31. E.R. Yendt and M. Cohanim, Prevention of calcium stones with thiazides, Kidney Int. 13:397 (1978).

32. C.D. Fetner, D.E. Barilla, J. Townsend, and C.Y.C. Pak, Effect of magnesium oxide on the crystallization of calcium salts in urine in patients with recurrent nephrolithiasis, J. Urol. 120:399 (1978).

33. B. Ettinger, Recurrent nephrolithiasis: Natural history and effect of phosphate therapy, Am. J. Med. 61:200 (1976).

34. M.J.V. Smith, Placebo versus allopurinol for renal calculi, J. Urol. 117:690 (1977).

35. J. Pietrek and F. Kokot, Treatment of patients with calcium-containing renal stones with cellulose phosphate, Brit. J. Urol. 45:136 (1973).

36. N.J. Blacklock and M.A. MacLeod, The effect of cellulose phosphate on intestinal absorption and urinary excretion of calcium, Br. J. Urol. 46:385 (1974).

37. C.Y.C. Pak, R. Tolentino, A. Stewart, and R.A. Galosy, Enhancement of renal excretion of uric acid during long-term thiazide therapy, Invest. Urol. 16:3:191 (1978).

38. D.S. Bernstein and R. Newton, The effect of oral sodium phosphate on the formation of renal calculi and on idiopathic hypercalciuria, Lancet 1105 (1966).

39. W.C. Thomas, Jr., Effectiveness and mode of action of orthophosphates in patients with calcareous renal calculi, Trans. Am. Clin. Climetol. Assoc. 83:113 (1971).

40. L.H. Smith, W.C. Thomas, Jr., and C.D. Arnaud, Orthophosphate therapy in calcium renal lithiasis, in:"Urinary Calculi International Symposium on Renal Stone Research," S. Karger, New York (1973).
41. B. Ettinger and F.O. Kolb, Inorganic phosphate treatment of nephrolithiasis, Am. J. Med. 55:32 (1973).
42. I. Melnick, R.R. Landes, A.A. Hoffman, and J.F. Butch, Magnesium therapy for recurring calcium oxalate urinary calculi, J. Urol. 105:119 (1971).

# INCREASED INCIDENCE OF NEPHROLITHIASIS (N) IN LIFEGUARDS (LG) IN ISRAEL

O.S. Better, M. Shabtai, S. Kedar, A. Melamud,
J. Berenheim and C. Chaimovitz

Rambam Medical Center and Technion School of Medicine,
Haifa,   Rothschild Hospital, Haifa  and
Beit Meir Hospital, Kfar Saba, Israel

ABSTRACT

Eleven of 45 (24%) LG had proven N.  This is approximately twenty times the incidence of N in the general population.  The present study was undertaken to determine the factors that contribute to this high incidence of N in LG.

On the job LG are exposed to heat and intense sunlight over almost their entire body surface, for at least 8 hr/d, 6 mo/yr. In an attempt to study the influence of these conditions on vitamin D and calcium metabolism the following were measured: mean serum 25-hydroxycholecalciferol (25-HCC) of the LG of $59\pm42$ (SD) ng/ml (n=34) was greater than the mean of $26\pm10$ in season and age matched controls (n=25, $p < .01$).  Mean serum iPTH of $421\pm234$ pg/ml in LG (n=33) was lower than mean of $566\pm175$ in matched controls (n=50, $p < .01$).  Mean urinary calcium of the LG of $308\pm45$ mg/24 hr was greater than mean control of $168\pm87$ mg/24 hr (n=20, $p < 0.001$).  Mean urinary Mg/Ca ratio (mEq/24 hr) of those LG who had N was lower than control values ($72.3\pm33.6$ vs. $125\pm63$, $p < 0.001$).  This was due to increase in calciuria rather than to reduced magnesuria in LG.   Daily urine volumes of the 11 LG who worked in the warm and arid Gulf of Eilat had mean daily urinary volumes of $856\pm270$ ml/24 hr, which was lower than in controls and lower than in LG and in controls from Northern Israel ($p < 0.01$).  Levels of total serum calcium, magnesium, and phosphate in LG were within normal limits.  There was a slight but statistically significant hyperuricemia in the LG.

The data show that LG have:  a) enhanced incidence of N; b) increase in serum 25-HCC, and decrease in serum iPTH, and

c) hypercalciuria.  It is postulated that excessive exposure to
sunlight induced a state of hypervitaminosis D in LG.  This led
to hyperabsorption of calcium from the gut, which partially suppressed the parathyroid glands.  Each of these factors contributed
to the hypercalciuria and to the high incidence of N in LG.
Relative oliguria in certain instances, and the low urinary Mg/Ca
ratio, as well as the hyperuricemia were additional independent,
potentially lithogenic factors in LG.

INTRODUCTION

Epidemiologic surveys suggest increased risk of kidney stones
in populations residing in regions with warm climate (1-5).  The
purpose of the present investigation was to study the occurrence
of nephrolithiasis in lifeguards (LG).  This professional group
works under conditions of extensive exposure to heat, dehydration,
and sunlight.

METHODS

Our study is comprised of 45 randomly selected LG who work
on the beach (out of a total of 120 LG in Israel).   34 LG were
from northern Israel (Mediterranean shore), and 11 were from the
arid Gulf of Eilat (Red Sea).  The work was carried out during
August-September.   The control population was matched for sex,
age and season.  Diagnosis of past and present occurrence of
nephrolithiasis was established by two urologic surgeons on the
basis of at least one of the following:  (1) History of an operation to remove a stone in the kidneys or urinary tract.
(2) History of spontaneous passage of stones or x-ray evidence
for the presence of stones.  Samples of blood and urine for determination of calcium (Ca), magnesium (Mg), phosphate (P), and
uric acid were done during work without interfering with work
or dietary habits.

Estimation of serum and urinary Ca and Mg were done by
atomic absorption (Perkins Elmer, model 290B).  Estimation of P
and uric acid were performed by colorimetric standard procedures.
Serum levels of 25-hydroxycholecalciferel (25 HCC) were performed
by competitive protein binding radio ligand assay (6,7).  Serum
iPTH was determined by radioimmunoassay by a method that estimated
both COOH and $NH_2$ terminals (7,8,9).  The urinary Mg/Ca ratio was
calculated using 24 h urinary excretion of cation expressed as
mEq/1.  The results are expressed as mean ± standard deviation
(SD).  Statistical analysis was performed using Student t-test.

RESULTS

A preliminary survey showed that LG are exposed on the job to heat and intense sunlight almost over their entire body surface for at least 8h/d, 6 mos/y. 8 of 34 LG in Northern Israel (23.5%), and 3 of 11 LG in the Gulf of Eilat (27.2%) had nephrolithiasis. This is more than tenfold increase in the incidence of kidney stones reported previously by others from this country (1.2% in Northern and 2.2% in Southern Israel (1) ).

The mean age of LG was 38 years (range 25-61 y). Those of the LG who developed kidney stones on the average have been at work longer than LG who did not form stones (15.6±4.5, (n = 11), vs 10.8±7.5, (n = 34) years, p<0.05).

Mean levels of plasma Ca, Mg, and P in the LG were not significantly different from controls (Table I). The LG, however, had a statistically significant hyperuricemia (Table I).

Mean serum levels of 25 HCC of the LG (n = 44) were elevated approximately two-fold as compared with controls (n = 26), (53.4±33.6 vs 26.1±9.7 ng/ml, p< 0.005). For comparison, mean levels of serum 25 HCC in a sample population of St. Louis, Missouri, U.S.A., which has a climate similar to ours, were 20.1 ng/ml (10).

Mean iPTH in the LG (n = 43), was significantly lower than in controls (n = 50), (421+234 vs 566+175 pg/ml, p<0.001). Mean 24 h urine volume in LG of Northern Israel (n = 45) was 1432+659 ml vs 1180±490 in controls (n = 20, NS). In contrast, LG in the Gulf of Eilat (n = 11) were oliguric (mean 859±269, p<0.001). The LG had hypercalciuria, which was statistically significant (Table I), (308±45 vs 168±87 mg/24 h, p<0.001).

LG who formed stones had higher mean daily calcium excretion and lower mean magnesium excretion than LG who did not form stones. Neither of these values were statistically significantly different. However, LG who were stone formers had significantly decreased mean Mg/Ca ratio in the urine (72.3±33.6 vs 116±63, p<0.001), (Table II).

DISCUSSION

The present study shows that work as an LG under our local weather conditions carries with it a risk of nephrolithiasis. This risk is approximately ten-fold greater than in the general population. Moreover, the morbidity with nephrolithiasis increases with the duration of work as LG.

In the present study we examined whether the environmental factors peculiar to the LG contributed to their increased susceptibility to nephrolithiasis. At least in Southern Israel, the oliguria secondary to exaggerated insensible water losses could have contributed to the tendency to form stones.

The pattern in the entire population of LG of increase in serum 25 HCC levels, decrease in iPTH levels, and their conspicuous hypercalciuria, all suggest hyperabsorption of Ca from the intestines.

The proximal cause of this absorptive hypercalciuria would be the increase in serum 25 HCC levels with suppression of PTH levels (augmentation of intestinal Ca absorption with suppression of renal tubular reabsorption of Ca). Others have previously shown that exposure to sunlight may be associated with calciuria (4). Moreover, such calciuria is accompanied by reduced urinary Mg/Ca ratio as seen in our series (4).

Urinary Mg has previously been shown to protect against formation of kidney stones. The fall in urinary Mg/Ca ratio, therefore, could enhance the risk of nephrolithiasis (11). Indeed, the only parameter which in our hands could discriminate between LG who formed stones and those who did not was the higher mean urinary Mg/Ca ratio of the latter.

The LG had hyperuricemia. The reason for that is not clear. It is speculated that solar damage to the skin increases epithelial turnover (in analogy to the hyperuricemia or psoriasis, a possibility suggested to us by Dr. Sam Thier of Yale).

The present study has the drawback that it gives an episodic account of mineral handling by the LG. Longitudinal studies, stretching over several seasons will be necessary to further elucidate the nature of the hypercalciuria of the LG. Moreover, absorptive type of hypercalciuria, although strongly suggested by our study, has not been proven.

In summary, work as LG in Israel is associated with enhanced risk of nephrolithiasis. Oliguria, secondary to dehydration, hyperuricemia, absorptive hypercalciuria secondary to increase in serum 25 HCC levels, probably all contribute to the susceptibility of LG to form kidney stones. Most of these risk factors are eminently correctible.

TABLE I

Mean Serum Levels of Ca, Mg, P and Uric Acid and
Mean Daily Calcium Excretion in Lifeguards and Controls.

|  | LG (n = 45) | CONTROLS (n = 20) | P |
|---|---|---|---|
| Ca mg/100 ml | 9.6±1.4 | 9.9±0.4 | NS |
| Mg meq/1 | 1.5±0.7 | 1.7±0.2 | NS |
| P mg/100 ml | 3.4±1.8 | 3.7±0.8 | NS |
| Uric acid mg/100 ml | 6.8±2.6 | 4.9±1.4 | < 0.001 |

|  | Mean Urine Values | | |
|---|---|---|---|
| Ca mg/24 h | 308±45 | 168±87 | < 0.001 |

TABLE II

24 h Urinary Mg/Ca Ratio

|  | Mg/Ca | n | P |
|---|---|---|---|
| Controls | 126±63 | 20 | NS |
| Controls with Stone | 105±58 | 20 | NS |
| Sample of Total LG | 105±59 | 40 |  |
| LG without Stones | 116±63 | 29 |  |
| LG with Stones | 72±34 | 11 |  |

| Normal Controls vs Controls with Stone | NS |
|---|---|
| Controls vs LG | < 0.02 |
| LG with Stones vs LG without Stones | < 0.001 |

REFERENCES

1.  M. Frank, A. Atzman and P. DeVries,  Epidemiological
        investigation of urolithiasis in the hot southern
        arid region of Israel.  Urolog Int'l 15:65, 1963.

2.  W.G. Robertson, J.C. Gallagher, D.H. Marshall, M. Peacock
        and B.E.C. Nordin,  Seasonal variations in urinary
        excretion of calcium.   Brit. Med. J. 4:1523, 1974.

3.  E.M. Bateson,  Renal tract calculi and climate.
        Med. J. Australia 2:3, 1973.

4.  B.S. Parry and I.S. Lister,  Sunlight and hypercalciuria.
        Lancet 1:1063, 1975.

5.  O.S. Better, A. Malamud, M. Shabtai, J. Bernheim and
        C. Chaimovitz,  Studies on the pathogenesis of increased
        incidence of nephrolithiasis in lifeguards in Israel.
        Clin. Res. 26:126A, 1978 (abstract).

6.  J.G. Haddad and J.C. Kyung,  Competitive protein binding
        radioassay for 25-hydroxycholecalciferel.
        J. Clin. Endocrinol. 33:992, 1971.

7.  R. Belsey, H.F. Deluca and J.T. Potts, Jr.  Competitive binding
        assay for Vitamin D and 25 OHD.  J. Clin. Invest. 33:554,
        1971.

8.  L. David and J. Bernheim,  La Parathermone: aspects modernes.
        Lyon Medical 232:425, 1974.

9.  J. Bernheim and L. David:  Le dosage radioimmunologique de la
        parathermone.  Lyon Medical 232:429, 1974.

10. L.V. Avieli and J.G. Haddad,  Vitamin D: current concepts.
        Metabolism 22:507, 1973.

11. D. Oreopulus,  Magnesium Excretion, in: Renal stone research
        symposium (Eds: A.Hodgkinson, B.E.C. Nordin, J.A. Churchill)
        London 1969, p.269.

UROLITHIASIS RESEARCH:    PROGRESS AND TRENDS

Nancy Boucot Cummings, M.D.

National Institute of Arthritis, Metabolism and
Digestive Diseases, National Institutes of Health,
Bethesda, Maryland  20205, USA

The complexities of the field of urolithiasis have hampered
advances in knowledge in this area until cross-disciplinary efforts
began to evolve.  The series of Urolithiasis Research meetings begun
in Leeds, England in 1968, followed every four years by those in
Madrid and in Davos, have led to increasingly effective communication
among investigators in widely disparate fields.  This overview of
research draws heavily upon research efforts supported by the
National Institute of Arthritis, Metabolism and Digestive Diseases
(NIAMDD) and assumes that this research is representative of the
broad field.

The NIAMDD initiated a broad study, published in May 1979,
Research Needs in Nephrology and Urology (1), which involved over
100 scientists in order to develop a rational basis for research
support.  The Urolithiasis Committee of this study provided a
lengthy list of recommendations for future research.

This committee identified three broad areas in which new
knowledge was needed:  basic science, epidemiology, and clinical
research.  Within basic science six major areas were identified
(Table 1).  The sub-categories within basic science include:  renal
physiology (Table 2); metabolism (Table 3); and physical chemistry
(Table 4).  There were five general areas identified within the
recommendations in the clinical research area (Table 5).  These
rather extensive recommendations provided the basis for the guidelines for new research listed in the NIAMDD announcement of
Specialized Centers of Research (SCOR) in Urolithiasis published
in November 1976.  In September 1977 five awards were made for
(SCORs) to:  The University of Chicago; the University of Florida;

Table 1.  Future Research in Urolithiasis - BASIC SCIENCE

I.     Site of Crystal Formation and Retention
       Within Kidney
II.    Chemical Nature, Source and Role of Matrix
III.   Chemical Nature, Source and Role of Inhibitors
       or Crystal Formation
IV.    Physical Chemistry
V.     Metabolism
VI.    Renal Physiology

---

Table 2.  Future Research in Urolithiasis
          VI.   RENAL PHYSIOLOGY

A.     Better Definition of Distal Tubular and
       Collecting Duct Function
B.     Continued Investigation of Renal Transport of
       Divalent Cations, Phosphorus, Uric Acid,
       Hydrogen, Bicarbonate, Ammonia and Oxalate
C.     Drug and Hormonal Effects

---

Table 3.  Future Research in Urolithiasis
          V.   METABOLISM

A.  Oxalate
    1.  Methods of Measuring Oxalate in Biological Fluids
    2.  Metabolic Inhibitors of Oxalate Synthesis
    3.  Oxalate Absorption in Health and Disease
B.  Calcium
    1.  Primary Mechanisms of Hypercalciuria
    2.  Renal Transport of Calcium
    3.  Hormonal Effect
C.  Phosphorus
    1.  Renal Transport of Phosphorus
    2.  Orthophosphate-Pyrophosphate Relationships
D.  Uric Acid
    1.  Renal Acid Handling
    2.  Mechanisms of Hyperuricosuria
E.  Hormone Metabolism
    1.  Role of Parathyroid Disorders in Urolithiasis
    2.  Vitamin D Metabolism in Urolithiasis

---

the University of Texas; Southwestern; the Mayo School of Medicine
and Yale University.

Table 4.  Future Research in Urolithiasis
          IV.  PHYSICAL CHEMISTRY

A.  Definition and Role of Heterogeneous Nucleation
    and Epitaxy
B.  For all Crystal Systems (Calcium Oxalate,
    Calcium Phosphate, Uric Acid/Urates, Struvite
    and Cystine)
    1.  Improved Methods for Measurement of
        Saturation Product, Formation Product,
        and Supersaturation
    2.  Nucleation, Aggregation and Growth
        Characteristics
    3.  Dissolution and Disaggregation
        Characteristics
    4.  Nucleation Phase and Phase Transformation
    5.  Surface Phenomenon in Urine

---

Table 5.  Future Research in Urolithiasis - CLINICAL RESEARCH

I.    Better Methods to Define Metabolic Activity
      of Stone Formation
II.   Systematic Evaluation of Crystalluria
III.  Infected Renal Lithiasis
      A.  Development of Dissolution Irrigating
          Solutions
      B.  Urease Inhibitors
IV.   Urolithiasis Surgery
      A.  Improved Intraoperative Roentgenographic
          Techniques
      B.  Improved Technique for Renal Hypothermia
      C.  Development of New Tools
          1.  Flexible Nephroscope
          2.  Ultrasound
          3.  Electrohydraulic Stone Destruction
V.    Patient Care

---

The breadth of studies included within the SCORs fall into
nine broad categories and these run the gamut from fundamental
disciplines such as physical chemistry, biochemistry and ultra-
structure, on one end, to clinical application covering topics
such as nutrition, epidemiology and ambulatory evaluation of
patients, at the other end.

Typical of the SCOR's composition is one center which includes
fifteen investigators, nine of whom are M.D.s and six who are Ph.D.s.
Their interests cover the areas of nephrology, pediatric nephrology,

urology, endocrinology, chemistry, biochemistry, crystallography,
physical chemistry, biophysics, mineral metabolism, protein
chemistry and gastroenterology.

An inclusive summary of all the studies cannot be given
but the major topics included in the SCOR support will be presented.
It is assumed that these topics are reflective of much of the
current research in urolithiasis.

Placing the clinical problem in perspective is this graph,
(Figure 1) adapted from a table of Coe's (2) which shows metabolic
and clinical disorders diagnosed in 460 consecutive calcium stone-
forming patients.  It is noteworthy that the two highest groups,
which were about twenty percent each, fell into the categories of
idiopathic hypercalciuria (IH) and of "no disorder found".  Hyperuricosuria with almost fifteen percent; marginal hypercalciuria,
and combined hypercalciuria and hyperuricosuria follow with about
11-1/2 percent each.  Other less frequent causes of calcium stones
fall between less than six percent and 0.5 percent of the total
group.

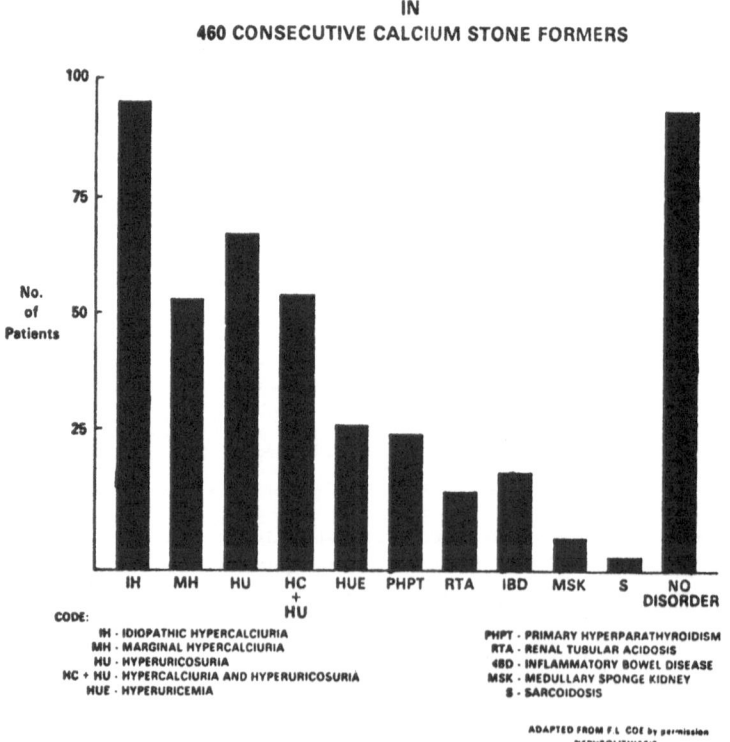

Figure 1.

Studies in physical chemistry (Table 6) include those of one center primarily involved with physical chemistry (3), which has twelve projects addressed to various aspects of whewellite behavior such as zeta potential determinations, effect of polymers on zeta potential, a mathematical model for precipitation, analysis of a peptide (4) representing over 60 percent of nitrogenous organic material in whewellite stones, porosity of whewellite, etc.

Table 6.  PHYSICAL CHEMISTRY

- Crystalluria Particle Size Analysis
- Physical Chemistry of Precipitation of Urine
- Physical Crystallization Chemistry of Urinary
    Stone Solutes
- Phase Transition of Uric Acid to Monosodium Urate and
    Heterogeneous Nucleation of Calcium Oxalate by
    Monosodium Urate

URINARY MACROMOLECULES AND INHIBITION

- Stone Matrix and Urinary Macromolecules
- Characterization and Purification of Peptide
    Inhibitors
- Promoters and Inhibitors of Crystallization
    of Stone-Forming Salts

---

Sergio Deganello (5), working with Coe, recently has identified the fundamental structure of calcium oxalate monohydrate, using a computer program analysis of about 5000 reflections of the crystal complex.  Knowledge of the fundamental arrangement of this crystal may aid in assessing at an analytical level how inhibitors work.

Studies of calcium activity products and uric acid saturation in urine indicate a tendency for calcium stone formation in urines of low pH.  Oversaturation is common in stone formers and treatment can reverse oversaturation.

In hyperuricosuria, Coe believes that low pH is caused by dietary factors, specifically the high sulfate content of meat. Pak (6) has confirmed that an oral purine load can induce hyperuricosuria and can facilitate spontaneous precipitation of calcium oxalate in urine in vitro.  The formation product decreases as the urinary saturation with monosodium urate increases.  Increasing amounts of "colloidal" urate were identified.  Urinary saturation of sodium urate increases with an increase in urinary sodium.  It is accompanied by a parallel decline in the limits of metastability of calcium oxalate in the urine of some patients with hyperuricosuric calcium oxalate nephrolithiasis.  Sodium urate plays a role in the genesis of oxalate stones.  Hence, there is a potential benefit of sodium restriction in management of hyperuricosuric calcium oxalate nephrolithiasis.

   The search for inhibitors and for promoters of renal stone formation has become an increasingly lively one.  1) Ito (8) and Nakagawa (9) have isolated a crystallization inhibitor which is probably a protein.  Chemically analagous compounds isolated from cell cultures appear to be glycoprotein macromolecules.  2) Pak has noted that varying fluid intake effects the crystallization of calcium salts in urine.  As the urine volume increases, there is a decline in the saturation of calcium phosphate and of calcium oxalate.  The limit of metastability (formation product ratio) increases upon fluid loading.  This is suggestive of a role of promoters which are diluted, since one would have anticipated that dilution of inhibitors would have decreased the limit of metastability.  This latter finding would provide a justification for forcing of fluids.  3) Pak also has found that certain muco-polysaccharides, such as heparin, were potent inhibitors of spontaneous precipitation of calcium oxalate.  Monosodium urate attenuates this inhibitory action of mucopolysaccharides upon calcium oxalate nucleation.  4) Smith has utilized an in vitro system to measure seeded crystal growth of calcium oxalate dihydrate. He has chemically isolated and identified a major inhibitor of this calcium oxalate crystal growth.  This major inhibitor is rich in uronic acid, has a uronic acid/protein ration of 1:1, and contains a sugar, suggesting that the inhibitor is a glycosaminoglycan.

   Physiologic studies cover absorptive hypercalciuria; intestinal calcium absorption; 1,25 dihydroxycholecalciferol (1,25 DHCC) parathyroid hormone (PTH), and phosphate handling by the tubule.  Knox and Dousa in elegant experiments utilizing stationary microperfusion and micropuncture have found that:  1) phosphate reabsorption is limited to the proximal convoluted and straight tubule; 2) phosphate transport is heterogeneous (10) with deep nephrons responding to physiologic phosphate balance, by a wider range of responses than do superficial nephrons, and 3) no demonstrable secretory flux for phosphate in the proximal con-voluted tubule or at terminal nephron sites.  Smith's group has noted that PTH and carbonic anhydrase (CA) inhibitors had additive effects upon phosphaturia.  Therefore, they concluded that the PTH effect is probably not mediated by CA.

   In a series of studies of patients with hypercalciuria, Pak has evaluated absorptive hypercalciuria (AH) and renal hypercalciuria (RH); measured intestinal calcium absorption; 1,25 DHCC levels and PTH, in addition to routine Ca, P, and electrolyte measurements. In preliminary studies he has found that sodium-induced hypercalciuria is associated with a rise in the circulating concentration of 1,25 DHCC and that intestinal calcium absorption is stimulated.

Intestinal hyperabsorption of calcium in RH may be Vitamin D dependent. Intestinal calcium absorption is correlated with circulating concentration of 1,25 DHCC, renal leak of calcium, and secondary HPTH. This can be corrected by thiazide treatment with a return of intestinal calcium absorption to normal and a parallel fall in the concentration of Vitamin D metabolites. On the other hand, in AH the circulating concentration of 1,25 DHCC is not correlated with intestinal calcium absorption. Only a minority of patients with AH had a decrease in phosphate concentration or in $T_mP$. Intestinal calcium absorption is not correlated with serum ($PO_4$) concentrations or with levels of 1,25 DHCC. Orthophosphate did not ameliorate intestinal hyperabsorption of calcium.

PTH excess may be demonstrable in RH by objective signs such as low bone density as measured by photon absorption, osteoporosis, high renal excretion of hydroxyproline, and negative calcium balance. Treatment with thiazides produces a normal urinary calcium, normal PTH function, and an intestinal calcium absorption commensurate with the drop in 1,25 DHCC. In AH, thiazide treatment does not abolish the hyperabsorption of calcium. RH responds to a glucose load with an exaggerated calciuria while AH does not.

Nephrogenous cyclic AMP was found to be elevated in 90-95 percent of a group of 135 patients with primary or secondary hyperparathyroidism, studied at Yale. Total urinary cyclic AMP was elevated in 90 percent of these patients while values were low in patients with absent or suppressed parathyroid function. The calcium tolerance test (CTT) has been developed as a diagnostic test for subtle primary hyperparathyroidism with intermittent hypercalciuria and is useful in categorizing those who do or do not have AH. Of this group, 65 percent had increased calcium absorption. Of those evaluated by the CTT, there was a good correlation between AH, the degree of hypercalciuria, and a history of renal stones. Rasmussen, using a $^{14}$C-oxalate absorption test, found an increase in total oxalate excretion in patients with AH.

Smith and his coworkers have made measurements and/or calculations of the state of saturation and inhibitor activity for calcium oxalate, calcium phosphate, and uric acid crystal systems in primary hyperoxaluria, primary hyperparathyroidism, enteric hyperoxaluria, and miscellaneous conditions including idiopathic hyperoxaluria. They have some leads in identification of the mechanisms of action of orthophosphates, thiazides, and parathyroid surgery in modification of the abnormalities and/or prevention of stone formation.

Coe (11) has presented evidence for a hereditary, possibly genetic disturbance of metabolism for IH. In a study of the families of nine hypercalciuric patients with IH, who formed recurrent calcium oxalate renal stones, 19 of 44 first degree relatives had IH and

formed stones, while none of the others formed stone.   Coe concluded
that there is a familial form of hypercalciuria which appears to be
transmitted as an autosomal dominant trait.   Species-dependent,
possibly hereditary IH has been described in the rat.   A subpopulation
of relatively hypercalciuric rats responded to dietary calcium restriction by reducing their calcium excretion.   It appears that
increased intestinal calcium absorption may be resonsible, although
the exact mechanism is unknown.   Gantt described DOCA escape
hypercalciuria in the rat and evidence for the impact of renal
hypercalciuria on parathyroid physiology in bone.

Using the CTT, Rasmussen has assessed the effect on calcium
excretion of a diet of 1000 mg of calcium as compared to 400 mg
calcium (Hypercalciuria is defined as excretion of calcium greater
than 4 mg/kg/day).   He found a strong correlation with the response
to CTT by an increase in calcium excretion in IH.   Dietary history
suggests that variations in sodium, protein, and carbohydrate intake
influence IH.   These dietary permutations may be potential "risk
factors" for calcium stone formation from a physico-chemical
viewpoint.

Further studies of oxalate metabolism test the hypothesis that
AH leaves less calcium in the gut to combine with oxalate, so that
more oxalate remains to be absorbed.   No significant difference in
urinary oxalate was noted in patients of high or low calcium diets.

Epidemiologic studies which can be elusive are being done in
three centers.   The Florida group is conducting field observations
on dietary habits of stone formers and of controls.   With the
Environmental Protection Agency (EPA), they are assessing the effect
of the water content of calcium, magnesium, sodium, and potassium
and the effect of these elements on renal stone disease.   "Water
hardness" is strongly correlated with protection against stones.
The correlation of the protective effect of potassium has a p value
of 0.01.

The Mayo group has assessed stone data for the Olmstead County,
Minnesota area from 1950 to 1974.   They have found that the incidence
of stones is 109/100,000 in men and 36/100,000 in women.   The
incidence of renal stone disease increased 50 percent in men over
this 25 year period while the incidence in women remained stable.
Their data suggest that about 12 percent of men and 5 percent of
women will have at least one symptomatic stone episode by age 70.
The Yale group is assessing the stone evaluation in an outreach
program in Danbury, Connecticut where there are over 60 patients
whose kindred are being followed also.   It was notable that the
routine follow-up included most tests that are important except
for the 24 hour urinary calcium and uric acid measurement which
were done in only 67 percent of patients.   Stone histories were
considered inadequate, renal tubular acidosis had not been ruled

out adequately, and in 28 percent of stone patients, adequate steps to rule out metabolic abnormalities had not been taken.

As this brief survey makes clear, there has been a rapid growth of interest and activity in urolithiasis research over the past 15 years. Without effort, one could pose more than a dozen questions to be answered of which a few are: What is the pathogenesis of stone formation in hypercalciuria? What mechanisms link hyperuricosuria to calcium oxalate stone formation? What causes hypercalciuria in distal RTA? What is the role of nutrition in renal stone formation? The fact that such a summary must be so condensed indicates the exciting possibilities in this field.

REFERENCES

1. "Research Needs in Nephrology and Urology", U.S. Department of Health, Education, and Welfare, DHEW Publication No. (NIH) 78-1481, Bethesda, Maryland (1978).
2. F. L. Coe, Nephrolithiasis, Pathogenesis and Treatment, Yearbook, Chicago (1978).
3. B. Finlayson, Physicochemical aspects of Urolithiasis, Kid. Int., 13:344 (1978).
4. P. J. Buscemi, W. Longo, W. A. Gilbert, B. Finlayson, and E. P. Goldberg. Calcium oxalate stone matrix: isolation and properties of a soluble low moleculor weight polypeptide.
5. S. Deganello and O. E. Piro, The crystal structure of calcium oxalate monohydrate, $Ca(CO_2)_2 \cdot H_2O$ (in press).
6. C. Y. C. Pak, D. E. Barilla, K. Holt, L. Brinkley, R. Tolentino, and J. E. Zerwekh, Effect of oral purine load and allopurinol on the crystallization of calcium salts in urine of patients with hyperuricosuric calcium urolithiasis, Am. J. Med., 65:593 (1978).
7. F. L. Coe, A. L. Strauss, V. Tembe, and M. S. Dunn. Uric acid saturation in calcium nephrolithiasis, Kid. Int. (in press).
8. H. Ito and F. L. Coe, Acidic peptide and polyribonucleotide crystal growth inhibitors in human urine, Am. J. Physiol., 233:455 (1977).
9. Y. Nakagawa, E. T. Kaiser, and F. L. Coe, Isolation and characterization of calcium oxalate crystal growth inhibitors from human urine. Biochem & Biophys (Res. Commun.), 84:1038 (1978).
10. J. A. Haas, T. Berndt, and F. G. Knox, Nephron heterogeneity of phosphate reabsorption, Am. J. Physiol., 234:287 (1978).
11. F. L. Coe, J. H. Parks, and E. S. Moore, Familial idiopathic hypercalciuria, N.E.J.M., 300:337 (1979).
12. M. J. Favus, and F. L. Coe, Evidence for spontaneous hypercalciuria in the rat, Mineral & Elec. Metab., 2:150 (1979).

# TOPICS ON PARATHYROID HORMONE

# THE UPTAKE OF IMMUNOREACTIVE PARATHYROID HORMONE BY PERIPHERAL ORGANS

Kevin Martin, Keith Hruska, Jeffrey Freitag, Ezequiel Bellorin-Font, Saulo Klahr, and Eduardo Slatopolsky

Department of Medicine, Renal Division
Washington University School of Medicine
St. Louis, Missouri  63110  U.S.A.

The demonstration that circulating immunoreactive parathyroid hormone (PTH) consists of a mixture of intact PTH and smaller molecular weight hormonal fragments by Berson and Yalow[1] led to intensive research by several laboratories into the origin, fate and significance of these fragments. Although much has been learned from these studies, some controversy persists and some observations remain unexplained. Thus, it is clear that the predominant species of circulating i-PTH in hyperparathyroidism are fragments of PTH from the carboxy-terminal portion of the PTH molecule[1-4]. Assays for PTH which detect these carboxy-terminal fragments provide better discrimination between normal subjects and those with hyperparathyroidism than assays which detect only the amino-terminal region of the PTH molecule[4-6]. However, it has been shown that the structural requirements for the biological activity of PTH reside within the first 34 amino acids of the amino-terminal position of the molecule[7]. It appears paradoxical, therefore, that carboxy-terminal assays for PTH, which measure biologically inactive PTH fragments in addition to intact hormone, are most useful in assessment of parathyroid activity and correlate well with osteoclast number and activity in bone[5,8].

## SECRETED SPECIES OF IMMUNOREACTIVE PTH

Early results in vitro suggesting a predominant secretion of parathyroid hormone fragments[9,10] were not confirmed in studies in vivo by Habener et al[2] who found that the intact hormone was the predominant form of i-PTH in the parathyroid gland venous effluent. Although many studies in vivo and in vitro have confirmed these observations, it is now clear that secretion of fragments of PTH does occur in vivo[11,12] and in vitro[13] particularly in the presence of hypercalcemia. Studies in our laboratory have confirmed the presence of small amounts of carboxy-terminal fragments, accounting for 10-20% of total i-PTH, in parathyroid gland venous effluent at the time of surgery in hyperparathyroid patients.

## METABOLISM OF PTH BY PERIPHERAL ORGANS

Although the secretion of PTH fragments by the parathyroid glands may contribute to the immunoheterogeneity of circulating i-PTH, there is strong evidence that metabolism of intact PTH by peripheral organs also plays an important role. Many studies have shown that PTH fragments appear in the circulation following single injection or constant infusion of labelled or unlabelled intact bovine PTH (b-PTH 1-84)[14-21]. The studies of Segre et al[14,17] have shown that [125]I b-PTH 1-84 undergoes rapid and specific cleavage following injection into rats and dogs. Some investigators have localized the site of cleavage of intact hormone to amino acid positions 33-34 and 36-37 by Edman degradation. This site of cleavage confirmed in cattle and man by radioimmunoassay techniques can potentially give rise to a biologically active amino-terminal PTH fragment[18-22]. Further evidence for the role of peripheral metabolism of intact PTH has been obtained by demonstrating that a synthetic PTH fragment, syn b-PTH 28-48, inhibits the degradation of simultaneously infused b-PTH 1-84[21]. The organs involved in the peripheral metabolism of PTH are discussed in the following sections.

## a) Renal Uptake of PTH

A prolonged disappearance of i-PTH from plasma following parathyroidectomy in patients with renal failure was described by Berson and Yalow in 1968[1]. Subsequently, these observation have been confirmed by many investigators[15,23-25]. Hruska et al[15] and Singer et al[23] demonstrated a 20% arteriovenous difference for i-PTH across the kidney following injection or infusion of b-PTH 1-84 to normal dogs. Further studies from our laboratory[24] have characterized the nature of the renal uptake of i-PTH, utilizing the maneuver of acute unilateral ureteral obstruction to reduce glomerular filtration while preserving renal plasma flow. Thus, a reduction of the A-V difference for i-PTH across the kidney from 20% to 15% during infusion of b-PTH 1-84 was interpreted to indicate uptake at peritubular sites.

Similar findings were obtained during infusion of syn b-PTH 1-34. However, following a single injection of b-PTH 1-84 in the

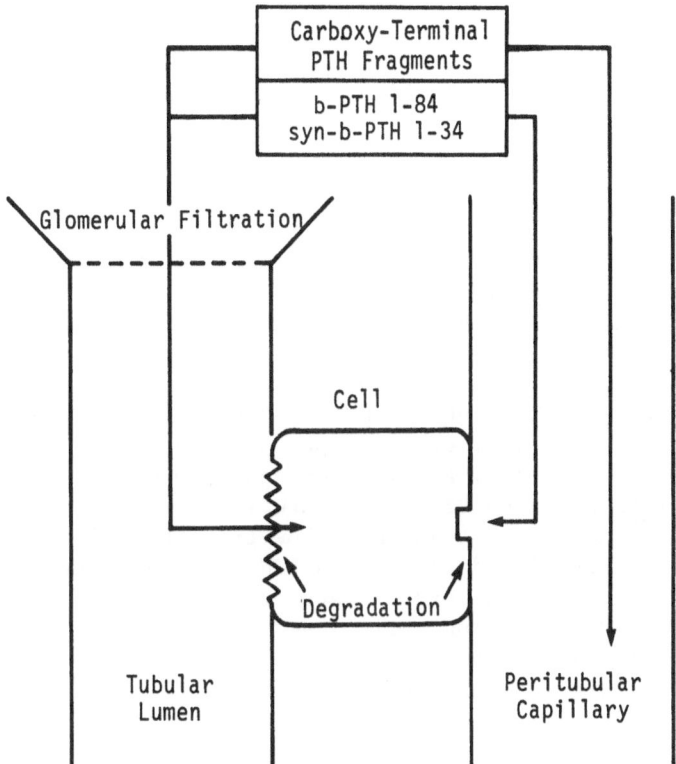

Figure 1.   Diagrammatic representation of the mechanisms for the
renal uptake of parathyroid hormone and its fragments
(adapted from J. Clin. Invest. 60: 808–814, 1977, with
permission).

presence of established ureteral obstruction, an A–V difference for
i-PTH across the kidney was observed only while biologically active
intact PTH persisted in the circulation (20 mins.).   Thereafter,
when plasma i-PTH consisted only of carboxy-terminal PTH fragments
no A–V difference across kidney was observed.   These observations
are summarized in Figure 1.   Biologically active forms of PTH
(b-PTH 1-84, syn b-PTH 1-34) are handled by peritubular uptake
whereas all forms of i-PTH undergo glomerular filtration and tubular
reabsorption (since minimal amounts of i-PTH appear in urine).
Glomerular filtration and tubular reabsorption appears to be the
only process whereby carboxy-terminal fragments are removed from
the circulation.   The studies of Kao and Maack[26] using [125]I-PTH
(biologically inactive) have shown that glomerular filtration is
the major mechanism of renal PTH uptake.   These observations with

biologically inactive $^{125}$I b-PTH 1-34 are not inconsistent with
the findings of our laboratory discussed above.  Further confirmation of these findings was demonstrated by Freitag et al[25] who
found that the elevated levels of i-PTH in renal failure patients
(predominantly carboxy-terminal fragments) decreased rapidly
following successful renal transplantation reaching 20% of initial
values in 24 hrs. without any change in serum calcium which could
have reduced PTH secretion.

In addition to removal of PTH and its fragments from the
circulation, the kidney also appears to be a source of these fragments.  Many studies have shown degradation of PTH by kidney tissue
in vitro[27-33].  In the isolated perfused dog kidney it has been
shown that b-PTH 1-84 is metabolized to fragments similar to those
found in the peripheral circulation of intact animals[34].  In addition, this process was influenced by perfusate calcium concentrations such that low calcium accelerated and high calcium retarded
the rate of fragment production.  The studies of d'Amour following
injection of $^{125}$I b-PTH 1-84 in rats show that the kidney contained
only minimal amounts of radioiodinated PTH fragments similar to
those found in the circulation[35].  However, it is to be noted that
the $^{125}$I b-PTH 1-84 is biologically inactive and it is possible
that these observations may not be totally representative of the
metabolism of unlabelled hormone.

b) Hepatic Uptake of PTH

Many studies have demonstrated that the liver is an important
organ in PTH metabolism.  Fang and Tashjian[33] demonstrated a
prolonged plasma disappearance time for i-PTH following partial
hepatectomy.  Canterbury et al[36] have shown that the isolated
perfused rat liver metabolizes b-PTH 1-84 giving rise to PTH fragments similar by gel filtration to those seen in peripheral blood.
In addition, it was noted that a PTH fragment was produced which
was active in the rat renal cortical adenylate cyclase system.
Furthermore, it appeared that the rate of metabolism of intact PTH
was related to perfusate calcium concentrations.  Thus, more fragments were produced at low calcium concentrations whereas high
calcium concentrations retarded the metabolism of b-PTH 1-84.
Studies from our laboratory[19] have examined the uptake of PTH by
the liver in vivo, using dogs with indwelling hepatic venous
catheters.  Following a single injection of b-PTH 1-84 the arteriovenous difference for i-PTH across the liver fell from 40% initially
to zero after 20-25 minutes in spite of persisting high levels of
carboxy-terminal i-PTH in plasma.  Gel filtration of arterial and
hepatic venous plasma early (6 min.) after injection of b-PTH 1-84
revealed a marked reduction in intact hormone and an increase in
carboxy-terminal PTH fragments in hepatic venous plasma (Figure 2).

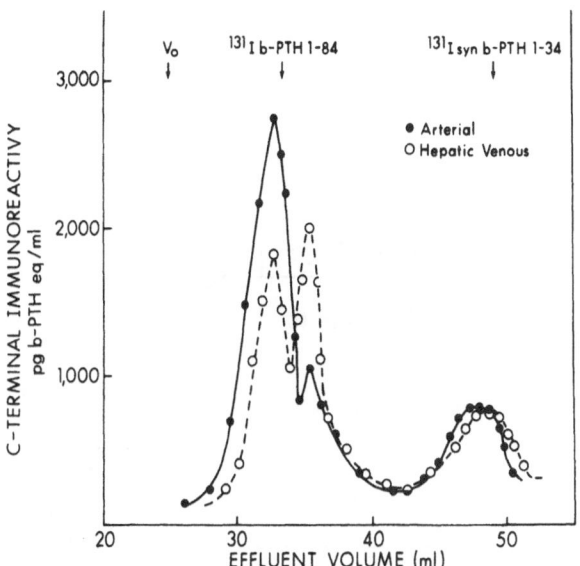

Figure 2.    Gel filtration of arterial and hepatic venous plasma
             5 minutes after single injection of b-PTH 1-84 to a
             normal dog.  There is an A-V difference for intact
             b-PTH 1-84 and the addition of a carboxy-terminal PTH
             fragment to hepatic venous blood.  (Reproduced from
             J. Clin. Invest. 58: 781-788, 1976, with permission.)

At later times (> 20 min. after injection of b-PTH 1-84), when no
A-V difference was present, circulating i-PTH consisted only of
carboxy-terminal fragments and arterial and hepatic venous samples
were identical.

     Additional studies failed to demonstrate any hepatic uptake
of i-PTH following injections of syn b-PTH 1-34.  Accordingly,
these studies were interpreted to indicate that the uptake of i-PTH
by the liver was selective for the intact hormone and that this
organ did not metabolize carboxy- or amino-terminal PTH fragments.
Recent studies by d'Amour et al[35] and Segre et al[37] suggest that
the Kupffer cells of the liver may be responsible for the metabolism
of intact PTH.

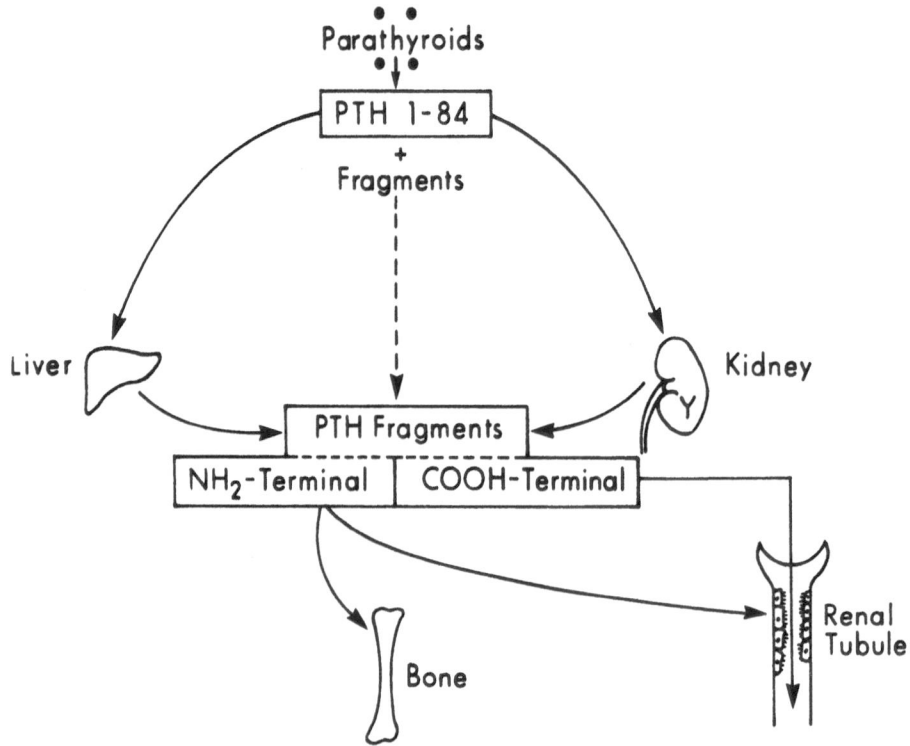

Figure 3.   Possible scheme for peripheral metabolism of parathyroid
            hormone.   For full description, see text.   (Reproduced
            from J. Clin. Invest. 62:   256–261, 1978 with permission.)

## c) Skeletal Uptake of PTH

In 1968 Parsons and Robinson[38] demonstrated that b-PTH 1-84 injected into a cat whose isolated tibia was being perfused with blood from the intact animal resulted in the release of calcium from bone. However, this effect was not seen when b-PTH 1-84 was injected directly into the bone so that the hormone did not enter the animal's circulation. These observations suggest that intact PTH must undergo some alteration in the intact animal before exerting its effect on bone.

Recent studies from our laboratory[39] have extended these findings utilizing an isolated perfused tibia preparation. These studies revealed a 36% arteriovenous difference for i-PTH across bone during infusion of syn b-PTH 1-34 whereas no significant uptake of i-PTH was demonstrable during infusion of b-PTH 1-84. These findings correlated with a biological effect in that cyclic AMP production was markedly increased by syn b-PTH 1-34 whereas b-PTH 1-84 had a minimal effect.

## COMMENT

The studies described above indicate that the characteristics of the uptake of i-PTH by liver, kidney and bone are different for each organ. The liver demonstrates a selective uptake for intact hormone, the bone a selective uptake for syn b-PTH 1-34, while all forms of i-PTH are metabolized by the kidney. A summary of our current interpretation of the above data is shown in Figure 3. PTH is secreted predominantly as intact hormone and undergoes metabolism in liver and kidney resulting in the production of carboxy- and amino-terminal PTH fragments. The carboxy-terminal fragments are further metabolized in the kidney by glomerular filtration and tubular reabsorption. Amino-terminal fragments produced by liver and kidney may act on the kidney and appear to mediate the effects of PTH on bone.

## REFERENCES

1.  S.A. Berson and R.S. Yalow, Immunochemical heterogeneity of parathyroid hormone in plasma, J. Clin. Endocrin. Metab. 28:1037 (1968).
2.  J.F. Habener, D. Powell, T.M. Murray, G.P. Meyer, and J.T. Potts, Jr., Parathyroid hormone: Secretion and metabolism in vivo, Proc. Natl. Acad. Sci. USA 78:2986 (1971).
3.  J.M. Canterbury, and E. Reiss, Multiple immunoreactive molecular forms of parathyroid hormone in human plasma, Proc. Soc. Exp. Biol. Med. 140:1393 (1972).

4.  R. Silverman, and R.S. Yalow, Heterogeneity of parathyroid
      hormone:  Clinical and physiologic implications, J. Clin.
      Invest. 52:1958 (1973).
5.  C.D. Arnaud, R.S. Goldsmith, P.J. Bordier, and G.W. Sizemore,
      Influence of immunoheterogeneity of circulating parathyroid
      hormone on results of radioimmunoassays of serum in man,
      Am. J. Med. 56:785 (1974).
6.  E. Slatopolsky, K. Hruska, K. Martin, and J. Freitag, Physio-
      logical and metabolic effects of parathyroid hormone, in:
      "Contemporary Issues in Nephrology," B. Brenner and J. Stein,
      ed., Churchill-Livingston, New York (In Press).
7.  G.W. Tregear, J. van Rietschoten, E. Green, H.T. Keutmann,
      H.D. Niall, B. Reit, J.A. Parsons, and J.T. Potts, Jr.,
      Bovine parathyroid hormone:  Minimum chain length of
      synthetic peptide required for biological activity, Endo-
      crinology, 93:1349 (1973).
8.  W.E. Rutherford, P. Bordier, P. Marie, K. Hruska, H. Harter,
      A. Greenwalt, J. Blondin, J. Haddad, N. Bricker, and
      E. Slatopolsky, Phosphate control and 25-hydroxycholecalci-
      ferol administration in preventing experimental renal
      osteodystrophy in the dog, J. Clin. Invest. 60:332 (1977).
9.  C.D. Arnaud, G.W. Sizemore, S.B. Oldham, J.A. Fischer, H.S.
      Tsao, E.T. Littledike, Human parathyroid hormone: Glandular
      and secreted molecular species, Am. J. Med. 50:630 (1971).
10. L.M. Sherwood, J.S. Rodman, and W.B. Lundberg, Evidence for a
      precursor to circulating parathyroid hormone, Proc. Natl.
      Acad. Sci. USA 67:1631 (1970).
11. J.D. Gleuck, F.P. DiBella, A.J. Edis, J.M. Kehrwald, and C.D.
      Arnaud, Immunoheterogeneity of parathyroid hormone in venous
      effluent serum from hyperfunctioning parathyroid glands,
      J. Clin. Invest. 60:1367  (1977).
12. G.P. Mayer, J.A. Keaton, J.G. Hurst, and J.F. Habener, Effects
      of plasma calcium concentration on the relative proportion
      of hormone and carboxyl fragment in parathyroid venous blood,
      Endocrinology, 104:1778 (1979).
13. D.A. Hanley, K. Takatsuki, J.M. Sultan, A.B. Schreider, L.M.
      Sherwood, Direct release of parathyroid hormone fragments
      from functioning bovine parathyroid glands in vitro,
      J. Clin. Invest. 62:1247 (1978).
14. G.V. Segre, H.D. Hiall, J.F. Habener, and J.T. Potts, Jr.,
      Metabolism of parathyroid hormone:  Physiologic and clinical
      significance, Am. J. Med. 56:774 (1974).
15. K.A. Hruska, R. Kopelman, W.E. Rutherford, S. Klahr, and
      E. Slatopolsky, Metabolism of parathyroid hormone in the
      dog.  The role of the kidney and the effects of chronic
      renal disease, J. Clin. Invest. 56:39 (1975).
16. W.F. Neuman, M.W. Newman, K. Lane, L. Miller, and P.J. Sammon,
      The metabolism of labeled parathyroid hormone:  V.  Collected
      biological studies, Calcif. Tiss. Res. 18:271 (1975).

17.  G.V. Segre, P. d'Amour, and J.T. Potts, Jr., Metabolism of
     radioiodinated bovine parathyroid hormone in the rat.
     Endocrinology, 99:1645 (1976).
18.  J.F. Habener, G.P. Mayer, P.D. Dee, and J.T. Potts, Jr., Meta-
     bolism of amino- and carboxyl-sequence immunoreactive
     parathyroid hormone in the bovine:  Evidence for peripheral
     cleavage of hormone. Metabolism, 25:385 (1976).
19.  K. Martin, K. Hruska, A. Greenwalt, S. Klahr, and E. Slatopolsky,
     Selective uptake of intact parathyroid hormone by the liver.
     Difference between hepatic and renal uptake, J. Clin.
     Invest. 58:781 (1976).
20.  W.H. Unziker, J.W. Blum, and J.A. Fischer, Plasma kinetics of
     exogenous bovine parathyroid hormone in calves, Pflugers
     Arch. 371:185 (1977).
21.  G.V. Segre, P. d'Amour, M. Rosenblatt, and J.T. Potts, Jr.,
     Heterogeneity and metabolism of parathyroid hormone, in:
     "Endocrinology of Calcium Metabolism," D.H. Copp and R.V.
     Talmage, ed., Excerpta Medica, Amsterdam (1978).
22.  G.V. Segre, J.F. Habener, D. Powell, G.W. Tregear, and
     J.T. Potts, Jr., Parathyroid hormone in human plasma.
     Immunochemical characterization and biological implications,
     J. Clin. Invest. 51:3163 (1972).
23.  F.R. Singer, G.V. Segre, J.F. Habener, and J.T. Potts, Jr.,
     Peripheral metabolism of bovine parathyroid hormone in
     the dog, Metabolism, 24:139 (1975).
24.  K.J. Martin, K. Hruska, J. Lewis, C. Anderson, and E. Slato-
     polsky, Renal handling of parathyroid hormone: Role of
     peritubular uptake and glomerular filtration, J. Clin.
     Invest. 60:808 (1977).
25.  J. Freitag, K.J. Martin, K.A. Hruska, C. Anderson, M. Conrades,
     J. Ladenson, S. Klahr, and E. Slatopolsky, Impaired para-
     thyroid hormone metabolism in chronic renal failure, New
     Engl. J. Med. 298:29 (1978).
26.  S.T. Kao, and T. Maack, Transport and catabolism of parathyroid
     hormone in isolated rat kidney, Am. J. Physiol. 223(5):
     F445 (1977).
27.  T.J. Martin, R.A. Melich, and M. DeLuise, Metabolism of para-
     thyroid hormone degradation of $^{125}$I-labeled hormone by a
     kidney enzyme, Biochem. J. 111:509 (1969).
28.  N. Kugai, F. DiBella, and C.D. Arnaud, Metabolism of parathy-
     roid hormone by isolated tubules and plasma membranes from
     rat kidney cortex:  Possible role and regulation of the
     production of "circulating fragments." Clin. Res. 22:618
     (1974).
29.  J.A. Fisher, S.B. Oldham, G.W. Sizemore, and C.D. Arnaud,
     Calcium regulated parathyroid hormone peptidase, Proc. Natl.
     Acad. Sci. 69:2341 (1972).
30.  H. Orimo, T. Fugita, H. Morii, and K. Nakao, Inactivation in
     vitro of parathyroid hormone activity by kidney slices.
     Endocrinology, 76:255  (1965).

31. B.D. Catherwood and F.R. Singer, Generation of a carboxyl-
    terminal fragment of bovine parathyroid hormone by canine
    renal plasma membranes, Biochem. Biophys. Res. Comm. 57:
    469 (1974).

32. L.L.H. Chu, L.R. Forte, C.S. Anast, and D.V. Cohn, Interaction
    of parathyroid hormone with membranes of kidney cortex:
    Degradation of the hormone and activation of adenylate
    cyclase, Endocrinology 97:1014 (1975).

33. V.S. Fang and A.H. Tashjian, Studies on the role of the liver
    in the metabolism of parathyroid hormone. I. Effects of
    partial hepatectomy and incubation of the hormone with
    tissue homogenates, Endocrinology 90:1177 (1972).

34. K.A. Hruska, K. Martin, A. Greenwalt, C. Anderson, S. Klahr,
    and E. Slatopolsky, Degradation of parathyroid hormone and
    fragment production by the isolated perfused dog kidney:
    Role of glomerular filtration rate and perfusate $Ca^{++}$ con-
    centrations, J. Clin. Invest. 60:501 (1977).

35. P. d'Amour, G.V. Segre, S.I. Roth, and J.T. Potts, Jr., Analysis
    of parathyroid hormone and its fragments in rat tissues:
    Chemical identification and microscopical localization,
    J. Clin. Invest. 63:89 (1979).

36. J.M. Canterbury, L.A. Bricker, J.S. Levey, P.L. Kozlovskis,
    E. Ruiz, J.E. Zull, and E. Reiss, Metabolism of bovine para-
    thyroid hormone: Immunological and biological characteris-
    tics of fragments generated by liver perfusion. J. Clin.
    Invest. 55:1245 (1975).

37. G.V. Segre, A. Perkins, L.A. Witters, and J.T. Potts, Jr.,
    Proteolysis of parathyroid hormone by isolated Kupffer
    cells, Clin. Res. 26:533A (1978).

38. J.A. Parsons, and C.J. Robinson, A rapid indirect hypercalcemic
    action of parathyroid hormone demonstrated in isolated
    perfused bone, in: "Parathyroid HOrmone and Thyrocalcitonin
    (calcitonin)," R.V. Talmage and L.F. Belanger, ed., Excerpta
    Medica Foundation, Amsterdam (1968).

39. K.J. Martin, J.J. Freitag, M. Conrades, K. Hruska, S. Klahr,
    and E. Slatopolsky, Selective uptake of the synthetic
    amino-terminal fragment of bovine parathyroid hormone by
    isolated perfused bone, J. Clin. Invest. 62:256 (1978).

EFFECT OF ACUTE ETHANOL LOADING ON PARATHYROID GLAND

SECRETION IN THE RAT

J.CHANARD, B.LACOUR, T.DRÜEKE,J.P.BRUNOIS
and J.C. RUIZ
Université de Reims and I.N.S.E.R.M. U.90
Paris - France
C.H.U. Service de Néphrologie. 51090 Reims

INTRODUCTION

Ethanol as well as other anesthetic agents such as methanol, chloral hydrate and urethane can induce hypocalcemia in the rat when ingested at anesthetic dosage (5).

The mechanism by which ethanol acts to cause hypocalcemia is still unclear. Ethanol prevents the calcium raising effect of exogenous parathyroid hormone (PTH) in normal and in parathyroidectomized rat (6,7) suggesting an inhibitory effect on calcium release at the bone level. However, a possible impairment of PTH secretion by ethanol is possible. Additionnally, Kravitt (3) has documented an inhibition of duodenal calcium transport and the inability of 1,25 dihydroxycholecalciferol to reverse the ethanol-induced inhibition of transport capacity.

The present study was designed to evaluate the effects of ethanol on PTH secretion  a) in vivo, in the hours following ethanol administration, and  b) in vitro using isolated rat parathyroid glands.

MATERIALS and METHODS

Animal studies

Sprague-Dawley rats weighing 200-300g were fed a normal diet that contained 1.5% calcium, 0.95% phosphorus and 200 I.U. of vitamin D.

Ethanol was administered via an intragastric tube. Absolute ethyl alcohol was diluted to 50% (v/v) with distilled water. A single oral dose of 6g ethanol per kg body weight, or saline (control) was administered. Blood samples were collected under light ether anesthesia by puncture of the jugular vein at its junction with the subclavicular vein through a small skin incision. During intravenous administration of disodium EDTA in animals anesthetized with nembutal, blood samples were drawn through a catheter inserted into the carotid artery. Blood samples were collected in heparinized syringes ; an aliquot of 0.5ml was kept at 4°C and after centrifugation the resulting plasma was frozen for PTH assay.

Two groups of rats were studied.

Group I : This group was designed to study the effect of ethanol administration on plasma calcium and immunoreactive PTH. Blood samples were collected before ethanol loading and at hourly intervals thereafter. However, to avoid blood loss (hematocrit decrease > 2%) each rat was used for two to three samples. In a subgroup of 4 rats blood samples were taken to measure ethanol concentration using an enzymatic method with alcohol deshydrogenase.

Groupe II : This group was designed to study the effects of disodium EDTA on PTH release in rats loaded with ethanol. Two hours after gavage with saline, control rats were injected intravenously with disodium EDTA, at a dose of 1.7mg/kg/min (0.02ml/min) and blood was sampled each 15 min for 90 min. In the experimental rats ethanol was administered in place of saline and the same schedule was used. As in group I, each animal had three blood samples.

In vitro studies

In vitro studies were designed to measure the direct effect of ethanol on PTH secretion. After surgery, each rat parathyroid gland was carefully cut into small pieces and incubated for 4 hours in MES buffer with 5mM/l glucose, 10% calf serum and $CaCl_2$ (final volume 1ml). Incubation was carried out in a Dubnoff apparatus at 37°C under 5% $CO_2$ in air. Each series of measurements included an equilibrum time of 1h with a calcium concen-

tration of 1.25 mmol/l. Then, the glands were divided
into two groups; the medium was withdrawn and replaced.
In one batch the medium contained 0.75mmol/l calcium
and in the other 3mmol/l calcium. In separate experi- ·
ments ethanol was added to the medium at concentration
of 0.05%, 0,5% and 5%. The effect of ethanol on PTH
secretion was determined on paired glands; distilled
water replaced ethanol in the medium for controls.

## Radioimmunoassay

Plasma levels and the medium concentration of immunoreactive PTH was measured as previously described
(1) using a chicken antiserum against bovine PTH (gift
from Dr.E.SLATOPOLSKY) that crossreacts with rat PTH.
Preabsorption of the antiserum with 5% ethanol did not
modify the displacement of bovine 125 I-PTH tracer binding to the antiserum after increasing the amount of
unlabeled b.PTH. Results were expressed as pg equivalents
of bovine PTH. In each sample where PTH was determined
calcium concentration was measured using atomic absorption spectrometry.

## Statistical analysis

The data obtained were analyzed using paired and
unpaired Student's t tests when appropriate. Values indicated are mean $\pm$ SD.

## RESULTS

### In vivo studies

As shown on figure 1, plasma calcium decreased significantly from a control value of 2.41 $\pm$ 0.10 mmol/l
to 2.16 $\pm$ 0.09 mmol/l 4 hours after ethanol loading
(P<0.001). This decrease was inversely correlated with
the increase in plasma ethanol concentration (r= -0.98).
Plasma immunoreactive PTH did not differ from the control in either ethanol or saline loaded groups and remained at the level of 80 $\pm$ 10 pg/ml.

To determine the responsiveness of the parathyroid
glands in ethanol loaded rats to a further decrease in
plasma calcium, disodium EDTA was infused intravenously
for 1 hour. Plasma calcium decreased in ethanol loaded
rats from 2.21 $\pm$ 0.18 mmol/l before disodium EDTA infusion to 2.05 $\pm$ 0.18 mmol/l and 1.80 $\pm$ 0.32 mmol/l, 30
mn and 60 mn respectively after starting the infusion
of the chelating agent. Thirty minutes after the comple-

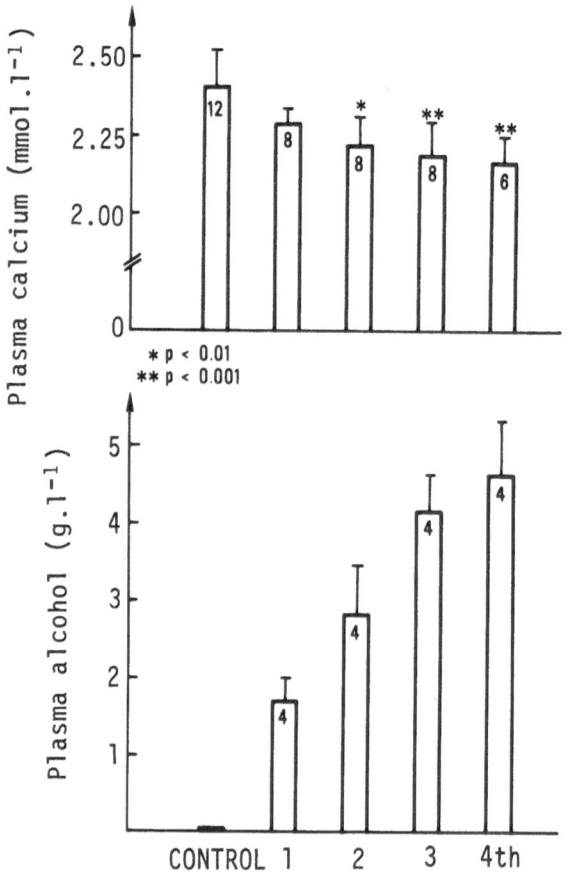

Fig. 1  Effects of intragastric ethanol administration (6g/kg bwt) on total plasma calcium and plasma alcohol concentration in normal rats.


tion of EDTA infusion, plasma calcium rose to 2.10 ± 0.30 mmol/l. A decrease in plasma calcium induced by EDTA was also observed in saline loaded control rats but the relative decrement from the pre-infusion value was greater. However, it was not significantly different from the ethanol loaded group. During disodium EDTA infusion, plasma immunoreactive PTH showed a significant increase (P<0.001) only in the control group. The decrease in plasma calcium brought about by disodium EDTA did not elicit any increase in plasma PTH in ethanol loaded animals (fig.2).

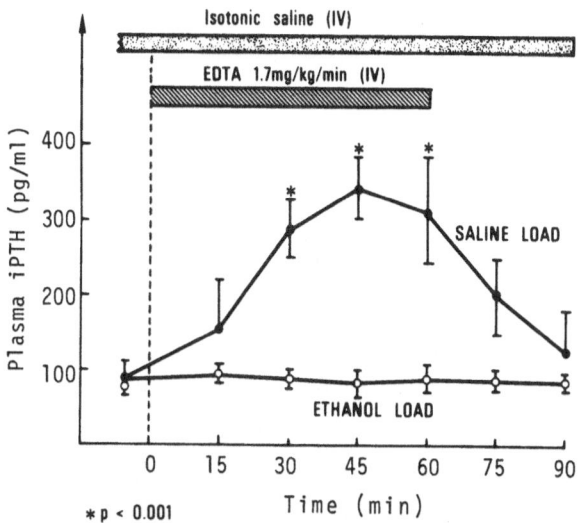

Fig. 2 : Plasma immunoreactive PTH concentration at the onset and during IV infusion of disodium EDTA in normal rats preloaded with ethanol (O) or saline (●).

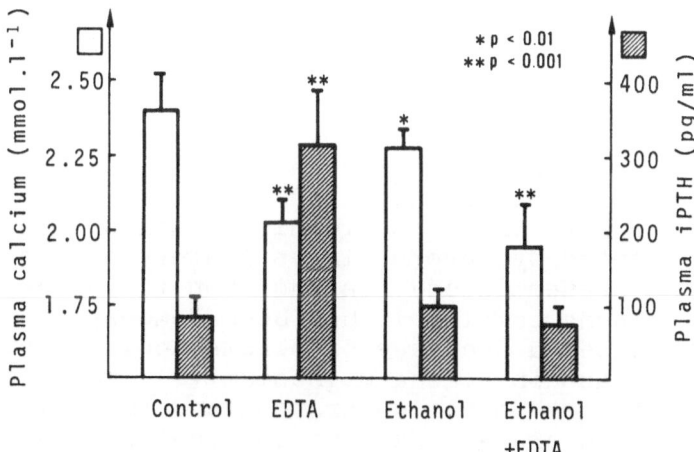

Fig.3 : Total plasma calcium and immunoreactive PTH concentration measured in rats two hours after preloading with saline (controls) and with ethanol. In rats infused with disodium EDTA, the parameters were measured two hours after gastric administration of either ethanol or saline and 1h after starting the IV administration of disodium EDTA.

Figure 3 summarizes the changes in plasma immunoreactive PTH in response to acute changes in plasma
calcium. Whatever the level of plasma calcium the PTH
level in control and ethanol loaded rats remains virtually unchanged.

## In vitro studies

During incubation, in vitro, parathyroid glands
responded to the decrease in calcium concentration of
the medium by a significant increase in PTH secretion.
Shifting the medium calcium concentration from 1.25 to
0.75 mmol/l resulted in a twofold increase in medium
PTH concentration. When calcium increased from 1.25 to
3.0 mmol/l the PTH secretion was only 40% of the basal
value (fig.4).

The stimulating effect of 0.75 mmol/l medium concentration of PTH secretion was selected to analyze
the effects of ethanol added to the culture medium.
With ethanol concentrations of 0.5% to 5% the PTH concentration did not change from the beginning to the
end of the experiment. Moreover, ethanol prevented significantly ( p< 0.001) the increase in PTH concentration observed in response to the hypocalcemic stimulus
that is normal in the absence of ethanol.

## DISCUSSION

The present study was designed to measure PTH
secretion in response to hypocalcemia induced by large
amounts of ethanol administered via an intragastric
tube in the rat. The hypocalcemic effect of ethanol has
been documented by several investigators and was confirmed in the present study. In addition to the decrease
of total plasma calcium it has been demonstrated that
ethanol induces a decrease of plasma ionized calcium
and an increase in plasma magnesium (7). The mechanisms
of these changes is not understood and the role of PTH
remains controversial. We have documented ethanol-induced inhibition of PTH secretion whereas others have
obtained opposite results (8,10).

Hypocalcemia induced by acute ethanol loading
could be the result of : 1) inhibition of parathyroid
gland secretion leading to a fall in plasma PTH ; 2)
excessive PTH catabolism in spite of a near normal parathyroid gland responsiveness to the hypocalcemic stimulus ; 3) decrease in bone resorption due to a direct

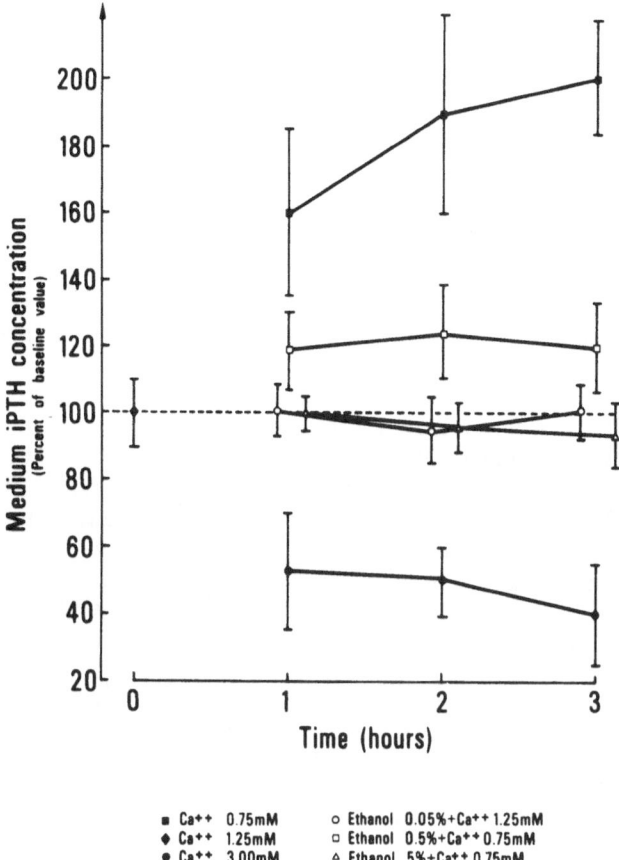

Fig. 4 : Time course of immunoreactive PTH secretion
measured in the medium where rat parathyroid glands
were incubated. Concentrations are expressed as percentage of the baseline value measured in all the experiments with a 1.25 mmol/l calcium concentration.
Ethanol was added to the medium which was replaced
hourly.

skeletal effect of ethanol ; 4) a combination of the
preceding hypotheses.

The ethanol-induced hypocalcemia in the rat could
result, at least in part, from a direct inhibitory effect on bone, because exogenous PTH cannot elicit an
increase in plasma calcium (7). However, we do not

known if this effect is associated with a decrease in
parathyroid gland secretion. We have documented a total
unresponsiveness of the gland in experiments lasting
five hours after administration of alcohol to the animals. The hypothesis of an increased catabolic rate of
PTH seems improbable. One could speculate a possible
interference of ethyl alcohol with hepatic PTH breakdown since ethanol decreases or inhibits several hepatic
enzymes. Ethanol could inhibit or decrease the activity
of proteolytic enzymes as has been demonstrated for
lipid oxidation and microsomal drug metabolism (4).

This in vitro study was in favour of a
direct effect of ethanol on parathyroid gland secretion.
The hypothesis derived from a previous in vivo study (7)
that hypermagnesemia occuring after ethanol loading
could inhibit PTH secretion cannot explain the present
findings. Recent study (8,10) has documented an increase in plasma PTH in man as well as an increased PTH secretion by bovine parathyroid glands in vitro in the
presence of ethanol. We were unable to measure such a
stimulatory effect of ethanol on PTH secretion. On the
contrary, in our experiments, ethanol suppressed the
PTH secretion even with a superimposed decrease in plasma calcium induced by infusion of disodium EDTA. The
discrepancy between the two studies could be due to
the different designs of the experiments.

We have no explanation for the suppressed PTH
secretion and hypocalcemia induced by ethanol. It seems
possible that ethanol acts simultaneously and directly
on numerous target cells including liver (4), brain (9),
intestine (3) and also bone and parathyroid gland, by
impairing cellular metabolism and especially membrane
transfer. In conclusion, the mechanisms of hypocalcemia
following acute ethanol ingestion remain  unknown. They
could be related to an inhibitory effect of calcium release at the bone level associated with an inhibition
of PTH secretion.

ACKNOWLEDGEMENTS

We gratefully acknowledge the technical assistance
of D.Coraboeuf and M.Lair and the secretarial assistance
of F. Probst. Our thanks are also due to Pr. M. Thevenin
for measurement of plasma ethanol concentration.

SUMMARY

Acute ethanol loading in the rat induces hypocalcemia and hypermagnesemia. In addition, hypocalcemia
is not corrected by exogenous PTH. In the rat the mechanism of these changes was investigated by measuring
plasma immunoreactive parathyroid hormone (PTH). PTH
was also measured in culture medium in which parathyroid glands were incubated. The addition of ethanol
to test tubes did not interfere with PTH measurement.

Absolute ethyl alcohol diluted to 50% with distilled water was administered via an intragastric tube.
It failed to induce an increase in plasma immunoreactive PTH level. Similarly, it prevented an increase in
plasma PTH after disodium EDTA injection. Thus in the
presence of ethyl alcohol plasma PTH failed to increase in spite of a significant decrease of plasma calcium.

In vitro studies showed that the decrease of
calcium concentration of the medium from 1.50 to 0.75
mmol/l was associated with a 3 to 5 times increase in
PTH secretion rate. This increase was suppressed when
ethanol was added to the culture medium.

In conclusion, ethanol loading via gastric tubing
induced : 1) decrease in plasma calcium ; 2) suppression of immunoreactive PTH secretion in the presence
of hypocalcemia. It is postulated that the acute hypocalcemic effect of ethanol loading is mediated by a
dual effect at the level of the bone and the parathyroid gland.

REFERENCES

1. CHANARD J, BLACK R., PURKERSON M., LEWIS J., KLAHR
S., SLATOPOLSKY E. 1977. : The effects of Colchicine
and Vinblastine on parathyroid hormone secretion in
the rat. Endocrinology, 101:1972

2. HOYUMAA A.M.Jr., BREEN K.J., SCHENKER S., WILSON F.
A. 1975. : Thiamine transport across the rat intestine. II. Effect of ethanol. J.Lab.Clin.Med, 86:803

3 . KRAWITT J.L., SAMPSON H.W., KATAGIRI C.A. 1975 :
Effect of 1,25-dihydroxycholecalciferol on ethanol me-
diated suppression of calcium absorption. Calcif.Tiss.
Res, 18:119

4. LIEBER C.S., TESCHKE R., HASUMURA Y., DECARLI L.M. 1975: Differences in hepatic and metabolic changes after acute and chronic alcohol consumption. Fed.Proc. 34: 2060.

5. PENG T.C. 1970: The hypocalcemic effect of urethane in rats. Fed.Proc. 29:782

6. PENG T.C., COOPER C.W., MUNSON P.L. 1972 : The hypocalcemic effect of ethyl alcohol in rats and dogs. Endocrinology 91:586

7. PENG T.C., GITELMAN H.J. 1974 : Ethanol-induced hypocalcemia, hypermagnesemia and inhibition of the serum calcium raising effect of parathyroid hormone in rats. Endocrinology, 94:608

8. SHAH J.H., BOWSER E.N., HARGIS G.K., WONGSURAWAT N., BANERJEE P., HENDERSON W.J., WILLIAMS G.A. 1978 : Effect of ethanol on parathyroid hormone secretion in the rat. Metabolism 27:257

9. SUN A.Y. 1976 : Alcohol-membrane interaction in the brain. Annals N.Y.Acad.Sci, 273:295

10. WILLIAMS G.A., BOWSER E.N., HARGIS G.K., KURREJA S.C., SHAH J.J., VORA N.M., HENDERSON W.J. 1978 : Effect of ethanol on parathyroid hormone and calcitonin secretion in man. Proc.Soc.exp.biol.med.159:187

# EFFECTS OF CIMETIDINE ON PARATHYROID HORMONE IN CHRONIC UREMIA

Jacques J. Bourgoignie, Allan I. Jacob, George Gavellas and Janet Canterbury

Laboratory of the Howard Hughes Medical Institute and Dept. of Medicine, University of Miami School of Medicine, Miami, Florida 33101

## INTRODUCTION

Recent case reports suggest suppression of immunoreactive parathyroid hormone (iPTH) with cimetidine in two patients with primary hyperparathyroidism. In both patients peptic ulcer disease led to medical treatment with cimetidine. In the first patient given oral cimetidine (800 mg then 400 mg daily) for 8 months, iPTH decreased from 20 times to 6 times normal [1]. No changes in serum calcium and phosphorus occurred, but inhibition of gastric acid secretion and ulcer healing were demonstrated. In the second patient, a woman with a parathyoid adenoma, cimetidine treatment (1200 mg daily) was associated with a decrease in iPTH levels from a value 2.5 times normal to a normal value [2,3]. Concommittantly, serum calcium decreased from 11.3 mg/dl to 10.3 mg/dl and serum phosphorus increased from 2.1 mg/dl to 2.7 mg/dl. One month after discontinuation of cimetidine therapy iPTH had rebounded to values thrice normal and serum calcium and phosphorus were 10.8 and 2.3 mg/dl, respectively.

These intriguing observations led us to evaluate the effects of cimetidine on uremic hyperparathyroidism. Acute experiments were performed in dogs with a decrease in renal mass and chronic studies were performed in patients with end-stage renal disease maintained on chronic hemodialysis.

METHODS

Dog Experiments

Acute clearance experiments were performed in five female
mongrel dogs weighing 13 to 20 kg. Renal insufficiency was induced by ligation of the majority of the branches of the renal artery on one side followed, two weeks later, by contralateral nephrectomy. This model has been described in detail [4]. During a period of stabilization varying from 3 to 7 months, the
dogs were fed ad libitum high protein dog Purina chow.

On the day of the experiment the animals were studied awake,
standing in a supporting sling, following a standard protocol [5].
A catheter was inserted into the bladder for quantitative urine
collection. Venous catheters were placed in the inferior vena cava
through a hind limb vein for infusion and blood sampling. After
injection of a priming dose of creatinine, a solution of isotonic
saline containing creatinine was infused at a rate of 0.3 ml/min
throughout the experiment. After a 60 min. period of equilibration,
three 20-min. control clearance periods were obtained. Thereafter,
100 mg cimetidine was administered intravenously as a bolus followed
by a maintenance dose of 40 mg/hour for 5 hours dissolved in the
isotonic saline infusion. Immediately after the bolus cimetidine
injection five 1-hr. experimental clearance periods were obtained.
At the end of each period, the bladder was washed with 30 ml of
sterile water to ensure complete urine collection. At the midpoint
of each period, a sample of blood was collected anaerobically for
determination of creatinine, sodium, potassium, phosphorus, ionized
calcium and iPTH.

Human Experiments

Seven patients with end stage renal insufficiency of various
etiologies were studied. All patients were undergoing chronic hemodialysis thrice weekly for at least three months. During the period
of study they received cimetidine orally at a dose of 300 mg twice
daily. Other medications were not changed. In particular, treatment
with aluminum hydroxide antacids was not modified. Samples of blood
for iPTH assay, ionized calcium, total magnesium and phosphorus were
drawn twice before starting cimetidine and weekly for four weeks and
at six weeks after initiation of cimetidine therapy. Blood specimens were drawn anaerobically immediately before hemodialysis.

Phosphorus and creatinine were measured in urine and blood by
a modified autoanalyzer method (Technicon AutoAnalyzer II). Serum ionized calcium concentration was determined with a flow-through
electrode system (Orion Biomedical, Model SS-20), serum magnesium
by atomic absorption spectrometry, and sodium and potassium by

flame photometry. Serum iPTH in dogs and in patients was quantitated by radioimmunoassay with antiserum CH 71 and CH-824, respectively, at a final dilution of 1:125,000. These antisera cross
react with intact hormone as well as with NH2- and COOH-terminal
fragments [6]. All samples were measured in duplicate at two widely varying dilutions. The coefficient of variation of replicate
samples was less than 10 percent. Assays showing a larger variation
of replicate samples were repeated. iPTH levels are reported in
arbitrary units ($\mu$leq/ml) relating the potency of the test serum to
that of a standard hyperparathyroid serum sample of the appropriate
species.

Data are expressed as means $\pm$ SEM. Statistical analyses were
performed with Student's t test for paired data. All patients gave
informed consent for the study.

RESULTS

Dog Experiments

The effects of peripheral intravenous infusion of cimetidine
on circulating iPTH of chronically uremic dogs with secondary
hyperparathyroidism are depicted in Fig. 1. In the first experiment performed, iPTH averaged 540 $\mu$leq/ml during the control clearance periods and decreased after cimetidine to 350 and 315 $\mu$leq/ml
at four and five hours respectively (a 35 and 41 percent decrease).
In four other experiments, iPTH at the fifth hour was 98, 94,
79 and 74 percent of control values. For all five experiments, administration of cimetidine was associated with a progressive decrease in circulating iPTH from a mean control value of 638 $\pm$ 95
$\mu$leq/ml to mean values of 532 $\pm$ 122 and 530 $\pm$ 114 $\mu$leq/ml at four
and five hours, respectively. The decrease in circulating iPTH at
four hours and five hours averaged 20.4 $\pm$ 8.0, and 19.2 $\pm$ 7.1 percent respectively and reached statistical significance at five hour
(p=0.05).

For the same experiments, the effects of intravenous administration of cimetidine on urine flow rate, creatinine clearance,
serum ionized calcium and phosphorus and absolute and fractional
urinary excretion of electrolytes are shown in Table I. After five
hours of cimetidine infusion, urine flow rate and creatinine clearance were significantly decreased (p < 0.001 and p < 0.05, respectively). In contrast, no significant changes occurred in serum
ionized calcium and phosphorus or in urinary phosphorus, potassium,
sodium or calcium excretion.

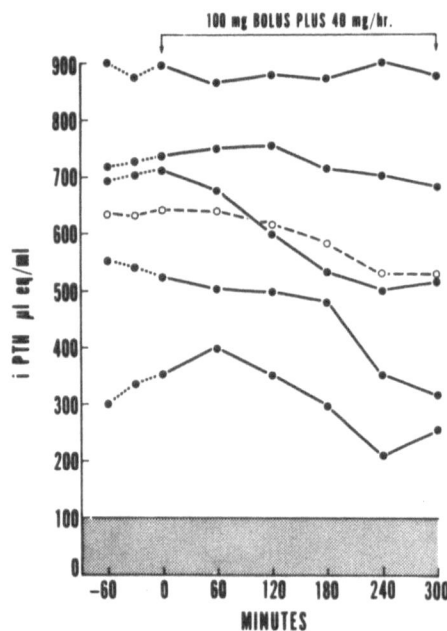

Figure 1.  Effects of intravenous cimetidine on iPTH in chronically uremic dogs.  Data for individual animals (●) and mean data (Ⓞ)
are presented.  Hatched area represent normal range for canine iPTH.

## Human Experiments

Data from a single patient are shown in Fig. 2.  Before cimetidine therapy, the mean serum iPTH, ionized calcium and phosphorus values averaged 715 μleq/ml, 4.66 mg/dl and 6.8 mg/dl, respectively.  One week after oral administration of 600 mg cimetidine
daily, circulating iPTH was 605 μleq/ml.  At four weeks of treatment iPTH had decreased to 210 μleq/ml and, at six weeks, to 190
μleq/ml.  This decrement in circulating iPTH occurred without marked changes in serum ionized calcium or phosphorus.

The average control values for circulating iPTH, phosphorus
and ionized calcium before and at six weeks of cimetidine therapy
are depicted in Fig. 3 for each of all seven patients studied.
Prior to cimetidine therapy the mean level of iPTH was 413 ± 68
μleq/ml.  After six weeks, the average iPTH value had fallen in
six of seven patients to a mean of 129. ± 29 μleq/ml (p < .01).

TABLE I. EFFECTS OF CIMETIDINE I.V. IN UREMIC DOGS (N=5)

| | CONTROL | 5 Hr. |
|---|---|---|
| UV ml/min | 1.9 ± 0.2 | 0.9 ± 0.2* |
| CREAT. CL. ml/min | 14.4 ± 2.7 | 12.7 ± 2.5* |
| SERUM $Ca^{++}$ mg/dl | 5.38 ± 0.10 | 5.32 ± 0.12 |
| SERUM P mg/dl | 5.4 ± 0.9 | 5.6 ± 0.8 |
| $U_P V$ µg/min | 182 ± 58.7 | 203 ± 62.5 |
| $FE_P$% | 26.9 ± 7.1 | 31.9 ± 7.2 |
| $U_K V$ µEq/min | 22.4 ± 7.7 | 17.1 ± 6.1 |
| $FE_K$% | 38.9 ± 12.2 | 35.2 ± 10.7 |
| $U_{Na} V$ µEq/min | 32.9 ± 15.1 | 22.8 ± 16.6 |
| $FE_{Na}$% | 1.7 ± 0.8 | 1.4 ± 0.9 |
| $U_{Ca} V$ µg/min | 12.1 ± 6.8 | 10.8 ± 5.1 |
| $FE_{Ca}$% | 2.1 ± 0.9 | 1.9 ± 0.7 |

*$p < 0.05$ or less.
Creat. Cl.= Clearance of exogenous creatinine
FE= Fractional excretion
Values for ionized calcium range from 4.16 to 5.25 mg/dl in normal
dogs. Canine normal range for iPTH is 35 to 85 µleq/ml

Concomitantly, the serum ionized calcium concentration fell from
a mean of 4.38 ± .20 mg/dl prior to therapy to 4.18 ± .29 mg/dl
at six weeks of therapy ($p < 0.05$), and serum phosphorus concentration rose insignificantly from 6.10 ±.5 mg/dl to 6.50 ± .7 mg/dl
($p < .2$). Serum magnesium concentration did not change significantly with mean values of 2.36 ± .2 before and 2.28 ± .54 meq/ml
after six weeks of cimetidine.

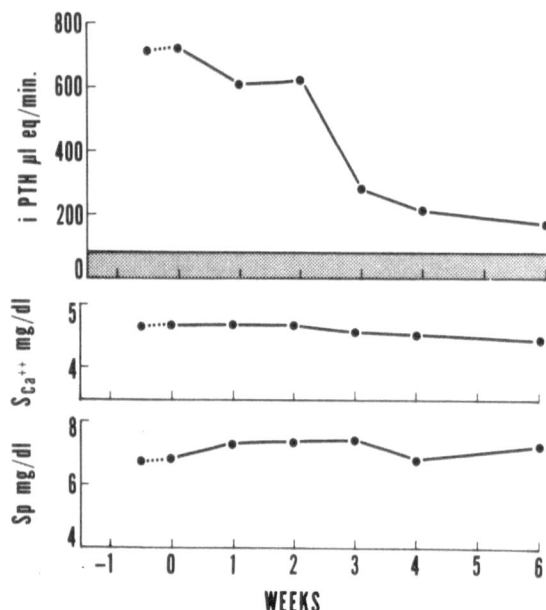

Figure 2.  Effects of cimetidine (300 mg po bid) on circulating
iPTH, ionized calcium and phosphorus in a patient with end stage
renal failure maintained on chronic hemodialysis.  Hatched area
represent normal range for human iPTH.

        To evaluate for a possible interference of cimetidine with the
radioimmunoassay for parathyroid hormone, cimetidine was added in
final concentrations of 1.5 and 4.5 μg/ml, equivalent to in-vivo
therapeutic concentrations, to a uremic hyperparathyroid serum sample.  The results, shown in Table II, demonstrate no interference
of the drug with the parathyroid immunoassay.

DISCUSSION

        Cimetidine, an histamine $H_2$ receptor antagonist, is a potent
inhibitor of gastric acid secretion.  It is used in the treatment
of peptic ulcer disease, Zollinger-Ellison syndrome, upper gastrointestinal hemorrhage, steatorrhea from pancreatic insufficiency,
and metabolic alkalosis induced by nasogastric drainage or protrac-

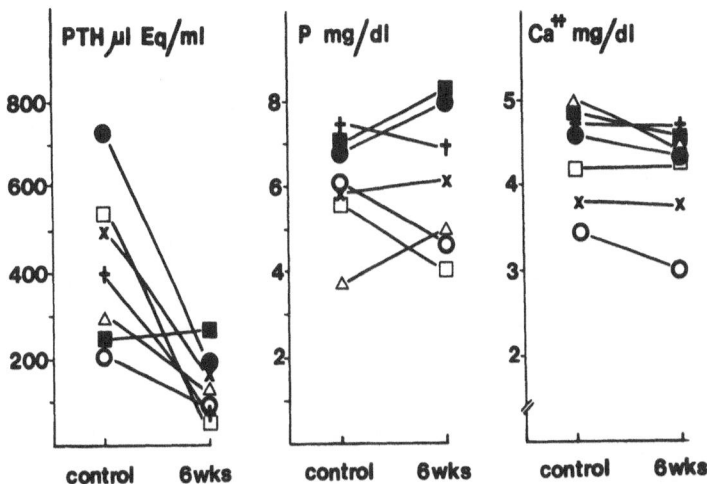

Figure 3. Circulating iPTH, phosphorus and ionized calcium before and at 6 weeks of cimetidine (300 mg po bid) in seven patients with end stage renal failure maintained on chronic hemodialysis.

ted vomiting [7,8]. It has become one of the one-hundred most often prescribed drugs in American hospitals. As the usage of cimetidine increases, a number of reports have appeared in the literature indicating biological effects of the drug other than inhibition of gastric acid secretion [9]. Subtle effects of cimetidine on the endocrine system have been described. In particular, it has an antiandrogenic effect. In rats and dogs, it decreases the weight of the prostate [10] and, in rats, it competes for binding to androgen cytosol receptors and blocks nuclear uptake of dihydrotestosterone [11]. In humans, small changes in the function of the hypothalamic-pituitary-gonadal axis have been reported: cimetidine may induce gynecomastia [13,14], reduce sperm count [12], reduce luteinizing hormone response to luteinizing hormone releasing factor [12], increase plasma testosterone [12,15] and stimulate prolactin [14,16]. Some of these alterations have not been uniformly observed [9] and their clinical importance presently remains undetermined.

We describe here another endocrine effect of cimetidine, i.e. suppression of circulating iPTH in dogs and patients with chronic renal insufficiency and secondary hyperparathyroidism.

TABLE II.   EFFECTS OF CIMETIDINE IN VITRO ON iPTH

|    | CONTROL SERUM | PLUS 1.5 µg/ml | PLUS 4.5 µg/ml |
|----|---------------|----------------|----------------|
| A. | 95            | 110            | 90             |
| B. | 105           | 115            | 95             |

Each value is average of triplicate samples.

Rows A and B are duplicate of each other.

In the chronically uremic dog, infusion of cimetidine was associated with a decrease in circulating iPTH of more than 20% in 3 of
5 animals.  For the group the decrease in iPTH was significant at
the fifth hour of administration of the drug.  This inhibition
occurred without significant changes in serum concentrations of
ionized calcium or phosphorus and without significant changes in
urinary excretion of sodium, potassium, calcium or phosphate.  In
the absence of timed control experiments, however, these observations in the dog with a decreased nephron mass are only suggestive
and do not conclusively, demonstrate an effect of cimetidine on
iPTH.

In contrast, oral administration of cimetidine for 6 weeks in
therapeutic dosages to patients with end stage renal failure resulted in a marked decrease in iPTH in 6 of 7 subjects.*  In several
instances, values for iPTH fell into well within the range seen in
euparathyroid subjects.  The inhibition of iPTH with cimetidine developed slowly and generally became evident only during the second
or third week of treatment.  The reason for this delayed effect is
unclear.  It is possible that a critical level of the drug is necessary to affect parathyroid gland function.  Cimetidine with a
molecular weight of 252 and little protein binding is dialyzable.
Hemodialysis clearance rates have been reported to range from 41

---

\* The patient who failed to suppress at 6 weeks was grossly over-
weight and, when the dose of cimetidine was then increased from
600 to 900 mg per day, a decrease in iPTH readily occurred.

to 76 ml/min [17]. Notwithstanding this substantial dialyzability, the total amount of cimetidine removed during four hours of hemodialysis constitutes only 8 to 14 percent of a 300 mg intravenous dose [17]. This suggests that cimetidine may slowly accumulate in patients with end stage renal failure and delay demonstrable effects.

The mechanism(s) whereby cimetidine decreases circulating iPTH is unknown. Hypercalcemia, which would suppress levels of iPTH, did not occur. Instead, serum ionized calcium tended to decrease rather than increase with cimetidine administration. Hypomagnesemia may lead to a blunted parathyroid gland response [18]; this mechanism was not operative in our patients as no significant changes in serum magnesium occurred. It is possible that cimetidine accelerates the degradation of inactive COOH-terminal fragments of PTH which are known to circulate for prolonged periods in uremic patients [19]. However, the radioimmunoassay used measures the active amino terminal of the whole PTH molecule as well as carboxyl terminal fragments suggesting that the major effect of cimetidine may be to impair either synthesis and/or release of the hormone from the parathyroid glands. This inhibition of iPTH may be the result of a direct effect of cimetidine on the parathyroid gland, or an indirect effect mediated through unknown mechanisms.

## ACKNOWLEDGEMENTS

This work was supported by the Howard Hughes Medical Institute, USPHS Grants Nos. 7 RO1 AM 19822 and IT 32 AM 07205 and through the generosity of Mr. and Mrs. Robert Chambers. Dr. J.J. Bourgoignie is an Investigator of the Howard Hughes Medical Institute. Dr. A. Jacob is a fellow of the National Kidney Foundation. The assistance of the personnel of the Dialysis Unit at Jackson Memorial Hospital is gratefully acknowledged.

## REFERENCES

1. B. Simon, A. Stiehl, G. Feurle and B. Kommerell. Erfolgreiche Ulkusbenhandlung mit cimetidin bei einem Patienten mit primarem Hyperparathyroidismus. Med. Klin. 73:1513-1516, (1978).
2. J. Sherwood, D. Reinhard, and M. Garcia. Does Cimetidine inhibit parathyroid hormone secretion? N. Eng. J. Med. 300:200, (1979).
3. D. Reinhard. Personal Communication.
4. J.M. Canterbury, G. Gavellas, J.J. Bourgoignie and E. Reiss. Metabolic consequences of oral administration of 24,25 $(OH)_2$ $D_3$ to uremic dogs. Proc. Fourth Workshop on Vitamin D, Berlin, West Germany, In Press.
5. M.A. Kaplan, J.M. Canterbury, J.J. Bourgoignie, G. Veliz, G. Gavellas, E. Reiss and N.S. Bricker. Reversal of hyperparathyroidism in response to dietary phosphorus restriction in

the uremic dog. Kidney Int. 15:43 (1979).

6.  J.M. Canterbury, L.A. Bricker, G.S. Levey, P.L. Kozlovskis, E. Ruiz, J.E. Zull, and E. Reiss. Metabolism of bovine pa- rathyroid hormone: Immunological and Biological characteris- tics of fragments generated by liver perfusion. J. Clin. Invest. 55:1245-1253, (1975).

7.  W. Finkelstein and K.J. Isselbacher. Cimetidine. N. Engl. J. Med. 299:992 (1978).

8.  N.D. Vaziri, C.H. Barton, R.L. Ness, K. Mirahmadi. Special uses of cimetidine. Ann. Intern Med. 88:266 (1978).

9.  R.J. Temple, J.K. Jones, and J.R. Crout. Adverse effects of newly marketed drugs. N. Engl. J. Med. 300:1046 (1979)

10. G.B. Leslie and T.F. Walker. A Toxicological profile of Ci- metidine. In Proc. Second Intern. Symposium on Histamine $H_2$-receptor antagonists. Excerpta Medica Amsterdam, p.24 (1977).

11. S.J. Winters, J.L. Banks, and D.L. Loriaux. The histamine $H_2$- antagonist cimetidine is an antiandrogen. Gastroenterology 76:504 (1979).

12. D.H. Van Thiel, J.S. Gavaler, W.I. Smith Jr. and G. Paul. Hypothalamic-pituitary-gonadal dysfunction in men using ci- metidine. N. Engl. J. Med. 300:1012 (1979)

13. W.H. Hall Breast changes in males on cimetidine. N. Engl. J. Med. 295:841 (1976)

14. G.D. Delle Fave, G. Tamburrano, C. Natoli, M.L. Santoro, R. Carratu, A. Torsoi and L. De Magistris. Gynaecomastia with cimetidine. Lancet 1:1319 (1977)

15. N.R. Peden, J.M. Cargill, Mc Browning. Male sexual dysfunction during treatment with cimetidine. Br. Med. J. 1:659 (1979).

16. A.M. Speigel, R. Lopatin, S. Peikin and D. Mc Carthy. Serum prolactin in patient receiving chronic oral cimetidine. Lancet 1:881 (1978).

17. N.D. Vaziri, R.L. Ness and C.H. Barton. Hemodialysis clear- ance of cimetidine. Arch. Intern. Med. 138:1685 (1978)

18. L.R. Chase, and E. Slatopolsky. Secretion and metabolic ef- ficacy of parathyroid hormone in patients with severe hypo- magnesemia. J. Clin. Endocrinol. and Metab. 38:363-371 (1974).

19. K.A. Hruska, R. Kopelman, W.E. Rutherford, S. Klahr, and F. Slatopolsky. Metabolism of immunoreactive parathyroid hor- mone in the dog: The role of the kidney and the effects of chronic renal disease. J. Clin. Invest. 56:39-48 (1975).

# PARATHYROID HORMONE DEPENDENT HYPERCALCIURIA IN CHRONIC

# METABOLIC ACIDOSIS

Daniel Batlle, M.D., Steven Hays, M.D., Jose A.L.
Arruda, M.D. and Neil A. Kurtzman, M.D.

University of Illinois Hospital – Section of
Nephrology – 840 South Wood Street – Chicago, Illinois
60680

## INTRODUCTION

Metabolic acidosis is well known to result in hypercalciuria
(6,8,9). The hypercalciuria of metabolic acidosis is
thought to be the result of a depression in calcium reabsorption
by the kidney (8,13). The role of parathyroid hormone (PTH)
in the calciuria of metabolic acidosis has not been completely
defined. Based on studies performed in humans with hypoparathyroidism, it has been suggested that PTH plays no role in
the hypercalciuria seen in metabolic acidosis (9). This
study was designed to investigate the effect of PTH on the
renal handling of calcium during chronic metabolic acidosis.

## METHODS

Experiments were performed on female mongrel dogs
weighing between 7 and 17 kg. utilizing clearance studies as
previously described by this laboratory (7). The following
issues were examined:

1. Effect of chronic metabolic acidosis on renal Ca
   excretion.

Five intact dogs were fed $NH_4Cl$ (6 mEq/kg body wt.) via
a nasogastric tube for three consecutive days. Three clearance
collections were obtained on the third day of $NH_4Cl$ feeding.

2. Renal handling of Ca in the intact control dog.

Three clearance collections were obtained as described

above using six non-acidotic dogs.

3.  Effect of thyroparathyroidectomy (TPTX) during chronic metabolic acidosis.

A total TPTX was surgically performed in 11 dogs fed $NH_4Cl$ as described above. Three clearance collections were obtained 24 or 48 hours after TPTX.

4.  Renal handling of Ca in TPTX control dogs.

Six dogs not given $NH_4Cl$ were studied 48 hours after TPTX in the same fashion as the TPTX acidotic animals.

5.  Effect of $CaCl_2$ infusion to TPTX dogs.

A $CaCl_2$ solution (8-10 μEq/kg body wt/min) was administered continuously for 90 minutes to the TPTX animals described above. Plasma total Ca was determined frequently to verify that a level between 4 and 5.5 mEq/l had been achieved. Six clearance collections were obtained.

6.  Effect of PTH administration to TPTX dogs with chronic metabolic acidosis and TPTX controls.

Upon completion of the clearance studies obtained during $CaCl_2$ infusion mentioned above, PTH was infused at a constant rate of 1 U/min for 1 hr. Six clearance collections were obtained.

Plasma ionizable Ca was determined using the Orion electrode. Filtered load of Ca and fractional Ca excretion were calculated by the formulas GFR x plasma Ca and clearance Ca/GFR, respectively, using the values of ionizable Ca.

RESULTS

Absolute Ca excretion of intact dogs made acidotic with $NH_4Cl$ feeding was significantly higher than in the intact control dogs (Fig. 1). This difference was observed despite similar levels of total plasma Ca and fractional Na excretion.

Absolute Ca excretion of TPTX acidotic dogs was not significantly different than that of TPTX controls (Fig. 1). This lack of difference in Ca excretion was observed at comparable levels of glomerular filtration rate (GFR) and fractional Na excretion. As a consequence of TPTX, plasma Ca levels were low in acidotic (total plasma Ca 3.18 ± 0.12 mEq/l) and non-$NH_4Cl$ loaded animals (total plasma Ca 2.33 ± 0.12 mEq/l). Since at these low levels of plasma Ca it

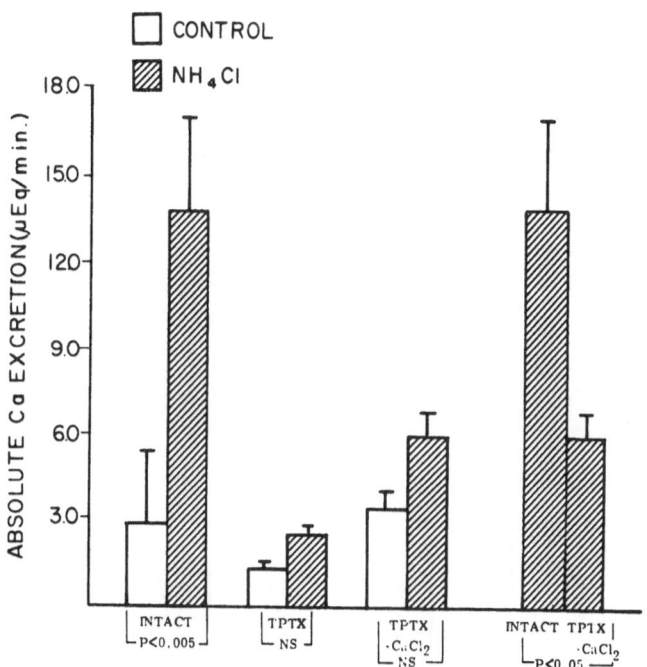

Fig. 1. The absolute Ca excretion of NH$_4$Cl treated dogs (shaded bars) is compared to non-NH$_4$Cl treated dogs (open bars). Observe that in the intact dogs, Ca excretion was higher in the NH$_4$Cl treated dogs than in the intact controls (right panel). After thyro-parathyroidectomy (TPTX), Ca excretion was not significantly different between NH$_4$Cl and non-NH$_4$Cl treated dogs either before or after CaCl$_2$ infusion (middle panels). The Ca excretion of TPTX acidotic animals infused with CaCl$_2$ was significantly lower than that of intact acidotic animals (left panel).

might not be possible to disclose any differences in renal Ca excretion between acidotic and control dogs, a CaCl$_2$ infusion was administered in order to restore the plasma Ca and the filtered load to normal levels. After CaCl$_2$ infusion,

the levels of total plasma Ca rose to the same extent in
acidotic and control animals (4.95 ± 0.12 and 4.44 ± 0.32
mEq/l, respectively).  Nonetheless, the absolute Ca excretion
was not significantly different between acidotic and control
TPTX dogs infused with CaCl$_2$ (Fig. 1).  Figure 1 illustrates
that the absolute Ca excretion of TPTX acidotic dogs infused
with CaCl$_2$ was significantly lower than in the intact acidotic
dogs.

   The administration of PTH to acidotic TPTX dogs resulted
in a significant increase in absolute Ca excretion (Fig. 2).

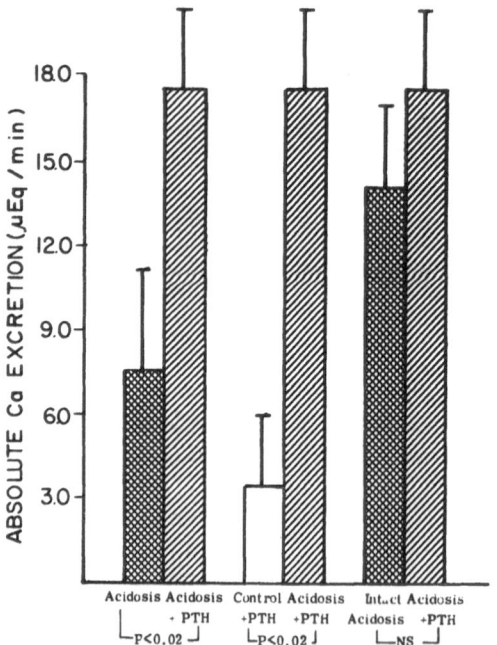

Fig. 2.  It is illustrated that the absolute Ca excretion of
         TPTX acidotic dogs replaced with PTH was higher than
         TPTX acidotic dogs without PTH (left panel) and TPTX
         controls with PTH (middle panel) but not significantly
         different from intact acidotic animals (right panel).

The filtered load of Ca and fractional Ca excretion also
increased significantly as a result of the PTH infusion.
During PTH infusion, however, at any given level of filtered
load of Ca, the fractional Ca excretion of the acidotic
dogs was higher than the controls.  No changes in GFR or Na
excretion were observed during PTH administration.

TPTX control dogs infused with PTH had an absolute Ca
excretion significantly lower than TPTX acidotic dogs infused
with PTH (Fig. 2).  However, when the absolute Ca excretion
of intact acidotic dogs was compared to that of TPTX acidotic
dogs replaced with PTH, no significant differences were found
(Fig. 2).

DISCUSSION

The results of the present study confirm and extend
numerous previous observations (6,8,9) that chronic metabolic
acidosis results in hypercalciuria.  The increased Ca excretion
that accompanies chronic metabolic acidosis could be the
result of several factors: changes in Na excretion or filtered
load of Ca, a change in PTH activity or effect, or an effect
of acidosis per se.  The results of the present study support
previous observations indicating that the hypercalciuria of
chronic metabolic acidosis can occur independently of changes
in Na excretion or changes in the filtered load of Ca (9,12).
The hypercalciuria therefore could arise either as a consequence
of acidosis per se or could be related to an effect of PTH.

The present studies clearly demonstrate that TPTX dogs
with chronic metabolic acidosis have a Ca excretion similar
to TPTX controls and significantly lower than that seen in
intact acidotic animals.  Therefore, these findings suggest
that PTH plays a critical role in the hypercalciuria of
chronic metabolic acidosis.

The demonstration that PTH administration to TPTX
acidotic dogs results in hypercalciuria while it fails to
elicit the same effect on non-acidotic TPTX dogs demonstrates
that acute administration of PTH is hypercalciuric only
during acidosis.  It appears therefore that the effect of PTH
on Ca excretion during chronic metabolic acidosis is opposite
to its effect under normal conditions of acid-base balance,
which is to enhance tubular Ca reabsorption (1,2,4,10,11).

The hypercalciuric effect of PTH during chronic acidosis
could have been the result of increased levels of plasma
ionizable Ca which would increase the filtered load of Ca.
The demonstration, however, that at any given level of
filtered Ca the renal Ca excretion is higher in the acidotic

than in the control dogs, shows that PTH depresses the
tubular reabsorption of Ca in the presence of acidosis.
Recent studies in man have also shown that PTH increases Ca
excretion during acidosis (5).

Our findings are in conflict with other studies showing
that metabolic acidosis inhibits tubular Ca reabsorption even
in the absence of PTH.  Lemann et al (9) did not find any
differences in renal Ca excretion between normal volunteers
and hypoparathyroid patients made acidotic with ammonium
chloride.  These authors concluded that the hypercalciuria of
chronic metabolic acidosis was independent of PTH based on
their findings of increased Ca excretion in four patients
with hypoparathyroidism.  The levels of PTH in these patients,
however, were not measured and it is possible that even small
amounts of this hormone can be sufficient to permit a high
rate of Ca excretion during acidosis.

The mechanism whereby PTH causes hypercalciuria during
chronic metabolic acidosis is not clarified by the present
study.  PTH is known to decrease the proximal reabsorption of
sodium bicarbonate and thereby increase its distal delivery
(3,7).  Recent findings have shown that sodium bicarbonate
administration is capable of enhancing the distal reabsorption
of Ca (13).  In metabolic acidosis the filtered load of
bicarbonate is low and therefore the distal delivery of
bicarbonate to the distal nephron by PTH is decreased compared
to non-acidotic subjects, and thus the distal reabsorption of
Ca would not be enhanced.  An alternative explanation is that
acidosis per se could modify the effect of PTH on distal Ca
transport so that Ca reabsorption would be depressed rather
than enhanced.

In conclusion, the present study demonstrates that TPTX
prevents the calciuric effect of chronic metabolic acidosis,
whereas PTH administration restores the hypercalciuria.  The
effect of PTH on Ca excretion during acidosis appears to be
the opposite to its effect under normal conditions of acid-
base balance; i.e. it increases renal Ca excretion during
acidosis.

REFERENCES

1.  Agus, Z.S., L.B. Gardner, L.H. Beck, and M. Goldberg.
    Effects of parathyroid hormone on renal tubular
    reabsorption of calcium, sodium and phosphate.  Am. J.
    Physiol.  224:1143-1148, 1973.

2.  Agus, Z.S., Peter, J.S.Chiu, and M. Goldberg.  Regulation
    of urinary calcium excretion in the rat.  Am. J. Physiol.
    232(6):F545-F549, 1977.

3.  Bank, N. and H.S. Aynedjian.  A micropuncture study of the
    effect of parathyroid hormone on renal bicarbonate reab-
    sorption.  J. Clin. Invest.  58:336-344, 1976.

4.  Burnatowska, M.A., C.A. Harris, R.A.L. Sutton, and J.H.
    Dirks.  Effects of PTH and cAMP on renal handling of
    calcium, magnesium, and phosphate in the hamster.  Am. J.
    Physiol.  233:F514-518, 1977.

5.  Chan, J.C.M. and F.C. Bartter.  Effect of metabolic
    acidosis and alkalosis on the renal response to parathyroid
    hormone infusion in normal man.  Kidney Int.  14:637,
    1978 (Abstract).

6.  Farquarson, R.F., W.T. Salter, D.M. Tibbetts, and J.C.
    Aub.  Studies of calcium and phosphorus metabolism.  XII.
    The effect of the ingestion of acid-producint substances.
    J. Clin. Invest.  10:221, 1934.

7.  Karlinsky, M., D. Sager, N.A. Kurtzman, and V.K.G.
    Pillay.  Effect of parathormone and cyclic adenosine
    monophosphate on renal bicarbonate reabsorption.  Amer.
    J. Physiol.  227:1226-1231, 1974.

8.  Lemann, J.Jr., J.R. Litzow, and E.J. Lennon.  The effects
    of chronic acid loads in normal man: further evidence
    for the participation of bone mineral in the defense
    against chronic metabolic acidosis.  J. Clin. Invest.
    45:1608, 1966.

9.  Lemann, J.Jr., J.R. Litzow, and E.J. Lennon.  Studies of
    the mechanism by which metabolic acidosis augments urinary
    calcium excretion in man.  J. Clin. Invest.  46:1318-1328,
    1967.

10. Massry, S.G., J.W. Coburn, L.W. Chapman, and C.R. Kleeman.
    Role of serum Ca, parathyroid hormone, and NaCl infusion
    on renal Ca and Na clearances.  Am. J. Physiol.  214:1403-
    1409, 1968.

11. Massry, S.G., J.W. Coburn, L.W. Chapman, and C.R. Kleeman.
    The interrelationship between serum calcium, sodium
    excretion and the parathyroids on renal handling of calcium.
    J. Clin. Invest.  46:1092, 1967.

12.  Stacy, B.D. and B.W. Wilson.  Acidosis and hypercalciuria:
     Renal mechanisms affecting calcium, magnesium and sodium
     excretion in the sheep.  J. Physiol.  210:549-564, 1970.

13.  Sutton, R.A.L., N.L.M. Wong, and J.H. Dirks.  Effects of
     metabolic acidosis and alkalosis on sodium and calcium
     transport in the dog kidney.  Kidney Int. Vol. 15:520-533,
     1979.

# THE PARATHYROID HORMONE RECEPTOR-ADENYLATE CYCLASE SYSTEM IN CHICKEN KIDNEY

R. A. Nissenson, N. Kugai and C. D. Arnaud

Endocrinology Section
Veterans Administration Medical Center
San Francisco, California 94121

## INTRODUCTION

There is a wealth of evidence that the renal actions of para-thyroid hormone (PTH) result, at least in part, from receptor-mediated stimulation of adenylate cyclase and a consequent increase in renal cell cyclic AMP. Thus, infusions of cyclic AMP (or its dibutyryl derivative) have been shown to reproduce the physiological effects of PTH on the kidney including inhibition of $PO_4$ reabsorption (1-4), stimulation of distal calcium reabsorption (1, 4) and increased production of $1,25(OH)_2D_3$ (5). Numerous studies have demonstrated PTH-stimulation of adenylate cyclase in renal tissue *in vitro*, and under certain circumstances nephrogenous cyclic AMP excretion can be used as a valid index of parathyroid function (6).

Nevertheless, fundamental questions remain concerning the de-tailed mechanism of target cell PTH action. First, very little is known about the interaction between PTH and its renal receptor. This has delayed progress in our understanding of pathological states as-sociated with altered renal PTH responsiveness (*e.g.* vitamin D defi-ciency, pseudohypoparathyroidism). A second question relates to the relative insensitivity of renal adenylate cyclase to PTH *in vitro* [$K_m \approx 10\text{-}100$ nM (7)] as compared to presumed physiological concen-trations (< 0.1 nM) *in vivo* (8). This discrepancy must be reconciled with the assumed role of cyclic AMP to mediate renal PTH action.

In the present study we identified and characterized chicken renal PTH receptors coupled to adenylate cyclase using the amino-terminal 1-34 peptide of bovine PTH [bPTH(1-34)] labeled by an elec-trolytic iodination procedure and purified by membrane adsorption. To determine whether the low sensitivity of the renal PTH receptor-

adenylate cyclase system might be an artifact due to tissue preparation *in vitro*, we also measured the plasma concentrations of
injected bPTH(1-34) required to produce increases in renal cyclic
AMP content *in vivo*.

METHODS

    Studies on PTH receptors and adenylate cyclase activation *in
vitro* were performed using highly purified chicken renal plasma
membranes isolated by a modification of the procedure of Fitzpatrick *et al*. (9) as described by DiBella *et al*. (7). Receptors
were identified using synthetic bPTH(1-34) radiolabeled by an
electrolytic iodination procedure (10, 11) and purified by receptor
adsorption, as previously described (12). Following incubation
with membranes for 30 minutes at 30°C, bound and free $^{125}$I-bPTH-
(1-34) were separated by filtration thru 0.2 μm cellulose acetate
Millipore filters at 4°C. Filters were washed 3 times with buffer
and counted in a gamma scintillation counter for $^{125}$I radioactivity.

    Adenylate cyclase was measured by the conversion of 0.1 mM
[α-$^{32}$P]ATP to [$^{32}$P] cyclic AMP, which was then isolated by the
double column procedure of Salomon *et al*. (13). For studies of
cyclic AMP production *in vivo*, various doses of bPTH(1-34) (0.3-
100 μg) in 0.4 ml of 0.9% NaCl + 0.1% BSA were administered into
brachial veins of thyroparathyroidectomized/ultimobranchialecto-
mized (TPTX/UBX) chickens. Precisely 90 seconds after hormone
administration, a blood sample was obtained from the left renal
portal vein. Two minutes after the administration of hormone,
liquid nitrogen was poured onto the right kidney, freezing it
instantly. The cyclic AMP content of the frozen tissue was then
determined by competitive protein binding assay (14).

    Immunoreactive PTH (iPTH) was measured in plasma samples by
radioimmunoassay, using an antibody that is highly specific for
the amino-terminal region of bPTH (antiserum GP-S). In this assay,
chloramine-T labeled $^{131}$I-bPTH(1-84) was used as labeled ligand and
bPTH(1-34) as standard.

RESULTS

    In initial experiments, we examined the binding of electro-
lytically labeled $^{125}$I-bPTH(1-34) to purified chicken renal plasma
membranes, and found very low binding values. Accordingly, we measured PTH binding to chicken renal plasma membranes both before and
after receptor purification of the labeled hormone. A typical competitive displacement experiment is shown in Figure 1. Receptor
purification resulted in a marked increase in initial $^{125}$I-bPTH(1-
34) binding, from 2.3% to 16.5%. This increase was not associated
with a change in the apparent affinity of the labelled hormone for

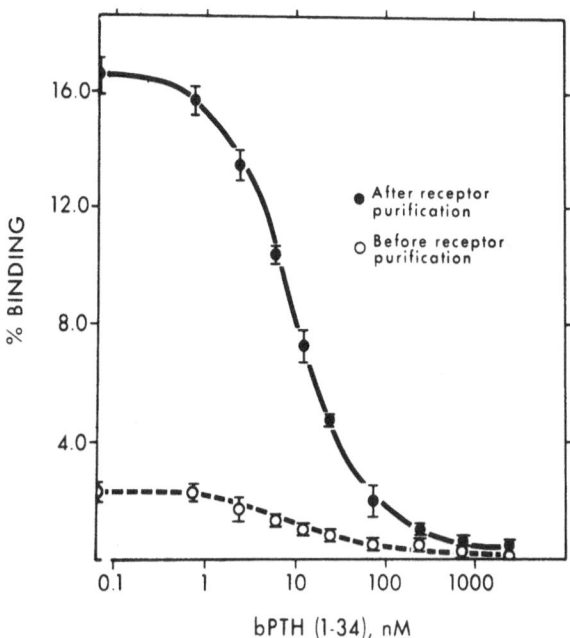

Figure 1.    $^{125}$I-bPTH(1-34) binding to chicken renal plasma membranes before and after receptor purification of the labeled hormone.  Binding was measured in the presence of 7,500 cpm (about 50 pg) of $^{125}$I-bPTH(1-34).  The percent binding of $^{125}$I-bPTH(1-34) is plotted as a function of the concentration of unlabeled bPTH(1-34) in the medium.  The final membrane concentration was 0.25 mg/ml (12).

membrane binding sites:  the concentration of unlabeled bPTH(1-34) giving 50% displacement of $^{125}$I-bPTH(1-34) was 7.3 nM and 9.0 nM before and after receptor purification, respectively.  Receptor purification of two additional preparations of electrolytically labeled $^{125}$I-bPTH(1-34) resulted in 5- and 9-fold increases in initial $^{125}$I-bPTH(1-34) binding.  In all cases, non-specific $^{125}$I-bPTH(1-34) binding to chicken renal plasma membranes [obtained in the presence of 2.5 μM unlabeled bPTH(1-34)] was virtually undetectable (< 0.5%).

The absence of significant non-specific binding of receptor purified $^{125}$I-bPTH(1-34) to chicken renal plasma membranes permitted us to use steady-state binding data to routinely estimate the

affinity and number of PTH binding sites by Scatchard analysis (15).
Figure 2A shows Scatchard plots of binding data obtained with three
different preparations of receptor-purified [125]I-bPTH(1-34).   The
equilibrium constant of dissociation ($K_d$) was calculated from the
negative reciprocal of the slopes of the lines and the number of
binding sites ($B_{max}$) was determined from the extrapolated x-inter-
cept of the plots.  Good agreement was obtained in the estimate of
binding site $K_d$ (7.4 - 10.1 nM) and number (4.2 - 5.2 pmol/mg of
protein) for different preparations of labeled hormone.  When these
binding data were analyzed in a Hill plot (Fig. 2B), a straight line
was obtained with a slope of 0.99, strongly suggesting the absence
of significant cooperative effects.

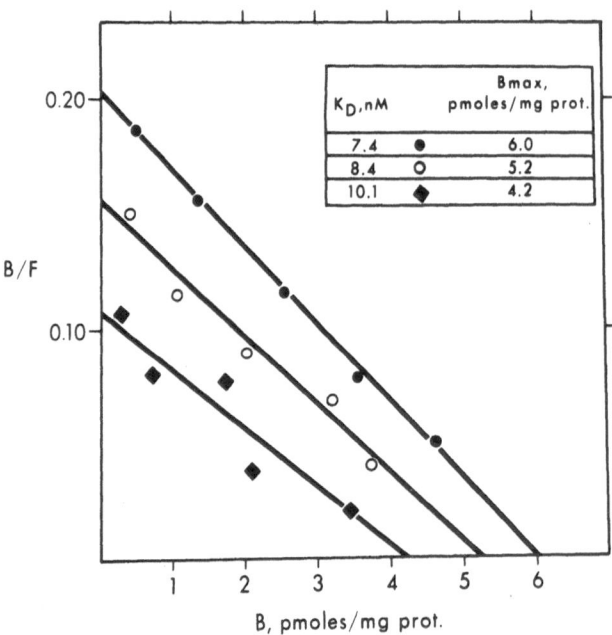

| $K_D$, nM | | Bmax, pmoles/mg prot. |
|---|---|---|
| 7.4 | ● | 6.0 |
| 8.4 | ○ | 5.2 |
| 10.1 | ◆ | 4.2 |

Figure 2A.   Scatchard plots of steady-state binding to chicken renal
            plasma membranes obtained with three preparations of
            receptor-purified [125]I-bPTH(1-34).   Equilibrium constants
            ($K_d$) and total number of binding sites ($B_{max}$) were deter-
            mined by least squares analysis (12).

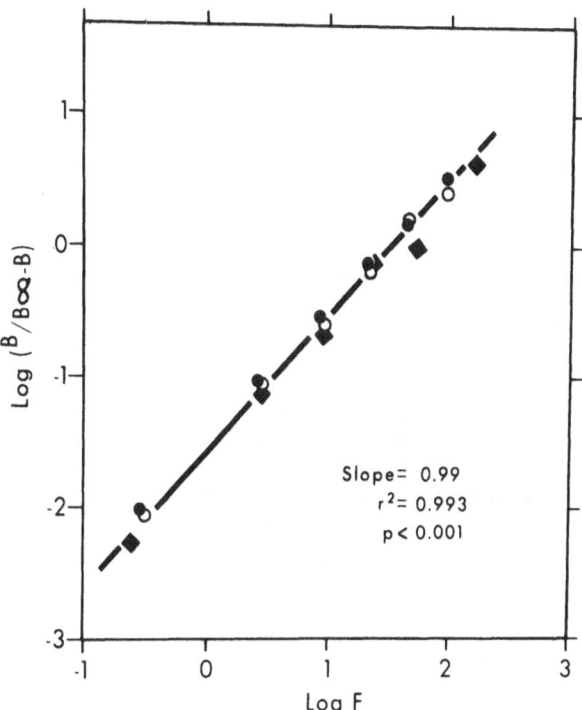

Figure 2B. Hill plot of steady-state binding data in 2A. The slope was determined by linear regression analysis. Free hormone is expressed as pmoles per mg of protein (12).

Inasmuch as the renal action of PTH is thought to be mediated via the adenylate cyclase-cyclic AMP system, occupation of true PTH receptors should be associated with adenylate cyclase activation. Figure 3 demonstrates a direct correlation between bPTH(1-34) binding and adenylate cyclase activation in chicken renal plasma membranes, when measured under identical conditions. Scatchard analysis of this binding data yielded an estimated $K_d$ value for the PTH binding site of 16 nM. This value is virtually identical to the apparent $K_m$ for bPTH(1-34)-stimulation of adenylate cyclase, 17 nM. The similarity of these values supports the notion that the observed PTH binding is coupled to adenylate cyclase activation in these membranes.

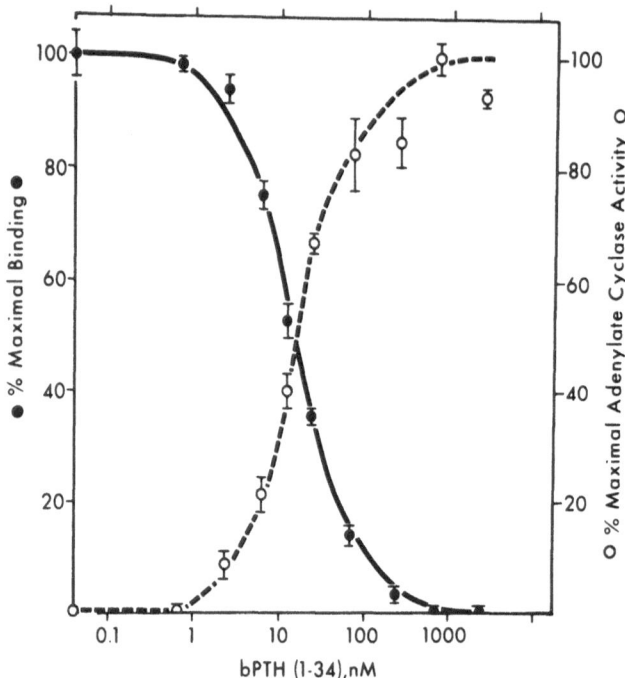

Figure 3.    bPTH(1-34) binding and activation of adenylate cyclase in
             chicken renal plasma membranes.  The binding of receptor-
             purified [125]I-bPTH(1-34) was measured under adenylate
             cyclase incubation conditions except that unlabeled ATP
             was used instead of [$\alpha$-[32]P]ATP.  Basal adenylate cyclase
             activity (223 pmole cyclic AMP/30 min/mg of protein) was
             subtracted from all cyclase values, which were then ex-
             pressed as a percent of maximal activity.  100% cyclase
             activity in this study was 1.06 nmole cyclic AMP/30 min/
             mg of protein (12).

        Further studies were done to compare the potencies of a series
of peptides in stimulating adenylate cyclase with their ability to
compete with receptor-purified [125]I-bPTH(1-34) for binding sites in
chicken renal plasma membranes.  Figure 4A shows that purified bPTH-
(1-84) was equipotent with bPTH(1-34), on a molar basis, in stimulating adenylate cyclase activity.  Despite its equal potency, bPTH-
(1-84) elicited 50% greater maximal cyclase response than did bPTH-
(1-34), an interesting effect which we have reported previously (7,
12).  A preparation of synthetic bPTH(1-34) was about 30 times less
potent whereas oxidized bPTH(1-34), salmon calcitonin, and pork

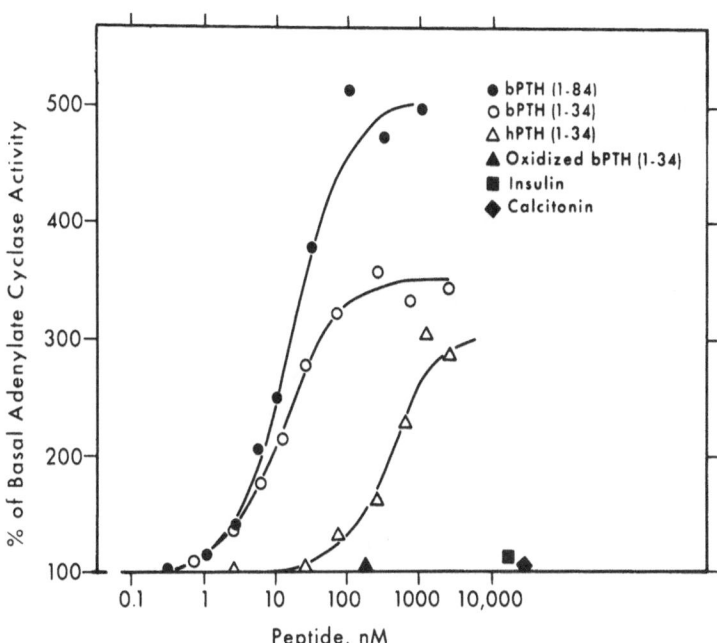

Figure 4A.   Peptide hormone stimulation of adenylate cyclase in
             chicken renal plasma membranes.  In this composite of
             4 experiments, basal adenylate cyclase activity was 174,
             180, 147 and 204 pmol cyclic AMP/30 min/mg of protein
             (12).

insulin were essentially inactive.  Similiar results were obtained
when the binding activities of these peptides were examined (Fig.
4B).  The close correlation between binding and cyclase activation
observed for this series of peptides (Table I) indicates that the
PTH binding site shows selectivity features expected of a PTH
receptor coupled to adenylate cyclase.  There was, however, one
discrepancy.  ACTH(1-24), although inactive in stimulating adenylate
cyclase activity, competed for PTH binding sites at concentrations
in excess of 1 μM.  Heath and  Aurbach (16) and Zull et al. (17)
also have reported that high concentrations of ACTH compete for PTH
binding sites in renal plasma membranes.  We found that the same
high concentrations of ACTH (> 1 μM) which competed for PTH binding
sites also inhibited PTH-stimulation of adenylate cyclase activity

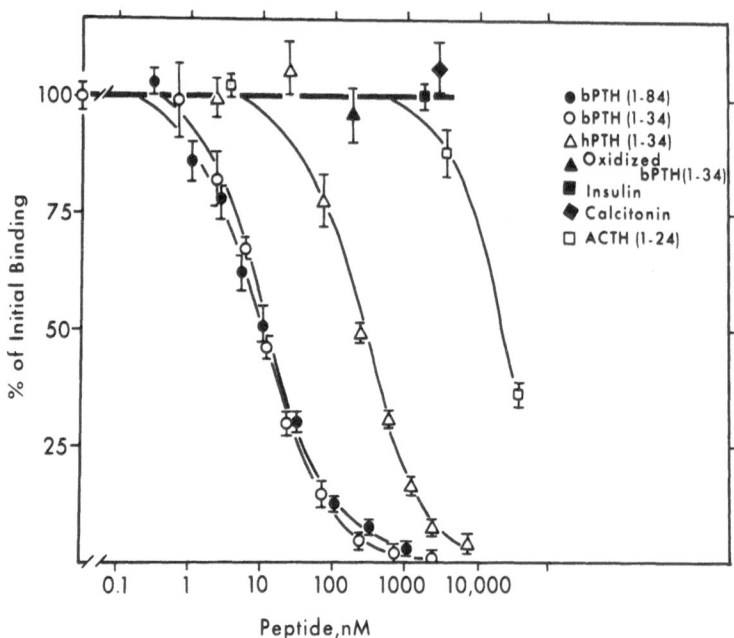

Figure 4B.    Competitive displacement of receptor-purified $^{125}$I-bPTH-
              (1-34) from chicken renal plasma membrane binding sites
              by various peptides (12).

(Fig. 5).  Thus, the occupation of PTH binding sites by ACTH was associated with decreased bPTH(1-34)-activation of adenylate cyclase,
exactly what one would predict if these binding sites represent PTH
receptors coupled to adenylate cyclase.

Although there is strong evidence that the observed PTH binding
sites represent physiologic receptors coupled to adenylate cyclase and
ultimate physiologic responses in renal cells, the $K_d$ value for these
receptors (7 - 10 nM) is at least 100 times greater that what is considered physiologic (8).  In order to estimate what a "physiologic"
plasma concentration of bPTH(1-34) might be in the chicken, we
designed experiments to determine the steady-state concentration of
infused bPTH(1-34) which rendered TPTX/UBX chickens normocalcemic
(Fig. 6).  After TPTX/UBX, mean plasma calcium decreased from 8.9
mg/dl to 5.3 mg/dl.  During continuous infusion of bPTH(1-34) into
these birds, plasma calcium increased and achieved steady-state values
after 16 hours.  There is a highly significant correlation (r = 0.85,
p <0.01) between plasma calcium and serum iPTH measured with a radioimmunoassay using an amino-region specific antiserum.  Plasma calcium
was restored to pre-TPTX/UBX values at plasma iPTH concentrations of

TABLE I

*Relative potencies of PTH analogs and other peptides in competing for PTH binding sites and stimulating adenylate cyclase in chicken kidney plasma membranes*

Relative $K_d$ values are expressed as a ratio of the molar concentrations of peptide/bPTH(1–34) required to reduce [125]I-bPTH(1–34) binding by 50%. Relative $K_m$ values for adenylate cyclase activation are expressed as a ratio of the concentrations of peptide/bPTH(1–34) required to stimulate adenylate cyclase activity half-maximally. bPTH Fraction C is a protein peak obtained from Bio-Gel P-10 gel chromatography of a bovine parathyroid gland extract, and contains partially purified (approximately 40%) bPTH(1–84)(12).

| Peptide | Relative binding $K_d$ | Relative cyclase $K_m$ |
|---|---|---|
| bPTH(1–34) | 1.0 | 1.0 |
| bPTH(1–84) | 1.0 | 1.0 |
| bPTH Fraction C | 2.2 | 2.5 |
| hPTH(1–34) | 25.0 | 30.0 |
| Oxidized bPTH(1–34) | | |
| Insulin | N.A.[a] | N.A. |
| Calcitonin | | |
| ACTH(1-24) | ~2500 | N.A. |

[a] N.A. = no activity at concentrations up to 2.0 $\mu$M for insulin, calcitonin, and ACTH(1-24), and 0.2 $\mu$M for oxidized bPTH(1–34).

about 0.5 nM. We compared this "physiologic" concentration to the concentrations of bPTH(1-34) required to increase the production of cyclic AMP in isolated renal tubules *in vitro*, and in renal tissue *in vivo* (Fig. 7). It is evident that the "physiologic" bPTH(1-34) concentration (0.5 nM) did not produce a significant increase in renal cyclic AMP either *in vivo* or *in vitro*. Half-maximal renal cyclic AMP production was produced at a bPTH(1-34) concentration of 22 nM *in vivo* and 55 nM *in vitro*. These values agree reasonably well with the $K_d$ for bPTH(1-34) receptor sites in chicken renal plasma membranes (16 nM). The data indicate that calcium homeostasis in chickens can be maintained at a plasma bPTH(1-34) concentration sufficient to occupy only a minute portion of the available renal PTH receptors.

DISCUSSION

The present results describe the use of receptor-purified [125]I-bPTH(1-34) in demonstrating and quantitating renal PTH receptors. Our ability to obtain highly reproducible estimates of PTH receptor number and affinity probably relate both to the purity of the receptor-

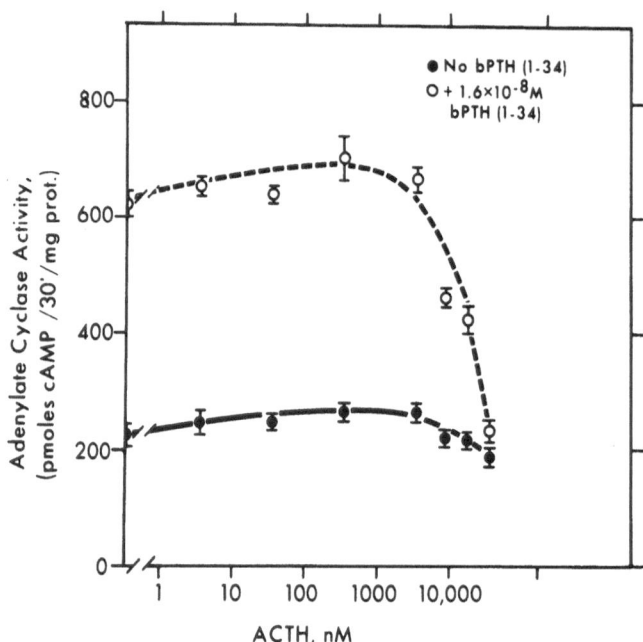

Figure 5.   The effect of ACTH(1-24) on basal (no added bPTH(1-34))
            and on bPTH(1-34)-stimulated adenylate cyclase activity
            in chicken renal plasma membrane (12).

purified tracer and to the high affinity of PTH binding sites in
chicken kidney, as compared to rat (18) and bovine kidney (16,17,
19).   It is uncertain why receptor purification of electrolytically
labeled $^{125}$I-bPTH(1-34) resulted in a 5- to 9-fold increase in specific PTH binding to chicken renal plasma membranes.   It seems likely
that a portion of the electrolytically labeled PTH was unable to bind
to the renal receptor, even though we observed no loss of biological
activity in various preparations of the labeled hormone.   Based on
the specific activity of the labeled peptide, we calculate that no
more than 25 to 50% of the bPTH(1-34) molecules are labeled by our
procedure.   It is doubtful that the bioassay system employed
(chicken renal adenylate cyclase assay) would be sensitive enough
to detect such a small loss of biological activity following the
iodinatio of PTH.   Thus, the issue of the biological activity of
electrolytically labeled bPTH(1-34) cannot be resolved until methods
are developed to separate labeled from unlabeled bPTH(1-34).

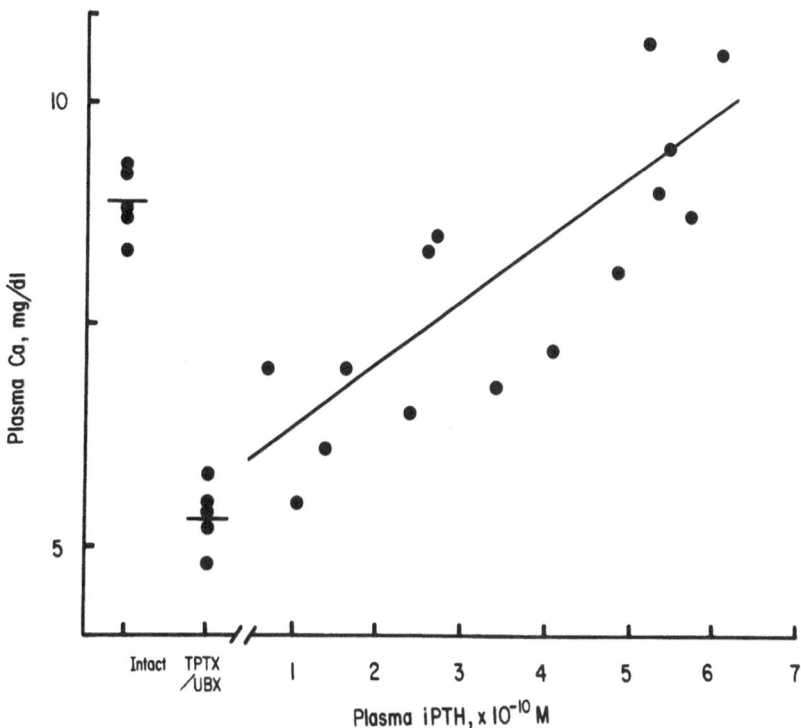

Figure 6.   Calcemic effect of infused bPTH(-34) in TPTX/UBX chickens.
            Four to six hours after TPTX/UBX, various amounts of bPTH-
            (1-34) were continuously infused (3 ml/hr) into the left
            jugular vein.   Blood samples were obtained from the right
            brachial vein before TPTX/UBX, just prior to bPTH(1-34)
            infusion, and 16 hours after commencing the PTH infusion,
            at which time plasma calcium had reached a steady-state
            level.   Samples were assayed for calcium and for ibPTH-
            (1-34).

     When we measured the affinity of the PTH binding site under ade-
nylate cyclase assay condition, the $K_m$ for bPTH(1-34)-activated adenylate cyclase was virtually identical to the calculated $K_d$ value for
bPTH(1-34) binding, suggesting that there is coupling of the binding
sites with adenylate cyclase.   The identification of these binding
sites as physiologic receptors is further supported by the observed
correlation between the binding and cyclase activities of a variety
of PTH peptides.   Thus, bPTH(1-84) was equipotent to bPTH(1-34) and
hPTH(1-34) was about 25 times less potent than bPTH(1-34) in binding
to chicken renal membrane receptors and in stimulating adenylate

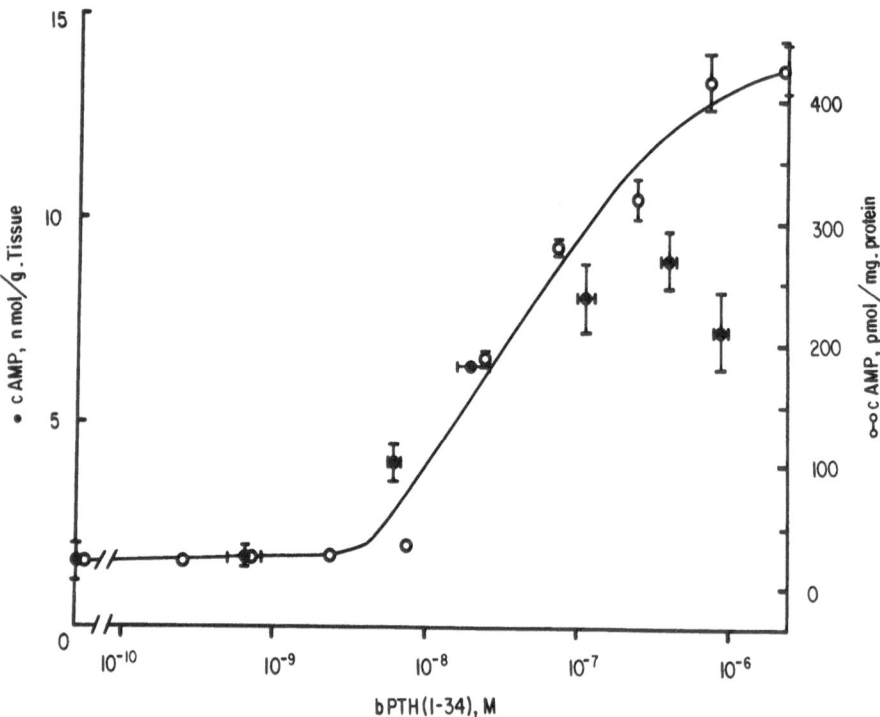

Figure 7.  Dose-response relationships of renal cyclic AMP production
by bPTH(1-34) in the chicken *in vivo* and in chicken renal
tubules *in vitro*.  *In vivo* results are expressed as cyclic
AMP content in kidneys as a function of plasma ibPTH(1-34)
2 min after the i.v. injection of the peptide.  Results *in
vitro* are expressed as cyclic AMP production by isolated
tubules as a function of the concentration of bPTH(1-34)
in the incubation medium.

cyclase.  Oxidized bPTH(1-34), salmon calcitonin and insulin did
not bind to PTH receptors, and did not stimulate adenylate cyclase.
High concentrations of ACTH(1-24) displaced PTH from membrane binding
sites, and also inhibited PTH-stimulation of adenylate cyclase.

The relatively low affinity of the PTH receptors in chicken renal
plasma membranes ($K_d \simeq 20$ nM) raises an important question concerning
their physiologic importance.  We therefore attempted to determine if
the renal adenylate cyclase system is more sensitive to PTH *in vivo*
than it is *in vitro*.  The plasma concentration of administered bPTH-
(1-34) which was required to half-maximally stimulate the renal

production of cyclic AMP *in vivo* was 22nM, suggesting that the renal
sensitivity to PTH *in vitro* is a reasonable reflection of the sensitivity *in vivo*. However, these concentrations of bPTH(1-34) are at
least 40 times that which might be considered physiologic based on
maintenance of normocalcemia in TPTX/UBX chickens.

Despite the relatively low sensitivity of the renal PTH receptor-
adenylate cyclase system *in vitro* and *in vivo*, the evidence that the
renal actions of PTH are mediated by cyclic AMP appear to be irrefu-
table (1-6). The present results, therefore, suggest that under physiologic conditions few of the available renal tubular PTH receptors
are occupied. Furthermore, it appears that calcium homeostasis can
be maintained at PTH concentrations that elicite minute increments in
renal cell cyclic AMP. It is likely that we will need to look beyond
cyclic AMP generation (*e.g.*, at the availability of renal cell protein
kinase) to discover the rate-limiting step(s) in the physiologic
actions of PTH on the kidney.

## ACKNOWLEDGEMENTS

The authors acknowledge the expert technical assistance of Ms.
Linda Zitzner. This work was supported by NIH Grant

## REFERENCES

1.  H. Rasmussen, M. Pechet and D. Fast, Effect of dibutyryl cyclic
    adenosine 3',5'-monophosphate, theophylline, and other nucleo-
    tides upon calcium and phosphate metabolism, J. Clin. Invest.
    47:1843 (1968).
2.  Z. S. Agus, J. B. Puschett, D. Senesky and M. Goldberg, Mode of
    action of parathyroid hormone and cyclic adenosine 3',5'-mono-
    phosphate on renal tubular phosphate reabsorption in the dog,
    J. Clin. Invest. 50:617 (1971).
3.  H. Kuntziger, C. Amiel, N. Roinel and F. Morel, Effects of para-
    thyroidectomy and cyclic AMP on renal transport of phosphate,
    calcium and magnesium, Am. J. Physiol. 227:905 (1974).
4.  M. A. Burnatowska, C. A. Harris, R. A. L. Sutton and J. H. Dirks,
    Effects of PTH and cAMP on renal handling of calcium, magnesium
    and phosphate in the hamster, Am. J. Physiol. 233(6):F514
    (1977).
5.  N. Horiuchi, T. Suda, H. Takahashi, E. Shimazawa and E. Ogata, In
    vivo evidence for the intermediary role of 3',5'-cyclic AMP in
    parathyroid hormone-induced stimulation of 1α, 25-dihydroxy-
    vitamin D synthesis in rats, Endocrinol. 101:969 (1977).
6.  A. E. Broadus, J. E. Mahaffey, F. C. Bartter and R. M. Neer,
    Nephrogenous cyclic adenosine monophosphate as a parathyroid
    function test, J. Clin. Invest. 60:771 (1977).
7.  F. P. DiBella, C. D. Arnaud and H. B. Brewer, Jr., Relative bio-
    logic activities of human and bovine parathyroid hormones and
    their synthetic, NH$_2$-terminal(1-34) peptides as evaluated *in*

*vitro* with renal cortical adenylate cyclase obtained from three different species, Endocrinol. 99:429 (1976).

8.  J. A. Parsons and B. Reit, Chronic response of dogs to para-thyroid hormone infusion, Nature 250:254 (1974).

9.  D. F. Fitzpatrick, G. R. Davenport, L. Forte and E. J. Landon, Characterization of plasma membrane proteins in mammalian kidney. I. Preparation of a membrane fraction and separa-tion of the protein, J. Biol. Chem. 244:3561 (1969).

10. P. J. Sammon, J. S. Brand, W. F. Neuman and L. G. Raisz, Meta-bolism of labeled parathyroid hormone. I. Preparation of biologically active $^{125}$I-labeled parathyroid hormone. Endocrinol. 92:1596 (1973).

11. W. F. Neuman, M. W. Neuman, P. J. Sammon and K. Lane, The meta-bolism of labeled parathyroid hormone. II. Methodological studies, Calcif. Tiss. Res. 18:241 (1975).

12. R. A. Nissenson and C. D. Arnaud, Properties of the parathyroid hormone receptor-adenylate cyclase system in chicken renal plasma membranes, J. Biol. Chem. 254:1469 (1979).

13. Y. Salomon, C. Londos and M. Rodbell, A highly sensitive adeny-late cyclase assay, Anal. Biochem. 58:541 (1974).

14. A. G. Gilman, A protein binding assay for adenosine 3',5'-cyclic monophosphate, Proc. Natl. Acad. Sci., USA 67:305 (1970).

15. G. Scatchard, The attraction of proteins for small molecules and ions, Ann. N.Y. Acad. Sci. 51:660 (1949).

16. D. A. Heath and G. D. Aurbach, Studies on the binding of $^{125}$I-parathyroid hormone to renal cortical membranes, in, "Calcium Regulating Hormones," R. V. Talmadge, M. Owen and J. A. Parsons, eds., Excerpta Medica, Amsterdam (1975).

17. J. E. Zull, C. C. Malbon and J. Chuang, Binding of tritiated bovine parathyroid hormone to plasma membranes from bovine kidney cortex, J. Biol. Chem. 252:1071 (1977).

18. C. C. Malbon and J. E. Zull, Interactions of parathyroid hormone and plasma membranes from rat kidney, Biochem. Biophys. Res. Commun. 56:952 (1974).

19. F. P. DiBella, T. P. Dousa, S. S. Miller and C. D. Arnaud, Para-thyroid hormone receptors of renal cortex: specific binding of biologically active $^{125}$I-labeled hormone and relationship to adenylate cyclase activation. Proc. Natl. Acad. Sci., USA 71:723 (1974).

# RENAL RECEPTORS FOR PARATHYROID HORMONE IN NORMAL,

# PARATHYROIDECTOMIZED AND VITAMIN D-DEFICIENT RATS

Nadine Loreau, Chantal Lajotte, Michèle Lafaye and
Raymond Ardaillou

INSERM 64
Hôpital Tenon, Paris, France

The physiological role of PTH and particularly its renal
effects have been extensively studied in the rat. However, since
PTH is rapidly degraded in the presence of rat renal tissue (1),
the first step of its action, namely binding to specific receptors,
has mainly been studied with chicken or bovine renal membranes
(2-5). The only binding studies using membranes from murine source
were reported by Malbon and Zull (6), but were limited to a single
incubation time and a single concentration of labelled PTH. Moreover, the physiological control of PTH binding to its receptors and
particularly the role of plasma PTH have not been till now analyzed.
We have recently prepared a biologically active tritiated derivative
of the synthetic 1-34 fragment of human PTH (7). Furthermore, we
have demonstrated that this tracer specifically binds to renal
membranes (7) and to glomeruli (8) isolated from rat renal cortex.
The present paper extends our earlier results obtained with rat
renal membranes and demonstrates that PTH binding and PTH-sensitive
adenylate cyclase activity are inversely related to plasma PTH
concentration.

## MATERIAL AND METHODS

### Animals

Male rats from the Sprague-Dawley strain were divided into
three groups : control, PTX and vitamin D-deficient rats. In the
PTX group, parathyroid glands were surgically removed eight days
prior to the experimental protocol. Efficiency was confirmed by
determination of plasma calcium (mean ± s.e.m = 1.44 ± 0.03 mmol/1).

In the vitamin D-deficient group, weaning  rats weighing 60 g were
maintened during one month in the darkness on a calcium and vitamin
D-deficient synthetic diet. Plasma calcium in these rats was 1.21
± 0.03 mmol/l. Normal rats weighing 180-200 g fed a laboratory chow
were used as control animals. Plasma calcium in this group was 2.54
± 0.10 mmol/l.

## Hormone and receptor preparations

    1-34 human PTH was a gift from Armour-Montagu (Paris). This
synthetic peptide corresponds to the sequence proposed by Niall et
al. (9). The method for labelling PTH with sodium $|^3H|$ borohydride
has been described in detail (7). The specific activity of the
labelled hormone measured by radioimmunoassay was 15 Ci/mmol. Its
biological activity estimated from stimulation of renal adenylate
cyclase was fully retained. 1-34 bovine PTH was purchased from
Beckman (Geneva). Renal tubular membranes were prepared from rats
of the three experimental groups according to Fitzpatrick et al.
(10). Their degree of purification was estimated by measuring the
specific activities of two enzyme markers, adenylate cyclase and
$(Na^+ + K^+)$-ATPase as previously described (11).

## Binding studies

    Binding studies were carried out at 22°C in a metabolic shaker
with 100 µg membrane protein in each tube. The incubation medium was
0.1 ml of 0.05 M Tris-HCl buffer, pH 7.5, containing 2 % bovine
serum albumin and 1 mM $CaCl_2$. $|^3H|$ 1-34 h PTH was added at a final
dilution of 2-5 nM. At the end of the incubation period, which
usually lasted 15 min, 3 ml of chilled 100 mM Tris-HCl buffer,
pH 7.5, containing 0.2 % Tween 20 were added. The total volume was
filtered through a Millipore filter (HAWP 0.45 µm) previously soaked
in 2 % Tween 20. Addition of Tween was necessary to obtain very low
blank values (approximately 0.2 % of total radioactivity). $|^3H|$
radioactivity was counted in 8 ml of Bray's solution (12) with a
Searle (Mark II) liquid scintillation counter. Non specific binding
onto membranes was measured in the presence of 10 µM 1-34 h PTH and
subtracted from total binding to obtain specific binding. Results
were expressed as fmol PTH bound per mg of membrane protein. Protein
determinations were carried out according to Lowry et al. (13). In
order to study degradation of $|^3H|$ 1-34 h PTH present in the incu-
bation milieu, its concentration as a function of time was measured
using a specific radioimmunoassay according to Desplan et al. (14).

## Enzyme studies

    Adenylate cyclase activity present in renal membranes was

measured in the presence of increasing concentrations of 1-34 h PTH.
100 μg  of membrane protein were incubated at 22°C with the hormone
in 100 μl of 0.1 M Tris-HCl buffer, pH 7.5, containing 10 mM MgCl$_2$
and a regenerating system for ATP as previously described (11).
ATP (1 mM, final concentration) was added after 20 min incubation.
The enzymatic reaction was stopped 10 min later by heating the
incubation medium at 100°C for 3 min after addition of 150 μl of
Tris buffer. The amount of 3'-5' cyclic AMP formed was measured by
radioimmunoassay using its $^{125}$I iodinated succinyl derivative as a
tracer. Adenylate cyclase activity was expressed as pmole of cyclic
AMP formed per 10 min and per mg of tubular membrane protein.


RESULTS


Binding studies

     $|^{3}H|$ 1-34 h PTH binding was measured as a function of time
with membranes prepared from the three groups of rats (Fig. 1). The
amount of hormone specifically bound increased with time and reached
a plateau after 10 min incubation. Approximately, 1-2 % of $|^{3}H|$ 1-34
h PTH was specifically bound at a concentration of 5 nM in the
incubation medium. Non specific binding was constant during the
same experiment but varied from 15 to 30 % of the total binding
observed at equilibrium when all the time-course studies performed
were considered. Binding was the greatest with membranes from PTX
rats and the lowest with those from vitamin D-deficient rats.

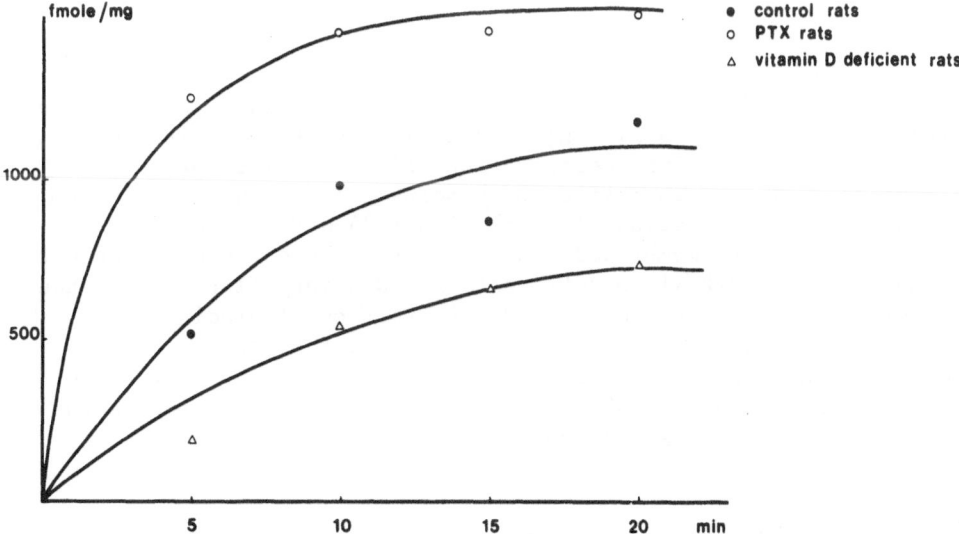

Fig. 1.   Time-course of binding of $|^{3}H|$ 1-34 h PTH to tubular
          membranes from control, PTX and vitamin D-deficient rats.
          Each point is the mean of duplicates.

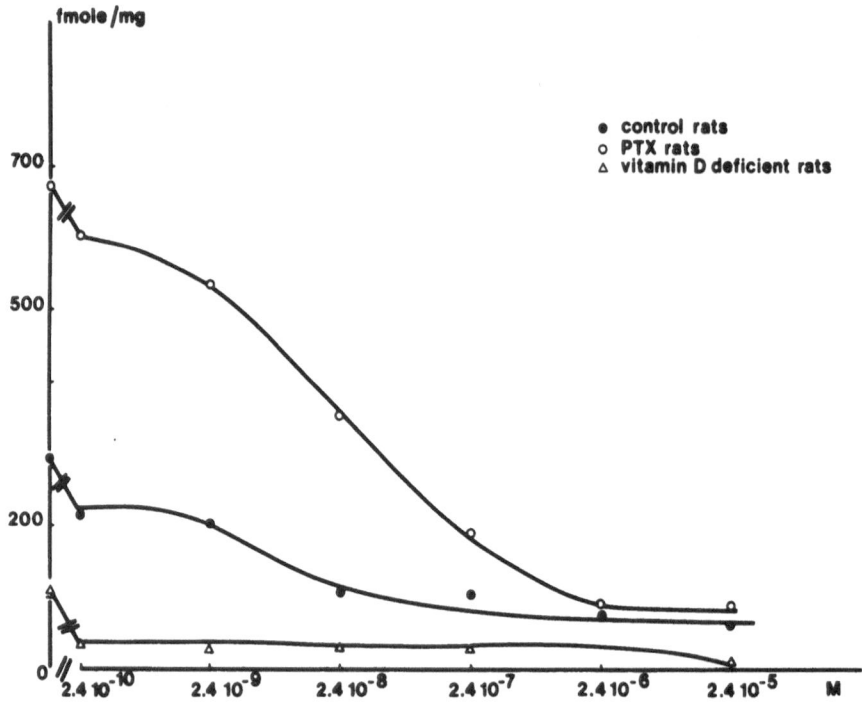

Fig. 2.   Competitive inhibition of binding of $|^{3}H|$ 1-34 h PTH to
         tubular membranes from control, PTX and vitamin D-
         deficient rats in the presence of increasing concentra-
         tions of unlabelled 1-34 h PTH. Each point is the mean
         of duplicates.

It was intermediary with membranes from control rats. Competitive
inhibition of binding of $|^{3}H|$ 1-34 h PTH was observed in the
presence of increasing concentrations of unlabelled hormone
(Fig. 2). Complete inhibition of binding was obtained above 2 µM.
At a given concentration of unlabelled 1-34 h PTH, binding was
the greatest with membranes from PTX rats. The curve obtained with
membranes from vitamin D-deficient rats was very flat even at the
lowest concentrations tested. 50 % inhibition of binding was
observed with membranes from both control and PTX rats at approxi-
mately 10 nM. Degradation of $|^{3}H|$ 1-34 h PTH estimated by radio-
immunoassay was negligible during the first 30 min of incubation
in the presence of rat membranes whatever their origins.


Enzyme studies

    Adenylate cyclase activity present in the renal membranes of
the three groups of rats was clearly stimulated by 1-34 h PTH

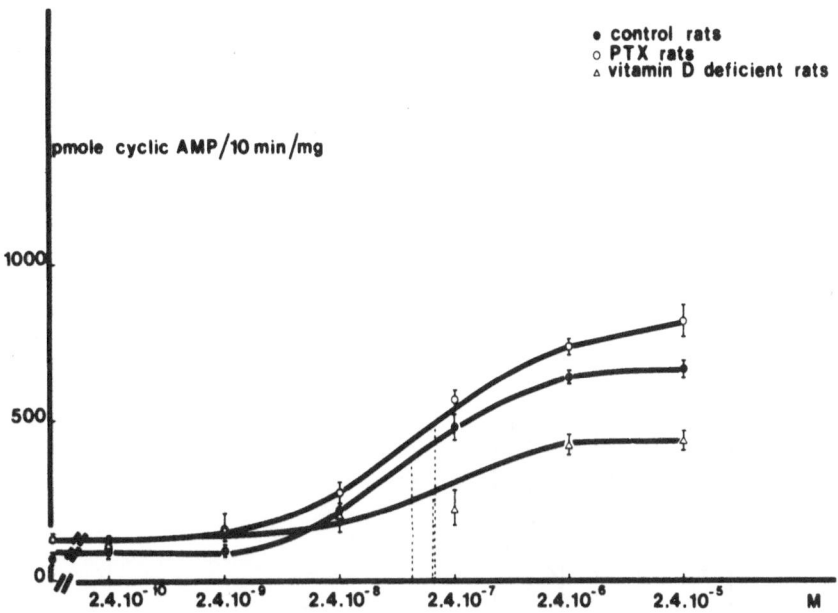

Fig. 3.   Adenylate cyclase activity in tubular membranes from
          control, PTX and vitamin D-deficient rats in the presence
          of increasing concentrations of unlabelled 1-34 h PTH.
          The dotted lines indicate the concentrations correspon-
          ding to 50 % of the maximum values. Each point is the
          mean of triplicates and each vertical bar twice the
          standard error of the mean.


(Fig. 3). Maximum stimulation was observed at 10 μM and corresponded
to 4 to 5 times basal activity. The apparent $K_m$ estimated from the
concentrations corresponding to 50 % of the respective maximum
activities were similar with the three preparations and close to
0.1 μM. On the contrary, maximum activities were clearly different.
The greatest value was obtained with the preparation from PTX rats
and the lowest with that of vitamin D-deficient rats. The value
corresponding to control rats was intermediary but closer to that
observed with PTX rats. Basal fluoride- and calcitonin-stimulated
adenylate cyclase activities were not significantly different with
the three preparations whereas PTH-stimulated activity measured
in the same experiments was markedly lower with membranes from
vitamin D-deficient rats ($p < 0.001$) and greater, but at a slighter
degree ($p < 0.05$), with membranes from PTX rats (Fig. 4).


DISCUSSION

    The data presented here confirm our previous results (7)

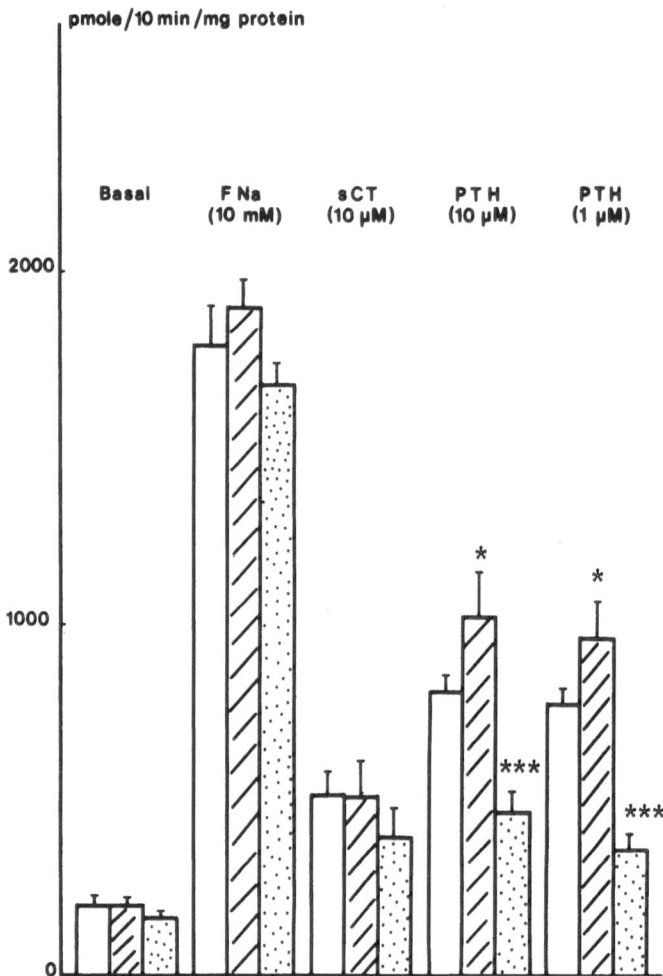

Fig. 4.   Adenylate cyclase activity in tubular membranes from
          control (open rectangles), PTX (cross-hatched rectangles)
          and vitamin D-deficient rats (dotted rectangles) under
          various conditions : basal, in the presence of 10 mM
          sodium fluoride or 10 µM salmon calcitonin or two different
          concentrations (10 µM and 1 µM) of 1-34 h PTH. The top of
          each rectangle indicates the mean of 10 individual values
          and each vertical bar the standard error of the mean.
          Results obtained in each experimental condition with
          membranes from PTX or vitamin D-deficient rats were
          compared with those obtained with membranes from control
          rats using Student's t test. * = p < 0.05 ; *** = p < 0.001

showing the presence of specific receptors for PTH in rat renal
membranes. Hormone degradation in our conditions was very small
compared to previously published studies (3, 4). This can be due
to the structure of the peptide used and is in agreement with the
results of Moseley et al. (1) who reported that 1-34 h PTH was less
rapidly degraded than 1-34 and 1-84 b PTH in the presence of renal
membranes. Thus, our study demonstrates that PTH binding to rat
renal membranes can be correctly studied and is inconsistent with
the results of Sutcliffe et al. (2) and of Mac Intosh et al. (3)
who concluded that species other than the rat must be used.

Our data showing a clear decrease in PTH-stimulated adenylate
cyclase activity of renal membranes in vitamin D-deficient rats are
in agreement with those observed by Forte et al. (15) and Kakuta
et al. (16). Furthermore, we have demonstrated that renal PTH-
stimulated adenylate cyclase activity was significantly increased
when preparations from PTX rats were tested. On the contrary, there
is no change in basal, fluoride- and calcitonin-stimulated adenylate
cyclase activity when preparations from the three groups of rats
are compared. This data clearly shows that renal PTH-stimulated
adenylate cyclase activity is inversely related to chronical modifications of plasma PTH. Hypocalcemia itself does not play a major
role since it is present both in PTX and vitamin D-deficient rats
which exhibit opposite responses. Down regulation of PTH-responsive
adenylate cyclase has also been demonstrated in vitro after exposition of isolated bone cells (17) or chick renal membranes (18) to
PTH. These studies left unprecised the molecular basis for the
PTH-induced refractoriness. The present report demonstrates that
changes in adenylate cyclase activity are related to parallel changes in PTH binding. Analysis of the competitive inhibition curves
and of the adenylate cyclase stimulation curves obtained in the
presence of increasing concentrations of 1-34 h PTH showed that
the apparent $K_D$ and $K_m$ were similar whatever the origin of the
membrane preparation. This suggests that the modifications of
adenylate cyclase activity and of PTH binding observed are rather
secondary to changes in the number of receptors. It is still
unknown whether or not PTH-induced sensitization and desensitization
require only binding or binding and adenylate cyclase stimulation.
Answer to this question will be facilitated by using inactive
analogs of PTH.

ACKNOWLEDGMENTS

This work was supported by grants from the "Délégation
Générale à la Recherche Scientifique et Technique" N° 7970204.

REFERENCES

1.  J.M. Moseley, T.J. Martin, C.J. Robinson, B.W. Reit and
    G.W. Tregear, Hormone metabolism and response of adenylate
    cyclase to parathyroid hormone in kidney, Clin. Exp.
    Pharmacol. Physiol. 2:549 (1975).

2.  H.S. Sutcliffe, T.J. Martin, J.A. Eisman and R. Pilczyk,
    Binding of parathyroid hormone to bovine kidney-cortex
    plasma membranes, Biochem. J. 134:913 (1973).

3.  C.H.S. Mac Intosh and R.D. Hesch, Characterization of the
    parathyrin receptor in renal plasma membranes by labelled
    hormone and labelled antibody binding techniques, Biochim.
    Biophys. Acta 426:535 (1976).

4.  J.E. Zull, C.C. Malbon and J. Chuang, Binding of tritiated
    bovine parathyroid hormone to plasma membranes from bovine
    kidney cortex, J. Biol. Chem. 252:1071 (1977).

5.  R.A. Nissensson and C.D. Arnaud, Properties of the parathyroid
    hormone receptor-adenylate cyclase system in chicken renal
    plasma membranes, J. Biol. Chem. 254:1469 (1979).

6.  C.C. Malbon and J.E. Zull, Interactions of parathyroid hormone
    and plasma membranes from rat kidney, Biochem. Biophys.
    Res. comm. 56:952 (1974).

7.  D. Chansel, J. Sraer, J.L. Morgat, R.D. Hesch and R. Ardaillou,
    Preparation of biologically active tritium labelled 1-34
    human parathyroid hormone, FEBS lett. 78:237 (1977).

8.  J. Sraer, J.D. Sraer, D. Chansel, H. Jueppner, R.D. Hesch and
    R. Ardaillou, Evidence for glomerular receptors for
    parathyroid hormone, Am. J. Physiol. 235:F96 (1978).

9.  H.D. Niall, R.T. Sauer, J.W. Jacobs, H.T. Keutmann, G.V. Segre,
    J.L.H. O'Riordan, G.D. Aurbach and J.T. Potts, The amino-
    acid sequence of the amino-terminal 37 residues of human
    parathyroid hormone, Proc. Natl. Acad. Sci. US 71:384 (1974).

10. D.F. Fitzpatrick, G.R. Davenport, L. Forte and E.J. Landon,
    Characterization of plasma membrane proteins in mammalian
    kidney. I. Preparation of a membrane fraction and separation
    of the protein, J. Biol. Chem. 244:3561 (1969).

11. N. Loreau, C. Lepreux and R. Ardaillou, Calcitonin-sensitive
    adenylate cyclase in rat renal tubular membranes, Biochem.
    J. 150:305 (1975).

12.  G.S. Bray, A simple efficient liquid scintillator for counting
     aqueous solution in a liquid scintillator counter, Anal.
     Biochem. 1:279 (1960).

13.  O.H. Lowry, N.J. Rosebrough, A.L. Farr and R.J. Randall,
     Protein measurement with the Folin phenol reagent, J. Biol.
     Chem. 193:265 (1951).

14.  C. Desplan, A. Jullienne, M.S. Moukhtar and G. Milhaud,
     Sensitive assay for biologically active fragment of human
     parathyroid hormone, Lancet 2:198 (1977).

15.  L.R. Forte, G.A. Nichols and C.S. Anast, Renal adenylate
     cyclase and the interrelationship between parathyroid
     hormone and vitamin D in the regulation of urinary phosphate
     and adenosine cyclic 3',5'-monophosphate excretion, J. Clin.
     Invest. 57:559 (1976).

16.  S. Kakuta, C. Sato, T. Suda, N. Kimura, N. Araki, Y. Ono and
     N. Nagata, Relationship between parathyroid hormone and
     adenosine 3',5'-monophosphate metabolism in the kidney of
     vitamin D-deficient rats, Biochim. Biophys. Acta 539:173
     (1978).

17.  G.L. Wong, Induction of metabolic changes and down regulation
     of bovine parathyroid hormone-responsive adenylate cyclase
     are dissociable in isolated osteoclastic and osteoblastic
     bone cells, J. Biol. Chem. 254:34 (1979).

18.  V.P. Michelangeli, N.H. Hunt and T.J. Martin, States of
     activation of chick kidney adenylate cyclase induced by
     parathyroid hormone and guanylnucleotides, J. Endocr. 72:69
     (1977).

# TOPICS ON BONE AND VITAMIN D

# WHAT IS OSTEOMALACIA ?

Robert K. Schenk and Attila J. Olah

Anatomisches Institut der Universität Bern
Bühlstrasse 26
CH 3012 Bern

## INTRODUCTION

A commonly accepted answer to this question given in many text-
books is 'softness of bones caused by an increase in the relative
amount of unmineralized bone matrix'. This definition is still valid,
but only as long as the physical characteristics of a softening of
bone are respected. The histological assessment of an increase in
the relative amount of osteoid alone is not sufficient as a diagnostic criterion. This limitation became obvious when reliable staining
procedures for the detection of osteoid in undecalcified sections
were introduced. Based on his experience with such specimens, Frost[1]
proposed a distinction between 'histological osteomalacia' and what
he called 'dynamic osteomalacia'. According to his definition, histological osteomalacia characterizes bone with more osteoid seams than
normal and therefore includes, besides such conditions where osteoid
accumulates because of a mineralization delay, a variety of states
with increased bone turnover such as thyrotoxicosis, hyperparathyroidism, Paget's disease etc. Histological osteomalacia corresponds
to 'hyperosteoidosis', a term used by Meunier and his group[2], and
with some restriction to 'osteoidosis' coined by Delling[3].
   The main features of Frost's dynamic osteomalacia[4] are
1) an increase in osteoid seams, 2) a prolonged osteon formation
time ( 2 times and more ) and 3) a marked decrease in the ratio of
resorption cavities to osteons with osteoid seams. In view of the
second and third statement one has to consider that Frost's concepts
are based mainly on Haversian remodeling in cortical rib bone, where
the dynamics of newly forming osteons = BMU's (Bone Metabolizing
Units) were analyzed after tetracycline labelling. Thus, the osteon

formation time includes not only the period of osteoid deposition
but also the period of osteoid mineralization. In a more generalized
way, Frost's concept of dynamic osteomalacia is compatible with the
formula, that osteomalacia represents an accumulation of osteoid
due to <u>continuing matrix production by osteoblasts</u> (at a normal,
decreased or increased ? rate) <u>combined with delayed or arrested</u>
<u>mineralization.</u>

MICROSCOPIC AND MORPHOMETRIC CRITERIA FOR OSTEOMALACIA

    In virtue of the above definitions, there are several possi-
bilities for a microscopic diagnosis of dynamic osteomalacia. One
is directed towards an assessment of the mineralization defect.
Tetracycline uptake in the mineralization front indicates, especially
after sequential application, a marked delay or an arrest of mineralization by a diffuse labelling or a complete lack of fluorescence[5].
Another distinction between normal and arrested mineralization has
been advocated by Bordier[6] on the basis of certain staining properties of the calcification front.
    The accumulation of osteoid is reflected by a number of histo-
morphometric parameters, such as osteoid volume, osteoid surface
and width of osteoid seams. These osteoid values, finally, can be
related to the extent of the bone surface covered by osteoblasts,
provided that the cells identified morphologically as osteoblasts
are indeed actively producing bone matrix.
    That the osteoid parameters alone are not sufficient for the
detection of dynamic osteomalacia has been recognized by most
authors working in this field. Meunier and coworkers[2,7] characterize
osteomalacia mainly by a marked increase in the width of osteoid
seams plus low calcification rate, determined by double tetracycline
labelling. Bordier[8] considered an increased osteoid surface combined
with a reduced calcification front as key symptoms, whereas in our
hands[9], the relation between osteoid volume and surface covered by
osteoblasts turned out to be the most sensitive parameter for the
detection of a mineralization deficiency. It is obvious that some
of the preferences listed above arise from differences in the
specific histological techniques used by various authors. Undecalcified sectioning requires plastic embedding, and the choice of
the plastic already has a decisive influence on the staining
properties of both matrix and cells. This is especially true for
Bordier's calcification front and for the differentiation of osteoblasts and other bone lining cells. Unfortunately, these pecularities
make a direct comparison of the individual parameters rather difficult. In the following discussion, we have to restrict ourselves
mainly to values which are preferentially used in our laboratory.
This, however, should not be taken as a prerogative of their
superiority.

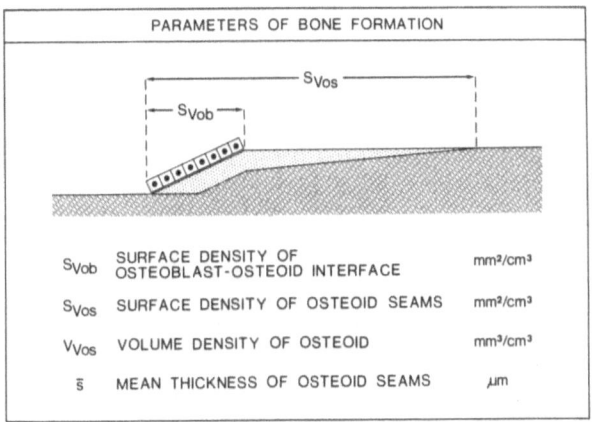

Figure 1.

HISTOMORPHOMETRIC EVALUATION OF BONE TURNOVER

The histological techniques used in these studies[10,11,12] allow an accurate distinction between mineralized and unmineralized bone matrix and a reliable differentiation of cells lining the bone surfaces. Measurements are carried out in the cancellous bone of the iliac crest within an identical area as chosen by Bordier, Delling, Meunier a.o. The parameters used for the evaluation of bone formation are given in Fig. 1. We use the definitions and notations adopted by most members of the International Society for Stereology (ISS). These relate relative volumes and surfaces of particular tissue components in terms of volume density ($mm^3.cm^{-3}$) and surface density ($mm^2.cm^{-3}$) to an unit total reference volume.

One important observation during the elaboration of the standard values from a collection of 120 random autopsy cases was the fact, that less than one third of the osteoid surface is normally lined by osteoblasts[9]. This confirmed similar preliminary findings of Shen et al.[13] in cortical bone. Even more striking was the surprisingly good correlation between osteoid volume density and surface density of osteoblasts (Fig. 2). At that time, this was taken as an indication of a coupling between osteoid deposition by osteoblasts and its subsequent mineralization. Since tetracycline labelling had shown that mineralization proceeds in healthy individuals at a remarkably constant rate of about 1 μm per day, this also confirmed the assumption that cells identified as osteoblasts are in fact producing matrix at a fairly constant rate.

Later on, this correlation turned out to be very suitable for a detection of mineralization deficiencies in different types of 'hyperosteoidosis'[14,15]. For this purpose, the regression line and

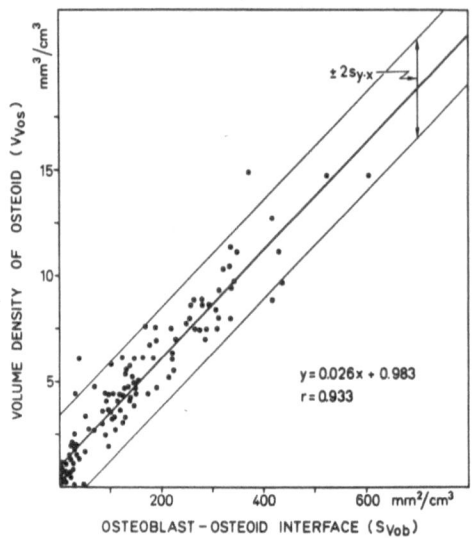

Figure 2. Correlation between osteoid volume and osteoblast surface
density in normal iliac crest cancellous bone[9]

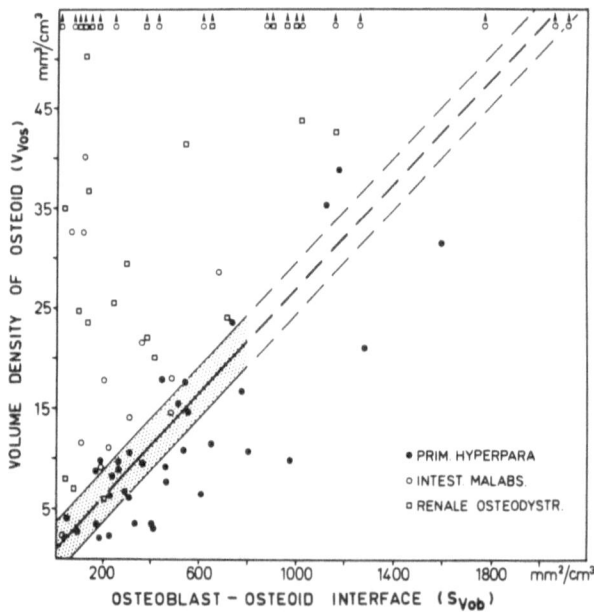

Figure 3. Correlation between osteoid and osteoblasts in biopsies
of primary hyperparathyroidism, intestinal malabsorption
and renal osteodystrophy. Dotted area = normal range[14].

confidence limits have to be prolonged hypothetically. But in most
cases with osteoid accumulation due to mineralization delay the
osteoid values are so far above the normal range, that any impli-
cation of this generalization can be neglected. The only possible
alternative to the supposed mineralization delay would be an acceleration of osteoid deposition, combined with normal mineralization.
But an increase in osteoid apposition rate, as it occurs in Paget's
disease[16] and occasionally in renal osteodystrophy[7] has always been
found to be coupled with a proportional acceleration of osteoid
mineralization.

CLASSIFICATION OF OSTEOMALACIA

Following the principle concept of dynamic osteomalacia, a histological classification of its various forms should be based on the
dynamics of bone remodelling. This is also of clinical importance,
since osteomalacic conditions are often combined with secondary
hyperparathyroidism, and under treatment, the mineralization defect
and the turnover alterations may react in a different way. The
guidelines for such a classification are simple. We differentiate
between low and high turnover types, and in view of new drug-induced
forms that are coming up, between substitional and appositional
osteomalacia.
      The difference between low and high turnover osteomalacia
can best be demonstrated in renal osteodystrophy. The bone changes
that occur in chronic renal disorders can be classified, according
to Delling[17], in type I (secondary hyperparathyroidism), type II
(osteomalacia) and type III (osteomalacia with secondary hyperparathyroidism). In our material (239 cases), type III is by far
the most frequent (67%). Type I was found in 13%, type II in 20%
(Olah, unpublished data). Again, the osteoid : osteoblast ratio
turns out to be very suitable for a discrimination of type I against
the osteomalacic forms II and III. The values for type I are high
but stay within the confidence limits of this correlation. In
biopsies of type II, the osteoblast surface density remains in the
normal range, but the accompanying osteoid volume is definitely
too high (Fig. 4). The normal or low turnover is reflected by the
low osteoclast index and the smaller surface extent of osteoblasts.
In contrast to this, biopsies of type III have augmented and often
very high osteoclast and osteoblast values, and always a high,
sometimes exorbitant osteoid volume density (Fig. 5). In both types,
but more pronounced in type III, the accumulating osteoid replaces
bone which was previously removed by osteoclasts in the remodeling
sites, and thus substitutes for mineralized bone matrix. The turnover may be low or high, but the changes in the resorptive and
formative activities tend to be proportional. It is tempting to
speculate that a high turnover osteomalacia as in type III may

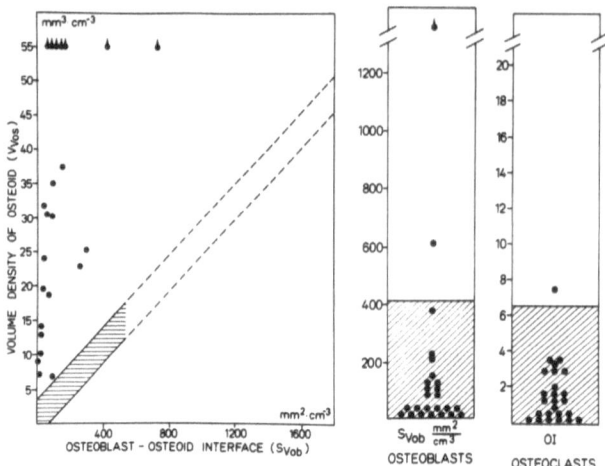

Figure 4. Osteoid : osteoblast ratio, osteoblast surface density
          and osteoclast index in renal osteodystrophy type II
          (hatched ares = normal range).

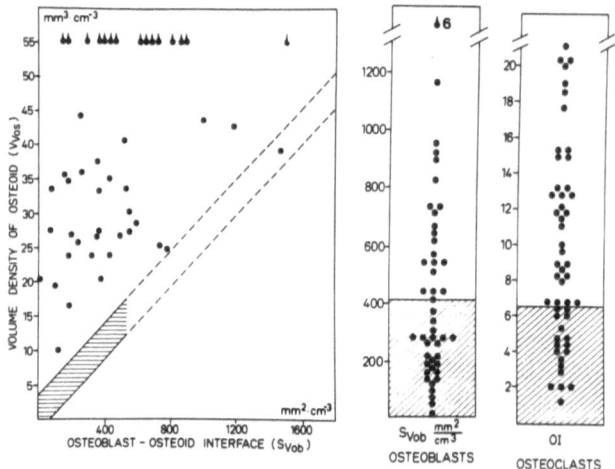

Figure 5. Osteoid : osteoblast ratio, osteoblast surface density
          and osteoclast index in renal osteodystrophy type III

result in a faster increase of osteoid and therefore in a higher
degree of 'softness' of bone. But the final amount of osteoid also
depends on the degree of the mineralization defect which may be
less severe in type III compared to type II.

     In contrast to substitutional osteomalacia, an <u>appositional</u>
<u>form</u> can be expected if a mineralization delay or mineralization

arrest is superimposed upon a turnover situation where the changes
in the rate of bone resorption versus osteoid apposition are
disproportional. This has been observed as a transient state under
the influence of certain compounds that were under investigation
in the recent years, namely sodium fluoride and certain diphosphonates. These compounds are supposed to improve the net balance
between resorption and formation, but they also cause a retardation
of osteoid mineralization, at least at higher dose levels. The
resulting changes in the bone structure thus mimic, to a certain
extent, an osteomalacic defect.

Sodium fluoride stimulates osteoblastic bone formation in
osteoporotic patients drastically at dose levels of 70 - 100 mg
per day, with only small concomitant changes in bone resorption
(19,20,21). But the amount of osteoid present after 6 - 12 months
clearly exceeds the values that can be expected from the osteoid :
osteoblast ratio (Fig. 6). The apparent delay of mineralization

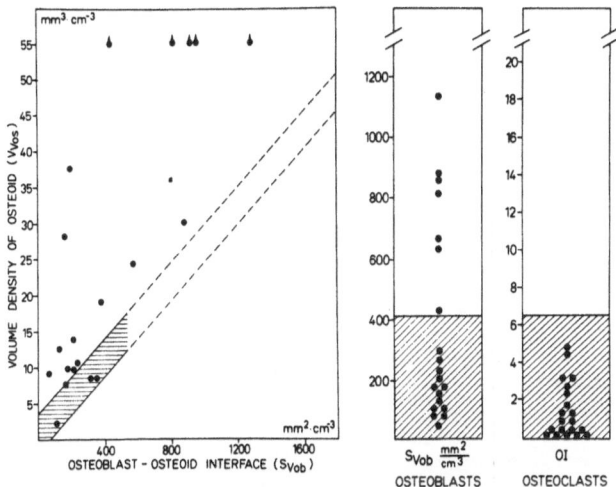

Figure 6. Osteoid : osteoblast ratio, osteoblast surface density
          and osteoclast index in osteoporotics treated with
          sodium fluoride, 70 - 100 mg / day

is confirmed by a diffuse labelling of the newly formed bone and
a defective calcification along the cement lines and in the lacunar
wall of the osteocytes. But this slowly mineralizing osteoid is
deposited upon all the trabecular surfaces, regardless of whether
resorption preceeded formation or not. The result is a net increase
in trabecular bone volume and mean trabecular diameter, first by
apposition of osteoid, followed by its gradual conversion into
mineralized bone. Besides its transitory character, this state
does not correspond to osteomalacia in terms of 'softness of bone',

since there is no real substitution of mineralized bone by osteoid.
        A transient 'appositional osteomalacia' also occurs in Paget's
disease under the influence of high doses of ethane-1-hydroxy-1,1-
diphosphonate ( EHDP ), 20 mg/kg/day. The mechanism of this osteoid
accumulation is again different. The initial effect of the drug is
an inhibition of bone resorption, first by suppression of the
activity of osteoclasts, followed by numerical reduction of these
cells. During this phase, the osteoblasts will continue to produce
osteoid for at least 4 - 6 months. Mineralization, however, is at
this dose level almost completely arrested and finally a large
amount of osteoid accumulates. At that time, the surface covered
by osteoblasts also decreases and the vascularity and fibrous
dysplasia in the bone marrow normalizes. But in spite of the
normalized bone turnover and marrow structure, a large extent of
bone surface remains coated by wide osteoid seams, which are deposited 'on top' of the original mineralized bone rather than repla-
cing it (Fig. 7). The interesting fact that this osteoid persists
for several months after withdrawal of the drug will be discussed
below.

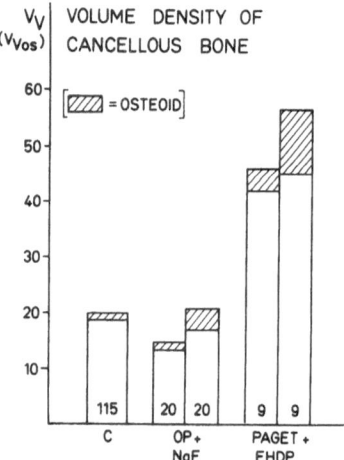

Figure 7. Volume density of mineralized bone and osteoid in
          115 random autopsy cases ( C ) and in 'appositional
          osteomalacia' resulting from sodium fluoride given to
          osteoporotic patients (OP + NaF) and Paget's disease
          treated with EHDP. The double columns compare the mean
          values in paired biopsies taken before and after
          6 - 12 months of treatment.

MECHANISM OF BONE AND CARTILAGE MINERALIZATION

Electronmicroscopic investigations have revealed two structural components that are thought to be involved in the precipitation of the first apatite crystals and their final arrangement in bone and cartilage. The apparent association of crystals to the cross striation pattern of collagen in bone has first attracted attention and generated a number of theories on the role of collagen as a biological nucleator[22]. Later on, matrix vesicles have been described, first in calcifying cartilage, then in bone (23,24,25). They now are considered as important candidates for primary nucleation in most mineralizing tissues. The current concepts and theories of mineralization are discussed in detail in Professor Fleisch's contribution to this volume. In this context, the following statements, which are mainly based on ultrastructural observations, have to be considered :

1 - The first step of mineral deposition in both bone and cartilage is triggered by matrix vesicles. The exact nature of their action is not clear, but since there is good evidence that matrix vesicles originate from the cytoplasm of osteoblasts and chondrocytes, this first step of mineralization is mediated by cells.

2 - In cartilage, the first clusters of mineral spread out into the interfibrillar spaces without any tendency to associate with collagen fibers (which may be 'protected' by a coat of proteoglycans). There are indications, however, for some association of mineral to remnants of proteoglycans[26].

3 - In bone, the vesicle induced mineralization is followed by a second step at the site of the calcification front. This step leads to the final association between mineral and collagen and may be governed by the same principles that act in vitro when collagen is used as a nucleator. This process is mainly of physico-chemical character and not directly mediated by cells.

Such a distinction between a cell-mediated, vesicle-induced first step of mineralization and a second, collagen-dependent phase has some interesting consequences for the pathogenesis and therapy of osteomalacic conditions. The mechanism of the mineralization disorder in D - deficient osteomalacia is still not clear, in spite of the numerous theories that range from a low calcium-phosphate product in the interstitial fluid to the production of a defective, not calcifiable matrix by the osteoblasts. Even less is known about the healing or recovery of osteomalacic bone defects, except that osteoid can persist for surprisingly long periods after the metabolic defect is corrected.

In this respect, some observations on the recovery pattern of severe mineralization defects induced by EHDP in rats are of

particular interest. In this experimental study[27], one single
injection of 30 mg P/kg proved to be sufficient to arrest bone and
cartilage mineralization for at least one week. Thereafter, the
first sites of resumed mineralization in the extremely widened
growth plates appeared at the normal distance from their epiphyseal
border and then spread out throughout the accumulated hypertrophic
cartilage towards the metaphysis. In areas where lamellar bone is
formed, i.e. along the periosteal and endosteal circumference of
the diaphysis, osteoid piled up throughout the first three weeks
after the one single injection. Again the first traces of recom-
mencing mineralization became visible at the site of the actual
mineralization front, i.e. about 7 μm below the osteoblast-osteoid
interface. As soon as the mineral in the calcification front
reappears, it spreads out rapidly into the deeper layers of accumulated osteoid. At this stage, the histological aspect often gives
the impression of a 'buried osteoid seam'. But after a couple of
days, a lower mineral density can only be detected along the cement
lines which correspond to the sites of the initial, EHDP - induced
arrest of calcification.

From these observations one can conclude that the mineralization
arrest produced by EHDP can only be overcome in areas where cells
are present that release new vesicles into the matrix. It seems
likely that vesicles, after being detached from the cells, have
only a limited time of functional competence. They have been found
throughout arrested calcifying cartilage as well as in accumulated
osteoid, but obviously had lost their nucleating capacity[25]. The
presence of osteoblasts lining the surface of accumulated osteoid
therefore is essential for the recovery of a mineralization defect,
at least under these experimental conditions.

On this background, some recent biopsy findings merit attention. One is the surprisingly long persistence of accumulated
osteoid in Pagetic bone after treatment with high doses of EHDP.
It has been shown that this osteoid remains unmineralized for
3 - 6 months after cessation of the drug and then disappears
suddenly. But almost nothing is known about the pattern of this
final mineralization. In view of this long persistence, the normalization of bone turnover has to be taken into account. After
6 months of treatment, the osteoclasts have almost disappeared, and
the osteoblasts have returned to values found in normal cancellous
bone ( 3 - 5 % of total trabecular surface ). This represents only
a small fraction of the osteoid surface which still amounts to
60 - 80 % at this moment. The chance, that new, functionally competent matrix vesicles are deposited upon this osteoid thus becomes
rather small. This offers an explanation for the long lag time
until bone mineralization is resumed and the accumulated masses
of osteoid disappear.

Similar observations have been made in recent studies on the effects of 1,25 - DHCC on the bone changes in chronic renal insufficiency (Olah et al, unpublished data ). The improvement of the metabolic situation, especially the increase in intestinal calcium absorption is reflected in the biopsies mainly by a normalization of the symptoms of secondary hyperparathyroidism, i.e. by a normalization of the turnover values, expressed in osteoclast numbers and osteoblast surface density. The amelioration of mineralization, however, is much less pronounced. There is a reduction in osteoid volume, but this is coupled with a decrease in the surface covered by osteoblasts. In most cases that could be analyzed by paired biopsies, the osteoblast-osteoid ratio shifts parallel to the regression line. In other words, the osteoid volume remains too high compared to the number of osteoblasts. At the first look, this would indicate that a high turnover osteomalacia simply has changed into a low turnover type, and the mineralization problem still persists. Another possible interpretation is that mineralization only normalizes in osteoblast-covered seams and the surplus osteoid stems from resting osteoid seams denuded of osteoblasts. This would be in favor of the supposition that osteoid which is no longer lined by osteoblasts, cannot simply undergo mineralization when the calcium : phosphate ratio is corrected and D - metabolites of known or unknown configuration become available. The reduction in osteoblast number that accompanies the normalization of the calcium and phosphate disorder also diminishes the chance, that new osteoid, furnished with functionally competent matrix vesicles is deposited on top of resting osteoid and that a restored calcification front can trigger the collagen associated mineralization step in the deeper layers. Such a hypothesis fits nicely with the biopsy findings in various kinds of treated osteomalacia and also helps to prevent disillusions resulting from exaggerated expectations due to an incomplete or erraneous concept of the mechanism of calcification.

CONCLUSIONS

Osteomalacia is characterized histodynamically as an accumulation of osteoid due to continuing matrix production by osteoblasts, combined with delayed or arrested mineralization. The histological diagnosis, therefore, is only possible by an assessment of the defective mineralization rate by tetracycline labelling or special staining methods of the calcification front, or by a correlation between the amount of osteoid present and the extent of bone surface covered by osteoblasts.

Dynamic osteomalacia can be classified according to the intensity of bone remodelling into a low and high turnover type. Substitutional osteomalacia is present when the changes in bone resorption and bone formation remain proportional and osteoid thus substitutes for mineralized bone. Appositional osteomalacia is described in conditions, where a mineralization defect is superimposed on a disproportional alteration in turnover, resulting either from a suppression of osteoclasts (e.g. by diphosphonates) or from a stimulation of bone formation (e.g. by sodium fluoride). The appositional type seems unlikely to cause osteomalacia in the classical sense of softness of bone, since it does not alter the amount of mineralized bone substance originally present.

In view of the mechanism of bone mineralization, two phases are considered. The initial step depends on the presence of matrix vesicles and is directly mediated by cells. In the second step, collagen induces the final association between crystals and fibrils, a process which is not directly cell dependent.

The mineralization defect in osteomalacia is thought to affect the initial process of cell-mediated, vesicle-induced mineralization. It is proposed that matrix vesicles have only a limited time of functional competence. This would explain why osteoid accumulated during periods of inhibited mineralization is unable to mineralize after correction of the metabolic situation, unless it is covered by osteoblasts which release new, functionally competent vesicles into the matrix.

The remarkably long persistance of osteoid after elimination of the cause of a mineralization deficiency may be partially attributed to the fact, that treatment often also corrects the abnormally high turnover and thus reduces the relative extent of osteoid surface that remains covered by osteoblasts.

REFERENCES

1. Frost, H.M., The bone dynamics in osteoporosis and osteomalacia, Thomas, Springfield, Ill. (1966)
2. Richard, O., L'histomorphometrie du tissu ostéoide. Son application au diagnostic des ostéomalacies et des états d'hyperostéoidose, Lyon (1976)
3. Delling, G. and Luhmann, H., Ineffectiveness of 1,25-DHCC treatment in a special type of renal bone disorder - a histomorphometric investigation, IVth Workshop on vitamin D, Berlin (1979)
4. Ramser, J.R., Frost, H.M., Frame, B., Arnstein, A.R. and Smith, R., Tetracycline-based studies of bone dynamics in rib of 6 cases of osteomalacia, Clin.Orthop. 46, 219 (1966)

5. Ritz,E., Malluche,H.H., Krempien,B. and Mehls,O., Bone histology
   in renal insufficiency, In:Calcium metabolism in renal failure
   and nephrolithiasis (Davis,S.D.,ed.), John Wiley & Sons,
   New York, 145 (1977)
6. Bordier,P.J. and Tun-Chot,S., Quantitative histology of metabolic
   bone disease, J.Clin.Endocr.Metabol. 1, 197 (1972)
7. Meunier,P., Edouard,C.,Bressot,J.-N.,Courpron,P. et Zech,P.,
   Histomorphométrie osseuse dans l'insuffisance rénale aiguë
   et chronique, J.Urol.Nephrol. 12,931 (1975)
8. Bordier,Ph.,Ryckwaert,A.,Marie,P.,Miravet,L.,Norman,A. and
   Rasmussen,H., Vitamin D metabolites and bone mineralization
   in man, In: VitaminD. Biochemical,chemical and clinical aspects
   related to calcium metabolism (Norman,A.W. et al.eds.),
   Walter de gruyter, Berlin, New York (1977)
9. Merz,W.A. and Schenk, R.K., A quantitative study on bone
   formation in human cancellous bone, Acta anat. 76,1 (1970)
10. Burkhardt,R., Präparative Voraussetzungen zur klinischen Histo-
    logie des menschlichen Knochenmark, 1. Mitteilung, Blut 13,
    337 (1966)
11. Schenk, R.K., Zur histologischen Verarbeitung von unentkalkten
    Knochen, Acta anat. 60, 3 (1965)
12. Olah,A.J., Simon,A., Gaudy,M., Herrmann,W. and Schenk,R.K.,
    Differential staining of calcified tissues in plastic embedded
    microtome sections by a modification of Movat's pentachrome
    stain, Stain Technol. 52, 331 (1977)
13. Shen,S., Villanueva,A.R., and Frost,H.M., Number of osteoblasts
    per unit area of seam in cortical human bone, Canad.J.Physiol.
    Pharm. 43, 319 (1964)
14. Olah,A.J., Histomorphometrie des Knochens, Verh.Dtsch.Ges.Path.
    58- 104 (1974)
15. Olah,A.J., Quantitative relations between osteoblasts and osteoid
    in primary hyperparathyroidism, intestinal malabsorption and
    renal osteodystrophy, Virch.Arch.Path.Anat. 358, 301 (1973)
16. Meunier,P., La maladie osseuse de Paget. Histologie quantitative,
    histopathogénie et perspectives thérapeutiques, Lyon Médical
    233, 839 (1975)
17. Delling,G., Endokrine Osteopathien, Gustav Fischer,Stuttgart
    (1975)
18. Olah,A.J., Jahn,H., Reutter,F.W.,König,R., Blumberg,A., Colombi,
    A., Histomorphometry of bone changes in renal osteodystrophy
    after treatment with 1,25-dihydroxycholecalciferol. Proc.
    IVth Workshop on Vitamin D, Berlin (in press)
19. Schenk,R.K.,Merz,W.A., Reutter,F.W., Fluoride in osteoporosis.
    Quantitative studies on bone structure and bone remodelling
    in serial biopsies of iliac crest. In: Fluoride in Medicine,
    (Vischer,Th- ed.) Hans Huber, Bern, 153 (1970)

20. Jowsey,J., Riggs,B.L., Kelly,P.J., Hoffman,D.L., Effect of
    combined therapy with dosium fluoride, vitamin D and calcium
    in osteoporosis, Am.J.Med. 53, 43 (1972)
21. Olah,A.J., Reutter,F.W. and Dambacher,M.A., Effects of combined
    therapy with sodium fluoride and high doses of vitamin D in
    osteoporosis. A histomorphometric study in the iliac crest,
    In: Fluoride and Bone (Courvoisier,B., Donath,A. and Baud,
    C.A., eds.) Editions Médicine et Hygiène, Genève (1978)
22. Glimcher, M.J., Molecular biology of mineralized tissues with
    particular reference to bone, Rev.Med.Physics 31, 359 (1959)
23. Bonucci,E., Fine structure of early cartilage calcification,
    J.Ultrastruc.Res. 20, 33 (1967)
24. Anderson, H.C., Vesicles associated with calcification in the
    matrix of epiphyseal cartilage, J.Cell Biol. 41, 59 (1969)
25. Schenk, R.K., Ultrastruktur des Knochens, Verh.Dtsch.Ges.Path.
    58, 72 (1974)
26. Bonucci, E. and Reurink,J., The fine structure of decalcified
    cartilage and bone : A comparison between decalcification
    procedures performed before and after embedding, Calc.Tiss.
    Res. 25, 179 (1978)
27. Hufschmied, P. and Schenk, R.K., Recovery of cartilage and
    bone mineralization after EHDP - induced calcification
    arrest in rats ( in preparation )

Acknowledgment

This work is supported by the Swiss National Science Foundation,
Grant No. 3.407 - 0.78 .

# MECHANISMS OF CALCIFICATION

H. Fleisch

Department of Pathophysiology
University of Berne
Murtenstrasse 35, 3010 Berne, Switzerland

## INTRODUCTION

Despite intensive investigations the calcification
process is still poorly understood.  The great number
of theories which have been and are still being proposed
reflect the complexity of the subject and the uncertainty
of our knowledge.  In this review  an attempt will be
made to sum up knowledge of the nature of the biological
mineral and the mechanism(s) of its formation.   Emphasis
will be placed on the inorganic part of the calcified
tissues, although it must be kept in mind that mineral
never deposits without an organic matrix which represents
an appreciable proportion of the total weight.

## CHEMICAL COMPOSITION OF MINERAL

To understand the mechanism of the calcification  process, it is necessary to have an exact knowledge of the
composition of the formed salts. It has been known for
more than 100 years that mineralized tissues contain
calcium and phosphate in a similar proportion as in
minerals in nature known under the name of apatite.
The apatitic structure was confirmed later by X-ray
diffraction.  While everybody still agrees that the
mineral phase of bone, dentine, enamel and pathological
calcifications is basically a hydroxyapatite
$Ca_{10}(PO_4)_6(OH)_2$ (1), it is now also clear that it is
not a pure hydroxyapatite.  Thus chemical analyses
have shown that the Ca/P ratio of these tissues is
usually below the value of 1.67 of hydroxyapatite.  The

mineral also contains many other constituents, especially about 5 % carbonate, 1 % citrate, 0.5 - 1 %
sodium and magnesium (2).  Furthermore, although
the X-ray diffraction pattern corresponds to that of
hydroxyapatite, the peaks are much less well resolved
than in synthetic salts.  The reasons for these discrepancies are complex, which explains the great number
of opinions about the exact character of biological
minerals.

The main mechanisms leading to these variations in
composition are the following:  a) Deficiencies of
certain compounds and substitutions by other ions,
b) incomplete crystallization and lattice imperfections,
c) the presence of other salts than hydroxyapatite, and
d) adsorption of ions on the surface.

a) The fact that the Ca/P ratio in biological apatites
is generally below the theoretical value of 1.67 led
to the concept of the Ca-deficient apatites (3).  While
it was initially thought that each Ca could be replaced
by 2 $H^+$ ions, the most commonly accepted suggestion
now is that for each missing $Ca^{++}$ one $H^+$ is added
and one $OH^-$ deleted, giving thus the formula
$Ca_{10-x}H_x(PO_4)_6(OH)_{2-x}$, x varying between 0 and 2 (4,5).
Since the $H^+$ ions lie between the $PO_4$ groups, some of
the $PO_4$ groups transform into $HPO_4^=$ which would explain
the fact that bone mineral gives pyrophosphate upon
heating, a transformation which indicates the presence
of $HPO_4^=$ ions (5).  The formula would thus become
$Ca_{10-x}(PO_4)_{6-x}(HPO_4)_x(OH)_{2-x}$.  Calcium can also be replaced by other cations such as strontium, radium and lead
(2) although in normal conditions the amounts are
negligible.

Besides calcium,the other components of the hydroxyapatite can also undergo substitution.  Thus phosphate
can be replaced by carbonate (6) both within the
lattice and on the crystal surface. Finally, $OH^-$ ions
can be replaced by fluoride, which alters both the
precipitation behaviour and the solubility of the
mineral.

b) These various substitutions, which are not surprising
in view of the complex milieu from which the mineral
precipitates, can lead to distorsion of the láttice and
defects within it, leading to a low "crystallinity" as
evaluated by X-ray diffraction.  The main ion leading
to these changes is probably carbonate  so that the
bulk of bone mineral appears to be a carbonate contain-

ing apatite with internal disorder (6,7), showing thus
a paracrystalline structure (8). With aging the
mineral ripens and slowly perfects its structure so
that the "crystallinity" will improve.

c) In addition to viewing biological mineral as a
Ca-deficient apatite with random deficiencies, it has
also been suggested to be a mixture of hydroxyapatite,
octocalcium phosphate ($Ca_8H_4(PO_4)_65H_2O$) (9), and perhaps
tricalcium phosphate. The latter have a structure and
an X-ray diffraction pattern very similar to that of
hydroxyapatite, making their detection in biological
systems difficult.

The fact that biological apatites do not have a sharp
X-ray diffraction pattern also led to the suggestion
that bone is a mixture of hydroxyapatite and an
amorphous calcium phosphate with no long range order
(10). This suggestion was supported by the fact that
when calcium phosphate is precipitated in vitro from
clear solutions, the first phase to form is amorphous
(10). Recently, however, X-ray radial distribution
function studies (7) showed that the changes in X-ray
diffraction pattern are due largely to the small size
of the crystals and to lattice distorsions induced by
the incorporation of other ions, such as carbonate.
Thus the amount of amorphous calcium phosphate in bone
and teeth is at best a few percent.

d) Finally, since the crystals of the biological
apatites have very small dimensions resulting in a
large crystal suface, estimated to be 100-200 $m^2/g$,
adsorbed compounds can influence bone composition to a
relatively large extent (2). Among these carbonate,
citrate, phosphate, and pyrophosphate as well as
calcium and magnesium should be mentioned.

Information on the nature of bone mineral can be found
in a series of reviews (2,3,5,11,12).

MORPHOLOGICAL ASPECTS

Significant information concerning the process of
calcification has been gained by means of electron
microscopy. Mineral seems to be deposited initially
both within the cells and extracellularly. Intracellularly it is seen in the mitochondria in osteoblasts,
osteocytes, osteoclasts and epiphyseal cartilage cells
(13,14) in the form of granules of up to 1000 Å dia-

meter.  It appears at least in the epiphyseal cartilage,
that the granules disappear at the onset of extracellular
calcification (13), so that it has been proposed that
the mineral is translocated in some way outside the
cell.

Extracellularly, precipitation starts in two locations.
Some is on and within the collagen fibrils, with an
axial periodicity related to the hole and the overlap-
ping regions of the collagen (14,15).  Some starts
to deposit in very close relation with extracellular
vesicles present in the extracellular matrix.  These
trilaminar bodies called matrix vesicles were first
described in the longitudinal septa of epiphyseal
cartilage and later found in other calcifying tissues
such as bone and dentine (16,17).  They are thought to
be originated from the cell membrane.  It appears that
in cartilage vesicles are the main inducing mechanism,
while in bone collagen plays the important role.
Detailed information on their formation, composition
and role can be found in two recent symposiums (18,19).

The mineral then develops into extracellular clusters,
suggesting that once deposition has started at a specific
site crystallization proceeds readily, mostly by increase in the number of crystals (20).  Later on the
clusters tend to coalesce into one mass of heavily
extracellular calcified tissue, within and outside the
collagen fibrils.

While there is general agreement that the biological
calcium phosphate crystals have a very small size, in
the range of a few hundred Å, discrepancy exists
as to their form.  Particles, rods, needles and plates
have been described (14,21,22,23).  Although the
needles are the most common element seen, it appears
that many are really plates cut transversally (20,23).
It is likely that all of the forms are encountered with
some being the precursors of the others.

PHASE TRANSFORMATION

While there is general agreement that the end stage in
the calcification process is the formation of a more or
less pure hydroxyapatite, some uncertainty still
exists, however, as to the way this end product is
formed.  In vitro during de novo precipitation the
first phase to be formed both under high and low
supersaturation is an amorphous calcium phosphate (10).
Whether in the presence of preformed crystals the first

mineral formed is also amorphous, or can be directly
crystalline is not known.  This amorphous precipitate
is thought to be composed of small clusters of about
9.5 Å diameter of $Ca_9(PO_4)_6$ closely packed into large
spherical particles of 300-1000 Å diameter with
water held in the interstices (7). This phase is
unstable and transforms spontaneously into a crystalline
material with a hydroxyapatite diffraction pattern
(10).  The process is first order and is regulated both
by the dissolution of the amorphous phase and the
autocatalytical nucleation, perhaps on the surface of
the amorphous material, of the hydroxyapatite.  Whether
in the process the clusters themselves are also dissolved or remain intact is not known.  The transformation
is inhibited by various compounds, among others magnesium, carbonate, pyrophosphate, ATP and diphosphonates
which act either by inhibiting the dissolution of the
precursor phase or by inhibiting the crystallization
process.

The question of whether an amorphous phase is also
first formed in vivo is not yet settled, although
electron microscopic data suggest that this can be the
case (24), especially in avian medullary bone with high
turnover (25).  Once formed, the amorphous phase is
rapidly transformed into a crystalline one, except for
specific locations such as inside the mitochondria.  It
is possible that an amorphous coat stabilized by
carbonate can also be maintained at the crystal surface
(26). If true, since amorphous calcium phosphate has a
higher solubility than hydroxyapatite, an explanation
would be given for the relatively high Ca x Pi product
in blood.

Uncertainty also exists as to the chronological
development of the crystalline phases formed.  In
vitro they are strongly dependent on the conditions
present, especially supersaturation and pH.  Thus
brushite ($CaHPO_4$ x $2H_2O$) is formed preferentially
at low pH and high supersaturation (6).  In vivo this
salt is thought to form in urine (27) but its formation
in bone has still to be proven. A great deal of attention has been given to octocalcium phosphate (9) as the
first crystalline phase.  In vitro octocalcium phosphate
has been shown to form and be transformed in a second
step into hydroxyapatite, both when the precipitation
occurs de novo through an amorphous phase (28,29) and
in a solution seeded with apatite crystals (30).  It
can occur in physiological conditions of supersaturation
and pH (30).  The formation of an octocalcium phosphate

phase in vivo is also supported by solubility studies
of bone powder at various pH's (31) and by the finding
of octocalcium phosphate in biological mineralized
tissues (32).  The in loco transformation of octocalcium
phosphate into hydroxyapatite would also explain the
plate-like habit of the bone crystals which is unusual
for a salt like apatite with a hexagonal structure, but
is consistent with the triclinic structure of octocalcium phosphate.

## ION CONCENTRATION NECESSARY FOR MINERAL FORMATION

It has been known for over 50 years that blood ultrafiltrate is supersaturated with respect to hydroxyapatite
(2).  This supersaturation is less accentuated but
nonetheless present with respect to bone powder (2,33),
suggesting that the surface of the bone crystals, or
the phase determining the solubility is not well
crystallized hydroxyapatite but a more soluble phase
such as a less perfect apatite, octocalcium phosphate
or an amorphous calcium phosphate.

Although plasma is supersaturated with respect to
existing bone mineral, the ion Ca and P concentrations
are below those necessary to form calcium phosphate de
novo.  Indeed this value, also called the formation
product, although depending on the conditions used, is
usually greater than the ion concentration in plasma
ultrafiltrate (2).  This gap between the formation
product and the solubility exists to some extent for
all salts, since the solubility of the small embryos
is greater than that of the larger stable crystals.
Thus, a higher energy is needed to form a solid phase
de novo, than in presence of already formed crystals.
In the calcium phosphate system the gap is specially
large, since the first phase formed is not hydroxyapatite but a precursor with a higher solubility.

The question therefore arises as to how precipitation
is induced in vivo under these circumstances.  Various
theories have been proposed.

## BOOSTER THEORY

The oldest theory, called the booster theory, is that
the calcium x phosphate ion product is increased locally up to the level of precipitation.  Various ways have
been suggested to obtain this rise in concentration.

One is that a phosphate ester would be hydrolyzed by

alkaline phosphatase increasing the inorganic phosphate
concentration (34).  This hypothesis was supported by
studies in vitro on calcifying cartilage showing that
inhibitors of glycolysis inhibited calcification,
but that addition of the intermediate below the block
restored it (35).  It would also provide an explanation
for the well known fact that alkaline phosphatase is
always present at sites of calcification.  However,
alkaline phosphatase is present in many other tissues
in addition to those which mineralize.  Furthermore,
the attempts to find an intermediate which would be in
concentrations high enough to lead to a sufficient
increase in Pi have been without success.  Finally,
findings by micropuncture showed that, at least in
calcifying cartilage, the Ca x Pi product is not
elevated (36).  Thus, if such a booster mechanism
exists, it would have to operate in a microenvironment.
Recently it has been suggested that the matrix vesicles
would fulfil this role, since they are rich in phosphatases, the substrate being perhaps a nucleotide (37).

Another possibility is that the Ca x Pi product is
increased locally by an active cellular pump.  One
possible example are the mitochodria, which are indeed
known to pump actively calcium into their interiors
(38). In vivo amorphous calcium phosphate deposits are
seen in these organelles (13), although this appears to
be the case not only in calcifying tissues. Another
candidate is the matrix vesicles, although the suggestion that they pump calcium (39) has not be proven.

NUCLEATION THEORY

A second theory, which emerged in the Macy conferences
in the late fifties, was that a local factor would
facilitate the precipitation.  In view of the presence
of an organic matrix in all calcified tissues, the
respective organic templates were the obvious candidates.  After an initial interest in glycosaminoglycans
in view of their strong affinity for calcium, attention
was directed mainly towards collagen (2,15).  Indeed in
the presence of collagen the minimum calcium x phosphate
product necessary to induce precipitation is greatly
decreased. This effect is explained by heterogenous
nucleation, a mechanism whereby precipitation is
induced in an otherwise stable supersaturated solution
by introduction of crystals of the salt to be formed,
or of other foreign materials, similar in structure
to the salt. It was therefore suggested that collagen
would bind either phosphate or calcium at locations

which would present some symmetry with their position
in the calcium phosphate crystal (2,15). This theory
was supported by electron microscopic findings that
bone crystals are in close relationship with the
collagen fibrils and often seem to first form on these
fibrils (14,15).

Other candidates as nucleators are lipids. The interest for a possible role of lipids in the calcification process was stimulated by histological findings
that lipids appear at the calcification front, but are
deficient in vitamin D rickets (40). The lipids
involved are thought to be mainly acidic phospholipids,
especially phosphatidyl serine and phosphatidyl inositol.
They are present in various calcified tissues, often in
the form of a calcium-phospholipid-phosphate complex
and are able to induce calcium phosphate precipitation
in vitro from metastable solutions through the formation of such a complex (41).

Other proteins, such as a phosphoprotein extracted from
dentine and the protein containing the newly described
amino acid γ carboxyglutamate, have been consider-
ated as nucleators too, but proof for such a role is
still lacking. The matrix vesicles have also been shown
to act in vitro as nucleators (42). Part of this
effect, although not all, might be due to the lipids
they contain (43).

Finally the last facet of the nucleator theory is the
fact that certain salts induce the precipitation of
salts of another kind. This mechanism is thought to
play a role, especially in the formation of urinary
stones, and explains why stones are often a mixture of
different salts (44,45).

INHIBITION THEORY

The fact that some of the nucleators such as collagen
are also present in non-mineralizing tissues raised the
question why more tissues do not calcify in vivo. A
possibility, which has received increasing attention in
these last years, is that soft tissues are protected in
vivo by inhibitors of crystallization, which are then
destroyed at the sites of calcification. Indeed
plasma, urine and other biological fluids contain
powerful crystallization inhibitors (46). The first to
be recognized and investigated was inorganic pyrophosphate, which inhbits precipitation at very low concentrations and is present in blood, urine, saliva and joint

fluid in concentrations sufficient to be active (46).
The hypothesis that pyrophosphate plays a role in vivo
was strengthened by the finding that this compound is
able to prevent ectopic calcifications induced in
animals by various means (46).  Since alkaline phosphatase is known to have pyrophosphate activity, this
enzyme might act by destroying the inhibitor and thus
allow the mineralization process to take place.  The
matrix vesicles possess strong pyrophosphatase and
ATPase activities (39,47) so that one of their modes of
inducing calcification could be through hydrolysis of
inhibitors such as pyrophosphate and ATP.  However,
since many tissues which do not calcify also contain
alkaline phosphatase, the pyrophosphate mechanism can
obviously not be the only one operating.

Indirect support for the pyrophosphate theory is
given by the studies on diphosphonates, compounds
closely related in structure to pyrophosphate but with
a P-C-P moiety instead of the P-O-P of pyrophosphate.
The diphosphonates have similar inhibitory properties
on calcium phosphate precipitation in vitro as pyrophosphate (48).  Like pyrophosphate, they are strongly
bound to the apatite crystals, the inhibition being
related to this binding. However, contrary to pyrophosphate, they are not broken down in vivo, the P-C-P bond
being totally resistant to enzymatic degradation at
least in mammals.  This property permits their use as
models for pyrophosphate activity in vivo.  They
inhibit, like pyrophosphate, ectopic calcifications,
but in contrast are also active when given orally, and
also unlike pyrophosphate, they inhibit mineralization
of bone, cartilage and dentine (48).  The effect on
ectopic calcifications has been used therapeutically in
man both against soft tissue calcification and dental
calculus.

Besides pyrophosphate, plasma and urine contain several
other inhibitors.  Among them citrate and magnesium are
present in active amounts (49).  Recently phosphocitrate
has also been proposed (50).  The relative importance
of these various compounds cannot be estimated since
the results depend greatly on the technique used.
Finally, saliva also contains one or several macromolecular inhibitors.  One of them, called statherin, has
recently been characterized as a polypeptide with
43 amino acids (51).

Besides these circulating inhibitors, local inhibitors
are also likely to be of importance. Recently attention

has been revived on the possible role of proteoglycans,
compounds which had been suggested but without adequate
proof to work as inhibitors many years ago.   Thus,
fluid of epipyhseal cartilage contains a high molecular
weight inhibitory fraction consisting of proteoglycans
in the aggregated form.   When this fraction is disaggre-
gated into subunits it looses its inhibitory activity
(36).   Therefore, part of the regulatory process, at
least in the epiphyseal cartilage, might consist of a
change in the aggregation of proteoglycans.   Furthermore,
an inhibitor of unknown structure with a molecular
weight of about 100,000 daltons has been extracted from
tendon (52).

CRYSTAL AGGREGATION

Besides crystal formation, another process, neglected
in the past, is likely to play a role in the formation
of mineralized tissues: crystal aggregation.   This
process, which permits the crystals to bind to each
other, might be involved in giving the calcified
tissues their physical texture.   It is also thought to
be one of the causes distinguishing people who simply
form crystals in their urine from those forming urinary
stones.   Both plasma and urine contain inhibitors of
calcium oxalate (53,54,55) and calcium phosphate (56)
aggregation.   Glycosaminoglycans, pyrophosphate and
citrate are all powerful inhibitors of crystal aggregation (54,55), although here too their relative importance cannot be estimated.   It is of interest that the
inhibitors are diminished in stone formers (53), who
also tend to have more calcium oxalate aggregates in
their urine than normal people.

More detailed information on inhibitors of crystal
growth and aggregation can be found in a recent review
(57).

CONCLUSIONS

The various mechanisms thought to govern calcium
phosphate precipitation and crystallization have been
reviewed.   Until now it cannot be stated whether one,
several, or all of them are operative in vivo.   From all
the data available, it appears likely that the calcification process is regulated by more than just one of
the factors proposed.   Different mechanisms might also
occur at various sites of calcification.   An integration
of the various proposed mechanisms  might in the future
be a fruitful approach.

## ACKNOWLEDGEMENTS

This work has been supported by the Swiss National Science Foundation (3.725.76), by the Procter & Gamble Company, USA, and by the Ausbildungs- und Förderungs- fonds der Arbeitsgemeinschaft für Osteosynthese (AO), Chur, Switzerland.

## REFERENCES

1. R. Klement und G. Trömel, Hydroxyapatit, der Hauptbestandteil der anorganischen Knochen- und Zahnsubstanz, Hoppe-Seylers Physiol.Chem. 213: 263 (1932).
2. W.F. Neuman and M.W. Neuman, "The Chemical Dynamics of Bone Mineral", The University Chicago Press, Chicago (1958).
3. A.S. Posner, Crystal chemistry of bone mineral, Phys.Rev. 49: 760 (1969).
4. L. Winand, Physico-chemical study of some apatitic calcium phosphate, in: "Tooth Enamel", M.V. Stack and R.W. Fearnhead, eds., John Wright & Sons Ltd., Bristol, (1965).
5. M.J. Dallemagne, Le calcium dans la squelette et les dents, in: "Handbuch der experimentellen Pharmakologie", Z.-M. Bacq, ed.,Springer-Verlag, Berlin (1964).
6. D. McConnell, "Apatite", Springer-Verlag, Wien and New York (1973).
7. A. S. Posner and F. Betts, Synthetic amorphous calcium phosphate and its relation to bone mineral structure, Acc.Chem.Res. 8: 273 (1975).
8. E.J. Wheeler and D. Lewis, An X-ray study of the paracrystalline nature of bone apatite, Calcif.Tiss. Res. 24: 243 (1977).
9. W.E. Brown, Crystal growth of bone mineral, Clin. Orthop. 44: 205 (1966).
10. E.D. Eanes, J.D. Termine, and A. S. Posner, Amor- phous calcium phosphate in skeletal tissues, Clin.Orthop.Rel.Res. 53: 223 (1967).
11. J.C. Elliott, The problems of the composition and structure of the mineral components and the hard tissues, Clin.Orthop.Rel.Res. 93: 313 (1973).
12. G. Montel, Constitutions et structure des apatites biologiques: influence de ces facteurs sur leurs propriétés, Biol.Cell. 28: 179 (1977).
13. J.H. Martin and J.L. Matthews, Mitochondrial granules in chondrocytes, osteoblasts and osteocytes, Clin.Orthop.Rel.Res. 68: 273 (1970).
14. H.J. Höhling, R. Kreilos, G. Neubauer, and A. Boyde,

Electron microscopy of electron microscopical measurements of collagen mineralization in hard tissues, Z.Zellforsch. 122: 36 (1971).

15. M.J. Glimcher, Composition, structure, and organization of bone and other mineralized tissues and the mechanism of calcification, in: "Handbook of Physiology, Section 7: Endocrinology, Vol. VII: Parathyroid Gland", R.O. Greep, E.B. Astwood, G.D. Aurbach and S.R. Geiger, eds., American Physiological Society, Washington (1976).

16. H.C. Anderson, Matrix vesicles of cartilage and bone, in: "The Biochemistry and Physiology of Bone, Vol. IV: Calcification and Physiology", G.H. Bourne, ed., Academic Press, New York (1976).

17. E. Bonucci, Fine structure and histochemistry of "calcifying globules" in epiphyseal cartilage, Z.Zellforsch. 103: 192 (1970).

18. Federation Proceedings, Volume 35, Number 2, 105 (1976).

19. Metabolic Bone Disease and Related Research, Volume 1, Numbers 2 and 3, 83 (1978).

20. W.J. Landis, M.C. Paine, and M.J. Glimcher, Electron microscopic observations of bone tissue prepared anhydrously in organic solvents, J.Ultrastruc.Res. 59: 1 (1977).

21. R.A. Robinson and M.L. Watson, Collagen-crystal relationships in bone as seen in the electron microscope, Anat.Rec. 114: 383 (1952).

22. T.W. Speckman and W.P. Norris, Bone crystallites as observed by use of the electron microscope, Science 126: 753 (1957).

23. D.S. Bocciarelli, Morphology of crystallites in bone, Calcif.Tiss.Res. 5: 261 (1970).

24. Z. Molnar, Development of the parietal bone of young mice. 1. Crystals of bone mineral in frozen-dried preparations, J.Ultrastruc.Res. 3: 39 (1959).

25. A.L. Miller and H. Schraer, Ultrastructural observations of amorphous bone mineral in avian bone, Calcif.Tiss.Res. 18: 311 (1975).

26. E.D. Eanes, The interaction of supersaturated calcium phosphate solutions with apatitic substrates, Calcif.Tiss.Res. 20: 75 (1976).

27. C.Y.C. Pak, E.D. Eanes, and B. Ruskin, Spontaneous precipitation of brushite in urine: Evidence that brushite is the nidus of renal stones originating as calcium phosphate, Proc.Nat.Acad.Sci. 68: 1456 (1971).

28. H. Füredi-Milhofer, B. Purgaric, Lj. Brecevic, and N. Pavkovic, Precipitation of calcium phosphates

from electrolyte solutions. I. A study of the precipitates in the physiological pH region, Calcif.Tiss.Res. 8: 142 (1971).

29. J.L. Meyer and E.D. Eanes, A thermodynamic analysis of the secondary transition in the spontaneous precipitation of calcium phosphate, Calcif.Tiss.Res. 25: 209 (1978).

30. M.B. Tomson and G.H. Nancollas, Mineralization kinetics: A constant composition approach, Science 200: 1059 (1978).

31. J. McGregor and W. Brown, Blood: Bone equilibrium in calcium homeostasis, Nature 205: 359 (1965).

32. E. Hayek, Die Mineralsubstanz der Knochen, Klin. Wochenschrift 45: 857 (1967).

33. J. McGregor and B.E.C. Nordin, Equilibration studies with human bone powder, J.Biol.Chem. 235: 1215 (1960).

34. R. Robinson, "The Significance of Phosphoric Esters in Metabolism", New York University Press, New York (1932).

35. A.B. Gutman and T.F. Yü, A concept of the role of enzymes in endochondral calcification, in: "Metabolic Interrelations", E.C. Reifenstein, ed., Josiah Macy, Jr. Foundation, New York (1950).

36. D.S. Howell and J.C. Pita, Calcification and growth plate cartilage with special reference to studies on micropuncture fluids, Clin.Orthop.Rel.Res. 118: 208 (1976).

37. H.H.T. Hsu and H.C. Anderson, Calcification of isolated matrix vesicles and reconstituted vesicles from fetal bovine cartilage, Proc.Nat.Acad.Sci. 75: 3805 (1978).

38. A.L. Lehninger, Mitochondria and calcium ion transport, Biochem.J. 119: 129 (1970).

39. S.Y. Ali, Analysis of matrix vesicles and their role in the calcification of epiphyseal cartilage, Fed.Proc. 35: 135 (1976).

40. J.T. Irving and R.E. Wuthier, Histochemistry and biochemistry of calcification with special reference to the role of lipids, Clin.Orthop. 56: 237 (1968).

41. A.L. Boskey, The role of calcium phospholipid-phosphate complexes in tissue mineralization, Metab.Bone Dis.& Rel.Res. 1: 137 (1978).

42. R. Felix, W. Herrmann, and H. Fleisch, Stimulation of precipitation of calcium phosphate by matrix vesicles, Biochem.J. 170: 681 (1978).

43. R.E. Wuthier, Lipids of matrix vesicles, Fed.Proc. 35: 117 (1976).

44. C.Y.C. Pak, Y. Hayashi, and L.H. Arnold, Hetero-genous nucleation with urate, calcium phosphate and

calcium oxalate, Proc.Soc.Exp.Biol.Med. 153: 83 (1976).

45. J.L. Meyer, J. Bergert, and L.H. Smith, Epitaxial relationships in urolithiasis: The brushite-whewellite system, Clin.Sci.Mol.Med. 52: 143 (1977).

46. H. Fleisch and R.G.G. Russell, Pyrophosphate and polyphosphate, in: "International Encyclopedia of Pharmacology and Therapeutics, Section 51: Pharmacology of the Endocrine System and Related Drugs", H. Rasmussen, ed., Pergamon Press, Oxford and New York (1970).

47. R. Felix and H. Fleisch, Pyrophosphatase and ATPase of isolated cartilage matrix vesicles, Calcif.Tiss. Res. 22: 1 (1976).

48. H. Fleisch and R.G.G. Russell, Experimental and clinical studies with pyrophosphate and diphosphonate, in: "Calcium Metabolism in Renal Failure and Nephrolithiasis, chapter 9", D.S. David, ed., John Wiley & Sons Inc., New York (1977).

49. S. Bisaz, R. Felix, W.F. Neuman, and H. Fleisch, Quantitative determination of inhibitors of calcium phosphate precipitation in whole urine, Min. Electrol.Metab. 1: 74 (1978).

50. J.E. Howard, Studies on urinary stone formation: A saga of clinical investigation, J.Hopkins Med.J. 139: 239 (1976).

51. D.H. Schlesinger and D.I. Hay, Complete covalent structure of statherin, a tyrosine-rich acidic peptide which inhibits calcium phosphate precipitation from human parotid saliva, J.Biol.Chem. 252: 1689 (1977).

52. C. Quittner and C.L. Wadkins, A macromolecular inhibitor of in vitro calcification of tendon matrix, Calcif.Tiss.Res. 25: 161 (1978).

53. W.G. Robertson, Physical chemical aspects of calcium stone-formation in the urinary tract, in: "Urolithiasis Research", H. Fleisch, W.G. Robertson, L.H. Smith, and W. Vahlensieck, eds., Plenum Press, New York and London (1976).

54. W.G. Robertson, F. Knowles, and P. Peacock, Urinary acid mucopolysaccharide inhibitors of calcium oxalate crystallization, in: "Urolithiasis Research", H. Fleisch, W.G. Robertson, L.H. Smith, and W. Vahlensieck, eds., Plenum Press, New York and London (1976).

55. R. Felix, A. Monod, L. Broge, N.M. Hansen, and H. Fleisch, Aggregation of calcium oxalate crystals: Effect of urine and various inhibitors, Urol.Res. 5: 21 (1977).

56. N.M. Hansen, R. Felix, S. Bisaz, and H. Fleisch, Aggregation of hydroxyapatite crystals, Biochim. Biophys.Acta 451: 549 (1976).
57. H. Fleisch, Inhibitors and promoters of stone formation, Kidney Int. 13: 361 (1978).

# INTERACTIONS OF HORMONES, IONS, AND DRUGS IN THE REGULATION OF OSTEOCLASTIC BONE RESORPTION

Lawrence G. Raisz and Joseph A. Lorenzo

University of Connecticut, School of Medicine
Farmington, CT 06032

There are an ever-increasing number of factors which have been identified as having direct effects on bone resorption (Table 1). In part this may be the result of the ease with which organ cultures of bone can be used to identify such factors. They include: 1) calcium regulating hormones, 2) systemic circulating factors, 3) local factors, which have been implicated in pathologic bone resorption, 4) ions, which interact with hormones in the regulation of bone resorption and 5) drugs, which have been used to elucidate mechanisms of bone resorption or as therapy of disorders in which bone resorption is increased such as hypercalcemia and Paget's Disease.

## CALCIUM REGULATING HORMONES

Although parathyroid hormone (PTH) can stimulate bone resorption in organ culture directly[1], the concentrations required are much larger than those which occur in vivo. While this discrepancy remains unexplained, several possibilities have been explored. Direct infusions of 1-84 PTH into isolated canine bone were found to be less effective in stimulating cyclic AMP responses than the 1-34 amino terminal active fragment [2], suggesting that cleavage may be required for maximal activity. However, studies comparing these two compounds in organ cultures have not demonstrated such a discrepancy[3]. Another possibility is that the hormone is inactivated in vitro by oxidation of methionine residues at positions 8 and 18. However, this also seems unlikely since we have found that the dose response curves for 1-34 bovine PTH and an analog in which the methionines are replaced with norleucine are approximately equipotent in the rat organ culture

Table 1.  Factors Influencing Bone Resorption in Vitro

| | ENHANCES | INHIBITS |
|---|---|---|
| CALCIUM REGULATING HORMONES | Parathyroid Hormone<br>Vitamin D Metabolites | Calcitonin |
| SYSTEMIC FACTORS | Thyroid Hormones<br>Epidermal Growth Factor<br>Other Serum Factors | Cortisol<br>Glucagon<br>Nerve Growth<br>Factor |
| LOCAL FACTORS | Prostaglandins<br>Osteoclast Activating Factor<br>Endotoxin | ?Collagenase<br>Inhibitors |
| IONS | Calcium<br>Hydrogen Ion<br>Magnesium | Phosphate<br>Pyrophosphate<br>Lithium |
| DRUGS | Phosphodiesterase<br>Inhibitors<br>Calcium Ionophores<br>Heparin<br>Poly-1-lysine<br>1-24 ACTH | Diphosphonates<br>Mithramycin<br>Colchicine<br>Membrane Stabilizers<br>?Carbonic Anhydrase<br>Inhibitors<br>Lysosomal Enzyme<br>Inhibitors |

system[4]. One explanation for relative insensitivity in organ culture may be that PTH is bound or degraded at sites other than the
biologically active receptor. Support for this concept comes from
recent studies showing that the addition of a basic peptide, poly-1-
lysine, which does not itself stimulate bone resorption, can enhance
the sensitivity of bone to low doses of PTH[5]. Similar effects have
been obtained by the addition of ACTH (Dominquez and Raisz, unpublished observations). Using these compounds it has been possible
to demonstrate substantial bone resorptive responses to $10^{-9}M$ PTH.
However, these concentrations remain much higher than those found
in vivo. 1,25 dihydroxy vitamin D remains by far the most potent
bone resorbing factor yet identified. Recent studies have identified a receptor selective for this compound in bone[9]. Stern and
her co-workers[6,7,8] have established some structure-activity relations which are important for the actions of a number of vitamin D
metabolites. These requirements appear to be relatively broad with
hydroxylation in the 1 and 24 or 25 position conferring the greatest
bone resorbing activity, and hydroxylation in the 3 position also
enhancing potency. There is a discrepancy between the structure-
activity relations for stimulation of bone resorption and inhibition
of bone collagen synthesis. 25 hydroxy and 24,25, hydroxy analogs
do not seem to affect the latter process. It is speculated that
bone may contain more than one vitamin D receptor with differing
specificities. Analysis of the relationship between PTH and vitamin
D in bone resorption has been difficult. Early studies showed synergism between 25 hydroxy vitamin D and PTH (11), however it has not
been possible to demonstrate a similar synergism using 1,25-dihydroxy
vitamin D (Stern, P.H. and Trummel, C.L., unpublished observations).
The two agents clearly act independently in organ culture, however
these systems use tissue obtained from animals exposed to both hormones in vivo.

   The osteoclast is presumably the major, if not the only, target
cell for calcitonin in bone. Calcitonin does not alter bone collagen
synthesis[12] and cell populations which are enriched in osteoblasts
and osteocytes do not show an increased cyclic AMP content in response to calcitonin[13]. A major unresolved question concerning calcitonin is the mechanism of the "escape" phenomenon[14]. Recent studies from Tashjian's laboratory[15] has suggested that this phenomenon
may be due to down regulation of the calcitonin receptor. However,
we have recently found that the inhibitory effect of dibutyryl cyclic
AMP (DBcAMP) on bone resorption is also followed by escape (Figure 1).
Of course, DBcAMP does not truly mimic calcitonin since it also
stimulates resorption slowly when given without PTH. It may be that
a new resistant cell population emerges during inhibition of resorption, since inhibitors of cell replication such as cortisol[16] and
radiation[17] can prevent escape. Whatever the mechanism, solution of
this problem is important clinically. Escape from calcitonin inhibition may explain why this agent has been so ineffective in the long
term treatment of hypercalcemia and hyper-resorptive states other
than Paget's Disease.

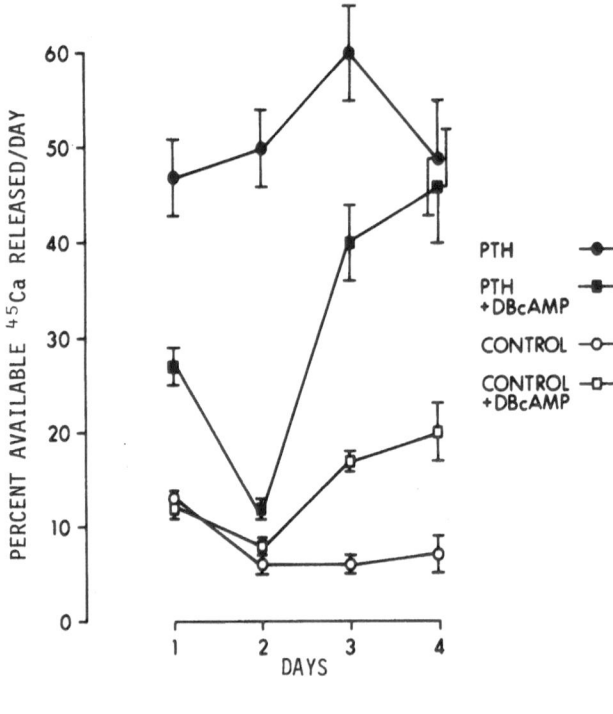

Figure 1

Effect of dibutyrl cyclic AMP (DBcAMP, $3 \times 10^{-4}$M) on the rate of $^{45}$Ca release from control and parathyroid hormone (PTH, $10^{-8}$M) stimulated fetal rat bones. Points are means and vertical lines S.E. for % of available $^{45}$Ca released during one day culture (n=6). Bones were precultured with or without PTH for 24 hours before adding DBcAMP.

SYSTEMIC FACTORS

There are a number of systemic hormones and, as yet unidentified factors which can affect bone resorption directly. Both thyroxin and tri-iodothyronin at low concentrations can stimulate bone resorption in vitro[18]. This effect is probably responsible for the hypercalcemia of thyrotoxicosis, associated with decreased parathyroid activity[19].

The effects of glucocorticoids on bone resorption are complex. In vitro they produce a variable inhibitory effect dependent on the agent stimulating resorption[16,20]. PTH-mediated bone resorption is particularly resistant to cortisol inhibition. In vivo, inhibitory effects of glucocorticoids are frequently overcome by secondary hyperparathyroidism. Another hormone which has been shown, both in vivo and in vitro, to inhibit bone resorption is glucagon [21]. However, its effect in vivo may be indirect as it also stimulates calcitonin secretion. Nerve growth factor (NGF) was recently shown to decrease PTH stimulated bone resorption in vitro [22]. This effect is probably dependent on the ability of the nerve growth factor complex to cause increased degradation of PTH, rather than to a direct effect of NGF on bone cells.

Epidermal growth factor (EGF) has been found to increase resorption of new born mouse calvaria by a mechanism which appeared dependent on prostaglandin synthesis [23]. However, we found using fetal rat long bones that both human and mouse EGF are potent direct stimulators of bone resorption independent of prostaglandin synthesis [24]. EGF not only causes increased resorption but also causes marked cellular proliferation in cultured bone. The relationship between these two phenomenon has not been elucidated. The EGF effect is of particular interest because this material is found in human urine (urogastrone) and may be related to the calcium-mobilizing peptides recently discovered in the urine of hyperparathyroid patients [25]

The presence of resorbing activity in serum[26] is a problem for workers in bone tissue culture because it results in variable control resorption which makes it difficult to compare similar experiments. Potent bone resorbing activity has been identified in certain batches of bovine serum albumin [27], as well as in fetal calf serum (FCS) (Table 2). The activity in FCS can be absorbed out with dextran-coated activated charcoal, is nondialyzable and elutes in the large molecular weight fractions on sephadex G-200 gel filtration [28]. Whether the fetal calf serum factor is new or a combination of already identified hormones remains to be determined. It is of interest that this activity is significant only in fetal calf serum and not in sera obtained from adult humans or post-natal calves in which growth and skeletal turnover are less rapid.


LOCAL FACTORS

Prostaglandins [29], osteoclast activating factor [20] and endotoxin [30] have all been implicated as potential pathologic factors which might produce local bone resorption in inflammatory or neoplastic disease. There is evidence from both animal and human studies that prostaglandins may act systemically to stimulate bone resorption in malignancy [31,32]. Nevertheless, the role of prostaglandins in either physiologic or pathologic bone resorption is far from established. A number of different pathways and metabolites have been implicated. Of the stable prostaglandins, $PGE_2$ and $PGE_1$ are the most potent bone resorbers; among metabolites the 13,14 dihydro-compounds are still quite active, while 15-keto metabolites

Table 2.  Effect of Various Sera Before and After Treatment With Dextran-
          Coated Charcoal (D-C) on Resorption of Cultured Fetal Rat Long
          Bones.

| Serum | $^{45}$Ca released | | Treated/control ratio |
|-------|---------|---------|------------------------|
|       | Before D-C | After D-C | |
| Fetal Calf | 75 ± 5* | 48 ± 3 | 1.56 ± .08* |
| Newborn Calf | 57 ± 7 | 46 ± 3 | 1.24 ± .13 |
| Adult Human | 52 ± 1 | 50 ± 5 | 1.04 ± .03 |

Values are means ± S.E. for 6 cultures maintained for 5 days.

*
Significant effect of D-C treatment.  p < .01.

are inactive [33,34]. There is also a rapid stimulatory effect of
prostaglandin endoperoxides on bone calcium release [34] but these
agents do not appear to be potent stimulators of resorption. Bone
can produce prostaglandins in response to a number of different
stimuli [35,36]. Antibodies to cell surface antigens combined with
complement cause prostaglandin mediated bone resorption which may
involve metabolites other than PGE [37]. Prostacyclin (PGI$_2$) is im-
licated since its metabolite 6-keto-PGE$_1$ is produced by complement-
treated bone; moreover PGI$_2$ as well as a stable analog, thia-
prostacyclin, can stimulate bone resorption in vitro. Since PGI$_2$
is produced by vascular endothelium this finding could explain the
close association between vascular invasion and bone resorption in
haversian canals and at the epiphyseal growth plate. Prostaglandins
not only resorb bone directly, but they may be an important intermediate in the production of osteoclast activating factor (OAF).
Mitogen stimulated T cells can not produce OAF in the absence of
macrophages [38] unless PGE$_2$ is added to the medium [39]. PGE produced by macrophages may also resorb bone directly. This effect
is probably more important in vivo than the ability of macrophages to resorb devitalized bone [40]. Thus, multiple interacting
prostaglandin effects may be involved in the hypercalcemia and
bone destruction of malignancy or inflammatory disease.

Although the pathologic role of OAF in hematologic malignancies
appears established [41] its physiologic role is still elusive. It
has been suggested that OAF is involved in bone marrow development.
Studies of osteopetrosis in experimental animals [42] show an abnormality of the osteoclasts which is unresponsive to all resorptive
stimuli although OAF production in these animals has been demonstrated.

Low concentrations of bacterial endotoxins can stimulate bone
resorption and these substances may play a role in the pathogenesis
of bone loss in osteomyelitis and periodontal disease. In recent
studies of gingival extracts from dogs with chronic periodontitis,
the activity of a bone resorbing factor could not be ascribed solely
to newly-synthesized prostaglandins [43] and may have been due in
part to bacterial endotoxin. However, we can not assess the importance of endotoxin in disease until we know the concentrations
actually reached in bone.

There is relatively little evidence concerning the role of
local inhibitors of bone resorption. The fact that uncalcified
cartilage or osteoid are not resorbed suggest that these tissues
may contain an inhibitor of chondroclasts or osteoclasts. A material has been extracted from cartilage at high concentrations[44]
which inhibits collagenase and can block bone resorption in vitro.

IONS

There is new evidence to support the concept [11,45] that an increase in intracellular calcium concentration may mediate hormonal stimulation of bone resorption. Increased intracellular calcium is thought to be responsible for the stimulation of bone resorption by calcium ionophores such as A23187 [46,47] and ionomycin [48] (Table 3). However, high concentrations of these agents are inhibitory and in one study A23187 was found only to inhibit bone resorption [49]. Recently some of the biochemical changes associated with bone resorption were produced by culturing bone cells at high calcium concentrations [50].

The major effect of hydrogen ion in the regulation of bone resorption appears to be on the dissolution of bone mineral [51]. There is a linear relationship between hydrogen ion concentration and calcium loss from devitalized bone in vitro. In contrast, cell-mediated bone resorption is little affected except at extremes of pH, above 7.5 or below 6.9. These effects are independent of whether pH is altered by changing bicarbonate or carbonic acid concentration, but a $CO_2$ requirement for bone resorption can be demonstrated at concentrations below 0.6% [52]. Inhibition of bone resorption by carbonic anhydrase inhibitors [53] suggests a role for this enzyme. The effect of high pH to inhibit cell-mediated bone resorption is not simply toxic since it is readily reversible. One possible explanation is that when the concentration of hydrogen ion is unusually low ionic calcium is more readily bound intracellularly or taken up by mitochondria so that a calcium dependent step in the stimulation of bone resorption is blocked.

Our understanding of the role of magnesium in regulating bone resorption has been clarified by in vivo studies which demonstrated that in magnesium depletion both the secretion of PTH and the response to PTH are impaired [54]. The latter effect presumably is due to impaired bone resorption [55], but may also be due to enhanced deposition of calcium which occur at low magnesium concentrations [56].

Lithium inhibits bone resorption [57] at concentrations of 3 to 10mM, levels only somewhat greater than those achieved clinically. There is also evidence that prolonged lithium administration may be associated with hyperparathyroidism [58].

PHOSPHATE

The ability of high phosphate concentrations to inhibit cell mediated bone resorption as well as dissolution of bone mineral [55]

Table 3. Effects of Ionomycin on Resorption of Cultured Fetal Rat Long Bones.

| Treatment | $^{45}$% Ca Released | Treated/control ratio |
|---|---|---|
| Control | 38 ± 3 | |
| Ionomycin $10^{-5}$ M | 19 ± 1* | 0.50 ± .03* |
| $10^{-6}$ M | 59 ± 5* | 1.54 ± .14* |
| $10^{-7}$ M | 55 ± 3* | 1.46 ± .09* |
| $10^{-8}$ M | 43 ± 3 | 1.12 ± .08 |

Values are means ± S.E. for 8 bones cultured for 5 days in BGJ medium with 1mg/ml bovine serum albumin (W.A. Soskolne and L.G. Raisz, unpublished observations).

*Significantly different from control, $p < .01$.

and to enhance bone mineralization and collagen synthesis [56], has
been demonstrated in vitro, but the mechanism of these effects is
unknown.  One explanation for the effects is physico-chemical;
high phosphate concentrations causes calcium phosphate to precipitate and decreases the ionized calcium concentration at the
surface of bone.  This would presumably impair the ability of osteoclasts to remove mineral.  Increased intracellular phosphate concentration could drive calcium into mitochondria and lower the
cytosol ionic calcium.  The effect of phosphate is certainly
different from that of other inhibitors of resorption (Table 4).
In contrast to the effect of calcitonin, there is no decrease in
lysosomal enzyme release and the inhibition of PTH stimulated bone
resorption is incomplete.  The inhibition of calcium release by
high phosphate concentrations does cause decreased collagen breakdown [59] presumably because mineralized collagen can not be attacked
by collagenolytic enzymes.  These results suggest that the inhibitory
effect of phosphate is on calcium transport and not on the cellular
induction of the resorptive response.


DRUGS

    Recent studies have suggested some new mechanisms of drug
action on bone resorbing cells and cast some doubt on the role
of cyclic AMP as the major second messenger for stimulation of
bone resorption [60].  It is difficult to reconcile the transient
cyclic AMP response to PTH and PGE with their prolonged effects on
resorption or with the slow direct effects of cyclic nucleotide
analogs (Table 5).  We have examined additional cyclic nucleotide
analogs and found that the action which correlates best with
potency as a stimulator of bone resorption was potency as an
inhibitor of cyclic AMP phosphodiesterase.  For example 8 pCl-
phenyl-thio-cyclic AMP which mimics cyclic  AMP in the kidney [61]
does not stimulate bone resorption, whereas 8-pCl-phenyl-thio-
cyclic GMP which can not mimic cyclic AMP directly but does inhibit cyclic AMP phosphodiesterase [62] stimulates bone resorption
at relatively low concentrations (Table 5).

    Recent studies have revealed two new classes of agents which
inhibit bone resorption; membrane stabilizers or local anesthetic
agents such as propanolol, diphenylhydantoin  and lidocaine [60,63]
and inhibitors of lysosomal enzyme release or action such as
chloroquine, stilbamidine, and dapsone (Table 6).  It is possible
that more than one active membrane system is involved in these
effects.  Transport across the ruffled border of the osteoclast
might be inhibited by local anesthetic agents, while the release
of lysosomal enzymes presumably involves interactions between
lysosomal and surface membranes.  All of these pharmacologic agents,
as well as calcitonin and colchicine [42] show inhibition of

Table 4. Effect of Increasing Medium Phosphate Concentration on $^{45}$Ca and Lysosomal Enzyme Release in Response to Parathyroid Hormone (PTH, 400 ng/ml) and Calcitonin (CT, 10 ng/ml) in Cultured Fetal Rat Bones.

| Treatment | % Total Bone $^{45}$Ca released | | B-Glucuronidase released –nM/hr | |
|---|---|---|---|---|
| | $PO_4$ 1mM | $PO_4$ 4mM | $PO_4$ 1mM | $PO_4$ 4mM |
| Control | 15 ± 1 | 6 ± 1* | 2.5 ± .2 | 1.9 ± .1 |
| CT | 12 ± 1 | 6 ± 1* | 1.8 ± .1 | 1.6 ± .1 |
| PTH | 28 ± 2 | 11 ± 1* | 3.4 ± .2 | 3.4 ± .3 |
| PTH + CT | 12 ± 1 | 6 ± 1* | 2.2 ± .1 | 1.9 ± .2 |

Values are means ± S.E. of four 24 hr cultures.

*Significant effect of high phosphate, p <.01.

Table 5.  Effect of 8 p-Cl Phenylthio Cyclic GMP and AMP (PCcGMP and
PCcAMP) on Resorption of Cultured Fetal Rat Long Bones.

| Treatment | $^{45}$ % Ca Release | Treated/Control Ratio |
|---|---|---|
| Control | 44 ± 3 | |
| PCcGMP 10$^{-4}$ M | 82 ± 7* | 1.86 ± .16* |
| 10$^{-5}$ M | 72 ± 4* | 1.64 ± .08* |
| 10$^{-6}$M | 43 ± 4 | 0.98 ± .09 |
| PCcAMP 10$^{-4}$M | 33 ± 9 | 0.75 ± .20 |
| 10$^{-5}$M | 51 ± 4 | 1.16 ± .10 |
| 10$^{-6}$M | 37 ± 3 | 0.84 ± .07 |

Values are means ± S.E. for 4 to 20 bones cultured for 5 days in BGJ with 5% fetal calf
serum.

*Significantly different from control, $p < .01$.

Table 6.  Effects of Chloroquine (Chlor, $10^{-5}$M) and Stilbamidine (Stilb, $10^{-5}$M) in Parathyroid Hormone (PTH, 100 ng/ml) Stimulated Resorption and B-glucuronidase (B-G) Release in Cultured Fetal Rat Long Bones.

| Treatment | %$^{45}$Ca released | % B-G released |
|---|---|---|
| Control | 19 ± 1 | 24 ± 1 |
| PTH | 36 ± 3* | 42 ± 2* |
| Chlor | 16 ± 1 | 18 ± 1 |
| Stilb | 22 ± 1 | 26 ± 1 |
| PTH + Chlor | 21 ± 1 | 21 ± 1 |
| PTH + Stilb | 20 ± 1 | 23 ± 1 |

Values are means ± S.E. for 8 to 12 bones cultured for 2 days in BGJ with 1 mg/ml bovine serum albumin.

*Significantly different from control, p < .01.

lysosomal enzyme release when they block bone resorption. Moreover, impaired resorption in micropthalamic mice is associated with impaired lysosomal enzyme release [42]. We still do not know precisely the function of these enzymes in resorption. Their early release is consistent with the presence of a material in bone which must be degraded before the bulk of mineral and collagenous matrix can be removed.

CONCLUSION

From this summary it is apparent that many hormones, ions, and drugs influence osteoclastic bone resorption. However, the identification of more factors and accumulation of data on their interactions has not clarified the fundamental processes involved. Progress has been hampered by our inability to study the biochemical changes in isolated osteoclasts while they are engaged in their complex tasks. Future research will depend on adding new methods which measure the function of specific cell types to our present techniques for measuring overall resorbing activity and biochemical changes.

1. L.G. Raisz, Bone resorption in tissue culture. Factors influencing the response to parathyroid hormone, J. Clin. Invest. 44:103 (1965).
2. K.J. Martin, J.J. Freitag, M.B. Conrades, K.A. Hruska, S. Klahr, and E. Slatopolsky, Selective uptake of synthetic amino terminal fragment of bovine parathyroid hormone by isolated perfused bone, J. Clin. Invest. 62:256 (1978).
3. M.P.M. Herrmann-Erlee, J.N.M. Heersche, J.W. Hekkelman, P.J. Gaillard, G.W. Tregear, J.A. Parsons, and J.T. Potts Jr., Effects of bone in vitro of bovine parathyroid hormone and synthetic fragments representing residues 1-34, 2-34, and 3-34, Endocrine Res. Commun. 3:21 (1976).
4. L.G. Raisz, J. Lorenzo, S. Gworek, B.E. Kream, and M. Rosenblatt, Effects of PTH analog on bone metabolism, Calc. Tissue Res. (In press).
5. L.G. Raisz, P.J. Bergmann, J.H. Dominguez, and M.A. Price, Enhancement of parathyroid hormone stimulated bone resorption by poly-1-lysine, Endocrinology (In press).
6. P.H. Stern, H.F. DeLuca, and N. Ikekawa, Bone resorbing activities of 24-hydroxy stereoisomers of 24-hydroxyvitamin $D_3$ and 24,25-dihydroxy vitamin $D_3$, Biochem. Biophys. Res. Commun. 67:965 (1975).
7. P.H. Stern, C.L. Trummel, H.K. Schnoes, and H.F. DeLuca, Bone resorbing activity of vitamin D metabolites and congeners in vitro: Influence of hydroxyl substituents in the A ring,

Endocrinology 97:1552 (1975).

8. P.H. Stern, T. Mavreas, C.L. Trummel, H.K. Schnoes, and H.F. DeLuca, Bone resorbing activity of analogues of 25-hydroxy-cholecalciferol: Effects of side chain modifications and sterioisomerization on responses of fetal rat bones in vitro, Mol. Pharm. 12:879 (1976).

9. B.E. Kream, A specific high-affinity binding macromolecule for 1,25-dihydroxyvitamin $D_3$ in fetal bone, Science 197:1086 (1977).

10. L.G. Raisz, D.M. Maina, S.C. Gworek, J.W. DIetrich, and E.M. Canalis, Hormonal control of bone collagen synthesis in vitro. Inhibitory effects of 1-hydroxylated vitamin D metabolites, Endocrinology 102:731 (1978).

11. L.G. Raisz, Physiologic and pharmacologic regulation of bone resorption. New Eng. J. Med. 282:909 (1970).

12. J.W. Dietrich, E.M. Canalis, D.M. Maina, and L.G. Raisz, Hormonal control of bone collagen synthesis in vitro: Effects of parathyroid hormone and calcitonin, Endocrinology 98:943 (1976).

13. G.L. Wong, and D.V. Cohn, Target cells in bone for parathormone and calcitonin are different: Enrichment for each cell type by sequential digestion of mouse calvaria and selective adhesion to polymeric surfaces, Proc. Nat. Acad. Sci. 72:3167 (1975).

14. J.A. Wener, S.J. Gorton, and L.G. Raisz, Escape from inhibition of resorption in cultures of fetal bone treated with calcitonin and parathyroid hormone, Endocrinology 90:752 (1972).

15. A.H. Tashjian, Jr., D.R. Wright, J.L. Ivey, and A. Pont, Calcitonin binding sites in bone: Relationships to biological response and "Escape", Rec. Prog. Hormone Res. 34:285 (1978).

16. L.G. Raisz, C.L. Trummel, J.A. Wener, and H.A. Simmons, Effect of glucocorticosteroids on bone resorption in tissue culture, Endocrinology 90:961 (1972).

17. N.S. Krieger, Calcitonin and parathyroid hormone interaction in bone: Irradiation-induced inhibition of escape, Prog. 61st Meeting of Endocrine Soc. Abst. 69 (1979).

18. G.R. Mundy, J.L. Shapiro, J.G. Bandelin, E.M. Canalis, and L.G. Raisz, Direct stimulation of bone resorption by thyroid hormones, J. Clin. Invest. 58:529 (1976).

19. L. Mosekilde, and M.S. Christensen, Decreased parathyroid function in hyperthyroidism: Interrelationships between serum parathyroid hormone, calcium-phosphorus metabolism and thyroid function, Acta. Endocrinol. 84:566 (1977).

20. L.G. Raisz, R.A. Luben, G.R. Mundy, J.E. Horton, and C.L. Trummel, Effect of osteoclast activating factor from human leukocytes on bone metabolism, J. Clin. Invest. 56:408 (1975).

21. P.H. Stern, and N.H. Bell, Effects of glucagon on serum calcium in the rat and on bone resorption in tissue culture, Endocrinology

87:111 (1970).

22. S.J. Teitelbaum, R.Y. Andres, N.E. Cooke, T.J. Hahn, and A.J. Kahn, Inhibition of parathyroid-hormone induced fetal rat bone resorption in vitro by nerve growth factor, Calc. Tissue Res. 26:203 (1978).

23. A.H. Tashjian, Jr., and L. Levine, Epidermal growth factor stimulates prostaglandin production and bone resorption in cultured mouse calvaria, Biochem. Biophys. Res. Commun. 85:966 (1978).

24. H.A. Simmons, E. Canalis, and L.G. Raisz, Effect of epidermal growth factor on resorption of fetal rat long bone in vitro, Prog. 1st Annual Meeting Amer. Soc. Bone & Min. Res. Abst. 14 (1979).

25. N. Nijs-De Wolf, N. DeNutte, H. Brauman, and J. Corvilain, Parathyroid hormone-like biological activity in urine, Clin. Science 54:349 (1978).

26. P.H. Stern, and L.G. Raisz, An analysis of the role of serum in parathyroid hormone induced bone resorption in tissue culture, Exper. Cell Res. 46:106 (1967).

27. P.H. Stern, J.C. Miller, S.F. Chen, and D.J. Kahn, A bone re-sorbing substance from bovine serum albumin, Calc. Tissue Res. 25:233 (1978).

28. J.A. Lorenzo and L.G. Raisz, Bone-resorbing activity in fetal calf serum, Prog. 1st Annual Meeting of Amer. Soc. Bone & Min. Res. Abst. 17 (1979).

29. D.C. Klein, and L.G. Raisz, Prostaglandins: Stimulation of bone resorption in tissue culture, Endocrinology 86:1436 (1970).

30. E. Hausmann, L.G. Raisz, and W.A. Miller, Endotoxin: Stimulation of bone resorption in tissue culture, Science 168:862 (1970).

31. E.F. Voelkel, A.H. Tashjian, Jr., R. Franklin, E. Wasserman, and L. Levine, Hypercalcemia and tumor-prostaglandins: The $VX_2$ carcinoma model in the rabbit, Metabolism 24:973 (1975).

32. H.W. Seyberth, G.V. Segre, J.L. Morgan, B.J. Sweetman, J.T. Potts Jr., and J.A. Oates, Prostaglandins as mediators of hypercalcemia associated with cancer, New Eng. J. of Med. 293:1278 (1975).

33. A.H. Tashjian, Jr., J.E. Tice, and K. Sides, Biological activities of prostaglandin analogues and metabolites on bone in organ culture, Nature 266:645 (1977).

34. L.G. Raisz, J.W. Dietrich, H.A. Simmons, H.W. Seyberth, W. Hubbard, and J.A. Oates, Effect of prostaglandin endoperoxides and meta-bolites on bone resorption in vitro, Nature 267:532 (1977).

35. L.G. Raisz, A. Sandberg, J.M. Goodson, H.A. Simmons, and S.E. Mergenhagen, Complement-dependent stimulation of bone resorption mediated by prostaglandins, Science 185:789 (1974).

36. A.J. Tashjian, J.L. Ivey, B. Declos, and L. Levine, Stimulation of prostaglandin production in bone by phorbol diesters and mellittin, Prostaglandin 16:221 (1978).

37. L.G. Raisz, J.Y Vanderhoek, H.A. Simmons, B.E. Kream, and K.C.

Nicolaou, Prostaglandin synthesis by fetal rat bone in vitro: Evidence for a role of prostacyclin, Prostaglandins (In press).

38. J.E. Horton, J.J. Oppenheim, L.G. Raisz, and S.E. Mergenhagen, Macrophage lymphocyte synergy in the production of osteoclast activating factor (OAF), J. Immunol. 113:1278 (1974).

39. T. Yoneda, G.R. Mundy, Prostaglandins are necessary for osteoclast-activating factor production by activated peripheral blood leukocytes, J. Exper. Med. 149:279 (1979).

40. G.R. Mundy, A.J. Altman, M.D. Gondek, and J.G. Bandelin, Direct resorption of bone by human monocytes, Science 196:1109 (1977).

41. G.R. Mundy, Calcium and cancer, Life Sciences 23:1735 (1978).

42. L.G. Raisz, H.A. Simmons, S.C. Gworek, and G. Eilon, Studies on congenital osteopetrosis in microphthalmic mice using organ cultures--impairment of bone resorption in response to physiologic stimulators, J. Exper. Med. 145:857 (1977).

43. R.M. Hopps, K. Nuki, and L.G. Raisz, Demonstration of bone resorptive activity in freeze-dried gingiva, J. of Dental Res. Special Issue C 58:1245 (1979).

44. J.E. Horton, F.H. Wezemann, K.E. Kuettner, Inhibition of bone resorption in vitro by a cartilage-derived anticollagenase factor, Science 199:1342 (1978).

45. L.G. Raisz, C.L. Trummel, and H.A. Simmons, Induction of bone resorption in tissue culture. Prolonged response after brief exposure to parathyroid hormone or 25-hydroxycholecalciferol, Endocrinology 90:744 (1972).

46. R. Dziak and P.H. Stern, Responses of fetal rat bone cells and bone organ cultures to the ionophore, A23187, Calc. Tissue Res. 22:137 (1976).

47. G. Eilon, and L.G. Raisz, Comparison of the effects of stimulators and inhibitors of resorption on the release of lysosomal enzymes and radioactive calcium from fetal bone in organ culture, Endocrinology 103:1969 (1978).

48. C.M. Liu, T.E. Hermann, Characterization of ionomycin as a calcium ionophore, J. of Biol. Chem. 253:5892 (1978).

49. J.L. Ivey, D.R. Wright, A.H. Tashjian, Jr., Bone resorption in organ culture, J. Clin. Invest. 58:1327 (1976).

50. G.L. Wong, G.N. Kent, K.Y. Ku, D.V. Cohn, Interaction of parathormone and calcium and hormone-regulated synthesis of hyaluronic acid and citrate dicarboxylation in isolated bone cells, Endocrinology 103:2274 (1978).

51. J.H. Dominguez and L.G. Raisz, The effect of $CO_2$, $HCO_3^-$, $H^+$ concentrations of bone resorption in vitro, Calc. Tissue Res. (In press).

52. A. Mahgoub and P.H. Stern, Carbon dioxide and the effect of parathyroid hormone on bone, Amer. J. Physiol. 226:1272 (1974).

53. C. Minkin, and J.M. Jennings, Carbonic anhydrase and bone remodeling: sulfonamide inhibition of bone resorption in organ culture, Science, 176:4038 (1972).

54. R.K. Rude, S.B. Oldman, F.R. Singer, Functional hypoparathyroidism

and parathyroid hormone end-organ resistance in human magnesium deficiency, Clin. Endocrinol. 5:209 (1976).

55. L.G. Raisz, and I. Niemann, Effect of phosphate, calcium and magnesium on bone resorption and hormonal responses in tissue culture, Endocrinology 85:446 (1969).

56. P.J. Bingham and L.G. Raisz, Bone growth in organ culture: Effects of phosphate and other nutrients on bone and cartilage, Calc. Tissue Res. 14:31 (1974).

57. H.M. Holak.and L.G. Raisz, Effect of lithium on bone metabolism in organ culture, Endocrinology 104:908, 1978.

58. L.I. Christensson, Lethium, hypercalcemia and hyperparathyroidism, The Lancet 2:144 (1976).

59. J.S. Brand, and L.G. Raisz, Effects of thyrocalcitonin and phosphate ion on the parathyroid hormone stimulated of bone, Endocrinology 90:479 (1972).

60. M.P.M. Herrmann-Erlee, and J.M. v.d. Meer, The effects of dibutyryl cyclic AMP, aminophylline and propanolol on PTE-induced bone resorption in vitro, Endocrinology 94:424 (1974).

61. D.A. Hall, L.D. Barnes, and T.P. Dousa, Cyclic AMP in action of antidiuretic hormone:  Effects of exogenous cyclic AMP and its new analogue, Amer. J. Physiol. 232:F368 (1977).

62. J.P. Miller, K.H. Boswell, A.M. Mian, R.B. Meyer, R.K. Robins and R.A. Khwaja, 2' derivatives of guanosine and inosine cyclic 3',5'-phosphates. Synthesis, enzymic activity and the effect of 8-substituents, Biochem., 15:217 (1976).

63. J.W. Dietrich, G.R. Mundy, and L.G. Raisz, Inhibition of bone resorption in tissue culture by membrane stabilizing agents, Endocrinology 104:1644 (1979).

# RECENT ADVANCES IN MANAGEMENT OF OSTEOPOROSIS

G. Donald Whedon, M.D.

National Institute of Arthritis, Metabolism, and
Digestive Diseases, National Institutes of Health
Bethesda, Maryland 20205, USA

Osteoporosis is defined as a condition of decreased total bone mass, that is, a decrease in amount of essentially normal bone tissue within an undiminished outer bone volume or envelope. The suggestion in recent years of a substitute term, "osteopenia," came from a desire to give a better indication of decreased bone mass. The degree of bone loss has not been specifically determined, but in concept it is that beyond which bones under stress are especially susceptible to fracture. Although the key word in the title of this paper is "management," some comments on etiology are important, because out of a broadening of our ideas of cause and development over the past 35 years have come suggestions for more intelligent management overall and even for potential treatment for milder or earlier forms.

Albright[1] in 1941 coined the term, "postmenopausal," for the most common form, recognizing the sex ratio of 4 to 1, women over men, and built a specific mechanism, decreased bone formation, and a recommendation for therapy into the definition, as though it was a specific disease. The condition in men, generally older when diagnosed, has been assigned the term "senile." Incidentally, the word "idiopathic" is an attractive trap for the unitiated since it implies lack of understanding, but for the regulars in the bone specialty, the term "idiopathic" is reserved for an unusual group of cases of early onset, usually in the 20s and 30s (years of age), and most frequently males.

The consensus today is that clinical osteoporosis is really a "syndrome" with a common physical state of bone atrophy resulting from any one or usually more of several potential causes or mechanisms.[2-4] As a temporary but practical aside from consideration of

the main aspects of the general disorder, the very first step in
clinical management is to rule in or out a major demineralizing
effect from other diseases or from drug therapies.[2,4]  The most
usual other diseases with associated osteoporosis are hyperparathyroidism, hyperthyroidism, hyperadrenocorticism ("Cushing's"
disease or syndrome), acromegaly, osteogenesis imperfecta tarda,
multiple myeloma, paralysis, long-time immobilization, diabetes, and
advanced renal disease.  Usually associated with localized demin-
eralization but occasionally generalized are rheumatoid and other
forms of arthritis and metastatic or advancing carcinoma.  The most
usual drugs associated with osteoporosis are corticosteroids,
heparin and alcohol.  Depending upon the degree of advancement of
the accompanying osteoporosis and the availability of therapy for
the original disease, dealing specifically with the original disease
may be effective, or somewhat effective, against the bone atrophy.

As may be inferred from the several different possible associated diseases, the bone pathology may be somewhat varied from case
to case, and some degree of osteomalacia may even be superimposed.

To understand the most common form of osteoporosis, so-called
postmenopausal or senile, it is useful to have a sense of the
physiological and pathophysiological processes within the skeleton.[5]
In the dynamics of bone tissue that lead to osteoporosis, bone
resorption must exceed bone formation.  Based mainly on histologic
observations and measurements, Parfitt[6] makes the case that in
involutional bone loss (loss with aging) depression of osteoblast
function is the major process, in other words, with advancing age
bone building and rebuilding simply slow down.  Clinical osteoporosis, however, must result from a rate of bone loss somewhat
greater than 0.5 to 1.0 percent per year, and this loss is visual-
ized as occurring through turned up bone resorption by osteoclasts,
not necessarily in steady fashion.  The systemic factors which
interplay, or reinforce one another, to bring about intensified bone
resorption are, in three classes, physical, nutritional and hormonal.

Just how the absence of physical stress brings about rapid bone
loss is uncertain,[7] whether by some interaction between decreased
direct physical or piezo-electric forces, diminished muscle pull on
periosteum or some combination of altered neurologic or circulatory
factors.  The net effect, however--as shown (Figure 1) in a study of
immobilized bed rest[8,9] on four healthy subjects carried out many
years ago--is gradually increasing urinary calcium to a plateau
double the control level and increased fecal calcium as well.  No
amount of vigorous exercise will prevent this mineral loss if weight-
bearing is not present, as attested by the balance studies[10] carried
out a few years ago on astronauts during the Skylab orbital space
flights; in those measurements the pattern and degree of calcium
loss for the duration of the flights of up to 3 months was very

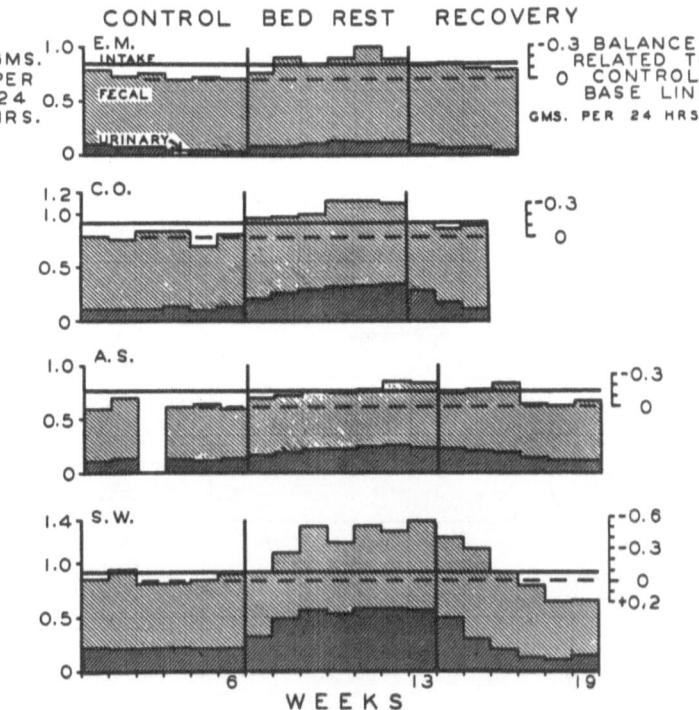

Fig. 1. Effect of immobilization on the calcium metabolism of four
normal male subjects. In each subject the daily calcium intake was
kept constant throughout all periods of the experiment. For each
subject the control base-line (interrupted horizontal line) is an
average of the total outputs of the last four control weeks. In
this graph the intake and output are plotted upward from the zero
base-line. (Reproduced by permission of Med. Clin. N. Amer.[9])

similar to that of immobilized bed rest. Lesser degrees of inactivity bring about lesser degrees of bone loss, as found in more recent
bed rest studies.[11]

In the class of nutritional factors, failure to maintain
calcium balance, whether by impaired intake or intestinal absorption
or by excessive loss, is a significant contributing factor to bone
loss over long periods of time. The basic logic of a central role
for the building block minerals, calcium and phosphorus, is displayed in a diagram (Figure 2) of the various metabolic processes of
calcium.[5] The key to the logic is that the body zealously maintains
the concentration of calcium in the miscible pool, including the
serum, within narrow limits, and if any deficit occurs from inadequate input or excessive excretion, bone mineral is sacrificed to
hold pool concentration at the proper level.

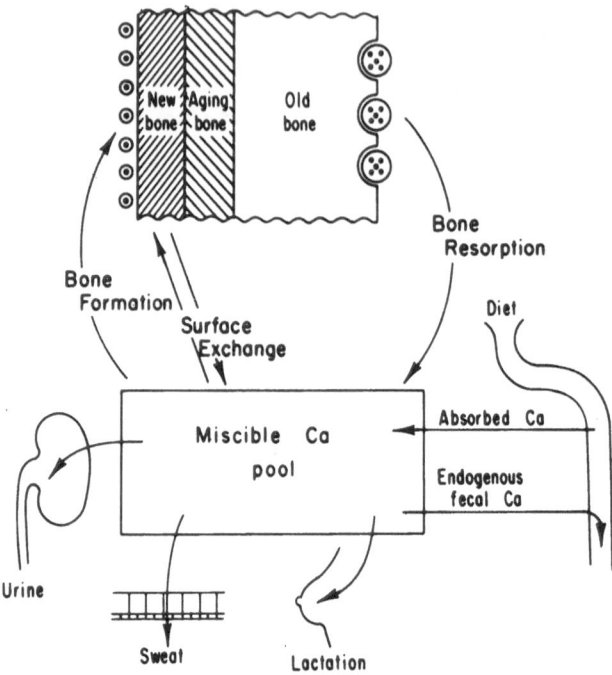

Fig. 2.   Schematic presentation of major metabolic processes of calcium homeostasis.   (Reproduced by permission of <u>Disease-a-Month</u>.[2])

Among the alterations in various input and output pathways which would affect calcium balance adversely, low customary dietary intake is the most obvious, and the correlation has been demonstrated--as in a graph (Figure 3) of the relationship between dietary calcium intake and balance in Heaney's study of 100 normal postmenopausal women[12] and Riggs' dietary survey[13] of normal versus osteoporotic women (Figure 4).

Customary low calcium intake may be associated with intestinal lactase deficiency in which patients will lower their milk intake to avoid gastrointestinal symptoms.  The association among this enzyme deficiency, low calcium intake and osteoporosis was first reported by Birge and others in our group at NIH several years ago.[14] Table 1 from Riggs' study of 139 osteoporotic women[13] illustrates a number of other influences on calcium balance.  In this table, besides low dietary intake are listed hypercalciuria, steatorrhea (which could increase endogenous fecal excretion or interfere with

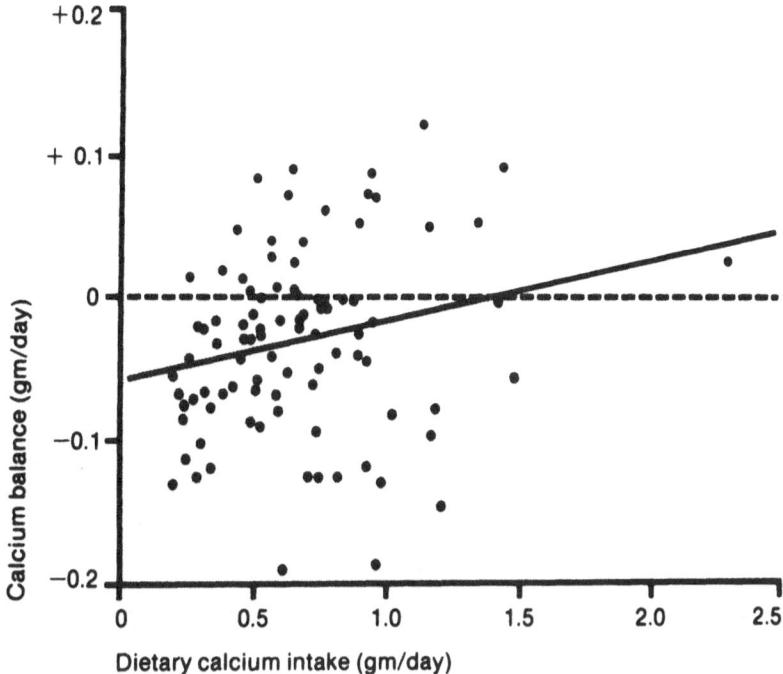

Fig. 3.   Relationship between calcium balance and dietary calcium intake in 100 postmenopausal women.[12]

absorption or both) and abnormal intestinal absorption (nearly 50 percent as measured in this small group).

Of particular interest to this audience would be the question of whether high dietary intakes of phosphorus or protein influence calcium balance adversely and thus contribute to the development of osteoporosis.  The effect of high protein intake to increase urinary calcium is well established[15-17] and adds another reason to decry the popular trend toward higher meat proportions in the diet to the one mentioned by Coe with regard to nephrolithiasis.[18]   Spencer,[19] on the other hand, recently reported that increasing the protein intake from 1 to 2 gm./kg./day, given as meat, did not raise the urinary calcium, attributing the lack of change to the high phosphorus content of the type of protein used.  As for phosphorus intakes, there is abundant animal data (notably from Clark[20]) to show that dietary calcium/phosphorus ratios below 1.0 tend to interfere with intestinal calcium absorption and cause osteitis fibrosa cystica and kidney damage, but Heaney in a recent review of studies *in humans* by Spencer[21] and by himself concluded that "variations in dietary phosphate intake have no apparent net effect on calcium balance."[22]

Estimated dietary calcium intake

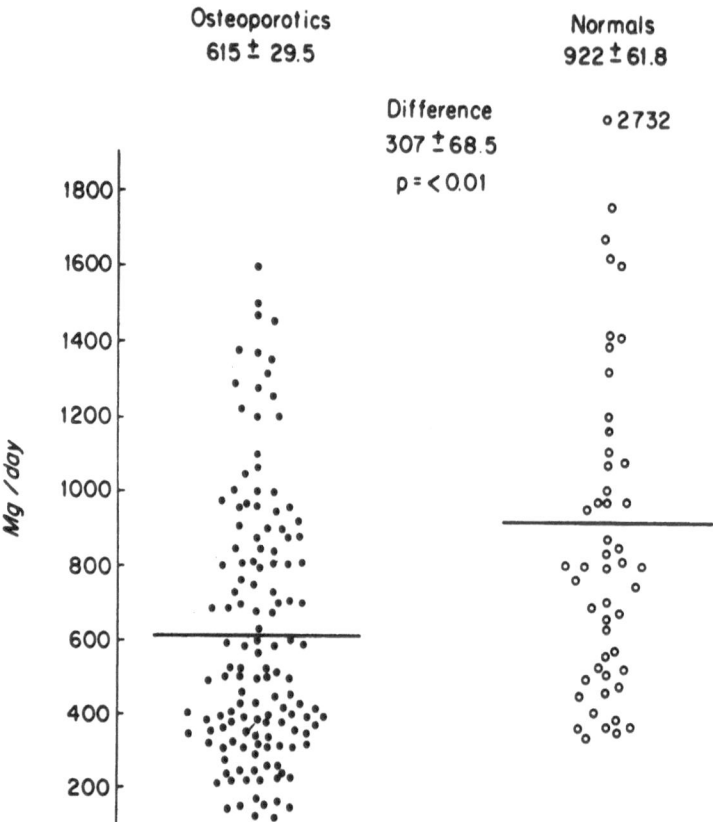

Fig. 4. Results of survey of dietary calcium intake of osteoporotic versus normal individuals, indicating significantly lower customary intake in those with osteoporosis.[13]

The association of alterations in hormone production, particularly of estrogen, with osteoporosis needs no formal exposition in this discussion, but some recent data bearing on this association should be of interest. Table 2 from a prospective study by Johnston[23] of rates of bone loss in females, using the Norland-Cameron technique on the radius, shows the effect of estrogen withdrawal after the menopause. Among the three different age groups, the rate of loss was much greater in the group shortly after menopause (mean 57 years) than in the groups with mean ages of 44 and 80 years. Heaney's observations[12] on a large number of pre-menopausal and post-menopausal women treated and untreated with estrogens showed that estrogen-deprived women, as compared with those with estrogens, have (1) a considerably higher calcium intake requirement for balance

Table 1.

**POSSIBLE ABNORMALITIES IN
CALCIUM METABOLISM**
139 Osteoporotic Patients

|  | Patients | |
| --- | --- | --- |
|  | No. | % |
| Low dietary intake (< 400 mg/da) | 49 | 35.3 |
| Hypercalciuria (> 250 mg/da) | 26 | 18.7 |
| Steatorrhea (> 10 gm/da) | 8 | 5.8 |
| Abnormal intestinal absorp. calcium[47] (31 cases studied) | 15 | 48.4 |

Table 2.  Prospective study of rates of bone loss in females

| Mean age (years ± SD) | No. of subjects | Midshaft bone loss (gm/cm/yr) ± SE | Distal bone loss (gm/cm/yr) ± SE |
| --- | --- | --- | --- |
| 44.5 ± 5.0 | 39 | −0.0049 ± 0.0027 | −0.0053 ± 0.0031 |
| 56.7 ± 4.5 | 89 | −0.0116 ± 0.0008* | −0.0147 ± 0.0011* |
| 80.5 ± 5.8 | 70 | −0.0015 ± 0.0015 | −0.0007 ± 0.0015 |

*P < .005

Adapted from C. C. Johnston, Jr.[23]

(Figure 5); (2) less effective intestinal calcium absorption; and (3) a higher mean 24-hour urinary calcium level by about 17 mg./day, a significant figure when cumulative over several years.

More specific data on recent advances in management or therapy, may be presented in three parts: firstly, data on agents or modalities intended to suppress bone resorption; secondly, data on efforts at actual bone repair or restoration with agents which are intended to increase bone turnover and formation; and, thirdly, brief progress notes on several new agents.

At center stage for a long time in the so-called "treatment" of postmenopausal osteoporosis have been various estrogen preparations, but firm support for their efficacy has only come forward within the past few years. Development of methods have long been awaited for measuring bone mineral content with sufficient precision and reproducibility to be applied to prospective therapeutic trials. A number of such methods have now arrived, and they along with microradiography for measurements of bone forming and resorbing surfaces, now make it possible to say clearly that estrogens are effective in suppressing bone resorption. Table 3 is from a study by Riggs[24] on the effects of 10 to 16 weeks of estrogen therapy in postmenopausal osteoporotic women. It shows no change in bone forming surfaces, a marked reduction in resorbing surfaces, the usual reduction in serum calcium and an increase in serum iPTH; the latter finding suggests that estrogen impedes or interferes with the action of PTH on bone and fits the concept that estrogen decline after the menopause facilitates development of osteoporosis by increased sensitivity of bone to the action of PTH. There is agreement among the results of the three principal studies on estrogens[25-27] in which bone mineral content and cortical bone thickness were measured; estrogen therapy slowed or prevented bone loss in postmenopausal women. Figure 6 from the study by Horsman et al.[27] shows the effectiveness of estrogens in protecting metacarpal cortical area; in fact, the data indicate a slight increase in this bone area measurement. The exact place of and best recommendation for estrogens in osteoporosis is now uncertain, however, at least in the United States, because of concern for their reported effects on blood coagulation and the recognized possibility that endometrial carcinoma may be stimulated by them. If estrogens *are* given to postmenopausal women, the consensus is that they should be given in small dose, in interrupted cyclical sequence with progestin and there be withdrawal of both hormones to allow periodic bleeding. Regular examinations should be made for early detection of endometrial neoplasm. Fortunately, this form of cancer is one of the easiest to recognize early and early treatment is generally effective. Over how many years estrogens should or may be given is in doubt; their action on bone more than just a few years after the menopause may not be as great, and it is possible that there is increased sensitivity of older individuals to estrogen.

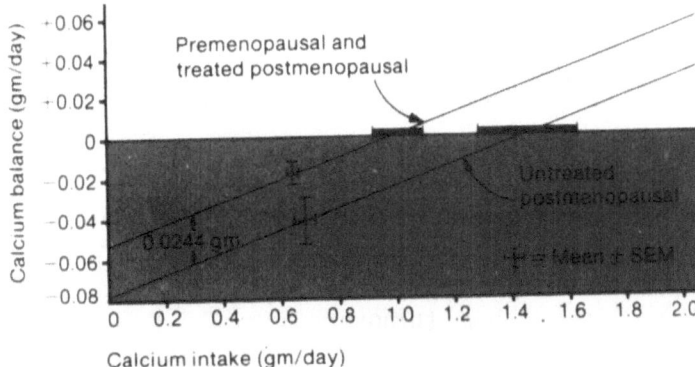

Fig. 5. Comparison of relationship between calcium balance and dietary calcium intake in estrogen-replete and estrogen-deprived women.[12]

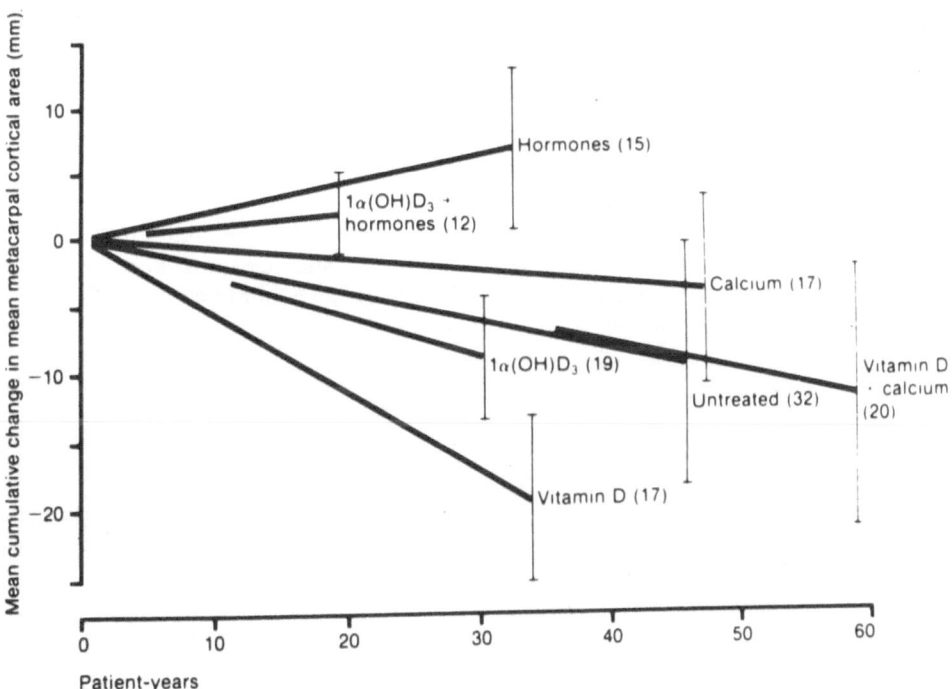

Fig. 6. Comparisons of effects of six different therapies on mean metacarpal cortical area in postmenopausal osteoporotic women;[27] cumulative change over patient-years. Figures in parentheses indicate numbers of patients.

| | Bone turnover (%total surface as assessed by microradiography) | | Serum levels | |
|---|---|---|---|---|
| | Formation | Resorption | Calcium (mg/dl) | i PTh (μl eq/ml) |
| Before treatment | 3.3 ± .5 | 13.0 ± .8 | 9.60 ± .07 | 24.7 ± 2.0 |
| After treatment | 3.3 ± .6 | 7.2 ± .6 | 9.14 ± .05 | 34.5 ± 3.6 |
| P value | NS | <.001 | <.001 | <.01 |

*iPTH levels measured in eight patients only

Table 3. Effects of 10- to 16-week course of estrogen therapy on bone turnover and serum calcium and immunoreactive parathyroid hormone (iPTH levels in 17* postmenopausal osteoporotic women

With regard to mineral supplements, the two major studies[26,27] agree that they are *also* effective in suppressing bone resorption in postmenopausal women though somewhat less so than estrogens. Figure 7 from the study of Horsman et al.[27] indicates that calcium supplementation effectively prevented increasing collapse of vertebrae in contrast to the result in untreated cases and, in fact, more effectively in this area of the skeleton than estrogens.

Concern is sometimes expressed with calcium supplementation as to possible increased risk of urinary tract stone formation from an increase in urinary calcium; fortunately, the degree to which urinary calcium is raised is slight. Data from Heaney indicated that for each gram of calcium added to the intake, the mean increase in urinary calcium was 69 mg.[28]; in an earlier study with a much smaller number of patients, Lutwak and Whedon found the increase even less, 46 mg. of urinary calcium for each gram of added calcium supplement.[2] Thus, unless the patient has a history of stone formation or an infected urinary tract, as long as adequate fluid intake and urine output are maintained, the risk of stone formation from calcium supplementation seems insignificant.

Experience with vitamin D and its analogues is limited and results in studies thus far are not conclusive, but Riggs found reduced serum levels of 1,25 dihydroxy-vitamin D in some patients with osteoporosis[29] and the correlation of this reduction with decreased intestinal absorption of calcium was significant.[30] A 6-month controlled trial of 1,25 dihydroxy-D in these patients improved calcium absorption and calcium balance.[31] Care must be taken, however, with administration of 1,25 dihydroxy-D since too high a dose may increase bone resorption.

Probably the most interesting, if not exciting, part of the story concerns the new agents which have been suggested as means of stimulating osteoid formation. Sodium fluoride (NaF) was first introduced for this purpose in the 1960s[32] but did not pick up real interest until it looked as though giving 1 gram/day of calcium supplement with the fluoride might prevent the bizarre, malacic architecture produced by fluoride alone.[33] As assessed by microradiography, on iliac crest biopsy samples,[34] NaF and Ca increase bone forming surfaces in relation to the dose of fluoride (Figure 8) and decrease bone resorbing surfaces in relation to the dose of oral calcium (Figure 9). Meunier[35] has found that NaF with Ca increased osteoid surfaces three-fold, increased resorption surfaces x 1.7 and also increased trabecular bone volume. Various investigators,[36] however, have cautioned about the use of fluoride, including Riggs,[37] who has written regarding his experience with a dosage of 40-60 mg. NaF daily:

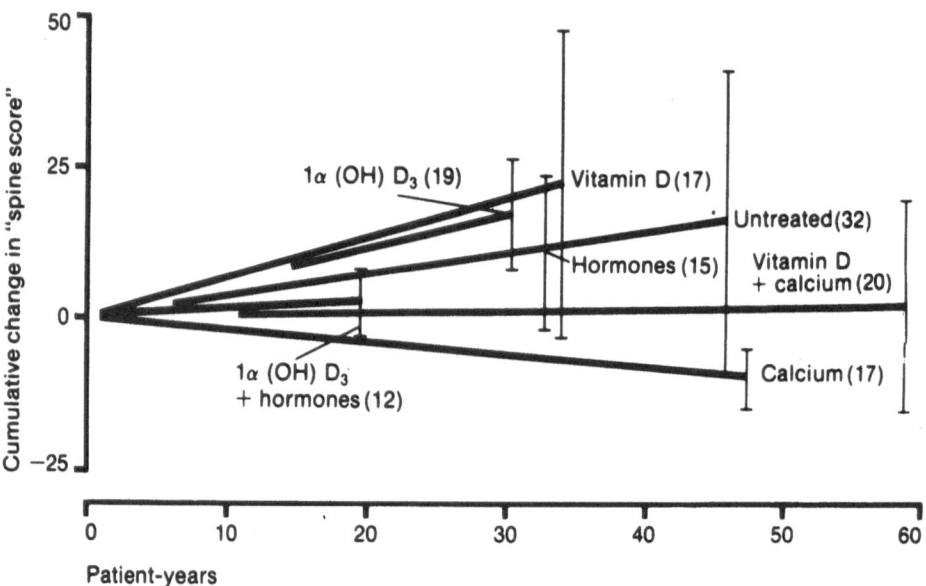

Fig. 7. Comparison of effects of six different therapies on "spine score" in postmenopausal osteoporotic women; cumulative change over patient-years. Negative change represents a favorable result.

"Many studies have shown that the breaking strength of bone
is highly related to bone mass. Fluoridic bone, however,
has increased crystallinity and decreased elasticity and,
thus, does not necessarily have normal strength. Several
studies (including our own unpublished data) indicate
that additional vertebral fractures occur even after up to
6 years of combined therapy with sodium fluoride and calcium
supplements. We have also found that significant side effects
(synovitis, recurrent, vomiting, painful plantar fascitis, and
anemia from gastrointestinal bleeding) may occur in up to 50%
of patients treated for 4 to 6 years. The true incidence of
side effects and the antifracture efficacy of combined therapy
with sodium fluoride and calcium for osteoporosis must await
a controlled prospective study, and at present fluoride should
be used only for investigational purposes ".

The second agent recently suggested (by Parsons[38]) as a possible stimulant to bone formation is parathyroid hormone (PTH) itself,
more particularly the 1-34 synthetic fragment. By giving small
enough doses it was thought that bone remodeling would be encouraged.
Indeed, not only are resorbing surfaces increased but also trabecular
osteoid surfaces. Preliminary studies in humans are, however, not
convincing and whether its administration along with other agents,
such as calcium supplements, will be useful awaits further study.

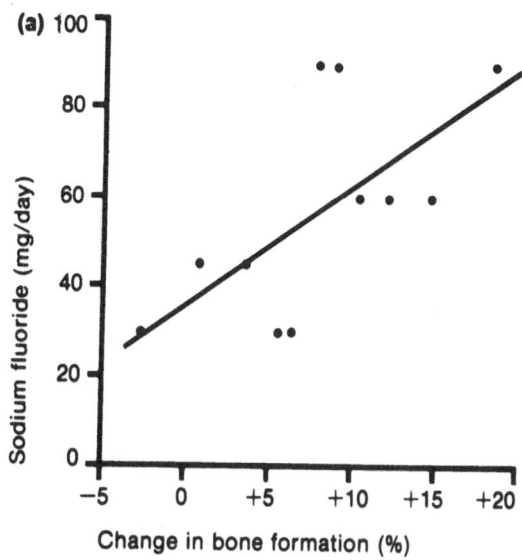

Fig. 8. Effect of combined therapy with sodium fluoride and calcium supplements on bone remodeling in 11 patients with osteoporosis: direct relationship of changes in bone-forming surfaces to dose of fluoride.[34,37]

A number of other substances have been suggested, particularly with suppression of bone resorption in mind: calcitonin, oral phosphate, the di-phosphonates (EHDP and $Cl_2MDP$), and a synthetic androgen, stanozolol. Except for oral phosphate which causes a considerable *increase* in bone resorbing surfaces and so is not regarded as a useful treatment alternative, these latter compounds have been insufficiently studied clinically to determine their possible value.

To epitomize only the most important points relative to management of osteoporosis at this time: an awareness of the three classes of factors (physical, nutritional and hormonal) affecting calcium balance is essential for understanding the pathogenesis of the diminished bone mass in osteoporosis and also for developing more effective management. With these factors in mind, prevention or early treatment are still the surest ways to maintain or obtain a sound skeleton, and even in this time of many new treatment ideas aimed at stimulating bone formation, the physician should not wait until osteoporosis is far advanced; from what we know now no treatment will bring back lost trabeculae. Specifically, the fundamentals

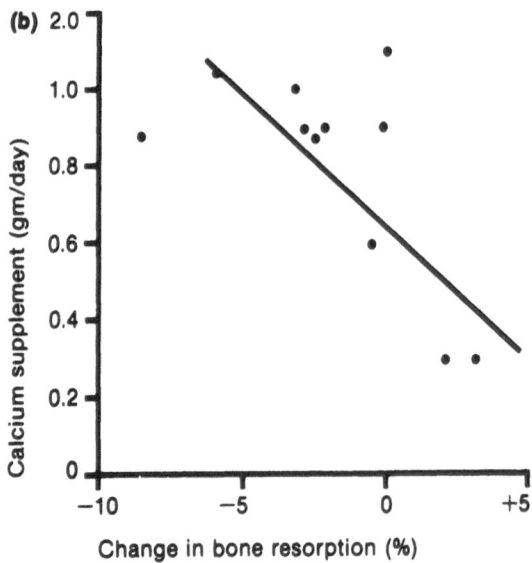

Fig. 9. Effect of combined therapy with sodium fluoride and calcium supplements on bone remodeling in 11 patients with osteoporosis: inverse relationship of changes in bone-resorbing surfaces to dose of oral calcium.[34,37]

of comprehensive management of osteoporosis still involve avoidance of physical inactivity, attention to dietary calcium and phosphorus early if not throughout life, addition of oral calcium supplements, administration of an appropriate vitamin D analogue when malabsorption of mineral is detected, and in those individuals identifiable as particularly at risk of osteoporosis, use of estrogen with suitable caution. Research on the management of clinical osteoporosis, however, is now in a high turnover stage (pun intended) with many new agents undergoing or awaiting more detailed and definitive study.

References

1. F. Albright, P. H. Smith and A. M. Richardson, Post-menopausal osteoporosis: its clinical features, J.A.M.A. 116:2465 (1941).
2. L. Lutwak and G. D. Whedon, Osteoporosis, Disease-a-Month, Year Book Med. Publ. Inc., Chicago, pp. 1-39 (April 1963).

3.  R. P. Heaney, A unified concept of osteoporosis, Am. J. Med.
    39:877-880 (1965).
4.  B.E.C. Nordin, The osteoporoses, in: "Metabolic Bone and Stone
    Disease," Williams and Wilkins Co., Baltimore, pp. 1-52
    (1973).
5.  G. D. Whedon, Osteoporosis, in: "Clinical Endocrinology, Vol.
    II," Astwood and Cassidy, eds., Grune and Stratton, Inc.,
    New York, pp. 349-376 (1968).
6.  A. M. Parfitt, Remodeling dynamics in osteoporosis, in:
    "International Symposium on Osteoporosis," St. John, Virgin
    Islands, October 25-27, 1978, sponsored by Marion Labora-
    tories, Inc., R. P. Heaney, ed., Biomed. Inf. Corp., New
    York, pp. 21-24 (1979).
7.  G. D. Whedon, Osteoporosis:  atrophy of disuse, in: "Bone as
    a Tissue," Rodahl, Nicholson and Brown, eds., McGraw-Hill,
    New York, pp. 67-82 (1960).
8.  J. E. Deitrick, G. D. Whedon and E. Shorr, Effects of immobili-
    zation upon various metabolic and physiologic functions of
    normal men, Am. J. Med. 4:3-36 (January 1948).
9.  G. D. Whedon, Management of the effects of recumbency, Med.
    Clin. N. Amer. 35, No. 2: 545-562 (March 1951).
10. G. D. Whedon, L. Lutwak, J. Reid, P. Rambaut, M. Whittle, M.
    Smith and C. Leach, Mineral and nitrogen metabolic studies
    on Skylab orbital space flights, Trans. Assoc. Am. Physi-
    cians 87:95-109 (1974).
11. C. L. Donaldson, S. B. Hulley, J. M. Vogel, R. S. Hattner,
    J. H. Bayers and D. McMillan, Effect of prolonged bed rest
    on bone mineral, Metabolism 19, No. 12: 1071 (December 1970).
12. R. P. Heaney, R. R. Recker and P. D. Saville, Menopausal changes
    in metabolic balance performance, J. Lab. Clin. Med. 92:953-
    963 (1978).
13. B. L. Riggs, P. J. Kelly, V. R. Kinney, D. A. Scholz and A. J.
    Bianco, Jr., Calcium deficiency and osteoporosis:  observa-
    tions in 166 patients and critical review of the literature,
    J. Bone & Jt. Surg. 49A, No. 5: 915-924 (July 1967).
14. S. J. Birge, Jr., H. L. Keutmann, P. Cuatrecasas and G. D.
    Whedon, Osteoporosis, intestinal lactase deficiency and low
    dietary calcium intake, N.E.J. Med. 276:445-448 (1967).
15. S. Margen, J.-Y. Chu, N. A. Kaufmann and D. H. Calloway,
    Studies in calcium metabolism I:  the calciuretic effect
    of dietary protein, Am. J. Clin. Nutr. 27:584-589 (1974).
16. H. M. Linkswiler, C. L. Joyce and C. R. Anand, Calcium reten-
    tion of young adult males as effected by level of protein
    and of calcium intake, Trans. N.Y. Acad. Sci. 36:333-340
    (1974).
17. L. H. Allen, E. A. Oddoye and S. Margen, Protein induced
    hypercalciuria:  a longer term study, Am. J. Clin. Nutr.
    32, No. 4: 741-749 (1979).

18.   F. L. Coe, Hyperuricosuric calcium nephrolithiasis, in:
      "Proceedings of Fourth International Workshop on Phosphate
      Metabolism," Strasbourg, June 22-24, 1979, Plenum Publ.
      Corp., New York.

19.   H. Spencer, L. Kramer, C. A. Gatza and M. Lender, Calcium loss,
      calcium absorption and calcium requirement in osteoporosis,
      in: "Osteoporosis II," Barzel, ed., Grune and Stratton, Inc.,
      New York, pp. 65-89 (1979).

20.   I. Clark and F. Rivera-Cordero, Effects of endogenous para-
      thyroid hormone on calcium, magnesium and phosphate
      metabolism in rats, Endocrinol. 96:360 (1974).

21.   H. Spencer, L. Kramer, D. Osis and C. Norris, Effect of
      phosphorus on the absorption of calcium and on the calcium
      balance in man, J. Nutr. 108:447-457 (1978).

22.   R. P. Heaney, Can an excessive dietary intake of phosphate or
      protein contribute to the development of osteoporosis? in:
      "International Symposium on Osteoporosis," St. John, Virgin
      Islands, October 25-27, 1978, sponsored by Marion Labora-
      tories, Inc., R. P. Heaney, ed., Biomed. Inf. Corp., New
      York, p. 28 (1979).

23.   C. C. Johnston, Jr., J. A. Norton, Jr., R. A. Khairi and C.
      Longcope, Age-related bone loss, in: "Osteoporosis II,"
      Barzel, ed., Grune and Stratton, Inc., New York, pp. 91-100
      (1979).

24.   B. L. Riggs, J. Jowsey, R. S. Goldsmith, P. J. Kelly, D. L.
      Hoffman and C. D. Arnaud, Short- and long-term effects of
      estrogen and synthetic anabolic hormone in post-menopausal
      osteoporosis, J. Clin. Invest. 51:1659-1663 (1972).

25.   J. M. Aitken, D. M. Hart and R. Lindsay, Oestrogen replacement
      therapy for prevention of osteoporosis after oophorectomy,
      Brit. Med. J. 3:515-518 (1973).

26.   R. R. Recker, P. D. Saville and R. P. Heaney, Effect of estro-
      gens and calcium carbonate on bone loss in postmenopausal
      women, Ann. Intern. Med. 87:649-655 (1977).

27.   A. Horsman, J. C. Gallagher, M. Simpson and B.E.C. Nordin,
      Prospective trial of estrogen and calcium in post-menopausal
      women, Brit. Med. J. 2:789-792 (1977).

28.   R. P. Heaney, Hazards, if any, of administering oral calcium
      supplements? in: "International Symposium on Osteoporosis,"
      St. John, Virgin Islands, October 25-27, 1978, sponsored by
      Marion Laboratories, Inc., R. P. Heaney, ed., Biomed. Inf.
      Corp., New York, p. 48 (1979).

29.   J. C. Gallagher and B. L. Riggs, Impaired production of 1,25
      dihydroxy vitamin D in postmenopausal osteoporosis, Clin.
      Res. 24:580A (1976).

30.   J. C. Gallagher, B. L. Riggs, J. Eisman, A. Hamstra, S. B.
      Arnaud and H. F. DeLuca, Intestinal calcium absorption and
      serum vitamin D metabolites in normal and osteoporotic
      subjects:  effect of age and dietary calcium, J. Clin.
      Invest. (in press, September 1979).

31. J. C. Gallagher and B. L. Riggs, Therapeutic role of vitamin D and its metabolites, in: "International Symposium on Osteoporosis," St. John, Virgin Islands, October 25-27, 1978, sponsored by Marion Laboratories, Inc., R. P. Heaney, ed., Biomed. Inf. Corp., New York, pp. 51-52 (1979).

32. C. Rich, J. Ensinck and P. Ivanovich, The effects of sodium fluoride on calcium metabolism of subjects with metabolic bone diseases, J. Clin. Invest. 43:545-556 (1964).

33. J. M. Burkhart and J. Jowsey, Effect of variations in calcium intake on the skeleton of fluoride-fed kittens, J. Lab. Clin. Med. 72:943-950 (1968).

34. J. Jowsey, B. L. Riggs, P. J. Kelly and D. L. Hoffman, Effect of combined therapy with sodium fluoride, vitamin D and calcium in osteoporosis, Am. J. Med. 53:43-49 (1972).

35. P. J. Meunier, Therapeutic role of sodium fluoride, in: "International Symposium on Osteoporosis," St. John, Virgin Islands, October 25-27, 1978, sponsored by Marion Laboratories, Inc., R. P. Heaney, ed., Biomed. Inf. Corp., New York, pp. 54-57 (1979).

36. S. J. Marx, L. Avioli, R. P. Heaney, C. C. Johnston, Jr., B.E.C. Nordin, W. A. Peck, L. Raisz, B. L. Riggs and G. D. Whedon, editorial: restraint in use of high-dose fluorides to treat skeletal disorders, J.A.M.A. 240:1630-1631 (1978).

37. B. L. Riggs, Therapeutic role of sodium fluoride, in: "International Symposium on Osteoporosis," St. John, Virgin Islands, October 25-27, 1978, sponsored by Marion Laboratories, Inc., R. P. Heaney, ed., Biomed. Inf. Corp., New York, pp. 52-54 (1979).

38. J. Reeve, R. Hesp, D. Williams, P. Hulme, L. Klenerman, J. M. Zanelli, A. J. Darby, A. W. Tregear and J. A. Parsons, Anabolic effect of low doses of a fragment of human parathyroid hormone on the skeleton in postmenopausal osteoporosis, Lancet 1:1035-1038 (1976).

THE ROLE OF VITAMIN D METABOLITES IN THE MANAGEMENT

OF BONE ABNORMALITIES IN RENAL DISEASE

Hartmut H. Malluche and Shaul G. Massry

Division of Nephrology and Department of Medicine
University of Southern California School of Medicine
Los Angeles, California  90033

Considerable progress has been made in recent years in the field of vitamin D metabolism (1-7). There is better understanding of the factors controlling the formation of the various metabolites of the vitamin and the role of these metabolites in calcium and phosphorus homeostasis. In addition, methods have been developed for the measurement of blood levels of the various vitamin D analogs (8-13). These advances have permitted us to better understand the role of vitamin D in the pathogenesis of bone abnormalities in renal disease and the requirement of the various compounds for the management of these derangements. Therefore, the indications for, and the optimal time for the initiation of therapy with the various vitamin D metabolites for the management of renal osteodystrophy should be reconsidered. Bone abnormalities occur in patients with renal disease and normal renal function (14), in those with mild to moderate renal insufficiency (15), as well as in patients with advanced renal failure (16-20). Although the severity of the bone disease may vary among these groups of patients, the nature and characteristics of bone pathology are similar.

BONE DISEASE IN PATIENTS WITH NORMAL RENAL FUNCTION

Pathologic bone changes in patients with renal disease and normal renal function have been reported in patients with nephrotic syndrome (14). Urinary losses of $25(OH)D_3$ represent the first pathogenetic event resulting in decreased blood levels of $25(OH)_2D_3$ (21-23). A deficiency of the latter sterole is also associated with reduced blood levels of both $1,25(OH)_2D_3$ and $24,25(OH)_2D_3$ (24). Serum levels of ionized calcium fall in these patients due to defective intestinal absorption of calcium and skeletal resistance to the calcèmic action of PTH (24). The hypocalcemia stimulates

615

the parathyroid glands leading to secondary hyperparathyroidism
(21). Thus, patients with nephrotic syndrome suffer from a state
of vitamin D deficiency and have elevated blood levels of PTH; both
of these events should exert a deleterious effect on bone. We
studied bone histology in six patients with nephrotic syndrome and
normal renal function. Evidence for abnormalities in bone mineralization and enhanced bone resorption were present (Table I and II).
All patients had a decrease in the fraction of mineralizing osteoid
seams and three had increased volume of osteoid. All patients
displayed an increase in the fraction of mineralized trabecular
surface covered by Howships Lacunae, and increased active osteoclastic resorption was present in three of the six patients.

The severity of the bone abnormalities is probably dependent
on the duration and magnitude of the losses of $25(OH)_2D_3$ in urine
and on the consequent changes in ionized calcium and parathyroid
gland activity. Therefore, supplementation of $25(OH)D_3$ seems to
be justified in all patients with longstanding nephrotic syndrome.
Studies on the therapeutic effectiveness of $25(OH)D_3$ are needed.
Also, it is conceivable that patients with renal failure and longstanding proteinuria in the nephrotic range might have more severe
osteopathy than others with comparable degrees of renal insufficiency
but without proteinuria. Histological documentation of such a
postulate is required.

BONE DISEASE IN MILD TO MODERATE RENAL FAILURE

Elevated blood levels of PTH have been noted in patients with
mild to moderate renal failure (25,26). Also, resistance to the
calcemic action of PTH (27) and decreased intestinal Ca absorption
was described by our laboratory (28). The PTH resistance could be
reversed by administration of vitamin D metabolites (29). These
findings point to a status of absolute or relative vitamin D
deficiency in mild to moderate renal failure. Indeed, our studies
of bone histology revealed signs of hyperparathyroid bone disease
and osteomalacia in patients with incipient to moderate renal
failure (15). On the other hand, Slatopolsky et al (30) and our
laboratory (unpublished observations) found normal levels of
$1,25(OH)_2D_3$ in patients with GFR greater than 35 ml per minute.
Also, $25(OH)_2D_3$ levels were found to be normal (31). To reconcile
between these normal measurements of $1,25(OH)_2D_3$ and the target
organ diseases, one must assume that either the requirement of
target organs for vitamin D metabolites is increased in renal
failure or the latter is associated with resistance to the action
of vitamin D. Therefore, a rational approach for therapy in
patients with mild to moderate renal failure would be the supplementation of small amounts of $1,25(OH)_2D_3$.

We treated three patients with mild to moderate renal failure
for 6 months with 0.5 µg of $1,25(OH)_2D_3$. They all had biochemical

Table I

Micromorphometric Results in Nephrotic Patients with Normal
Renal Function

| Patient | $V_V$ | $V_{vos}$ | S/V | OS | $SV_{oci}$ | HL |
|---------|-------|-----------|-----|-----|------------|-----|
| | % | % | mm²/mm³ | % | mm²/mm³ | % |
| 1 | 16.1 | 0.53 | 21.7 | 4.2 | 10.40 | 19.9 |
| 2 | 24.4 | 0.39 | 21.9 | 2.8 | 15.60 | 22.7 |
| 3 | 30.9 | 4.67 | 15.5 | 22.3 | 36.40 | 20.2 |
| 4 | 24.1 | 2.34 | 15.6 | 21.9 | 36.40 | 31.5 |
| 5 | 24.9 | 0.31 | 20.6 | 9.3 | 5.20 | 15.3 |
| 6 | 22.2 | 1.06 | 21.0 | 15.8 | 62.41 | 23.9 |
| Normal mean±2 SD | 22.1 | 0.58 | 20.8 | 9.2 | 20.3 | 6.5 |
| | ±12.2 | ±0.29 | ±8.2 | ±10.9 | ±14.4 | ±7.2 |

*Abbreviations used in this table:* HL, fraction of Howship's lacunae, indicating the fraction of mineralized (nonosteoid) trabecular surface covered by resorption lacunae (active and inactive); OS, fraction of osteoid seams, representing the fraction of trabecular surface covered by osteoid seams; S/V, specific surface, i.e., the ratio of trabecular surface to trabecular volume; this ratio falls as trabecular diameter rises; $SV_{oci}$, surface density of bone-osteoclast interface (active osteoclastic lacunae); $V_V$, volumetric density of bone (indicating the fraction of spongiosal volume occupied by bone matrix); $V_{vos}$, volumetric density of osteoid (indicating the fraction of spongiosal volume occupied by osteoid).

Table II

Histomorphometric Parameters of Bone Formation
and Mineralization

| Patient | $^F$min | $^M$double | $^M$diffuse | $^M$total |
|---------|---------|------------|-------------|-----------|
|         | %       | $\mu m/d$  | $\mu m/d$   | $\mu m/d$ |
| 1       | 48      | 0.5        | 0.6         | 0.6       |
| 2       | 48      | 0.6        | 0.7         | 0.7       |
| 3       | 46      | 0.8        | 0.9         | 0.9       |
| 4       | 30      | 0.6        | 1.2         | 1.0       |
| 5       | 37      | 0.5        | 0.7         | 0.7       |
| 6       | 41      | 0.6        | 1.0         | 0.9       |
| Normal  | >60     |            |             | 1.1±0.45  |

*Abbreviations used in this table*: $^F$min, fraction of mineralizing osteoid seams, indicating fraction of osteoid seams with tetracycline double label. $^M$double, appositional rate of bone formation sites with double tetracycline uptake. $^M$diffuse, appositional rate of bone formation sites with diffuse tetracycline uptake. $^M$total, appositional rate of total bone formation sites.

and histological signs of bone disease before treatment.  The bone
abnormalities consisted of osteoid accumulation and increased active
or inactive osteoclastic bone resorption.  Under fluorescent light,
the percentage of appositional fronts taking up tetracycline in a
double fashion was decreased.  A repetitive bone biopsy after 6
months of treatment with 0.5 µg $1,25(OH)_2D_3$ revealed complete
healing of the osteopathy.  These results suggest that a state of
relative vitamin D deficiency does exist in patients with moderate
renal failure and long-term therapy with low doses of $1,25(OH)_2D_3$
could prevent the development of bone disease and its progression.

BONE DISEASE IN ADVANCED RENAL FAILURE

The bone disease that invariably occurs in patients with
advanced renal failure has been described in detail by many investigators (16-20).  Various degrees of osteomalacia and hyperparathyroid bone disease comprise the two main findings at the bone
level.  Although some investigators found that $25(OH)D_3$ could be
low in patients with chronic uremia, most of these patients have
normal $25(OH)D_3$ levels while on a nutritionally adequate diet (31).
In contrast, the blood levels of $1,25(OH)_2D_3$ are low or undetectable
(8).  Therefore, $1,25(OH)_2D_3$ should exert a major beneficial effect
in the treatment of bone abnormalities in this stage of renal
function.

Currently, there is information on the effect of $1,25(OH)_2D_3$
on bone histology in 105 uremic patients.  The dose of $1,25(OH)_2D_3$
employed varied from 0.14 to 2.0 µg per day.

We studied 12 dialysis patients before and after 6 months of
treatment with $1,25(OH)_2D_3$.  In our study we obtained two bone
specimens before treatment to overcome the issue of variance in
bone histology and we employed tetracycline double labeling (14).
Our results and those of others indicate that therapy with this
metabolite for several months could be associated with decrease in
bone resorption (32-37).  However, such an effect was not universal
and only in a few patients did bone resorption return to normal
(33,34,37).  This is not surprising since such an effect of the
metabolite is mediated through the reduction in serum concentrations
of PTH which have been found to return to normal levels only in a
small percentage of the patients.  Endosteal fibrosis was either
markedly reduced or even disappeared during therapy with $1,25(OH)_2D_3$
(32,34,36,37), irrespective of whether the serum levels of PTH were
decreased or not (37).  This finding raises the possibility that
endosteal fibrosis is not entirely the result of excess PTH but
could also be related to vitamin D deficiency as well.

The data on the effects of $1,25(OH)_2D_3$ on uremic osteomalacia
are variable.  Coburn et al (38) reported that therapy with this
sterol failed to exert a beneficial effect on bone in patients with

pure osteomalacia and normal serum levels of PTH. Delling et al
(39) also reported no improvement in histological parameters in
patients with osteomalacia and no evidence of hyperparathyroid bone
disease. On the other hand, other investigators reported improvement or healing of osteomalacia (33,36,37,40) in patients who displayed evidence of both osteomalacia and enhanced bone resorption.
In our study, osteomalacia healed in seven, improved in three and
did not change in two patients after 6 months of treatment.

Despite the improvement in bone mineralization, many investigators believe that $1,25(OH)_2D_3$ may not be adequate for the treatment of osteomalacia of renal osteodystrophy (32,43,36). Bordier
et al (32) reached this conclusion based on their studies in 3
patients treated for 3 weeks because $1,25(OH)_2D_3$ failed to produce
a reduction in serum alkaline phosphatase and osteoid volume. It
also has been reported that defective mineralization in patients
with normal renal function and vitamin D deficiency osteomalacia
is normalized by therapy with $25(OH)D_3$ and not by $1,25(OH)_2D_3$ (41).
This observation suggests that $25(OH)D_3$ is more critical for the
healing of osteomalacia and that $1,25(OH)_2D_3$ may not be necessary
for this purpose. Although these data may seem to be in direct
conflict with our results in renal failure patients, an alternative
interpretation may explain the apparent discrepancies; it is possible that both metabolites are needed for the healing of osteomalacia and the effectiveness of one or the other may depend on
the relative or absolute deficiency of either in any particular
subject. Thus, in patients with advanced renal failure who have
normal blood levels of $25(OH)D_3$ and low concentrations of $1,25(OH)_2D_3$
the supplementation of the latter is adequate for the healing of
osteomalacia. On the other hand, patients with normal renal function and vitamin D deficiency osteomalacia have low blood levels
of $25(OH)D_3$ but have either low or normal levels of $1,25(OH)_2D_3$.
Treatment of these patients with $25(OH)D_3$ alone will provide both
$25(OH)D_3$ and $1,25(OH)_2D_3$ and heals the osteomalacic lesions but
supplementation of $1,25(OH)_2D_3$ alone will not be adequate. According to this hypothesis it is worthwhile to measure blood levels
of $1,25(OH)_2D_3$ and $25(OH)D_3$ in order to know whether one or both
metabolites are needed for optimal therapy.

Other explanations for the lack of full responsiveness to
treatment with $1,25(OH)_2D_3$ in some patients include the necessity
of more prolonged therapy and/or higher doses of $1,25(OH)_2D_3$, a
certain critical level of bone turnover for healing of osteomalacia,
and possibly other metabolites which may be required for the
healing of osteomalacia and/or the suppression of the parathyroid
overactivity.

Recent evidence shows that $24,25(OH)_2D_3$ has an effect on bone
metabolism and may be needed for the maintenance of skeletal integrity (42). We studied 40 vitamin D deficient chicks, supplemented

with $1,25(OH)_2D_3$ and $24,25(OH)_2D_3$ singly or in combination at low or high doses (43). It was found that accumulation of osteoid could be avoided by $24,25(OH)_2D_3$ as well as by $1,25(OH)_2D_3$. Also, production of endosteal fibrosis was suppressed by either metabolite. These observations show that $24,25(OH)_2D_3$ exerts a direct effect on bone. Whether this metabolite would have a beneficial effect in the management of renal osteodystrophy awaits further studies.

## REFERENCES

1. J.W. Blunt, Y. Tanaka, and H.F. DeLuca, The biological activity of 25-hydroxycholecalciferol, a metabolite of vitamin $D_3$, Proc. Natl. Acad. Sci. 61:1503 (1968).
2. G. Ponchon, and H.F. DeLuca, The role of the liver in the metabolism of vitamin D, J. Clin. Invest. 48:1273 (1969).
3. D.R. Fraser and E. Kodicek, Unique biosynthesis by kidney of a biologically active vitamin D metabolite, Nature 228:764 (1970).
4. L.F. Myrtle and A.W. Norman, Vitamin D: A cholecalciferol metabolite highly active in promoting intestinal calcium transport, Science 171:79 (1971).
5. M.F. Holick, H.K. Schnoes, H.F. DeLuca, T. Suda, and F.J. Cousins, Isolation and identification of 1,25 dihydroxycholecalciferol: A metabolite of vitamin D active in intestine, Biochem. 10:2799 (1971).
6. A.W. Norman and R.G. Wong, Biological activity of the vitamin D metabolite 1,25-dihydroxycholecalciferol in chickens and rats, J. Nutrit. 102:1709 (1972).
7. K.W. McNutt and M.R. Haussler, Nutritional effectiveness of 1,25-dihydroxycholecalciferol in preventing rickets in chicks, J. Nutrit. 103:681 (1973).
8. P.F. Brumbaugh, D.H. Haussler, R. Bressler, and M.R. Haussler, Radioreceptor assay for $1\alpha,25$ dihydroxyvitamin $D_3$, Science 183:1089 (1974).
9. J.A. Eisman, A.J. Hamstra, B.E. Kream, and H.F. DeLuca, A sensitive, precise, and convenient method for determination of 1,25-dihydroxyvitamin D in human plasma, Arch. Biochem. Biophys. 176:235 (1976).
10. P.H. Stern, A.J. Hamstra, H.F. DeLuca, and N.H. Bell, A bioassay capable of measuring 1 picogram of 1,25-dihydroxyvitamin $D_3$, J. Clin. Endocrinol. Metab. 46:891 (1978).
11. T.L. Clemens, G.N. Hendy, R.F. Graham, E.G. Baggiolini, M.R. Uskokovic, and J.L.H. O'Riordan, A radioimmunoassay for 1,25-dihydroxycholecalciferol, Clin. Sci. Molec. Med. 54:329 (1978).
12. P.C. Schaefer, and R.S. Goldsmith, Radioimmunoassay of vitamin D metabolites, in "Vitamin D - Basic Research and Its Clinical Application" A.W. Norman, K.V. Schaefer, D. Herrath, H.G. Grigoleit, J.W. Coburn, H.F. DeLuca, E.B. Mawer, and T. Suda, ed., Walter de Gruyter, Berlin, New York (1979).

13.  R.L. Horst, R.M. Shepard, N.A. Jorgensen, and H.F. Deluca,
     Assays for vitamin D and its metabolites, in "Vitamin D –
     Basic Research and Its Clinical Application" A.W. Norman,
     K.V. Schaefer, D. Herrath, H.G. Grigoleit, J.W. Coburn,
     E.B. Mawer, and T. Suda, ed., Walter de Gruyter, Berlin,
     New York (1979).

14.  H.H. Malluche, D.A. Goldstein, and S.G. Massry, Osteomalacia
     and hyperparathyroid bone disease in patients with nephrotic
     syndrome, J. Clin. Invest. 63:434 (1979).

15.  H.H. Malluche, E. Ritz, J. Kutschera, H.P. Lange, V. Seiffert,
     and W. Schoeppe, Bone histology in incipient and advanced
     renal failure, Kidney Internat. 9:355 (1976).

16.  E. Ritz, H.H. Malluche, J. Bommer, O. Mehls, and B. Krempien,
     Metabolic bone disease in patients on maintenance hemodialy-
     sis, Nephron 12:393 (1974).

17.  V. Binswanger, D. Sherrard, C. Rick, and K.F. Curtis, Dialysis
     bone disease, Nephron 12:1 (1974).

18.  J.B. Eastwood, P. Bordier, and H.E. deWardener, Comparison of
     the effect of vitamin D and calcium carbonate in renal
     osteomalacia, Quart. J. Med. 40:569 (1971).

19.  S.A. Duusma, W.J. Visser, and L. Nijo, A quantitative histolo-
     gical study of bone in 30 patients with renal insufficiency.
     Cal. Tiss. Res. 9:216 (1972).

20.  J. Jowsey, S.G. Massry, J.W. Coburn, and C.R. Kleeman, Micro-
     radiographic studies of bone in renal osteodystrophy, Arch.
     Intern. Med. 124:539 (1969).

21.  D.A. Goldstein, Y. Oda, K. Kurokawa, and S.G. Massry, Blood
     levels of 25 hydroxyvitamin D in nephrotic syndrome. Studies
     in 26 patients, Ann. Intern. Med. 87:664 (1977).

22.  H. Schmidt-Gayk, W. Schmitt, C. Grawunder, E. Ritz,
     W. Tschoeppe, V. Pietsch, K. Andrassy, and R. Bouillon,
     25 hydroxyvitamin D in nephrotic syndrome, Lancet  II:105
     (1977).

23.  J.M. Barragry, M.W. France, N.D. Carter, J.A. Auton, M. Beer,
     B.J. Boucher, and R.D. Cohen, Vitamin D metabolism in
     nephrotic syndrome, Lancet II:626 (1977).

24.  D.A. Goldstein, B. Haldimann, A.W. Norman, and S.G. Massry,
     Blood levels of 25(OH)D$_3$, 1,25(OH)$_2$D$_3$ and 24,25(OH)$_2$D$_3$,
     intestinal calcium absorption and calcemic response to PTH
     in patients with nephrotic syndrome with normal renal
     function, Proc. 12th Annual Meeting, Am. Soc. Nephrol.,
     Boston, p. 150A, (1979).

25.  E. Reiss, J.M. Canterbury, and A. Kanter, Circulating parathy-
     roid hormone concentration in chronic renal insufficiency,
     Arch. Intern. Med. 124:417 (1969).

26.  H.H. Malluche, E. Ritz, H. Kutschera, G. Krause, E. Werner,
     A. Gati, V. Seiffert, and G.P. Lange, Calcium metabolism
     and impaired mineralization in various stages of renal insuf-
     ficiency, in "Vitamin D and Problems Related to Uremic Bone
     Disease" A.W. Norman, K. Schaefer, H.G. Frifoleit, D. Herrath
     and E. Ritz, ed., Walter de Gruyter, Berlin, New York (1975).

27. F. Llach, S.G. Massry, F.R. Singer, K. Kurokawa, J.H. Kaye
    and J.W. Coburn, Skeletal resistance to endogenous parathy-
    roid hormone in patients with early renal failure.  A possible
    cause for secondary hyperparathyroidism, J. Clin. Endocrin.
    Metab. 41:339 (1975).
28. H.H. Malluche, E. Werner, and E. Ritz, Intestinal absorption
    of calcium and whole body calcium retention in incipient and
    advanced renal failure, Miner. Elect. Metab. 1:263 (1978).
29. S.G. Massry, R. Stein, J. Garty, A.I. Arieff, J.W. Coburn,
    A.W. Norman, and R.M. Friedler, Skeletal resistance to the
    calcemic action of parathyroid hormone in uremia.  Role of
    1,25(OH)$_2$D$_3$.  Kidney Internat. 9:467 (1976).
30. E. Slatopolsky, R. Gray, N.D. Adams, J. Lewis, K. Hruska,
    K. Martin, S. Klahr, H.F. DeLuca, and J. Lemann, Low serum
    levels of 1,25(OH)$_2$D$_3$ are not responsible for the development
    of secondary hyperparathyroidism in early renal failure,
    Proc. 11th Annual Meeting, Am. Soc. Nephrol. 11:99A (1978).
31. G. Offermann, D. Herrath, and K. Schaefer, Serum 25-dihydroxy-
    cholecalciferol in uremia, Nephron 13:269 (1974).
32. P. Bordier, J. Zingraff, J. Gueris, P. Jungers, P. Marie,
    M. Pechet, and H. Rasmussen, The effect of 1$\alpha$(OH)D$_3$ and
    1$\alpha$25(OH)$_2$D$_3$ on the bone in patients with renal osteodystrophy.
    Am. J. Med. 64:101 (1978).
33. K.Y. Ahmed, M.R. Wills, Z. Varghese, E.A. Meinhard, and E.A.
    Moorhead, Long-term effects of small doses of 1,25-dihydroxy-
    cholecalciferol in renal osteodystrophy, Lancet I:629 (1978).
34. A.S. Brickman, D.J. Sherrard, J. Jowsey, F.R. Singer, D.J.
    Baylink, N. Maloney, S.G. Massry, A.W. Norman, and J.W.
    Coburn, 1,25-dihydroxycholecalciferol effect on skeletal
    lesions and plasma parathyroid hormone levels in uremic
    osteodystrophy, Arch. Intern. Med. 134:883 (1974).
35. D.J. Sherrard, J.W. Coburn, A.S. Brickman, D.J. Baylink,
    A.W. Norman, and N. Maloney, A histologic comparison of
    1,25(OH)$_2$ vitamin D treatment with calcium supplementation
    in renal osteodystrophy, in "Vitamin D, Biochemical, Chemical
    and Clinical Aspects Related to Calcium Metabolism" A.W.
    Norman, K.V. Schaefer, J.W. Coburn, H.F. DeLuca, D. Fraser,
    H.G. Grigoleit and D. Herrath, eds., Walter de Gruyter,
    Berlin, New York (1977).
36. A.M. Pierides, M.K. Ward, F. Alvarez-Ude, H.A. Ellis, K.M.
    Peart, W. Simpson, D.N.S. Kerr, and A. Norman, Long-term
    therapy with 1,25(OH)$_2$D$_3$ in dialysis bone disease, in
    "Dialysis Transplantation Nephrology" Moorhead, Mion and
    Baillod, ed., Pitman Medical, Kent (1976)
37. H.H. Malluche, D.A. Goldstein, and S.G. Massry, Management of
    renal osteodystrophy with 1,25(OH)$_2$D$_3$, Miner. Elect. Metab.
    2:48 (1979).
38. J.W. Coburn, A.S. Brickman, D.J. Sherrard, F.R. Singer,
    D.J. Baylink, E.G.C. Wong, S.G. Massry, and A.W. Norman,
    Clinical efficacy of 1,25-dihydroxyvitamin D$_3$ in renal

osteodystrophy, in "Vitamin D, Biochemical, Chemical and Clinical Aspects Related to Calcium Metabolism" A.W. Norman, K.V. Schaefer, J.W. Coburn, H.F. DeLuca, D. Fraser, H.G. Grigoleit and D. Herrath, eds. Walter de Gruyter, Berlin, New York (1977).

39.  G. Delling, H. Luhmann, M. Bulla, C. Fuchs, H.V. Henning, J.L.J. Jansen, W. Kohnle, and W. Schulz, The action of 1,25(OH)$_2$D$_3$ in turnover kinetic remodeling surfaces and structure of trabecular bone in chronic renal failure, Contributions to Nephrology (in press).

40.  H.A. Ellis, and K.M. Peart, Iliac bone marrow mast cells in relation to the renal osteodystrophy of patients treated by hemodialysis, J. Clin. Path. 29:502 (1976).

41.  P. Bordier, H. Rasmussen, P. Marie, L. Miravet, J. Gueris, and A. Ryckwaert, Vitamin D metabolites and bone mineralization in man. J. Clin. Endocrin. Metab. 48:284 (1978).

42.  A. Ornoy, D. Goodwin, D. Noff and S. Edelstein, 24,25 dihydroxy- lated D is a metabolite of vitamin D essential for bone formation, Nature 276:517 (1978).

43.  H.H. Malluche, H. Henry, W. Meyer-Sabellek, D. Sherman, S.G. Massry, and A.W. Norman, Effects and interactions of 24R,25 dihydroxycholecalciferol and 1,25 dihydroxycholecalciferol on bone, Am. J. Physiol. (in press).

ANTAGONISTIC EFFECTS OF 25(OH)Vitamin $D_3$ AND PEPTIDE HORMONES ON
THE ACTIVATION OF ADENYLATE CYCLASE/CYCLIC AMP SYSTEM IN RENAL
TISSUE IN VITRO

Hanna Wald and Mordecai M. Popovtzer

Nephrology Services, Hebrew University-Hadassah
School of Medicine, Jerusalem, Israel

INTRODUCTION

Previous studies from this laboratory demonstrated blunting
effect of 25(OH)vitamin $D_3$ (25(OH)vit $D_3$) on the phosphaturic
response to parathyroid hormone and calcitonin in parathyroidectomized rats (1, 2). The antiphosphaturic action of
25(OH)vit $D_3$ was associated with reduced urinary excretion of
cyclic AMP, suggesting interference of the vitamin with the
hormone-induced activation of adenylate cyclase/cyclic AMP system
in the kidney (2, 3). The observed changes in the rate of urinary
excretion of the nucleotide, however, could not be attributed with
certainty to a direct renal effect 25(OH)vit $D_3$, as other extrarenal systems were equally exposed to the action of the tested
substances.

To further explore the possible role of the kidney as a target
organ for the interaction between the peptide hormones and vitamin
D, we studied their effects on renal adenylate cyclase/cyclic AMP
system in vitro.

MATERIALS AND METHODS

Kidneys were obtained from male rats of the Hebrew University
strain, weighing 180-250 g, that had been maintained ad libitum on
Purina Laboratory chow. Parathyroidectomy (4) was performed 2-5
days prior to the in vitro studies.

Adenosine triphosphate (ATP)was obtained from Sigma Chemical
Co., St. Louis, Mo., U.S.A., c-AMP assay kit from the Radiochemical
Center, Amersham, Buckinghamshire, England, Parathormone (PTH) from

Eli Lilly & Co., Indianapolis, Ind., U.S.A., Pitressin (ADH) from Parke, Davis & Co., Detroit, Mi., U.S.A., Calcitonin from Armour-Montagu Laboratories, Paris, France, and 25-hydroxycholecalciferol (25(OH)vit $D_3$) from Hoffmann-La Roche & Co., Basle, Switzerland.

## Assay of Adenylate Cyclase

Adenylate cyclase (AC) activity was measured by a modification of the procedure of Chase and Aurbach (5). Kidney tissue was homogenized in 50 mM Tris buffer, pH 7.5 and the membrane fraction was isolated by centrifugation twice at 2.200 g. The membrane fraction was incubated for 10 min with ATP (1.23 mM) and the amount of cAMP formed was assayed. Any phosphodiesterase (PDE) activity that might have been present in the membrane preparation was inhibited by theophylline (10 mM). The cAMP generated during the incubation was measured by a radiochemical method using a cAMP radioassay kit (binding protein from bovine muscle). Enzyme activity was expressed in picomoles cAMP synthesized per milligram tissue protein per minute.

## Experimental and Control Incubations

1.   The effect of 25(OH)vit $D_3$ on PTH-induced activation of renal AC in vitro. The activity of renal cortical AC was assayed in the following incubations: (a) control (without PTH and without 25(OH) vit $D_3$), 10 experiments, (b) with 1 U/ml of PTH, but without 25(OH) vit $D_3$, 10 experiments, and (c) with 1 U/ml of PTH and with 50 U/ml of 25(OH)vit $D_3$. The results were evaluated by comparing (a) with (b) and (b) with (c).
2.   The effect of 25(OH)vit $D_3$ on calcitonin-induced activation of renal AC in vitro. The activity of renal cortical AC was assayed in the following incubations: (a) control (without calcitonin and without 25(OH)vit $D_3$), 12 experiments, (b) with 0.1 U/ml of calcitonin, without 25(OH)vit $D_3$, 12 experiments, and (c) with 0.1 U/ml of calcitonin and 50 U/ml of 25(OH)vit $D_3$, 12 experiments. The results were evaluated by comparing (a) with (b) and (b) with (c).
3.   The effect of 25(OH)vit $D_3$ on ADH-induced activation of renal AC in vitro. The activity of renal cortical AC was assayed in the following incubations: (a) control (without ADH and without 25(OH) vit $D_3$), 10 experiments, (b) with 0.1 U/ml of ADH, without 25(OH) vit $D_3$), 10 experiments, and (c) with 0.1 U/ml of ADH and 50 U/ml of 25(OH)vit $D_3$, 10 experiments. The results were evaluated by comparing (a) with (b) and (b) with (c).

Statistical analyses were performed with the Student's t-test. Data in the text and figures are presented as the mean $\pm$ SE.

RESULTS

## Dose Response Curves, for the Effects of the Hormones on the Activity of Renal Cortical AC

Fig. 1. shows the activation of renal cortical AC by PTH. The activation was gradual and failed to reach a plateau at concentrations of 5.0 U/ml of PTH. Fig. 2 shows the activation of renal cortical AC by calcitonin. 0.1 U/ml of calcitonin caused already maximal activation which persisted at 0.5 and 1.0 U/ml but declined markedly with a further increase in the concentration of calcitonin to 5.0 and 10.0 U/ml. Fig. 3 shows the activation of renal cortical AC by ADH. In this case the activation was maximal with the concentration of 0.002 U/ml. The plateau persisted through all tested concentrations unto 1 U/ml of ADH.

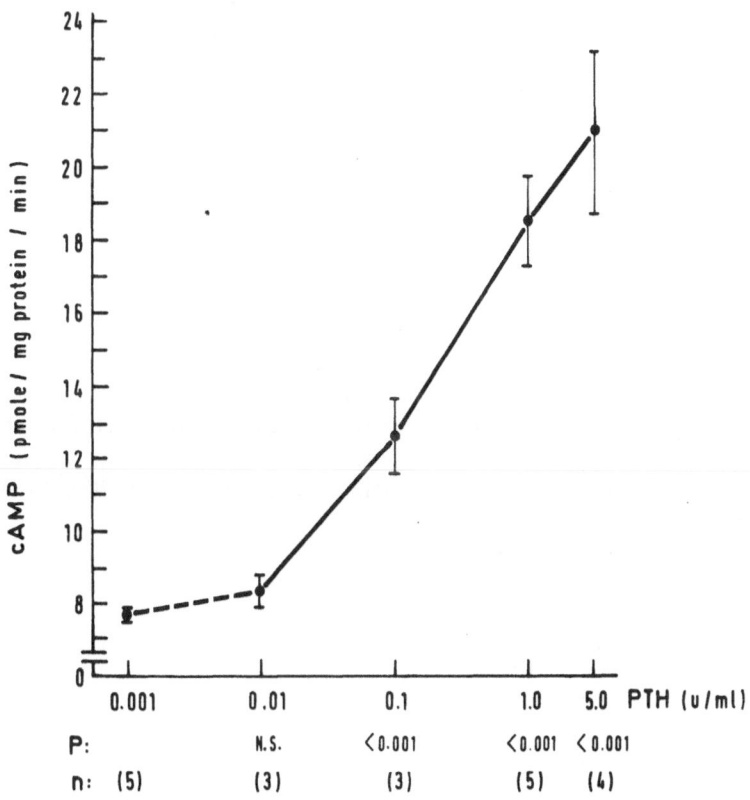

Figure 1.  The effect of PTH on renal cortical AC activity. Dose response curve. p refers to the difference between the minimal dose (0.001 U/ml) and each of the higher doses.

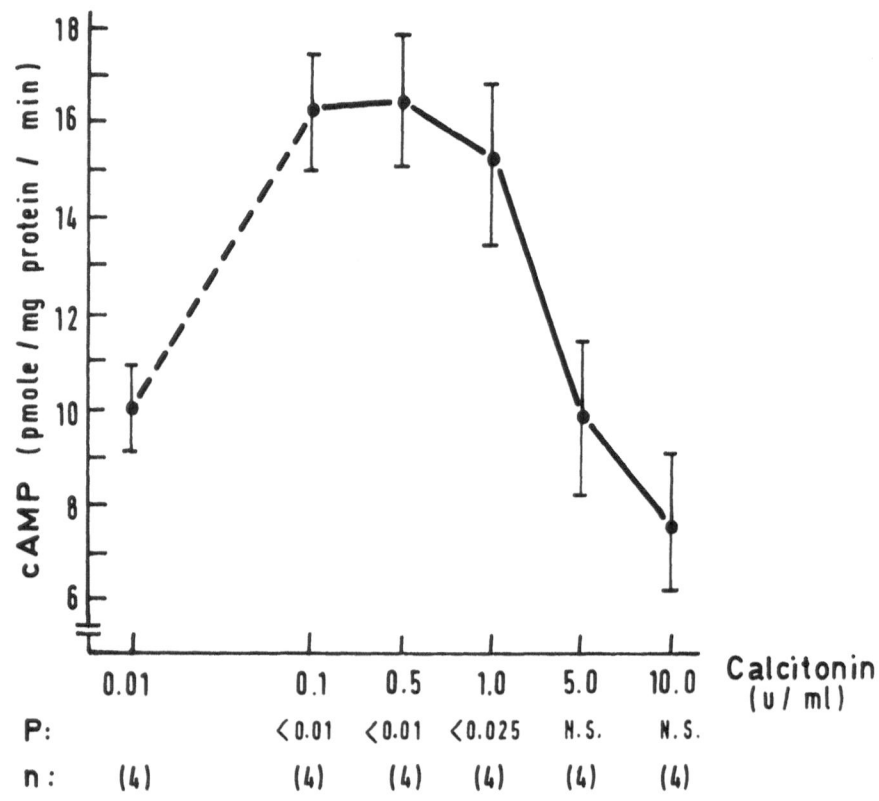

P:                    <0.01   <0.01   <0.025   N.S.    N.S.

n :      (4)          (4)     (4)     (4)      (4)     (4)

Figure 2.   The effect of calcitonin on renal cortical AC. Dose
            response curve. p refers to the difference between the
            minimal dose (0.01 U/ml) and each of the higher doses.

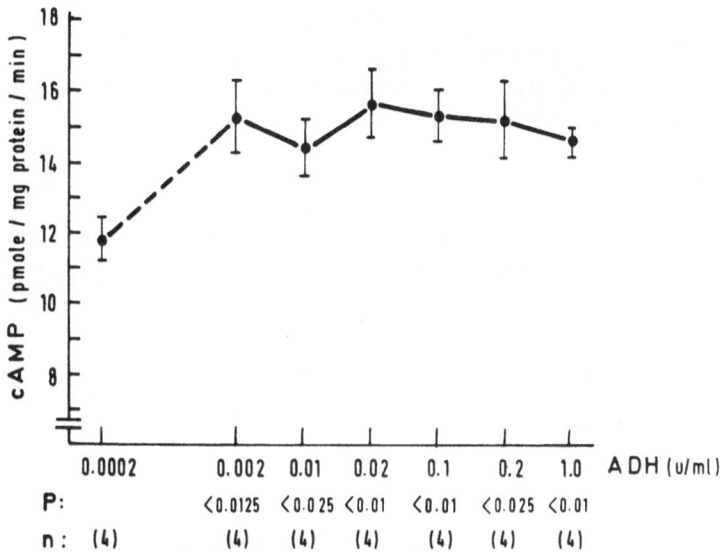

Figure 3.  The effect of ADH on renal cortical adenylate cyclase.
Dose response curve. p refers to differences between the
minimal dose and each of the higher doses.

1.   The effect of 25(OH)vit D$_3$ on PTH-induced activation of renal
AC.  Fig. 4 shows the effect of PTH and PTH + 25(OH)vit D$_3$ on AC
activity. PTH increased AC from a control value of 5.9 + 0.5 to
14.4 $\pm$ 1.5 (p< 0.001); the addition of 25(OH)vit D$_3$ to PTH reduced
AC activity from 14.4 + 1.5 to 10.5 $\pm$ 1.0 (p< 0.025) pmole/mg
protein/min of cAMP. 25(OH)vit D$_3$ in the absence of PTH did not
change AC activity in comparison to control.
2.   The effect of 25(OH)vit D$_3$ on calcitonin-induced activation
of renal AC.  Fig. 5 shows the effect of calcitonin and calcitonin
+ 25(OH)vit D$_3$ on AC activity. Calcitonin increased AC from a
control value of 6.1 $\pm$ 0.5 to 15.1 $\pm$ 0.5 (p< 0.001); the addition
of 25(OH)vit D$_3$ to calcitonin reduced AC activity from 15.1 $\pm$ 0.5
to 12.3 $\pm$ 0.8 (p< 0.01) pmole/mg protein/min of cAMP.
3.   The effect of 25(OH)vit D$_3$ on ADH-induced activation of renal
AC.  Fig. 6 shows the effect of ADH and ADH + 25(OH)vit D$_3$ on AC
activity. ADH increased AC from a control value of 5.9 + 0.5 to
8.0 + 0.7 (p< 0.025) pmole/mg protein/min of cAMP. The addition of
25(OH)vit D$_3$ failed to change the activation of AC by ADH.

DISCUSSION

     The results of the present study demonstrated, that at the
concentrations of the substances that were tested, 25(OH)vit D$_3$
suppressed the activation of renal cortical AC by PTH or by
calcitonin. 25(OH)vit D$_3$ failed to alter the ADH-induced activation
of AC. The latter could be interpreted as either indicating
specificity of this reaction with regard to the peptide hormone
that interacts with the vitamin, or lack of sensitivity because of
inadequate selection of the concentrations of the agents in the
incubation media.

     The dose response curves demonstrated marked variability in
the response of AC activity to increasing concentrations of the
three peptide hormones. In the case of calcitonin it is noteworthy
that the dose response curve assumed a bellshaped form. By contrast,
the curves of PTH and ADH showed either continuous climbing or
levelling-off of the AC activity in response to increasing
concentrations of the respective hormones. The biological significance of these responses cannot be defined by our present
observations.

     The present in vitro results are consistent with our previous
in vivo clearance data (2, 3). These experiments demonstrated that
25(OH)vit D$_3$ blunted the phosphaturic effects of PTH and of
calcitonin and that this suppression was associated with a
commensurate fall in the urinary excretion of cyclic AMP. Taken
together, the previous clearance studies (2, 3) and the present
results of in vitro experiments support the contention that the
mechanism that underlies the antiphosphaturic action of 25(OH)vit D$_3$

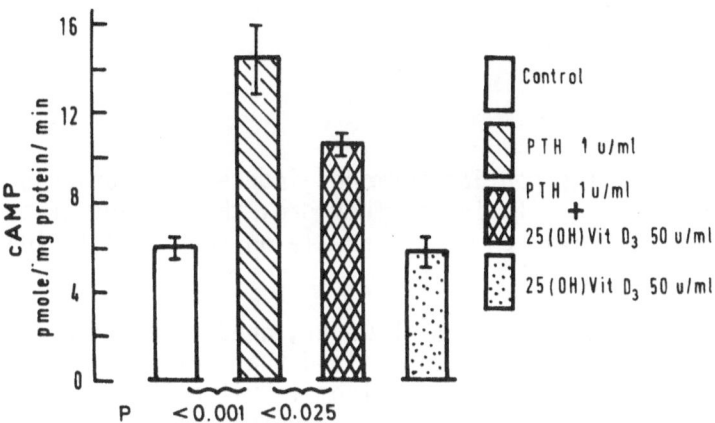

Figure 4.   The effect of 25(OH)vit D$_3$ on PTH-induced activation
of renal cortical AC.

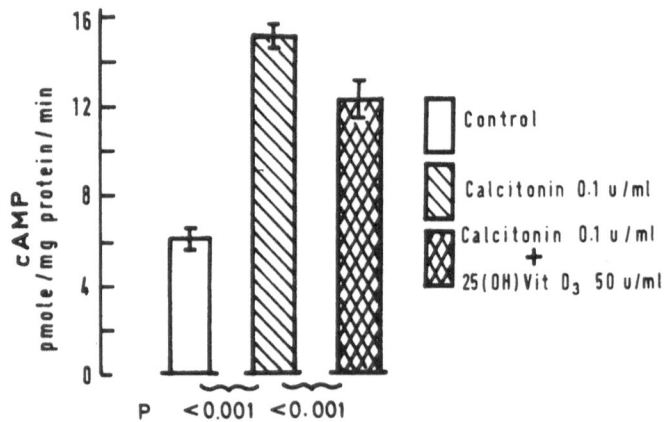

Figure 5.  The effect of 25(OH)vit D₃ on calcitonin-induced
           activation of renal cortical AC.

is inhibition of the peptide hormones-induced activation of renal
cortical AC, by the vitamin. Furthermore, the present experiments
suggest that 25(OH)vit D₃ acts directly on the renal tissue to
exert its effect.

     All above considerations, however, need to be viewed with
great caution. It has to be emphasized that arriving at definite
conclusion through extrapolation from in vitro to in vivo situation
may be unwarranted. In addition the physiological importance of the
present results has to be questioned because of using of
pharmacological doses of the tested substances.

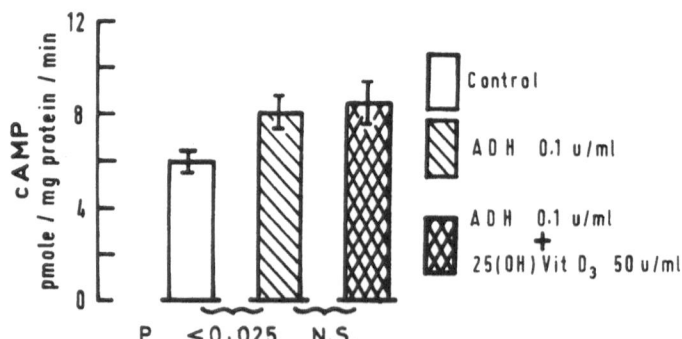

Figure 6.  The effect of 25(OH)vit D₃ on ADH-induced activation of
           renal cortical AC.

REFERENCES

1. M. M. Popovtzer, J. Robinette, H. DeLuca, and M. F. Holick, The acute effect of 25-OH-Cholecalciferol on renal handling of phosphorus: Evidence for parathyroid hormone dependent mechanism, J Clin Invest 53:913 (1974).

2. M. M. Popovtzer, R. S. Flis, and M. Blum, The effect of 25(OH) vit D$_3$ on renal handling of phosphorus: Evidence of interference with the phosphaturic action of calcitonin, Am J Physiol 232:515 (1977).

3. M. M. Popovtzer, and J. B. Robinette, The effect of 25-OH-vitamin D$_3$ on renal handling of phosphorus: Evidence for inhibition of cyclic monophosphate formation, Am J Physiol, 229:907 (1975).

4. M. M. Popovtzer, S. G. Massry, M. Villamil, and C. R. Kleeman, Renal handling of phosphorus in oliguric and non-oliguric mercury induced acute and renal failure in rats, J Clin Invest 50:2347 (1971).

5. L. R. Chase, and G. D. Aurbach, Renal adenyl cyclase: anatomically separate sites for parathyroid hormone and vasopressin, Science 159:545 (1968).

EFFECT OF UREMIC SERA ON PARATHYROID HORMONE (PTH) MEDIATED
RELEASE OF CALCIUM FROM NORMAL RAT EMBRYONAL BONE MAINTAINED
IN TISSUE CULTURE

Joseph M. Letteri and Syed Asad and Jeff Olmer

Nassau County Medical Center, East Meadow, L.I.
State University of New York
Stony Brook, New York

INTRODUCTION

Chronic renal failure is commonly associated with hypocalcemia
but the mechanisms responsible for the sustained decrease in plasma
ionized calcium are not clearly understood.  Two major hypotheses
have evolved to explain the hypocalcemia of chronic renal disease.
Slatopolsky and Bricker attribute the decrease in ionized calcium
in uremia to secondary hyperparathyroidism and retention of
inorganic phosphorus (1).  Massry and co-workers argue that
hypocalcemia and secondary hyperparathyroidism occur independently
of changes in serum inorganic phosphorus in acute and chronic
renal failure (2).  For Massry, altered Vitamin D metabolism
resulting in a relative deficiency of $1,25 (OH)_2D_3$ or other
metabolites and skeletal resistance to calcemic action of
parathyroid hormone are the principal determinants of hypocalcemia
in renal failure.  Other possible explanations for the hypocalcemia
of uremia include an increased volume of distribution of ionized
calcium due to increased transfer of calcium ions into cells and
altered distribution of ionized calcium between bone extracellular
fluid and plasma.  It is likely that the hypocalcemia of renal
failure is of multifactoral origin and that phosphorus retention,
secondary hyperparathyroidism, deficiency of $1,25 (OH)_2D_3$ and
impaired skeletal response for calcium release to increase
parathyroid hormone levels are contributing to the sustained
hypocalcemia in uremia.

Our studies were designed to test the hypothesis that the
sera of hypocalcemic uremic patients contains factors which inhibits
the release or is deficient in factors which are necessary for the
release of calcium from normal rat embryonal bone maintained in a

tissue culture system.  Each portion of a pair of rat calvaria, pre-
labeled during pregnancy with $^{45}$Ca, were maintained in tissue culture containing either twenty-five percent uremic sera or twenty-
five percent normal sera.  The amount of $^{45}$Ca released into the
media containing uremic sera was significantly lower than values
obtained in media containing normal sera.  This difference persisted
despite addition of PTH to media containing uremic or normal sera.
The impaired release of $^{45}$Ca in media with uremic sera was only
partially restored by addition of 1,25(OH)$_2$D$_3$ and 24,25(OH)$_2$D$_3$ but
not by 1,25(OH)$_2$D$_3$ and 25OHD$_3$.  These findings indicate that uremic
sera contains factors which inhibit the calcium mobilizing properties of bovine PTH added to a fetal rat embryonal tissue culture
system.  Deficiency of 1,25(OH)$_2$D$_3$ and 24,25(OH)$_2$D$_3$ may be, in part,
responsible for the defect in calcium mobilization noted in the
system.

METHODS

    The techniques used in this study consisted of modifications of
the usual methods employed to study bone reabsorption in tissue culture as described by Raisz (3), Reynolds (4), and Biggers (5).
Pregnant rats are injected with $^{45}$Ca, 50 uci/100 mg., on the 17th
day of gestation.  On the twentieth day the rats are sacrificed and
the fetus removed aseptically.  The calvaria of each fetus is removed and cut in two down the line of the median suture.  Each pair
is cut to identical size by placing one piece on top of the other
and trimming off any excess.  Explants are washed three times with
culture media and are cultured for 48 hours with high humidity and
5 percent CO$_2$.  $^{45}$Ca is counted in a 0.5 ml aliquot of the culture
with 10 ml insta-gel in a beta counter using an internal window
(O-$\alpha$).  The bone is then washed and dried to a constant weight.
Values are expressed as counts per milligram of bone released into
the media.  The culture media employed was modified GIBCO BGJ$_B$ (75%)
as described by Biggers (5) to which was added 25 percent normal AB
serum or 25 percent uremic serum from undialyzed hypocalcemic
patients.  All sera is heat inactivated at 37ºC for thirty minutes
in a water bath.  Culture media and sera were diluted with water to
which was added 1.75 grams of sodium bicarbonate, 1% Penicillin and
5000 units of Streptomycin.

    Paired samples of calvaria of the same fetus are maintained
in the culture system containing either 25 percent normal AB sera
or 25 percent uremic sera.  The phosphorus concentration of the
media containing normal AB sera was adjusted by adding buffered
sodium monohydrogenphosphate to the media so that the final concentration of phosphorus in the media equals the measured concentration of inorganic phosphorus in the uremic media.  The phosphorus
concentration of uremic sera varied from 3 mg/dl to 11.4 mg/dl
while the serum calcium varied from 4.7 mg/dl to 8.9 mg/dl.  The
amount of $^{45}$Ca released from the rat embryonal bone maintained

TABLE 1

THE EFFECT OF UREMIC SERUM ON THE CALCIUM MOBILIZING PROPERTIES OF HIGHLY PURIFIED PARATHYROID HORMONE ADDED TO EMBRYONAL RAT BONE MAINTAINED IN TISSUE CULTURE

| EXPERIMENT | N | BONE IN NORMAL SERUM | BONE IN UREMIC SERUM | p VALUE | N/U RATIO | p VALUE |
|---|---|---|---|---|---|---|
| | | CPM/MG DRY BONE | | | | |
| No Treatment | 31 | 8203 $\pm$5205 | 3984 $\pm$2668 | $p < .01$ | 2.11 $\pm$0.39 | ------ |
| PTH (0.5 unit/ml) | 5 | 19,748 $\pm$1390 | 11,697 $\pm$1652 | $p < .001$ | 1.70 $\pm$0.16 | $p < .01$ |
| PTH (1.0 unit/ml) | 8 | 18,209 $\pm$11,885 | 10,581 $\pm$8279 | $p < .05$ | 2.14 $\pm$.59 | NS |
| PTH (1.5 unit/ml) | 8 | 12,334 $\pm$2420 | 8258 $\pm$1788 | $p < .01$ | 1.48 $\pm$0.14 | $p < .01$ |
| PTH (3.0 unit/ml) | 2 | 14,668 $\pm$372 | 8234 $\pm$1104 | $p < .01$ | 1.80 $\pm$0.30 | $p < .01$ |

TABLE 2

THE EFFECT OF UREMIC SERUM ON THE CALCIUM MOBILIZING PROPERTIES OF PTH AND METABOLITES OF VITAMIN D ADDED TO EMBRYONAL RAT BONE MAINTAINED IN TISSUE CULTURE

| EXPERIMENT | N | BONE IN NORMAL SERUM | BONE IN UREMIC SERUM | N/U RATIO | p VALUE* |
|---|---|---|---|---|---|
| | | CPM/MG BONE | | | |
| $25$ (OH) $D_3$ | 7 | 16,194 +2267 | 8067 +1113 | 2.00 +0.21 | NS |
| $1,25$ (OH)$_2D_3$ | 7 | 7395 +3242 | 3672 +1896 | 2.11 +0.42 | NS |
| $24,25$ (OH)$_2D_3$ | 3 | 4612 + 430 | 2436 + 197 | 1.90 +0.25 | NS |
| PTH + $25$ (OH) $D_3$ | 8 | 3474 +1065 | 1756 + 439 | 1.95 +0.26 | NS |
| PTH + $1,25$ (OH)$_2D_3$ | 10 | 5471 +3633 | 3144 +2099 | 1.90 +0.35 | NS |
| PTH + $25$(OH)$D_3$ + $1,25$ (OH)$_2D_3$ | 10 | 6773 +1756 | 3383 + 879 | 2.00 +0.08 | NS |
| PTH + $24,25$ (OH)$_2D_3$ + $1,25$ (OH)$_2D_3$ | 9 | 3901 +1413 | 2420 + 770 | 1.58 +0.17 | p < .01 |
| PTH + $24,25$ (OH)$_2D_3$ | 2 | 19,399 +1844 | 10,454 + 824 | 1.85 +0.03 | p < .01 |

PTH = 1.0 units/ml of media
24,25 (OH)$_2D_3$ = 0.05 ug/ml of media
25 (OH)D$_3$ = 1.0 ug/ml of media
1,25 (OH)$_2D_3$ = 0.05 ug/ml of media

*p value calculated by students t test and estimate the statistical significance of the difference between untreated cultures (N/U ratio = 2.11 + 0.39) and the experiments listed.

in normal sera was compared to counts obtained from media containing uremic serum. In an additional series of experiments, the amount of $^{45}Ca$ released into media containing normal or uremic serum was measured when the following agents were added to the culture system:

a) parathyroid hormone (0.5 u/ml, 1.0 u/ml, 1.5 u/ml, 3.0 u/ml)
b) 1,25(OH)$_2$D$_3$ (0.05 ug/ml)
c) 25 OHD$_3$ (1.0 ug/ml)
d) 24,25(OH)$_2$D$_3$ (0.05 ug/ml)
    or in the following combinations:
e) parathyroid hormone (1.0 units/ml) and 1,25(OH)$_2$D$_3$ (0.5 ug/ml)
f) parathyroid hormone (1.0 units/ml) and 24,25(OH)$_2$D$_3$ (0.05 ug/ml)
g) parathyroid hormone (1.0 units/ml) and 25 OHD$_3$ (1.0 ug/ml)
h) parathyroid hormone (1.0 units/ml) and 25 OHD$_3$ (0.5 ug/ml) and
   1,25(OH)$_2$D$_3$ (0.05 ug/ml)
i) parathyroid hormone (1.0 units/ml) and 1,25(OH)$_2$D$_3$ (0.05 ug/ml)
   and 24,25(OH)$_2$D$_3$ (0.05 ug/ml)

The parathyroid hormone employed was highly purified bovine parathyroid hormone (Inolex Corp.) which was dissolved in de-ionized water titrated to a pH of 4.5 - 5.0 with acetic acid to which was added bovine serum albumin 1.5 mg/liter and L-Cysteine 5 mg/ml. The 1,25(OH)$_2$D$_3$, the 24,25(OH)$_2$D$_3$ and the 25 OHD$_3$ used in this study were kindly supplied by the Upjohn Company.

RESULTS

Table 1 & 2 list the results of experiments in which the $^{45}Ca$ released into the media containing normal serum (N) is compared to the $^{45}Ca$ released into the media containing uremic serum (U) with or without the addition of the bone calcium mobilizing factors 1,25(OH)$_2$D$_3$, 25 OHD$_3$, 24,25(OH)$_2$D$_3$ and PTH either alone or in combination to each pair of cultures containing either normal or uremic serum. Cultures in which bone were maintained in uremic serum consistently had lower $^{45}Ca$ (cpm/mg bone) than cultures with normal sera. The ratio of $^{45}Ca$ measured in the media containing normal sera to $^{45}Ca$ measured in the media containing uremic sera (N/U) averaged 2.11±0.39 in unstimulated cultures. A significant change in this ratio i.e., $^{45}Ca$ measured in cultures containing normal sera to $^{45}Ca$ measured in cultures containing uremic sera, when embryonal bone reabsorption is stimulated by the addition of calcium mobilizing/humoral factors to each pair of bones in cultures is an estimate of the responsiveness of the normal rat embryonal bone system. A significant decrease in the N/U ratio in stimulated cultures as compared to unstimulated cultures represents an increase in the responsiveness in the rat embryonal bone maintained in uremic sera. With stimulation of resorption by the addition of calcium mobilizing factors to the cultures maintained with uremic sera, a significant decrease in the N/U ratio was noted with a) increasing concentrations of bovine PTH were added to each pair

of cultures; b) PTH, 24,25(OH)$_2$D$_3$ and 1,25(OH)$_2$D$_3$ were added to
each pair of cultures (Table 2). No significant change from the
unstimulated N/U ratio was noted with the addition of 25 OHD$_3$,
1,25(OH)$_2$D$_3$ and 24,25(OH)$_2$D$_3$ alone or in the following combinations: PTH and 25(OH)D$_3$ ; PTH and 1,25(OH)$_2$D$_3$; PTH and 1,25(OH)$_2$D$_3$
and 25 OHD$_3$. Despite the lack of a significant change in the N/U
ratio in these stimulated cultures, the $^{45}$Ca released into the
media was always much greater in cultures containing normal sera
than in uremic sera. Since a change in the N/U ratio with the
addition of stimulators of bone resorption could result from a
decrease responsiveness of bone maintained in normal serum relative
to little or no change to that of bone maintained in uremic serum,
we tested the responsiveness of bone by adding PTH or 1,25(OH)$_2$D$_3$
to one of the pair of bones maintained in tissue culture containing
normal serum and compared this response to the PTH or 1,25(OH)$_2$D$_3$
added to one of a pair of bones maintained in cultures containing
uremic sera. PTH added to one of the pair of bones maintained in
culture containing normal sera results in a 77% increase of $^{45}$Ca
released into the media. PTH added to one of the pair of bones
maintained in culture containing uremic serum increased $^{45}$Ca by only
30 percent. The response of bones to PTH maintained in normal cultures was therefore, significantly higher than that observed in bone
maintained with uremic sera. The response of the embryonal bone to
1,25(OH)$_2$D$_3$ with normal sera was less impressive with a 47 percent
increase in $^{45}$Ca released in cultures with normal sera as compared
to a 17 percent increase in cultures with uremic sera.

Inhibitors of parathyroid action at the bone calcium mobilizing
site may exist in significant quantities in uremic serum. Thyrocalcitonin (TCT) inhibits the bone calcium mobilizing properties of
PTH. Increased immunoreactive thyrocalcitonin has been measured in
uremic plasma. The decreased release of $^{45}$Ca noted in tissue culture with uremic serum could be related to increased levels of TCT.
We, therefore, studied the effects of PTH added to cultures containing uremic serum obtained from a totally thyro/parathyroidecto-
mized uremic patient. It is presumed that there is little, if any,
PTH and TCT in this patient's sera. The addition of PTH to one of
a pair of bones maintained in uremic serum from this thyro-parathyroidectomized uremic patient stimulated the release of $^{45}$Ca into
the medium, but not to the same extent as observed in the other
bone pair maintained in the culture with normal sera. The N/U
ratio was 1.85. This ratio is not significantly different from
the N/U ratios noted in experiments with serum obtained from normal
and uremic patients with intact thyroid and parathyroid glands.

DISCUSSION

The direct measurements of the calcium mobilizing properties
of PTH in tissue culture indicate that uremic plasma is deficient
in or contains factors which inhibit calcium release from normal

embryonal fetal bone.  These observations could be related to a
number of factors and further studies are obviously required to
elucidate the mechanisms responsible for the inhibition of the
bone calcium mobilizing properties of PTH by uremic sera.  Uremic
serum does contain increased quantities of immunoreactive TCT which,
if biologically active, could inhibit PTH mediated release of calcium from bone.  The PTH response of fetal bone maintained in uremic
sera obtained from a thyro-parathyroidectomized uremic patient was
impaired.  The response noted with sera from this patient was not
significantly different from the PTH response noted in embryonal
bone cultures containing uremic sera from patients with intact
thyroid and parathyroid hormones.  Therefore, it appears unlikely
that an excess TCT in uremic serum is an adequate explanation for
our observations.  Another possible explanation for the observed
decreased release of calcium into the media containing uremic serum
with the addition of PTH to the bone culture system could be the
presence in high concentrations of non-specific proteases in uremic
serum which hydrolyze the added PTH in the culture system and inhibit its effect at the calcium mobilizing site.  This seems unlikely
because all sera were heat inactivated at $37^\circ$ prior to the addition
of the sera to the culture system.  The studies utilizing pharmacological quantities of $24,25(OH)_2D_3$ alone and in combination with
$1,25(OH)_2D_3$ and PTH strongly support the contention of Massry and
co-workers that these metabolites are necessary for the skeletal
effect of PTH.  This presumes that a deficiency of $24,25(OH)_2D_3$
and $1,25(OH)_2D_3$ existed in the patients we studied.  Direct measurements of the plasma concentration of these metabolites were not
made during these experiments and further studies are required to
validate this thesis.  Although the decreased calcium mobilizing
response to PTH of bone maintained in uremic plasma appears to be
partially corrected by the addition to the uremic media of either
$24,25(OH)_2D_3$ alone, or in combination with $1,25(OH)_2D_3$, it should
be noted that the amount of $^{45}Ca$ released by PTH stimulated bone
into the media containing uremic serum and the Vitamin D metabolites
was significantly decreased below values observed when PTH,
$1,25(OH)_2D_3$ and $24,25(OH)2D3$ were added to cultures containing
normal serum.  These observations strongly support the contention
that uremic serum _per se_ added to the media appears to impair the
calcium mobilizing properties of PTH.

The response of the rat bone to increasing concentration of
PTH added to uremic cultures (Table 1) suggests that part of the
differences observed with normal and uremic sera could be related
to receptor inter-reaction with biologically inactive PTH fragments
or other substances in uremic serum.  The addition of increasing
quantities of bovine PTH to cultures containing uremic and normal
sera was associated with a greater percentage increase in the
release of calcium into the media containing uremic sera than cultures containing normal sera suggesting that increasing quantities
of active bovine PTH may have displaced inactive fragments of PTH

from the receptors on the normal embryonal bone maintained in uremic sera. Another possible explanation for the impaired skeletal response to PTH in uremia could be the development of auto-antibodies to receptor proteins. The decreased calcium mobilizing properties to added PTH of bone maintained in tissue culture may be related to the uremic serum containing auto-antibodies to PTH receptor proteins on bone which share a common configuration with receptors on rat fetal calvaria.

Regardless of the explanation offered to partially explain the observations noted in our studies, we conclude that uremic sera contains factors or is deficient in factors which decrease the mobilization of bone calcium when active PTH is added to the bone culture system.

SUMMARY

1. $^{45}Ca$ released from embryonal fetal rat bone into a tissue culture system containing uremic serum was lower than $^{45}Ca$ measured in culture media containing normal sera.
2. With stimulation of bone calcium mobilization by the addition of PTH, $1,25(OH)_2D_3$, $24,25(OH)_2D_3$ and $25(OH)_2D_3$, the $^{45}Ca$ released into media containing uremic serum was significantly lower than measured in cultures containing normal serum.
3. Addition of PTH in combination with $24,25(OH)_2D_3$ or with $24,25$ $(OH)_2D_3$ and $1,25(OH)_2D_3$ to bone cultures containing uremic serum increased the $^{45}Ca$ released into the media when compared to cultures containing uremic serum and PTH.

CONCLUSION

1. Uremic sera is deficient in or contains factors which impair the calcium mobilizing properties of normal rat bone maintained in tissue culture.
2. Uremic serum impairs the calcium mobilizing properties of parathyroid hormone, $24,25(OH)_2D_3$, $25 OHD_3$ of normal rat embryonal bone maintained in tissue culture.
3. Pharmacologic quantities of $24,25(OH)_2D_3$ and $1,25(OH)_2D_3$ and $24,25(OH)_2D_3$ partially restores the calcium mobilizing properties of PTH added to bone cultures maintained in uremic serum.

REFERENCES

1.  E. Slatopolsky, S. Calgar, J.P. Pennell, D.B. Taggart, J.M. Canterbury, E. Reiss, and N.S. Bricker, On the pathogenesis of hyperparathyroidism in chronic experimental renal insufficiency in the dog, J. Clin. Invest. 50:492 (1971).

2.  S. Massry, Skeletal resistance to the calcemic action of
    parathyroid hormone in uraemia:  a mechanism for the hypocal-
    cemia and secondary hyperparathyroidism of chronic renal
    failure, Clin. Endocrinol. 5 (Suppl):317 (1976).

3.  L.G. Raisz, Bone resorption in tissue culture factors influenc-
    ing the response to parathyroid hormone, J. Clin. Invest. 44:103
    (1965).

4.  J.J. Reynolds and J.T. Doyle, A sensitive in vitro method for
    studying the induction and inhibition of bone resorption.
    Calc. Tissue Res., 4:339 (1970).

5.  J.D. Biggers, "Cells and Tissues in Culture", Vol. 3, E.N.
    Wilmer, ed., Academic Press, New York, (1965).

MULTIVARIATE ANALYSIS OF THE VITAMIN D ENDOCRINE SYSTEM: EVIDENCE
FOR THE ESSENTIALITY OF BOTH 24R,25-DIHYDROXYVITAMIN $D_3$ AND 1α,25-
DIHYDROXYVITAMIN $D_3$

ANTHONY W. NORMAN

Department of Biochemistry
University of California
Riverside, California 92521

INTRODUCTION

The secosteroid vitamin D plays an essential role in calcium
(Ca) and phosphorus ($P_i$) homeostasis and serves as a precursor of
a minimum of eight hydroxylated metabolites. Of these the two
dihydroxylated derivatives produced by the kidney, particularly
1α,25-dihydroxyvitamin $D_3$ [1,25(OH)$_2$D$_3$] and 24R,25-dihydroxy-
vitamin $D_3$ [24,25(OH)$_2$D$_3$] appear to be the most biologically relevant. Figure 1 presents a summary of the well documented actions
of these metabolites. The principal sites of regulation of Ca and
$P_i$ metabolism are the intestine, bone, and kidney. It is to be
anticipated that the relative contributions of these organs to Ca
and $P_i$ homeostasis will change in an endocrine-coordinated fashion
throughout growth and development, pregnancy and lactation (mammals)
or egg production (birds), and aging in a sex dependent fashion to
reflect changes in the Ca and $P_i$ requirements of the animal.

Extensive studies in the past decade have documented the
impressive biological potency of 1,25(OH)$_2$D$_3$[1,2] for intestinal Ca
absorption and bone Ca mobilization[1,3] and its clinical efficacy
in renal osteodystrophy. An important component of the biological responses mediated by 1,25(OH)$_2$D$_3$ is believed to occur as
a consequence of its interaction with a cytosol-nuclear receptor
in target tissues. This results in the utilization of new genetic
information coding for proteins, including a calcium binding
protein, related to the biological responses of vitamin D.[4]

In contrast to the accumulated knowledge regarding the
short-term actions of 1,25(OH)$_2$D$_3$,[1,2] relatively little is known
of the biological function of 24,25(OH)$_2$D$_3$. Henry et al.[5] have

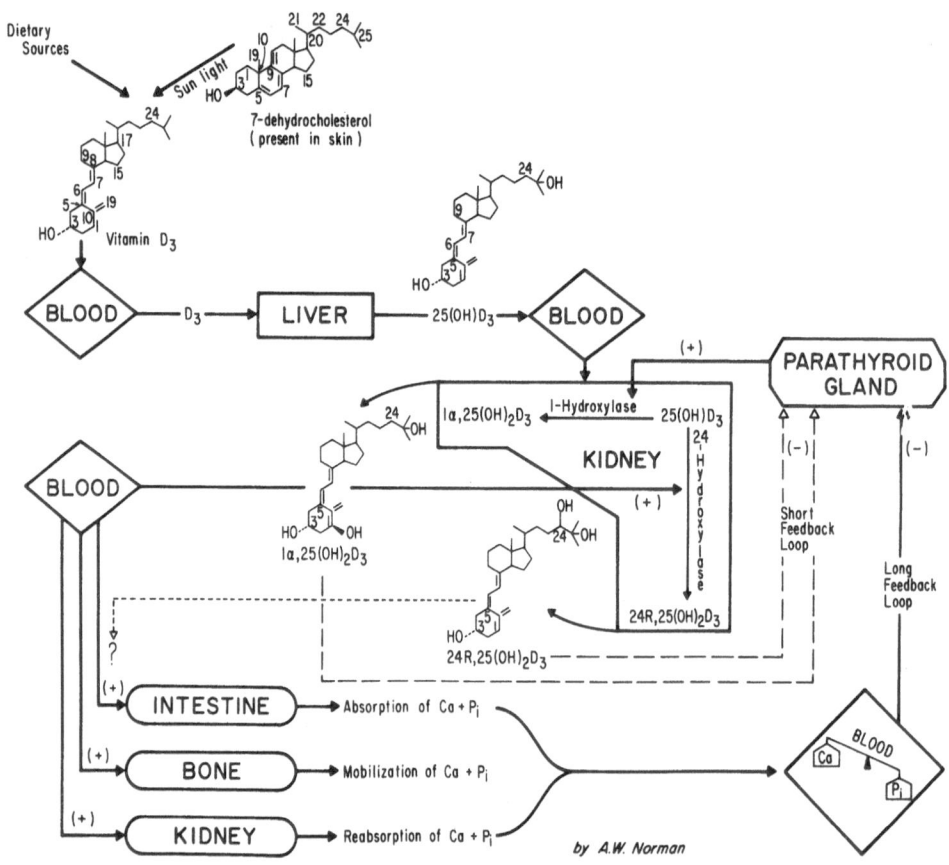

Fig. 1.   Metabolic pathway leading to known biological functions of
1,25(OH)$_2$D$_3$ and 24,25(OH)$_2$D$_3$.

shown that the regression of chicken parathyroid glands, which had
undergone hypertrophy and hyperplasia due to vitamin D deficiency,
required the simultaneous short-term presence of both 1,25(OH)$_2$D$_3$
and 24,25(OH)$_2$D$_3$.  Also, Henry and Norman[6] demonstrated that when
hens are raised to sexual maturity from hatching with 1,25(OH)$_2$D$_3$
as their sole source of vitamin D$_3$, their fertile eggs were
incapable of hatching.  However, when the hens received a combination of 24,25(OH)$_2$D$_3$ and 1,25(OH)$_2$D$_3$, hatchability equivalent to
that with hens given vitamin D alone was obtained.  These results
support the view that 24,25(OH)$_2$D$_3$ in the presence of 1,25(OH)$_2$D$_3$
is essential for the production of certain vitamin D-dependent
biological responses.  Also, Canterbury et al.[7] have shown effects

of acute administration of both $24,25(OH)_2D_3$ and $1,25(OH)_2D_3$ on the secretion of immunoreactive parathyroid hormone in the dog.

An alternative view concerning the role of $24,25(OH)_2D_3$ is that this dihydroxylated metabolite may lead to a catabolic pathway which diverts seco-steroids away from the production of $1,25-(OH)_2D_3$. As yet there are no convincing data to support this premise.

Reported in this paper are the results of two experiments designed to evaluate the ability of $24,25(OH)_2D_3$ and $1,25(OH)_2D_3$ singly and in combination to duplicate the effects of vitamin $D_3$ in effecting Ca and $P_i$ homeostasis. Presented in Figure 2 is a summary with regard to serum Ca, serum $P_i$ and intestinal phosphate absorption of the relative ability of $1,25(OH)_2D_3$ and $24,25(OH)_2D_3$ alone or in combination, to duplicate the response achieved by vitamin $D_3$ under three differing dietary levels of Ca and P. This experiment was carried out only over a 14 day interval. It is apparent that only the combination therapy of $24,25(OH)_2D_3$ + $1,25(OH)_2D_3$ most closely approached the responses achieved by vitamin $D_3$. This is particularly evident with regard to normalization of serum $P_i$ and stimulation of intestinal $P_i$ absorption. This suggests that $24,25(OH)_2D_3$ in combination with $1,25(OH)_2D_3$ may have important actions on phosphate metabolism.

Results from the experiment summarized in Figure 2 suggested the value of a longer term experiment in which the relative abilities of $1,25(OH)_2D_3$ and $24,25(OH)_2D_3$ alone and in combination to permit normal growth and sexual development would be assessed. White Leghorn hens were raised from the time of hatching through sexual maturity to the period (28-35 weeks of age) of steady state egg production on a standard chick rearing diet, devoid of vitamin $D_6$ and containing 1.2% Ca, 2.0% P (weeks 1-27) and 3.0% Ca, 2.0% P (weeks 28-35). Male chicks were raised similarly for a period of 5 weeks. At 5 weeks, groups of 5 males and 5 females were killed, while additional groups of 4-6 females were carried through week 35. After 36 weeks the hens received tetracycline hydrochloride (20 mg/kg body wt) for 3 days and were sacrificed on the fourth day. The right tibia was obtained immediately, fixed in alcohol, embedded in methyl methacrylate, and evaluated by previously described procedures of quantitative bone histology. All non-bone related measurements were carried out as described by Henry and Norman.[6,10].

Table 1 lists the doses of vitamin $D_3$ and dihydroxylated metabolites that were given orally every day over a 36-week period. The nmoles of steroid were adjusted weekly for changes in body weight. The two doses of $1,25(OH)_2D_3$ and $24,25(OH)_2D_3$ employed in this study and referred to throughout this paper as "low" and "high" were selected to represent less than optimal and near

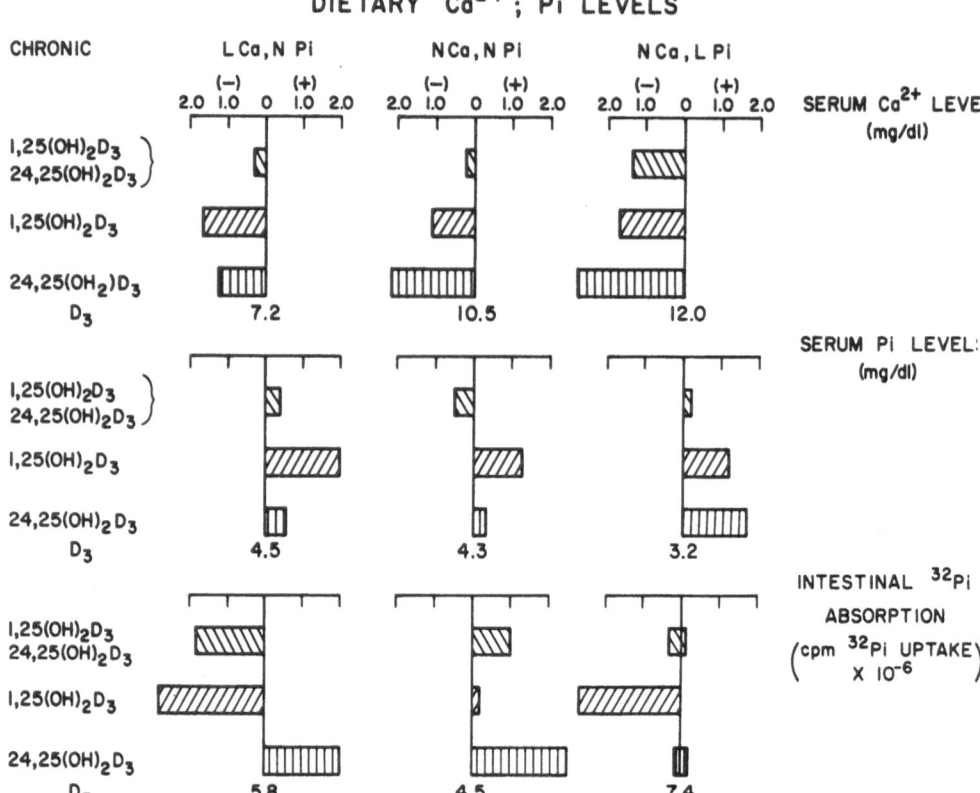

Fig. 2. Comparison of the biological responses to 1,25(OH)₂D₃ and 24,25(OH)₂D₃, alone and in combination, in relation to vitamin D₃ as a function of different levels of dietary Ca and P. Groups of hatchling chicks (10 birds/group) fed a standard vitamin D-deficient diet (3) containing 0.06% Ca, 0.4% P for 21 days. They were then switched for 14 days to diets containing different levels of Ca and P. Low Ca = 0.1%; Normal Ca = 1.0%; Normal P = 1.0%; low P = 0.05%. During the 14 day interval they received oral daily doses of vitamin D₃ 10.0 nmol/kg of body weight; 1,25(OH)₂D₃, 1.2 nmol/kg, 24,25(OH)₂D₃ 16.0 nmol/kg. One group received both 24,25(OH)₂D₃ and 1,25(OH)₂D₃, 10.0 and 1.2 nmol/kg respectively. On day 14 a 0.2 ml dose of 3 moles of HPO₄, pH 7.4 containing 10 μCi of ³²P was placed in an intestinal duodenal loop. Thirty minutes later the extent of absorption of ³²P was assessed by measurement of the ³²P remaining in the duodenal loop. The absolute results for serum Ca²⁺, serum P₁ (mg/100 ml) and ³²P absorption for the D₃-treated group are shown. Only the relative response for the other treatment groups is shown in relation to the D₃-response.

Table 1. Effect of daily doses of vitamin $D_3$ and its dihydroxyl-ated metabolites on adult hen weight and egg production. Vitamin D and the dihydroxylated metabolites were given orally daily from hatching in 0.2 ml of Wesson oil.

| Dose (nmole kg$^{-1}$ day$^{-1}$) | | | Body weight at 34 weeks* (g) | Eggs per group per week† | Eggshell thickness‡ (mm x 10$^2$) | Age at established egg laying§ (weeks) |
|---|---|---|---|---|---|---|
| Vitamin $D_3$ | 1,25-(OH)$_2$-$D_3$ | 24,25-(OH)$_2$-$D_3$ | | | | |
| 10* | 0 | 0 | 1680 ± 100 | 30 | 39.3 ± 2.6 | 26 |
| 0 | 0.24 | 0 | 1240¶± 100 | 12 | 31.0 ∓ 5.2 | 29 |
| 0 | 1.2 | 0 | 1670 ± 80 | 27 | 35.4 ∓ 4.9 | 27 |
| 0 | 0 | 16.0 | 1140¶± 40 | 5 | 34.5 ∓ 2.7 | 30 |
| 0 | 0.24 | 3.2 | 1250¶± 130 | 11 | 35.9 ± 5.5 | 29 |
| 0 | 0.24 | 16.0 | 1540 ± 100 | 31 | 36.0 ∓ 4.3 | 29 |
| 0 | 1.2 | 3.2 | 1590 ± 180 | 28 | 38.2 ± 3.1 | 27 |
| 0 | 1.2 | 16.0 | 1540 ± 130 | 30 | 38.3 ± 2.4 | 27 |

*Body weights are the mean of five hens per group ± the standard deviation. †The total number of eggs produced by a group of five hens during a representative week following established egg hatching. ‡The mean thickness of all eggs produced by the group in a week is given. §The age at which the hens in each group reached a plateau of egg production. *Ten nanomoles of vitamin $D_3$ per kilogram of body weight per day is equivalent to 154 I.U. per kilogram per day; 1.0 I.U. of vitamin $D_3$ is 65 pmole or 25 ng. ¶Significantly different from the control group that received vitamin $D_3$ (P<.001). (See reference 6 for details.)

optimal respectively.[6] The terms "low" and "high" therefore are only relative and have no pharmacological connotation.

Table 1 also shows that the hens receiving the higher dose of 1,25(OH)$_2$D$_3$ reached the same adult weight as those hens given the parent vitamin D$_3$; this indicates that no obvious growth retardation occurs in the absence of 24,25(OH)$_2$D$_3$.

Egg laying was initiated between 24 and 30 weeks.[6] Distinct differences were noted in the time required for establishment of steady-state egg production between the various groups (see Table 1). Hens receiving vitamin D$_3$ or the combination doses of high levels of 24,25(OH)$_2$D$_3$ and 1,25(OH)$_2$D$_3$ initiated egg production at weeks 26 to 27 while hens receiving the high dose of 24,25-(OH)$_2$D$_3$ or low dose of 1,25(OH)$_2$D$_3$ alone were delayed to week 29 to 30.[3] Steady-state egg production was established in all groups by week 30. At the beginning of week 34, and again a week later, hens were artificially inseminated with a pool of semen collected from 15 normal White Leghorn roosters.  Eggs were collected and stored at 12°C until the end of the 2-week period of fertility.

The nonbone-related variables include measurement at week 5 of body weight (g); measurement over weeks 30-36 of number of eggs layed per bird per week (for two separate 2-week intervals); the average thickness of the egg shell (mm); the percent hatchability of fertile eggs collected after artificial insemination; and measurement at week 36 (time of sacrifice) of body weight (g), serum $Ca^{2+}$ and $P_i$ level (mg/100 ml) amount of vitamin D-dependent calcium binding protein (CaBP) in the intestine and kidney ($\mu$g/mg protein).  The bone related variables, all measured at week 36, include:  percent bone ash, tibial length (cm), tibial diameter (mm), volumetric density of cancellous bone ($mm^3/cm^3$), volumetric density of osteoid ($mm^3/cm^3$), volumetric density of endosteal fibrosis (%), osteocytic index or number of osteocytic lacunae per unit volume of calcified trabecular bone, volumetric density of osteocytes (%), surface density of osteocytes ($mm^2/mm^3$), bone appositional rate in medullary and cortical bone (mm/day), and their ratio.

Separate measurements for all 22 variables were carried out individually in all birds included in the experiment.  The data was processed by a multivariate analysis computer program[11] and the results for each bird were plotted on a two dimensional figure with canonical variable #1 as the abscissa and canonical variable #2 as the ordinate.  In panel A the coordinates of each bird in each group are plotted with the coordinates of the mean indicated by an asterisk, while in panels B, C, and D the computed mean coordinates of the group are indicated by the group number. For panel A the equation employed to plot canonical variable #1 $CV_1$ = -7.6 - 0.19 (Vol. den. osteoid) + 0.23 (bone formation rate ratio) + 0.05 (% egg hatchability) + 0.01 (intest. CaBP) + 0.01 (body wt. 5 wk, g) and the equation for canonical variable #2 is $CV_2$ = -11.3 - 0.02 (% egg hatchability) - 0.056 (volume density osteoid) - 0.12 (bone formation rate ratio) + 0.05 (body wt. 5 wk) + 0.22 (intest. CaBP).

Presented in figure 3 are the contrasting results in the male versus female 5 week old chickens as analyzed by multivariate discriminant analysis for the seven treatment groups and control vitamin $D_3$ treated (group 1).  The abscissa and ordinate in each figure are respectively canonical variables 1 and 2.  Canonical variables are obtained from multivariate statistical analysis and represent a linear equation describing the weighted interrelationships existent in the experimental groups[12] which contribute to dispersion or heterogeneity of the cluster.  It is quite evident that the selected dose levels of the two metabolites produced very different responses in the male vs. female chicks.  In the female bird the two canonical variables were dominated by the level of

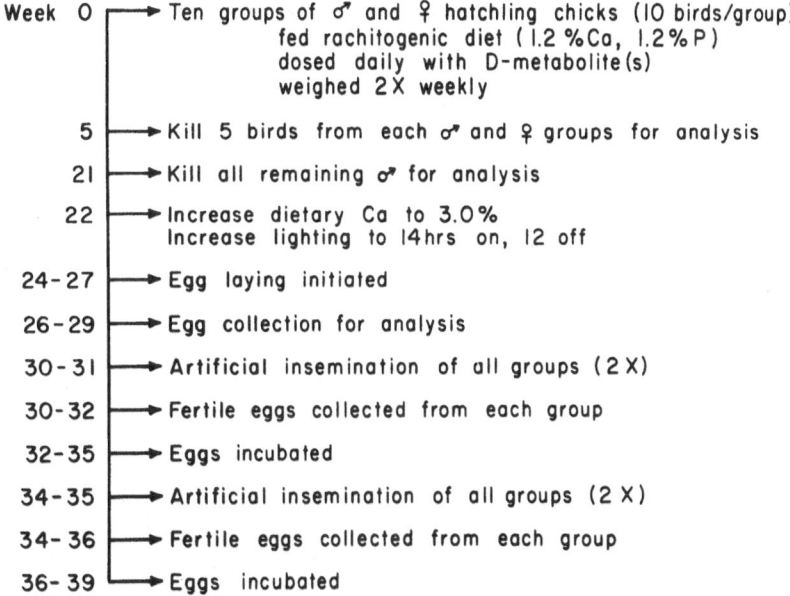

Week 0 ⟶ Ten groups of ♂ and ♀ hatchling chicks (10 birds/group)
              fed rachitogenic diet (1.2 % Ca, 1.2 % P)
              dosed daily with D-metabolite(s)
              weighed 2 X weekly

5 ⟶ Kill 5 birds from each ♂ and ♀ groups for analysis

21 ⟶ Kill all remaining ♂ for analysis

22 ⟶ Increase dietary Ca to 3.0%
         Increase lighting to 14 hrs on, 12 off

24-27 ⟶ Egg laying initiated

26-29 ⟶ Egg collection for analysis

30-31 ⟶ Artificial insemination of all groups (2 X)

30-32 ⟶ Fertile eggs collected from each group

32-35 ⟶ Eggs incubated

34-35 ⟶ Artificial insemination of all groups (2 X)

34-36 ⟶ Fertile eggs collected from each group

36-39 ⟶ Eggs incubated

Fig. 3. Experimental protocol of 35-week experiment to assess the effects of $1,25(OH)_2D_3$ and $24,25(OH)_2D_3$ alone and in combination to duplicate the effects of vitamin $D_3$ treatment.

intestinal CaBP and bone ash while in the male birds the canonical variables were determined largely by the level of renal CaBP and serum $P_i$ levels. Also it is evident that the group clusters of the female birds are more dispersed than are the treatment group clusters for the male birds. At the five week time point it is difficult to document the relative merit of combinations of the dihydroxylated metabolites over appropriate administration of either metabolite alone.

Shown in figure 4 are the integrated results obtained after 35 weeks of treatment with $1,25(OH)_2D_3$ or $24,25(OH)_2D_3$ alone or in combination. Specifically described here is the integrated operation of the vitamin D endocrine system as quantitated by individual measurement in all birds of 22 variables related to "vitamin D status" and as evaluated by the procedure of multivariate discriminate analysis.[11,12] Twelve of these variables

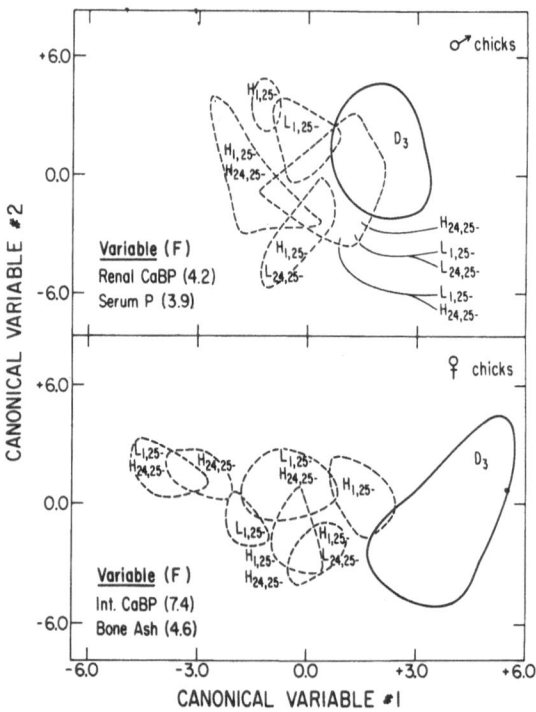

Fig. 4. Multivariate analysis of the vitamin D endocrine system in five week old male and female chicks. The experiment was conducted exactly as described in the legend to figure 3. Groups of birds (4-6) were sacrificed at 5 weeks and the following measurements determined on each individual bird, body wt. (g), level of vitamin D-dependent calcium binding protein (CaBP) in the intestine and kidney ($\mu$g/mg protein), serum $Ca^{2+}$ and $P_i$ (mg/100 ml) percent bone ash. Only the perimeters of each group are indicated.

are determined via detailed analysis of the bone including quantitative histology[13,14] and the 10 other variables reflect various manifestations of vitamin D action, e.g. serum $Ca^{2+}$ and $P_i$ levels, vitamin D-dependent calcium binding protein (CaBP), egg productivity, etc.[10]

Figure 5 presents four panels describing the multivariate analysis of differing combinations of the 22 variables related to the vitamin D endocrine system.  As evaluated by the multivariate analysis, it is clear that both $1,25(OH)_2D_3$ and $24,25(OH)_2D_3$ are simultaneously required for normalization of calcium and phosphorus homeostasis as evaluated over this 36 week period for the 22 reported variables.  It is apparent upon evaluation of Figure 5A (which includes analysis of all 22 variables) that the seven treatment groups of $1,25(OH)_2D_3$ and $24,25(OH)_2D_3$ singly and in combination all were distributed into individual clusters.  Only group 6, representing birds which received the combination of low $1,25(OH)_2D_3$ plus high $24,25(OH)_2D_3$ doses showed overlap with the control (group 1) which received vitamin $D_3$.  The experimental groups receiving the separate doses of $24,25(OH)_2D_3$ (group 4) and either low (group 2) or high (group 3) $1,25(OH)_2D_3$ alone were all distinctly separated from the control $D_3$-treated group.  The dominant components of the first canonical variable are percent egg hatchability, the volume density of the osteoid and the ratio of the bone appositional rates and of the second canonical variable are the body weight at week 5 and level of intestinal calcium-binding protein at week 36.

One useful feature of the multivariate statistical approach is the ability to exclude some variables from the analysis procedure and to ascertain the consequences of this deletion on the canonical variables, i.e. to observe changes in the relative positions (x,y coordinates) to one another of the various clusters. Such evaluations are reported on panels B, C, and D of Figure 5. Panel B reports the multivariate analysis of only the 12 bone parameters while panel C describes the evaluations of the 10 non-bone related parameters.  Striking differences are apparent in the relative positions of the metabolite treatment groups in relation to one another as well as to the vitamin $D_3$-treated group 1. Again a combination dose of $1,25(OH)_2D_3$ + $24,25(OH)_2D_3$ most clearly duplicated the consequences of vitamin $D_3$ treatment.

A detailed evaluation of panel 5B suggests for the 12 vitamin D-related bone parameters that the combination dose of high $24,25(OH)_2D_3$ + high $1,25(OH)_2D_3$ was most effective in normalizing all bone parameters as expressed by the two canonical variables. The dominant components of the two canonical variables are the ratio of the bone appositional rates of medullary and cortical bone, the tibial length and the volume density of the osteoid. The total amount of osteoid present in bone at any given time is

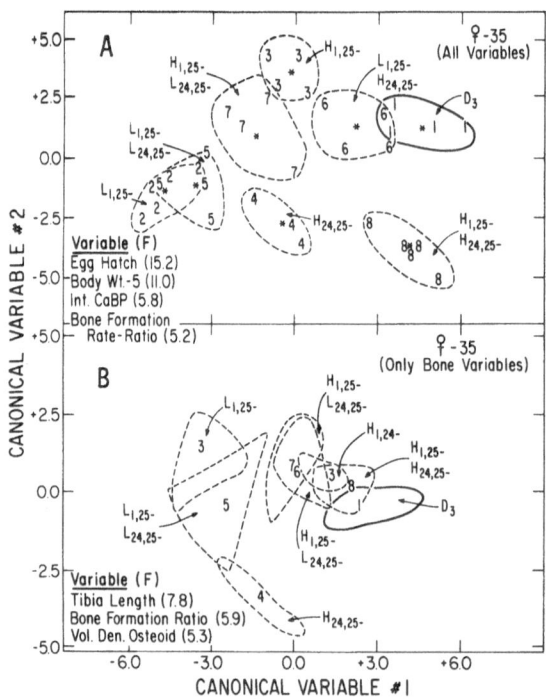

Fig. 5. Multivariate analysis of the vitamin D endocrine system.
The four panels (A-D) of this figure present the results of multivariate discriminant analysis[12] of differing sets of variables related to the vitamin D endocrine system over a 36 week study of
White Leghorn hens.  Panel A includes multivariate analysis of 22
vitamin D-related variables, including 10 nonbone-related variables
and 12 bone-related variables.  Panel B presents multivariate analysis of only the 12 bone variables.  Panel C presents analysis of
only the 10 nonbone-related variables while Panel D presents analysis of the 6 nonbone-related variables excluding any egg-related variables.  The birds were raised from the time of hatching through sexual
maturity to the period of steady state egg production on a standard

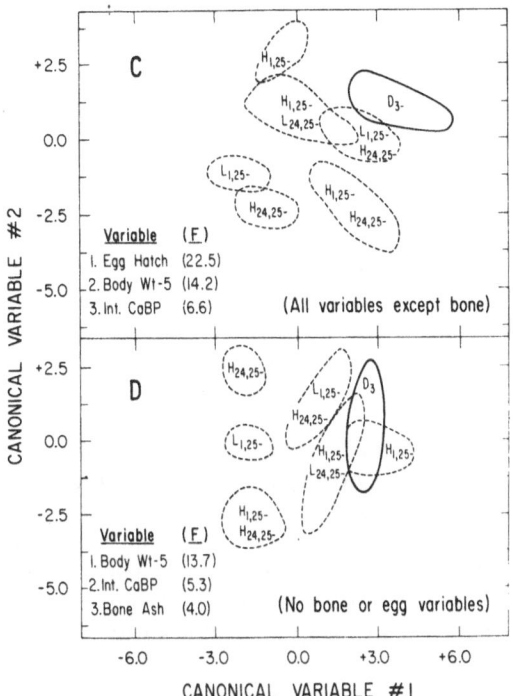

Fig. 5. continued

chick rearing diet containing 1.2% CA$^{2+}$, 2.0% P (weeks 1-27) or
3.0% Ca$^{2+}$, 2% P, (weeks 27-36) with no added vitamin D$_3$.    They
were divided into eight groups of 4-6 female birds which received
for 36 weeks either 10 nmol/kg/day of vitamin D$_3$ (group 1) or
1,25(OH)$_2$D$_3$ and 24,25(OH)$_2$D$_3$ alone or in combination as follows:
L-1,25 (group 2), H-L,25 (group 3); H-24,25 (group 4); L-1,25,
L-24,25 (group 5); L-1,25, H-24,25 (group 6); H-1,25, L-24,25
(group 7); or H-1,25, H-24,25 (group 8).    The two doses of
1,25(OH)$_2$D$_3$ and 24,25(OH)$_2$D$_3$ employed in this study and referred
to throughout the paper as "low" and "high" therefore are only
relative and have no pharmacological connotation. For 1,25(OH)$_2$D$_3$,
the low (L) dose was 0.24 and the high (H) dose was 1.2 nmol/kg/
day.    For 24,25(OH)$_2$D$_3$ the low dose was 3.2 and the high dose
16 nmol/kg/day.    For 24,25(OH)$_2$D$_3$ the low dose was 3.2 and the
high dose 16 nmol/kg/day.    After 36 weeks the hens received tetracycline hydrochloride (20 mg/kg body wt) for 3 days and were sacrificed on the fourth day.    The right tibia was obtained immediately, fixed in alcohol, embedded in methyl methacrylate, and
evaluated by previously described procedures of quantitative bone
histology.[9,18]    All non-bone related measurements were carried
out as described previously.[6,10]

a balance between the activation frequency of bone formation (birth rate of osteoid) and the rate of osteoid mineralization (disappearance of osteoid).   An increase in osteoid volume may occur if there is a perturbation in either of these processes. Disappearance of osteoid by mineralization is believed to be due to vitamin D and/or its metabolites,[9] while the formation of osteoid is thought to be governed by parathyroid hormone (PTH),[15] vitamin D metabolites, and other factors.[16]   Similarly the bone appositional rate is dependent upon the presence of both metabolites.   These results collectively emphasize not only that $24,25$-$(OH)_2D_3$ is necessary for normal bone as stated by Ornoy[17] and further elaborated on by Malluche et al.,[13] but that the simultaneous presence of both dihydroxylated metabolites is required for the multitude of steps related to bone formation and mobilization.

Only in the multivariate analysis presented in panel D which excludes 12 bone-related variables and 4 egg-related variables is there clear evidence that the high dose of $1,25(OH)_2D_3$ alone (group 3) can effectively duplicate the vitamin $D_3$ treatment. This suggests that those variables of the vitamin D endocrine system excluded from this analysis, (egg production and bone formation) are those that require the combined presence of both metabolites.

Figure 6 presents a summary statistical analysis according to the F-matrix of the probability of a significant difference between the vitamin $D_3$-treated group versus the other seven treatment groups.   While it is apparent that none of the treatment groups was totally indistinguishable from the vitamin $D_3$ group, group 6, which received the low dose of $1,25(OH)_2D_3$ + high dose of $24,25(OH)_2D_3$, was statistically not different at $p<0.05$ from the $D_3$-treated group in 3 out of 5 multivariate analyses.   Certainly neither the treatment regimen of $1,25(OH)_2D_3$ alone nor $24,25(OH)_2D_3$ was capable over the duration of this long term experiment of maintaining normal $Ca + P_i$ homeostasis.   The inability of $1,25(OH)_2D_3$ alone in the present study to supply all the biological responses produced by the parent vitamin $D_3$ is in marked contrast to our earlier report;[2] however that study was of only 4 weeks duration and included measurement of only 3 of the 22 variables reported in this study.

These results collectively emphasize the complexity of the interactions of $1,25(OH)_2D_3$ and $24,25(OH)_2D_3$ (or metabolites derived from them) in terms of their many sites of interaction in the vitamin D endocrine system.   It is not known at the present time whether the biological responses reported for these two dihydroxylated metabolites is due to them directly or further daughter metabolites; there is abundant evidence that both $1,25$-$(OH)_2D_3$ and $24,25(OH)_2D_3$ are subject to further metabolism.[18]

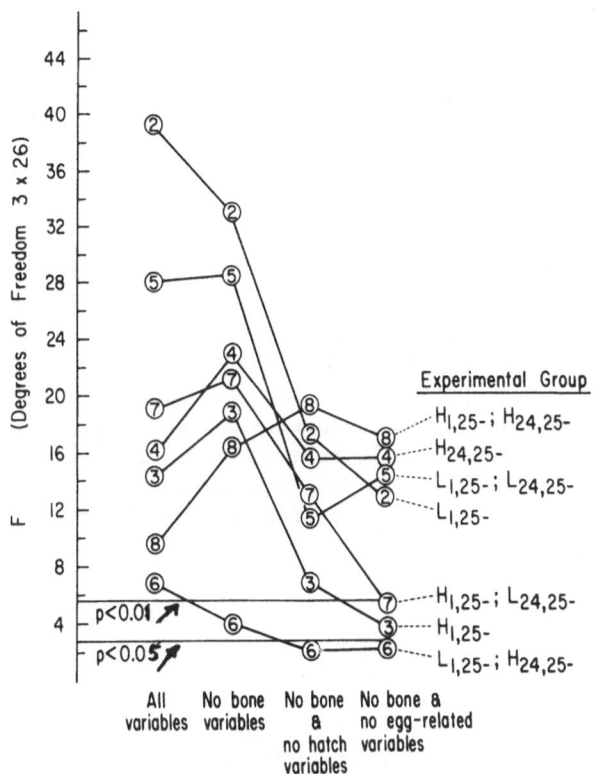

Fig. 6. Integrated statistical evaluation of the vitamin D endo-crine system. This figure presents a statistical evaluation of the vitamin $D_3$-treated group (#1) versus all other treatment groups (see legend to figure 5 for experimental details). The F-values obtained from the multivariate analysis computations[12] are shown for selected groupings of variables. Listed on the figure is the "cut-off" for $p < 0.05$ and $p < 0.01$. The F-values are used to test the distance (in the multivariate space) between each pair of groups and it is analogous to the Students t-test which tests the difference (difference in the univariate line) between two groups or pairs of groups.

It is also possible that the apparent requirement for the combined
presence of both dihydroxylated D-metabolites is the result of
sequential steps that individually require each of the metabolites
alone.  However, it now is established that both dihydroxymetabo-
lites are essential not only for bone but also for many other
variables indispensable for the integrated operation of calcium
and phosphorus homeostasis.  Future efforts to biochemically
characterize the actions of $24,25(OH)_2D_3$ or $1,25(OH)_2D_3$ need to
take cognizance of this fact.

ACKNOWLEDGMENTS

I wish to acknowledge the many fruitful discussions and
incisive comments provided by my colleague Dr. Helen L. Henry over
the course of this study.  I am indebted to Dr. Harmut H. Malluche
and his laboratory for carrying out the measurements associated
with the quantitative bone histology.  This project would have
been impossible without the dedicated assistance of Mr. B. Thuman,
Mr. R. Ochoa and Ms. J. E. Bishop in rearing and dosing the birds
employed in this experiment.  Special thanks are also due to
Mr. C. K. Huszar, Statistics Department, University of California,
Riverside for his careful introduction to multivariate discrimination analysis.  This work was supported in part by USPHS grant
AM-09012-014 and a grant-in-aid from Hoffmann LaRoche, Nutley, NJ.

References

1.  A. W. Norman, "Vitamin D: The Calcium Homeostatic Steroid
     Hormone", Academic Press, New York (1979).
2.  A. W. Norman, and R. G. Wong, The biological activity of the
     vitamin D metabolite 1-25-dihydroxycholecalciferol in
     chickens and rats, J. Nutr. 102:1709 (1972).
3.  A. W. Norman, J. W. Coburn, and K. Schaefer, Recent advances
     in the endocrinology of vitamin D and implications for
     renal failure, in: "Contributions to Nephrology," S.
     Karger, Basel (1978).
4.  A. W. Norman, and H. L. Henry, Vitamin D to 1,25-dihydroxy-
     cholecalciferol: Evolution of a steroid hormone, Trends in
     Biochem. Sci. 4:14 (1979).
5.  H. L. Henry, A. N. Taylor, and A. W. Norman, Response of
     chick parathyroid glands to the vitamin D metabolites,
     1,25-dihydroxycholecalciferol and 24,25-dihydroxycholecal-
     ciferol, J. Nutr. 107:1918 (1977).
6.  H. L. Henry, and A. W. Norman, Vitamin D: Two dihydroxylated
     metabolites 'are required for normal chicken egg hatch-
     ability, Science 201:835 (1978).
7.  J. M. Canterbury, S. Lerman, A. J. Claflin, H. Henry, A. W.
     Norman and E. Reiss, Effects of vitamin D metabolites on
     parathyroid hormone secretion, J. Clin. Invest. 61:1375
     (1978).

8. H. F. DeLuca and H. K. Schnoes, Metabolism and mechanism of action of vitamin D, Ann. Rev. Biochem. 45:631 (1976).

9. D. A. Goldstein, H. Malluche, and S. G. Massry, Management of renal osteodystrophy with 1,25(OH)$_2$D$_3$, J. Mineral and Electro. Metab. 2:48 (1979).

10. E. J. Friedlander, H. L. Henry and A. W. Norman, Studies on the mode of action of calciferol XII. Effects of dietary calcium and phosphorus on therelationship between the 25-hydroxyvitamin D$_3$-1$\alpha$-hydroxylase and production of chick intestinal calcium binding protein, J. Biol. Chem. 252:8677 (1977).

11. W. J. Dixon (ed.), "Biomedical Computer Program," University of California Press, Berkeley (1975).

12. R. E. Blackith and R. A. Reymet, "Multivariate Morphometrics," Academic Press, London and New York (1971).

13. H. H. Malluche, A. Meyer-Sabellek, H. L. Henry, S. G. Massry, and A. W. Norman, Effects of 1,25 dihydroxycholecalciferol and 24,25 dihydroxycholecalciferol on bone: A histologic study of micromophometric and dynamic parameters of bone, J. Clin. Invest. (in press).

14. E. Ritz, H. H. Malluche, B. Krempien and O. Mehls, in: "Calcium Metabolism in Renal Failure and Nephrolithiasis," D. S. David (ed.), John Wiley and Sons, New York (1977).

15. J. Parsons, Parathyroid physiology and the skeleton, in: Bourne: "The Biochemistry and Physiology of Bone," Vol. IV, Academic Press, New York (1976).

16. M. Parfitt, The actions of parathyroid hormone on bone: relation to bone remodeling and turnover, calcium homeostasis and metabolic bone disease, Metab. 25:809, 905, 1157 (1976).

17. A. Ornoy, D. Goodwin, D. Noh, and S. Edelstein, 24,25-Dihydroxyvitamin D is a metabolite of vitamin D essential for bone formation, Nature (London) 276:517 (1978).

18. A. W. Norman and F. P. Ross, Vitamin D seco-steroids: unique molecules with both hormone and possible membranophilic properties, Life Sci. 24:759 (1979).